Advances in Experimental Medicine and Biology

Volume 1229

Advances in Experimental Medicine and Biology provides a platform for scientific contributions in the main disciplines of the biomedicine and the life sciences. This series publishes thematic volumes on contemporary research in the areas of microbiology, immunology, neurosciences, biochemistry, biomedical engineering, genetics, physiology, and cancer research. Covering emerging topics and techniques in basic and clinical science, it brings together clinicians and researchers from various fields.

Advances in Experimental Medicine and Biology has been publishing exceptional works in the field for over 40 years, and is indexed in SCOPUS, Medline (PubMed), Journal Citation Reports/Science Edition, Science Citation Index Expanded (SciSearch, Web of Science), EMBASE, BIOSIS, Reaxys, EMBiology, the Chemical Abstracts Service (CAS), and Pathway Studio.

2018 Impact Factor: 2.126.

More information about this series at http://www.springer.com/series/5584

Junjie Xiao
Editor

Non-coding RNAs in Cardiovascular Diseases

Springer

Editor
Junjie Xiao
Institute of Cardiovascular Sciences, School of Life Science
Shanghai University
Shanghai, China

ISSN 0065-2598 ISSN 2214-8019 (electronic)
Advances in Experimental Medicine and Biology
ISBN 978-981-15-1670-2 ISBN 978-981-15-1671-9 (eBook)
https://doi.org/10.1007/978-981-15-1671-9

This Springer imprint is published by the registered company Springer Nature Singapore Pte Ltd.
The registered company address is: 152 Beach Road, #21-01/04 Gateway East, Singapore 189721, Singapore

Contents

Part I

Overview

An Overview of Non-coding RNAs and Cardiovascular System

1

Iram Mushtaq, Ayesha Ishtiaq, Tahir Ali, Muhammad Ishtiaq Jan, and Iram Murtaza

Abstract

Cardiovascular disease management and timely diagnosis remain a major dilemma. Delineating molecular mechanisms of cardiovascular diseases is opening horizon in the field of molecular medicines and in the development of early diagnostic markers. Non-coding RNAs are the highly functional and vibrant nucleic acids and are known to be involved in the regulation of endothelial cells, vascular and smooth muscles cells, cardiac metabolism, ischemia, inflammation and many processes in cardiovascular system. This chapter is comprehensively focusing on the overview of the non-coding RNAs including their discovery, generation, classification and functional regulation. In addition, overview regarding different non-coding RNAs as long non-coding, siRNAs and miRNAs involvement in the cardiovascular diseases is also addressed. Detailed functional analysis of this vast group of highly regulatory molecules will be promising for shaping future drug discoveries.

Keywords

Non-coding RNA · Cardiovascular diseases · Molecular medicines · Biomarker

1 Background

Non-coding RNA (ncRNA) can be defined according to their operational length of transcripts [1]. They can be divided into Short non-coding RNA and Long non-coding RNA.

Among the 98% of protein non-coding regions in human genome, 80% of them transcribed to RNAs. These non-coding RNAs were used to regard as Transcriptional "noise" for a longer period of time when their expression, mechanism and function were unknown. During the recent advancements in the field of molecular medicine these ncRNAs have drawn wide attention. Encyclopedia of DNA elements (ENCODE) and the Functional Annotation of the Mammalian Genome (FANTOM) major findings revealed that genome which is transcribed, produces large number of ncRNAs [2–4]. Therefore, it is believed now that number of non-coding RNAs is a determining parameter to understand the degree of complexity of specie than with number of protein coding genes [5]. Like protein coding regions, non-coding RNAs effect the normal physiological functions of the body including development, differentiation and regulation of gene expression both at transcriptional and trans-

I. Mushtaq · A. Ishtiaq · T. Ali · M. I. Jan
I. Murtaza (✉)
Department of Biochemistry, Signal Transduction Laboratory, Faculty of Biological Sciences, Quaid-i-Azam University Islamabad, Islamabad, Pakistan
e-mail: irambch@qau.edu.pk

J. Xiao (ed.), *Non-coding RNAs in Cardiovascular Diseases*, Advances in Experimental Medicine and Biology 1229, https://doi.org/10.1007/978-981-15-1671-9_1

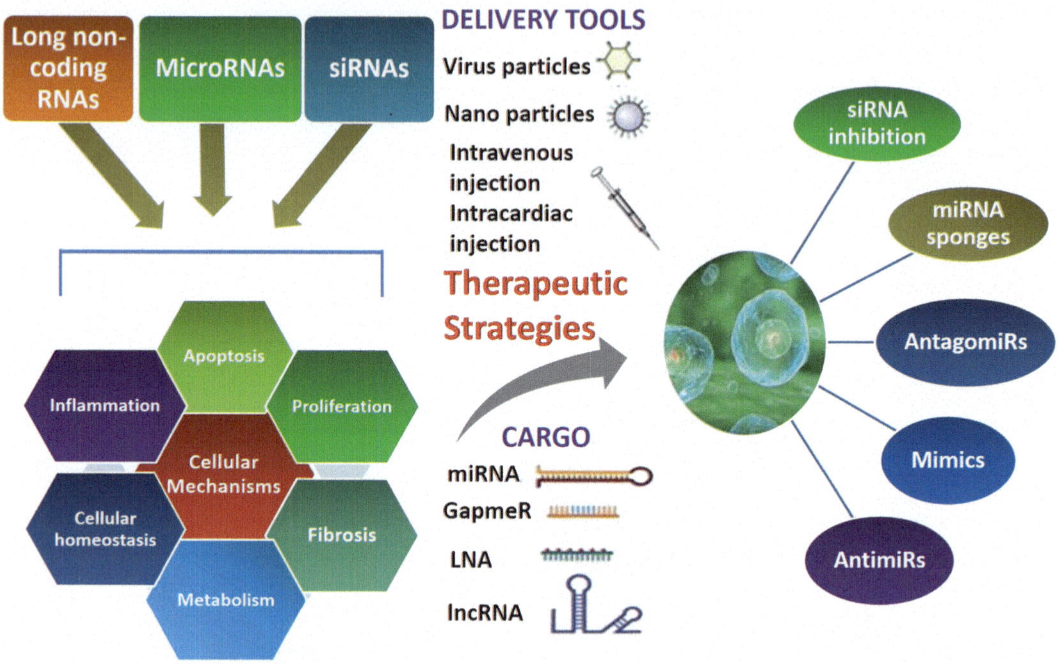

Fig. 1.1 An overview of non-coding RNAs and therapeutic strategies

lational level. Aberrant ncRNAs expression e.g., mutations in the genome are major contributory factors leading towards human diseases and serve as biomarkers in different pathologies like cancer, cardiovascular disease etc [6, 7]. Thus discovery of these non-coding RNAs revolutionized the field of molecular medicine and plays major role in enhancing our understanding in the mammalian genome organization and mechanistic regulation involved in pathophysiology of different diseases (Fig. 1.1) [8].

1.1 Discovery of Non-coding RNAs

58,000 long non-coding RNAs have been identified but among them very less are characterized in respect to their cellular structure, functions and their role in disease development. Their unique features as regulatory RNA molecules are to control the normal physiological functions of the body [9, 10]. Non-coding RNAs discovery period can be divided into three major eras.

(1) Before and during the 1950s, (2) 1960s to 1980s (3) 1990s to present. The discovery of double stranded DNA in 1950 by James Watson and Francis Crick laid the foundation of molecular biology. They described the mechanisms of flow of genetic information [11]. After that scientist found that organisms size and complexity is not much dependent upon amount of DNA [12, 13]. C value paradox phenomena described that more simpler and primitive animals like salamander have 15% larger genomes than humans [14]. The paradox phenomena described those genomic parts which are non-protein coding or not involved in regulatory functions termed as "junk DNA" [13, 15]. Functional analysis of junk DNA revealed that it is involved in maintenance of genome integrity, gene regulation and mRNA procession [16–19]. Discovery of different forms of RNAs "heterogeneous nuclear RNAs, small nuclear RNAs (snRNAs), small nucleolar RNAs (snoRNAs) suggested that junk DNA is much complicated [20–22]. High-through-put whole genome analysis techniques developed more accurate mechanism to understand the transcription. Among the transcribed RNA, 68% is long non-

coding RNA [2, 23, 24]. In the early 1990s, some non-coding RNAs were identified like H19 and X inactive specific transcript (Xist) [25–27]. Non-coding RNAs including micro RNA, circular RNA were discovered and classified by using High-through-put sequencing techniques [4, 28].

1.2 Types of Non-coding RNAs

Short Non-coding RNAs

Non-coding RNA transcripts comprising around 200 nucleotides are termed as short ncRNAs. Examples include microRNAs (19–23), short interfering RNA (21–25 bp), transfer RNAs (74–95), endogenous RNA, small nuclear RNAs (100 bp), small nucleolar RNAs (100–300 bp) and piwi interacting RNA (24-30 bp) that negatively regulates gene expression [29–33].

Micro RNAs

Micro RNA can be defined as short non-coding endogenous RNAs ranging in length, 18–25 nucleotides long that regulates mammalian gene expression by binding specific targeted transcripts [33, 34]. Micro RNA transcribed from miRNA loci and their host genes implicates enhancers, transcription factors and epigenetic regulators which are major components of transcriptional machinery [31]. Biogenesis of miRNA involves three major steps. (i) Transcription (ii) Nuclear and cytoplasmic processing (iii) RNA-induced silencing complex (RISC) assembly [8]. The long transcript which is generated by RNA polymerase II is spliced, capped, and acts as polyadenylated mRNA [35]. Primary miRNA comprehends one single or constellation of numerous miRNAs which get further mature by two major processing events. Formation of short hairpin precursor pri-miRNA involves splicing by nuclear microprocessor complex comprising of Drosha (known as RNase III enzyme) and its cofactor DGCR8 (DiGeorge syndrome critical region 8) [36]. Mature miRNA: miRNA∗ complex is generated by cytoplasmic RNase III dicer along with trans-activation-responsive RNA-binding protein. From this duplex RISC (RNA-induced silencing complex) is formed by the assembly of guide RNA along with argonaute proteins. Micro RNA targets are identified by binding of miRNA seed sequence in the 3′ UTR regions or in the coding region of messenger RNA. Therefore, it provokes the gene silencing by two mechanisms either by repressing the translational machinery or mRNA degradation. One micro RNA can influence the genetic and cellular functions of various distinct targets by these regulatory mechanisms [34].

Long Non-coding RNAs

Long ncRNAs transcripts comprising more than 200 nucleotides are called as long non-coding RNAs as ribosomal RNAs or like ribosomal RNAs [34, 37–39].

1.3 Classification of Long Non-coding RNAs

Currently there is no concise nomenclature for long non-coding RNA classification. The most distinctive method to classify them is according to their size, biogenesis, genomic proximity to protein coding genes, location and function [40]. Long non-coding RNAs can be divided into sense, antisense, intronic, intergenic, bidirectional lncRNAs, enhancer-associated RNAs (eRNAs) and promoter associated long RNAs (PALRs) [41].

Those non-coding RNAs which overlap with the exons or introns of the messenger RNA are called sense long non-coding RNA. Antisense non-coding RNAs arise from the contrasting strands of protein coding genes. BACE1-AS is an antisense long non-coding RNA which protects β amyloid-cleaving enzyme 1 (BACE1) mRNA from degradation [42]. BACE1-AS transcription is carried out in antisense direction from the intron of β-secretase 1 gene. This long non-coding RNA is of greater interest in the study of pathogenesis of Alzheimer's disease [43].

1.3.1 Classification of Long Non-coding RNAs According to Structural Organization

Structurally different non-coding RNAs regulating tissue developmental stage expression in mammalian cells are called circular RNAs

Table 1.1 Structural Characterization of non-coding RNAs

Characterization	Non-coding RNA	Reference
Antisense	BAC1-AS (β-secretase 1)	[42]
Circular RNAs	CDR1-AS	[132]
Natural antisense transcripts	Kcnq1ot1 or Airn	[40]
Nuclear noncoding RNA	ANRIL	[48]
	XIST	[25–27]
	HOTAIR	[49]
	Fendrr	[50]
	Bvht	[50]
	Half-STAU1	[51, 52]
	lincRNAp21	[51, 52]
	MALTA1	[53]
Competeing endogenous RNA	LINCMD1	[54]

(circRNAs). These endogenous RNAs are covalently closed, conserved, stable, and resistant to RNase R produced from exonic or intronic sequences [44, 45]. Enhancer RNAs transcribed from DNA sequences of enhancer regions can regulate gene expression. Splicing events of protein coding regions generate these covalently closed loops. Those long non-coding RNAs which are encrypted between the coding genes and transcribed independently are called intergenic RNAs. Long Intergenic RNA genes are present between the coding and non-coding regions. Intergenic regions related very long non-coding RNA ranging in length from 50 kb to 1 Mb. Examples include Kcnq1ot1 or Airn [40]. Those non-coding RNAs that are produced through transcription from the same promoter proceeding in opposite direction of coding genes are called as bidirectional RNAs [46, 47]. NATs (natural antisense transcripts) are originated from the antisense strand. These may be convergent or divergent (NATs) that results in sense/anti-sense pairs overlapping at 3′- or the 5′-end, respectively [3]. Brief overview of the structural characterization of non-coding RNAs is described in Table 1.1.

1.3.2 Functional Classification of Long ncRNAs

Long ncRNAs that are characterised according to their function and mechanism of action are epi-long ncRNAs [55, 56]. Nuclear long ncRNAs regulate gene expression in cis and trans genes in neighbouring loci and are involved in epigenetic and transcriptional regulation. Antisense non-coding RNA in the INK4 locus (ANRIL) recruits polycomb repression complex 2 (PRC2) and polycomb-assosiated proteins, influence gene expression both in cis and trans acting mechanisms [48]. These types of RNAs can temporarily or permanently activate or repress genes along with chromosomal regions by recruiting chromatin modification enzymes. Xist is the example of prototype chromatin remodelling, a long non-coding RNA which recruits polycomb repressive complexes (PRC) 2, and is expressed only on inactive X chromosome [53, 57]. HOX transcript antisense RNA (HOTAIR) is another example of non-coding RNA which binds to PRC1 and PRC2 and carry out tri-methylation (H3K27me3) at the promoter regions of target genes [49]. During embryonic development LncRNA H19 imprinted maternally expressed transcript acts as modifier of histone H3 methylation [58]. Cardiac expressed non-coding RNAs include FOXF1-adjacent noncoding developmental regulatory RNA (FENDRR) and braveheart long noncoding RNA (BVHT) that interact with PRC2 are key players in cardiac lineage commitment [50]. Cardiac hypertrophy associated myosin heavy-chain-associated RNA transcript (MHRT) long coding RNA expression is controlled by SWI/SNF related, matrix associated, Actin dependent regulator of chromatin, subfamily A, member 4 (BRG1)-mediated chromatin modification (SMARCA4) [59]. Half-STAU1-binding site RNAs and lincRNA-p21 regulate gene expression transcriptionally, by modulating translation and stability of target mRNA by long non-coding RNA and mRNA base pairing [51, 52]. Metastasis-associated lung adenocarcinoma transcript 1 (MALAT1) is associated with precursor mRNA splicing, regulates the distribution of serine/arginine-rich (SR) proteins [53]. Competing endogenous RNA (ceRNA) is another type of endogenous RNA function as sponges of micro RNA and other regulatory factors. Example of this type of non-coding RNA is long intergenic non-protein coding RNA, muscle differentiation

1 (LINCMD1) [54]. Genomic proportions lacking protein coding information never translated into mature peptides [60, 61]. These non-coding RNAs are classified according to their nucleotide number into different groups. Long non-coding RNAs are generally large heterogeneous groups and present shared characteristics with coding transcripts like, existence of intronic sequences, presence of epigenetic markers depicting differential expressions, specifically expressing splice variants [62]. Non-coding RNAs exists both in polyadenylated and non-polyadenylated forms thus characterizes as biomorphic [4]. Long ncRNAs share homology with the genomic structures and relationship with the coding transcriptome. Among them many are mutated pseudogene copies of coding regions representing them non-coding [63]. Data from previous findings suggested that 20% of long non-coding RNAs overlap the coding regions of human transcripts as entire gene or part of it exists as sense-antisense pairs [64–66]. Long intergenic non-coding RNAs (lincRNAs) does not lie within or overlapping coding regions [4]. Discovery of circular RNA depicted that transcripts usually not tend to be linear although transcribed from the coding regions [45, 67]. All the forms of RNA delineated from that genome are characterized not only on linear arrangement of transcriptional units but also contains a complex landscape of intertwining and coinciding transcripts. These transcripts either present on same strands or on the opposite strand while no clear distinction can be made between splice variants, overlapping and neighbouring genes [68].

2 Methods to Study Non-coding RNAs

RNA sequencing is the most widely used approach to study RNA detection. Some other approaches are also used:

Direct RNA sequencing Method:
In this method a library is prepared for sequencing of native RNA [69]. This method is more efficient to study low abundance transcripts, genetic variants, and isoforms differentiation. Due to low abundance, non-coding RNAs exhibit tissue specific patterns [70].

Cap assisted Gene expression sequencing method:
This sequencing method is followed for profiling of 5′ cap and has the accuracy of mapping the transcript at 5′ end [71].

Serial Analysis of Gene Expression and Paired-end Tagged Expression:
These methods are used to study poly A tailing mechanisms in non-coding RNAs [72].

Global run-on sequencing Method:
This assay is a nuclear run-on assay which is used to profile the nascent transcription [40, 73].

Profiling Microarrays:
Commercially available microarrays have the probes to study the species protein coding as well as non-coding transcripts. This method is more rapid, accurate and efficient in comparison to RNA sequencing method [74–76].

CRISPRi (CRISPR interference)-based libraries:
CRISPER interference is now an emerging approach to study long non-coding RNA. CRISPER interference based libraries are developed and > 16,000 non-coding RNAs are studied in cell lines, induced pluripotent stem cells and these RNA are required for study of robust cellular growth. Structural approaches are also studied to screen transcription factors interacting with non-coding RNAs. Recently a non-coding RNA named as RNA component of mitochondrial RNA processing endoribonuclease (Rmrp) is identified as an imperative interacting factor in (T-helper 17) responses found to be directly interacting RAR-related orphan receptor gamma (RORγt) [77].

Cross-linking or RNA immunoprecipitation Techniques:
Cross-linking and RNA immunoprecipitation techniques are accustomed to study RNA interactions of binding proteins [78, 79].

Long non-coding RNAs which are expressed at low levels required a specialized caveat as they possess tenfold lower expressions than their protein coding parts [80]. Directional libraries are prepared to study the standard orientation of antisense non-coding RNA transcripts in comparison to coding transcripts. Single cell sequencing approaches are used but limitation is the need of extensive amplification results in background noise. Different non-coding RNAs exhibit unique patterns. Some are polyadenylated, some are not like Enhancer RNA (eRNAs). These patterns affect the methods for development of library preparation for sequencing. Northern blotting and strand specific qRT-PCR are also used to study the long non-coding RNAs [81].

3 Mechanisms of Non-coding RNAs Regulation

Non-coding RNAs mechanism of action can be studied both at transcriptional and translational level. At transcriptional level these RNAs modify and regulate chromosomes that alter the gene expression. Post transcriptional levels involves RNA degradation in which non-coding RNA work as competing endogenous RNA and miRNA source.

3.1 The Transcriptional Regulation Control

Gene expression studies revealed that non-coding RNA localize in nucleus and can regulate genetic expression at transcriptional level [82, 83]. Scaffolding of non-coding RNAs in nucleus recruits different regulatory proteins that orchestrate the shape of chromosome through binding within the chromatin by site specific methods of three dimensional proximity, regulates gene expression either by activating or supressing the genes or altering the methylation status of the chromatin. X chromosome inactivation (XCI) phenomena is studied by Xist [84, 85]. It expresses only on inactive chromosomes (Xi) but do not express on active X chromosomes (Xa) [86]. During X chromosome inactivation, Xist expression recruits SMRT/HDAC1-associated repressor protein (SHARP), it binds with chromatin by scaffold attachment factor A (SAFA), promotes histone deacetylation by histone deacetylase 3 (HDAC3) on X chromosomes. This deacetylation escorted by demethylation of H3K4 disgorges the RNA polymerase II. All chromatin modifications lead towards the inactivation of X chromosomes [87–89]. Polycomb repressive complex 1 (PRC1) and PRC2 protein complexes are also recruited by Xist that triggers the methylation of H3K9 and H3k27 on histones [65, 90].

3.2 The Post-transcriptional Regulation Control

Post transcriptional regulation involves either RNA splicing or RNA degradation by directly or indirectly regulating miRNA functions. Non-coding RNAs regulate gene expression directly through RNA splicing or by RNA degradation in which precursor messenger RNA (pre-mRNA) is transcripted to mRNA. In RNA splicing, the introns are removed from precursor messenger RNA (pre-mRNA) and exons again ligated through spliceosome. Formation of splicing variants effects the maturation of mRNA. Non-coding RNAs sequences base paired with the pre-mRNAs and blocked the splicing of pre-mRNAs. For example, In Zinc Finger E-Box Binding Homeobox 2 (Zeb2) gene intronic sequence is located at 5′-UTR, an antisense non-coding RNA NAT binds and prevents the splicing of intron. Maintenance of this intronic sequence activates the expression of Zeb 2 because it contains internal ribosome entry site (IRES) necessary for expression of this gene [91]. Transcriptome-wide 18,871,097 analysis revealed that long non-coding RNA–RNA base pairing in human regulates the degradation of mRNA. Processing, stability control, and functions of 57,303 transcripts can be studied by these interactions [92]. For example, in

Alzheimer's disease antisense of beta-secretase-1 (BACE1-AS) basepairs with BACE1, alleviates the BACE1 mRNA, and endorses the generation of amyloid-beta 1-42 thus exacerbates disease [93].

Formation and proper functioning of miRNA to regulate gene expression is strongly influenced by non-coding RNAs. Many lncRNA genes contain entrenched miRNA sequences in their introns or exons, which harbours miRNAs. Long non-coding RNA originates miRNA like 172,713 DCL1-dependent small RNAs in Arabidopsis [94]. H19 is the firstly studied imprinted non-coding RNA precursor for miR-675 [95]. Long non-coding RNAs control the formation of miRNAs as host genes. ceRNA is a non-coding RNA that reduces the concentrations of miRNAs. Long non-coding RNAs negatively regulate the function of miRNAs, contain complementary binding sites to certain miRNAs, which exude the target miRNAs and result in the diminution of miRNA functions in cells [96]. Research from recent years found that a bulk of lncRNAs act as miRNA sponge.

3.3 miRNA-Independent mRNA Degradation

Long non-coding RNAs also modulate gene expression by direct degradation of mRNA at certain levels. Example include Staufen 1 (STAU1) that undergoes nonsense mediated mRNA decay (NMD) by directly recognising a binding motif in the 3′UTR of mRNAs [97]. For instance, STAU1 can bind to a double-stranded RNA motif and form stem loop structure within the 3′UTR of ADP-ribosylation factor 1 (ARF1) [98]. Serpin peptidase inhibitor, clade E member 1 (SERPINE1) follows Staufen-mediated mRNA decay mechanisms contain only single-stranded binding site within the 3′UTR and not form stem loop structure. mRNAs targeted by these non-coding RNAs form imperfect binding between non-coding RNA to mRNA due to presence of single complementary binding site and forming a double-stranded binding motif for STAU [51], which is named as half STAU1 binding site RNA (1/2-SBS1RNA). Terminal differentiation-induced ncRNA (TINCR) is another non-coding RNA that recruits STAU1 to mRNA PGLYRP3 (peptidoglycan recognition protein 3) in epidermis. This interaction does not lead towards NMD. Data from above findings suggested that outcomes are also influenced by recruitment of additional factors [99].

3.4 Transient lncRNA Transcribed from Active Enhancers

Transcription of genes is dependent on the interaction between the promotor sequences and enhancer elements. Enhancers are positioned away from transcriptional start site that binds with transcription factors and regulate differential gene expression [100]. Combinatorial effects of one or more enhancers control the expression of gene in tissues or at developmental stage. NODAL gene expression is controlled by at least five enhancers during developmental stages. RNAP11 is a polymerase necessary to study interaction between the active enhancer and promoter [101].

3.5 eRNA as Enhancer in Calcium Signalling

Kim et al. studied active enhancers in mouse neurons that were activated by calcium signalling of a noncoding RNA of around 2 kb and is bi directionally transcribed from active enhancers and its expression was correlated with the activity of enhancer [102, 103]. The functional properties of this eRNA that it may be polyadenylated or non polyadenylated is depicting instability in later case. However, data from studies suggested it might be functional. Matrix metallopeptidase 9 (MMP9) gene transcription is regulated by nuclear receptors NRD1 and NRD2 by preventing eRNA expression is transcribed from a MMP9 enhancer [104]. These finding suggested that eRNAs play crucial roles in chromatin remodelling, chromatin accessibility and DNA loop stabilisation. For example, chromatin at the

Forkhead box C1(FOXC1) locus is steadied by a complex formed by estrogen receptor alpha (ERa) along with its ligand and a FOXC1 enhancer-transcribed eRNA [49].

4 LncRNA Genes with Enhancer-like Activity

Long non-coding RNAs have similar function like eRNAs but they are stable, spliced and polyadenylated transcripts. Sharing common features with DNA enhancers and eRNAs genes also require changes in chromosomal conformation to deliver ncRNA to the locus close to the promoter of its target gene. This is usually mediated by a mediator complex that links the enhancer-like element to the promoter of a target gene [105, 106].

5 Micro RNAs as a Source of Non-coding RNA

Formation of mature miRNA by primary transcript is carried out by two enzymes, Drosha and DiGeorge syndrome chromosomal region 8 (DGCR8). These enzymes cut the pri-miRNA in the nucleus into a precursor (pre-miRNA) of 60 nucleotides and export to cytoplasm processed by an enzyme complex Dicer/TAR RNA protein (TRBP). These series of events finally produces mature miRNA of 20–23 nucleotides [29, 107]. Pri-miRNAs greater than 1 kb in length regarded as a form of long non-coding RNAs [107]. Two major sources of pri-miRNAs are in the genome. First that embedded with in another gene and expression is linked with the parent transcript and second is transcribed independently from intergenic regions of miRNA genes containing promoter sequences that regulate transcription by RNA polymerase II (RNAPII) in similar fashion of mRNA [30]. Around 50% of miRNAs are formed from non-coding transcripts [30, 108]. Surprisingly, in common with those entrenched in coding genes, many miRNAs within non-coding genes are also to be found within introns. Finding from genome organisation advocates that host non-coding RNA not only act as pri-miRNA but also possess additional roles by the exons. Deleted In Lymphocytic Leukemia 2 (*DLEU2*), is host gene of the tumour suppressor miR-15a/16.1 cluster located within its third intron harbours intronic miRNA [109, 110]. Long non-coding RNAs harbour intronic miRNA and are mostly down-regulated in leukaemia. For example, expression of miR-15a/16.1 regulated by host gene promoter bound by transcription factor MYC and paired box 5 (PAX5; previously also known as B-cell-specific activator protein, BSAP) in adult chronic lymphocytic leukaemia [111]. Methylation assay data from childhood acute myeloid leukaemia indicates miRNA cluster is regulated mostly independent of its host gene [112]. Another example is tumour suppressor miR-31 mostly downregulated in breast cancer.

Transcription of many genes are regulated by the methylation state of host gene promoter like *MIR-31* gene is entrenched within an intron of non-coding RNA lncRNA LOC554202. Data from previous finding suggested that vey less long non-coding RNA-entrenched miRNAs lie not within introns but also within the exon of the spliced lncRNA [113]. Long non-coding RNAs also named for the miRNA which they encode. Examples includes (MIR155HG; earlier known as B-cell integration cluster, BIC) is host gene for miR-155 anchorages an exonic miRNA region which shows strongest cross species conservation [114, 115]. Mir-22 is encoded by MIR22HG with in its second exon. Another example is a gene MIR17HG which anchorages cluster of six miRNAs within its second exon [116]. The foremost discovered and extensively studied long non-coding RNA H19 harbours miR-675 within its first intronic region [95]. H19 transcript expression is more pronounced in mouse embryo but miR-675 is restricted to placenta. These findings indicates that binding of RBP human antigen R (HuR) to a site located upstream region of miR-675 blocks Drosha processing of the primary transcript and release of miR-675 is introverted. The discrepancy between H19 and miR-675 expression proposes that H19 not only function as pri-miRNA but also has additional functions [117].

5.1 Micro RNA as Negative Regulator of Gene Expression

miRNAs negatively regulates gene expression. Binding of a short 7-nt to miRNA response element that is not perfectly complementary, targets number of transcripts [118]. Computational data suggested hundreds of transcripts may be targets of a single miRNA. Discrepancies may exists between the actual targets and predicted targets [119]. Long non-coding RNAs containing predicted miRNA binding sites regulate gene expression by sequestering miRNAs and reducing their pool in the cell. Through these types of mechanisms long non-coding RNAs act both as positive and negative regulators of gene expression. This hypothesis is named as "competing endogenous RNA (ceRNA)" hypothesis [120]. Examples of such interactions are that miR-145 in pluripotent embryonic stem cells (ESCs) is inhibited by intergenic lincRNA-ROR [121]. Pluripotent transcription factors, Nanog homeobox, SRY (sex determining region Y)-box 2 and octamer binding transcription factor 4 (OCT 4) activates expression of lincRNA-ROR. These specific transcription factors are targeted by miR-145. A feedback loop network is created by this long non-coding RNA in pluripotent gene network. Expression of OCT4 is upregulated in hepatocellular carcinoma while miR-145 acts as a tumour suppressor in these cells [122]. Non-coding POU Class 5 Homeobox 1 Pseudogene 4 (OCT4-pg4) is pseudogene of OCT4 and co-expressed with OCT4. It become endogenous competitor of OCT4, thus it protects OCT-4 from miR-145-mediated degradation [123]. Pseudogenes are non-coding genes expressed as lncRNAs, sharing a degree of homology with coding gene, and many of its micro RNA response element (MRE) becomes good candidates acting as ceRNAs [63, 124, 125]. Lower expression of long non-coding RNAs relative to their respective mRNA shows that any change in these non-coding sequences will have very less influence on miRNA availability and will become ineffectual as a competitor [126].

Ectopic over expression of ceRNAs at artificially evaluated levels is studied and it provides better explanation to study undefined transcripts although its biological significance may be restricted [127, 128]. mRNA would act more better as ceRNA because it can regulates the expression of other mRNA so it is not only limited to non-coding RNAs. Coding genes mRNA also has protein-independent non-coding function acting as non-coding RNA. Examples of this expression narrates that 3′ UTR sequences of over 1500 human mRNAs independently expressed to coding parts of the respective transcript. Experimental data from mice showed that expression patterns of independent 3′UTRs are different from coding parts of the parent transcript [120, 129]. H19 is the well explained example of long non-coding RNA effective as ceRNA. Expression of this non-coding RNA is more in undifferentiated muscle cells but becomes less in differentiated cells and about the same time miRNA let-7 expression increases. In mouse C2C12 muscle cells, siRNA induced depletion of H19 has reduced the manifestation of let-7 target genes and enhanced expression of markers of muscle differentiation thus depicting that H19 have let-7 binding sites [130]. H19 also binds to the miR-17-5p seed family. During myoblast differentiation, expression level of H19 target mRNA suggests that this non-coding RNA is competing for miR-17-5p. Thus H19 has dual roles in one miRNA as primary transcript and as ceRNA for number of others [131].

6 Circular RNAs (CircRNAs) as Non-coding RNAs

CircRNAs are cytoplasmic having nuclear localisation and play role in post transcriptional gene regulation. CircRNAs can act as ceRNAs because they are potentially stable and do not undergo exonuclease digestion. Cerebellar degeneration-related protein 1 (CDR1-A), also named as ciRS-7 gene antisense transcript is the superlatively characterized circRNA, highly articulated in mouse hippocampus and neocortex overlays with miR-7 expression domains [132–134]. CDR1-AS has large number of miR-7 binding sites, regulate its targets genes expression in vitro by depleting miR-7. This makes CDR1-AS gene resistant to miRNA-mediated degradation, rendering it a competitor because the pool of ceRNA is not dwindling. Mir-761 negatively regulates gene expression because the binding sites within CDR1-AS are nearly or perfectly complementary to microRNA [132]. (ElcircRNAs) exon–intron circRNAs is a class of RNAs that retain both introns and exons and have the ability to increase transcription of parent coding genes by RNAPII need U1 small nuclear RNA (snRNA) [135]. The examples of these Long non-coding RNAs include X-chromosome inactivation (XIST) and H19, both types of lncRNA expressed from inactivated chromosome and has a dual relationship with its coding region controlled by a cis-acting master control region [136].

7 Non-Coding RNA Functions

7.1 Functions of Long Non-coding RNAs

Long non-coding RNAs functions are not fully understood yet. Differential gene expression and folding of non-coding RNAs into secondary structure makes them versatile. Therefore, their functions are highly diverse and reflect their binding specificity to large number of substrates. Their expression patterns are dynamically upregulated or downregulated to modulate gene expression [55, 137–139]. Long non-coding RNAs regulate gene expression in major cellular functions including cell proliferation, apoptosis, differentiation, metabolism, maintenance of pluripotency, cell cycle and also play significant role in chromatin modification [137]. They act as molecular scaffolds, binds with epigenetic machinery like histone-modifying enzymes and DNA methyltransferases and promote their interaction to DNA loci [140]. They can affect the transcriptional regulation of genes by binding or inhibiting the binding of transcriptional factors and mediators to the promotor sequences [141, 142]. RNA processing mechanisms including RNA splicing and mRNA decay are also influenced by these non-coding RNAs [51, 143].

7.2 Micro RNAs as Non-coding RNAs in Cardiovascular Diseases

Cardiovascular diseases are the emerging cause of morbidity and mortality worldwide. Chronic activation of remodelling processes in response to external stresses leads to increased fibrosis and hypertrophic responses of heart consequently results in myocardial infarction [144]. Altered miRNA expression profiles in different heart pathologies showed distinctive regulation pattern of microRNAs in different cardiovascular diseases. Different microRNAs regulate different functions like promotion or inhibition of apoptotic pathways, post ischaemic neovascularization and regulates cardiac fibrosis [145]. Upon halting microRNA biogenesis by dicer deletion, it leads to dilated cardiomyopathy, maladaptive cardiac remodelling and endothelial dysfunction. Endothelial dysfunction was well studied by endothelial knockout models and it proved micro RNAs as key regulator in endothelial physiology [146–148]. Some microRNAs are considered as key regulators in vascular development and angiogenesis like miR-24 expression is significantly upregulated in cardiac ischemia. GATA-4 endothelium-enriched-transcription factor and p21-activated kinase PAK4 are the targets of miR-24 and blockage of this non-coding RNA reduces myocardial infarct size, enhances vascularity and inhibits apoptosis in cardiomyocytes [149]. MiR-126-3p is pro-angiogenic factor mediates endothelium dysfunction and atherosclerosis [150]. Knockout mouse model studies show morphological changes in cardiomyocytes including multifocal haemorrhages, systemic edema and ruptured blood vessels. It shows angio-protective role through CXCL12-CXCR4 pathway and over expression of miR-24 lowers atherosclerosis [151]. Mir-208 regulates the expression of certain cardiac transcription factors and gap junction protein connexin 40 (Cx43). This non-coding RNA is strongly expressed in autopsy samples of infarcted heart tissues obtained from patients with myocardial ischemia and dilated cardiomyopathy. Knock down of miR-208 showed no hypertrophic mass or fibrosis in response to pressure overload stimulus. It is considered as strong predictor of clinical outcome [152–155]. Mir-15 family include miRNAs that are elevated in myocardial ischemia. Down-regulation of miR-15 by anti-miR oligonucleotides lowers the infarct size after ischemia–reperfusion injury in cardiac tissues of both pigs and mice by reducing the expression of antiapoptotic protein Bcl-2 and the mitochondrial protecting factor ADP-ribosylation factor-like protein 2 and regulates gene expression [156]. Mir-150 interacts directly with the cardio specific long non-coding RNA. ZFAS1 acts as miRNA sponge, induces cardiomyocyte apoptosis through C reactive protein in acute myocardial infaraction. Downregulation of miR-150 is related to the pathology of ventricular rupture and regulates adeno-receptor beta 1 and C Reactive Protein (CRP) genes linked to heart remodelling [157–159]. Neurologic-enriched miRNA miR-212/132 family regulated cardiac gene expression by targeting forkhead box O3 (FoxO3), a pro-autophagic and anti-hypertrophic transcription factor activates pro-hypertrophic calcineurin/NFAT signalling pathway [160, 161]. Mir-21 is considered as paracrine mediator of cardiomyocyte hypertrophy when it is transferred through fibroblast derived exosomes and its altered levels are involved in cardiac hypertrophy, ischaemic heart disease, proliferative vascular disease and heart failure. It regulates expression of genes transforming growth factor b1 receptor III (TbRIII) and matrix metalloprotease-2 (MMP2) and promotes cardiac fibrosis [162–165]. Mir-1 is considered as important regulator of cell cycle, conductive system, cellular differentiation and is known as mediator of fibroblast to cardiomyocyte reprogramming [166–168]. It is abundantly expressed in heart, regulates calcium uptake through endoplasmic reticulum by cardiac Serca2a and attenuates cardiac hypertrophy in intact heart and cultured cardiomyocytes by modulating the calmodulin calcium signalling components [169]. Mir-1 and its primary target Estrogen-related receptor beta (ERR-β) regulate cardiac hypertrophic response by decreasing the cardiac fetal gene program and its expression is down-regulated in early stage cardiac hypertrophy [70, 170]. In case of myotonic dystrophy patients due to increase in expression of its target genes, i.e., calcium voltage gated channel subunit alpha1C (CAV1.2) and Connexin 43 (Cx43), while decrease in miR-1 expression leads to arrhythmia [168]. Mir-1 and mir-133 grouped together on two chromosomes. On mouse chromosome 2 they are separated by 9.3 kb while on chromosome 18 separated by 2.5 kb [171]. Despite of driving from the same polycistron and transcribing together they pose antagonistic effects on cardiac muscle development [172]. Mir-1 increases myogenic differentiation while miR-133 prompts myoblast proliferation [173]. MiRNA-133 is downregulated through Ras homolog family member A (RhoA) and cell division control protein 42 homolog (Cdc42) genes in human and mouse models of cardiac hypertrophy and plays significant role in cardiac fibrosis by regulating the expression of connective tissue growth factor [174]. Inotropism is affected by miR-133 by controlling the expression of multiple components of the b1-adrenergic signalling cascade [175]. Hypertrophic biomarkers miR-212, miR-132 and miR-512 expressions were studied in both mouse models as well as in cardiomyocytes cell cultures upon administration of hypertrophic stimulants endothelin −1 and Isoproterenol. These all non-coding RNAs were significantly upregulated, while downregulation of miR-142 was observed under the same conditions [176]. MiR-541 is known to reduce cardiac hypertrophy in response to angiotensin II treatment in transgenic mouse model, thus negatively regulates gene expression [177]. MiR-23a is known as pro-hypertrophic miRNA, expression of this non-coding RNA is regulated by nuclear factor of activated T cells (NFATc3) transcription factor. Data from previous findings revealed that its expression is upregulated in response to hypertrophic stimulants isoproterenol and aldosterone. Knock down mouse model of miR-23 attenuated

Table 1.2 Functional roles of non-coding RNA in cardiovascular system

MicroRNA	Targeted cardiovascular pathology	Targeted genetic location	References
miR-24	Vascular development angiogenesis	GATA-4	[149]
		P21 activated kinase 4 (PAK4)	
miR-126-3p	Mediates endothelial dysfunction	CXCL12-CXCR4 pathway	[150]
	Atherosclerosis		
miR-208	Myocardial ischaemia	Cardiac transcription factors gap junction connexion 40 (CX43)	[152]
	Dilated cardiomyopathy		
miR-15	Myocardial ischaemia	Bcl-2	[156]
		ADP-ribosylation factor-like protein 2	
miR-150	Myocardial infraction	CRP (C reactive protein) genes	[157–159]
miR-21	Cardiac hypertrophy	Transforming growth factor b1 receptor III (TbRIII)	[162–165]
		Matrix metalloprotease-2 (MMP2)	
miR-1	Cardiomyocyte reprogramming	Serca2a	[70, 170]
	Cardiac arrhythmia	Estrogen-related receptor beta (ERR-β)	
miR-133	Cardiac muscle development	Ras homolog family member A (RhoA)	[174]
		Cell division control protein 42 homolog (Cdc42) genes	
miR-23a	Cardiac hypertrophy	Nuclear factor of activated T cells (NFATc3) transcription factor.	[178]
miR-214	Promotes apoptosis in Valvular heart disease	Drp1 (Dynamin related protein-1)	[179]
miR-761	Inhibits apoptosis in cardiomyocytes	Mitochondrial Fission Factor (MFF)	[180]
miR-512	Cardiac hypertrophy	Brain Natriuretic Peptide (BNP)	[176]
miR-184	Modulates apoptotic pathway	Bcl-xL	[181]
		Bcl-w	
miR-30	Mitochondrial fission and fusion	P53	[182, 183]
miR-421	Promotes apoptosis in cardiomyocytes	PINK 1	[184, 185]
miR-140	Mitochondrial survival pathway	Mito-fusin II	[186, 187]

hypertrophy confirms it a pro-hypertrophic non-coding RNA [178].

Dysregulated mitochondrial network causes membrane potential depolarization and disturbs the intricate balance between the mitochondrial fission and fusion. Upregulation of miR-214 and its putative target Dynamin related protein 1 (DRP1) gene was observed in valvular heart disease confirms apoptosis in cardiomyocytes [179]. Mitochondrial fission factor (MFF) is the direct target of miR-761, thus this non-coding RNA inhibits apoptosis in cardiomyocytes regulating mitochondrial dynamics network [180]. Functional modalities of different miRNAs are also mentioned in Table 1.2.

7.3 Role of Long Non-coding RNA in Cardiovascular Diseases

Highthrough-put sequencing data revealed that in comparison to miRNA and mRNA altered expression profiles, long non-coding RNA changing their molecular expression patterns are more susceptible to heart failure aetiologies [188]. Klattenhoff et al. firstly identified *Braveheart(Bvht) as* first long non-coding RNA in mouse heart development. This long coding RNA interrelates with Polycomb Repressive Complex 2 Subunit SUZ12, part of PRC2 complex and plays crucial roles in cardiomyocyte differentiation. Chast ('cardiac hypertrophy–associated transcript') is a long non-coding RNA that is associated with cardiac remodelling and hypertrophy in mouse model. Pathological cardiac remodelling attenuation and gain and loss function phenomena was observed in in-vivo mouse model where antisense mediated degradation of Chast was carried out [189]. Long non-coding RNA, MALAT1 has dual roles in cancer as well as in cardiovascular disease. In mouse model of hind limb ischemia and diabetic neuropathy it lowers the capillary growth. MALAT1- derived mascRNA (MALAT1-associated small cytoplasmic RNA) role is associated with viral myocarditis and cardiovascular innate immunity [190, 191]. GAS5 (growth arrest–specific 5) is another long non-coding RNA expressed and regulates endothelial cells and cardiac smooth muscles through b-catenin signalling. Expression profile studies shows that in hypertension, its expression is significantly downregulated [192]. CARL is cardiac apoptosis-related non-coding RNA and plays role in maintenance of mitochondrial homeostasis and regulator of cell death in cardiomyocytes [193]. Long non-coding RNA which is considered as important regulator of pathological cardiac remodelling and cardiac development is Novlnc6. Its expression is down regulated in response to hypertrophic response by angiotensin II in cardiomyocytes. Knockdown mouse model studies showed synergistic decrease in expression of Novlnc6 along with two important factors BMP10 and NKX2.5 that are the regulators of cardiac growth and function. It showed upregulated expression in human heart failure samples and transverse aortic constriction mouse model. It directly de-represses Myd88, which is a direct target of miR-489, regulates cardiac hypertrophy and acts as miRNA sponge [194, 195]. Polymorphism studies in long non-coding RNA myocardial infarction–associated transcript (MIAT) is considered as risk factor of myocardial infarction and dilated cardiomyopathy. This long non-coding RNA is highly expressed in fetal brain tissues and heart and present at lower levels in platelets of patients suffering from myocardial infarction. High levels were observed in patients of dilated cardiomyopathy already suffering from Chagas disease [196–198]. CARMEN (Cardiac mesoderm enhancer-associated noncoding RNA) is expressed in cardiac precursor cells during cell proliferation, differentiation and specification. It is considered as important regulator of miR-143 and miR-145. Knockout model studies showed that it interacts with two major components of PRC2 complex, SUZ12 and EZH2 and prevents cardiac differentiation in cardiac precursor cells [194]. FOXF1-adjacent noncoding developmental regulatory RNA (Fendrr) is cardiac-specific non-coding RNA, expressed in embryonic lateral mesoderm and binds with PRC2 induces trimethylation of H3 at lysine 27 and lysine 4. It modifies the chromatin landscape of cardiomyocyte encoding genes and transcription factors GATA binding protein 4 (GATA-4), Forkhead box (FoxF1), T-box 3(Tbx3), Iroquois homeobox 3(Irx3), NK2 homeobox 5 (Nkx2-5) and paired like homeodomain 2 (Pitx2) [199]. Myh7 locus termed myosin heavy-chain-associated (Myheart or Mhrt) RNAs is another example of cardiac expressed non-coding RNA whose target is Brg1, a stress-activated chromatin-remodelling factor leading towards cardiac myopathy and altered gene expression. It functions by negative feedback mechanism; binds with the helicase domain of Brg1 and inhibits gene regulation and chromatin remodelling encoded by Brg1 [59]. The steroid receptor RNA activator 1(SRA1) is gene which is dependent on alternative splicing and generates many isoforms. SRA and the steroid receptor RNA activator protein (SRAP) coding transcript both act as non-coding RNA. Experimental data from in vivo and in vitro experiments showed that it is the co-activator of MyoD and regulates skeletal myogenesis. Inhibition of SRA1 impairs the normal function of heart in ventricular chambers examined at 72 h post fertilization [200, 201]. Ppp1r1b-lncRNA is involved in the development of cardiovascular system in which heart undergoes a critical process named as extra-uterine life called 'perinatal circulatory transition' [202]. Transcriptomic analysis at different time periods of mouse heart development and cardiomyocyte terminal differentiation showed that Ppp1r1b-lncRNA plays important role in these developmental stages of mammalian heart. It is paired with its neighbouring gene Tcap and its expression is inversely correlated in myogenic differentiation and perinatal process. It encodes muscle specific proteins associated with cardiomyocyte sarcomere organization and silencing of this non-coding RNA excites Tcap expression [203]. ENSMUST00000117266 is an important regulator of proliferative growth and its activity decreases in late gestation. This non-coding RNA in oxidative stress and hypoxic stimuli loses its activity from p1 to p7. Silencing studies in mouse cardiomyocytes suggested that it in G2/M phase, it lowers the number of cardiomyocytes and move them from hyperplastic to hypertrophic growth transition [204, 205].

7.4 Long Non-coding RNA in Myocardial Infarction and Atherosclerosis

Coronary artery disease is the major cause of formation of fatty streaks, atherosclerotic plaques and atheromas leading toward myocardial infarction [206]. Long non-coding RNA regulates the function of endothelial cells, vascular and smooth muscles cells, macrophages, metabolism and inflammation. Therefore, these are the key players to develop atherosclerotic plaques in arteries. ANRIL, MIAT and H19 are considered as important regulators of progression in myocardial infarction [48].

7.5 Non-Coding RNAs in Apoptosis Linked Cardiovascular Pathologies

7.5.1 Micro RNAs as Regulator of Apoptosis

Cell death network is regulated by three major cellular mechanisms: apoptosis, necrosis and autophagy [207, 208]. Programmed cell death is one of the conserved mechanisms that regulate intricate signalling cascades by extrinsic death receptor and intrinsic mitochondrial pathways. The structural changes in these pathways demolish the cellular morphology by causing cell shrinkage, nuclear condensation, DNA fragmentation and membrane blebbing [209]. Extrinsic pathway of apoptosis is regulated by binding of plasma membrane death receptor (Fas, TNFR) with its ligand (FasL, TNF-α) and forms the death-inducing complex (DISC) that triggers caspase 8. Subsequent activation of downstream effector caspase 3 and 7 by caspase 8 degrades proteome and promotes cell death [210]. Intrinsic mitochondrial pathway is activated by intracellular stress signals including hypoxia, oxidative stress, acidosis and DNA damage. These signals stimulate the pro-apoptotic signals Bax and Bak in the outer membrane while releases cytochrome c in to the cytosol [211, 212]. Sequentially, downstream caspase 9 and its effector caspases 3 and 7 are activated. These caspases changes the morphology of mitochondria, initiates death cascade and disorders of genetic expression leads towards cardiovascular pathologies [182, 213]. Micro RNA as a class of short non-coding RNA is an important contributor in cell death signalling cascades involved in the pathogenesis and progression of cardiovascular diseases [214].

MiR-1 is the example of non-coding RNAs whose expression is downregulated in infarcted heart. Under oxidative stress conditions, cardiomyocytes undergoes apoptosis due to upregulation of miR-1 and by reducing the activity of anti-apoptotic gene Bcl2 [215]. Knock down model of miR-1 showed that it can supresses cardiac arrhythmia [216]. Mir 133 is another example of apoptosis linked biomarker. Mir -133 antagonize apoptotic cascades by negative regulation of caspase 9 which is triggered by H_2O_2 exposure to cardiomyocytes [217]. Over expression studies of micro RNA 133a studies revealed that it protects the heart from fibrosis [218]. Mir-181c is also a regulator of apoptotic pathway by targeting Bcl-2 through TNF-α-induced signalling pathways [219]. Differentially regulated other micro RNAs include miR-30, miR-320, miR-21 and miR-199a. They target apoptosis related proteins in the heart and modulate apoptotic program [220–223].

Modulation of apoptotic pathways by oxidative stress is the contributory factor in development of ROS induced lesions in myocardial tissues [224]. Interestingly, mouse model of myocardial infarction study depicted that modified miR-184 mis-recognises two important mitochondrial genes Bcl-xL and Bcl-w which are not proved as native targets of miR-184 [181].

Mitochondrial fission and fusion maintains the balance between the cell death and cell survival and both phenomena are under the control of different micro RNAs [225, 226]. Therefore, mitochondrial dynamics regulates different genes related to cardiac function and injury [209]. Dynamin related protein-1 (Drp1) is required for mitochondrial fission can reduce infract size in knockdown mouse models of ischemia/reperfusion injury. Expression of apoptosis linked marker P53, which is target of Drp1 is regulated by miR-30 by downregulating its expression in cardiomyocytes [182, 183]. Mir-499 expression is downregulated in the heart of ischemic injury but overexpression of this non-coding RNA prevents from myocardial infarction by inhibiting the dephosphorylation of Drp1 through calcineurin pathway [227]. Mitofusin1 (Mfn1) I is important regulator of mitochondrial survival pathway that prevents the cell from apoptotic signals. Mouse model studies showed that miR-140 supresses Mfn1 by directly targeting its 3′ UTR region [186, 187]. Dysregulated mitochondrial dynamic studies revealed that interplay of Pink1 is a Ser/Thr kinase, E2F1 and miR-421, is responsible for apoptosis in cardiomyocytes. This micro RNA supresses PINK 1 translation and induces mitochondrial fragmentation, myocardial infarction and apoptosis [184, 185]. Mtfr 1 (mitochondrial fission regulator 1) contributes in abnormal mitochondrial function by targeting NFAT/-324-5p/ [228]. Over expression of this non-coding RNA reduced apoptosis in ischemia reperfusion model and also reduces infract size in mouse injury model. Although microRNAs are considered as key regulators of mitochondrial network but still many mechanisms remained unexplored. Numbers of microRNAs have been identified that protects the heart from the doxorubicin (DOX) induced cardiomyocyte death in congestive heart failure [229, 230]. Data from previous findings revealed that cardiotoxicity and DOX-induced apoptosis is addressable by antagomir- based silencing mechanism of miR-532-3p and miR-208a [231, 232]. Further, over expression of miR- 21 and miR-30 prevents doxorubicin induced apoptosis in cardiomyocytes [233, 234]. These therapeutic strategies open better avenues to prevent doxorubicin induced cardiotoxicity.

7.5.2 Long Non-coding RNAs in Apoptosis

Long non-coding RNAs such as circular RNAs are considered as new regulators of apoptotic signalling cascades in cardiovascular diseases. These non-coding RNAs comprises a class of RNA having more than 200 nucleotides are present in the whole genome [235]. Cellular functions displayed by circular RNAs include capturing miRNAs, directing transcription factors, modification of three dimensional structure of chromatin, genomic imprinting and cell fate determination [236–239]. Two important non-coding RNAs; Braveheart and FOXF1 adjacent non-coding developmental regulatory RNA are key players of cardiomyocyte differentiation [196, 199]. CARL is apoptosis linked non-coding RNA executed as endogenous miRNA sponge directly targets prohibitin 2 (PHB2). PBH2 expression inhibits mitochondrial fission and apoptosis reduces the infarct size in ischaemia reperfusion mouse model [195]. Mitochondrial fission and apoptosis is inhibited by CARL by miR-539/PHB2 pathway. Another class of non-coding RNA is identified as a close loop that join together at 3′ and 5′.These circular RNAs acts as sponge to miRNAs and participates in multiple major cellular processes [134]. HRCR (heart-related circRNA) is a circular non-coding RNA considered as modulator of apoptosis pathway. This specific non-coding RNA acts as miRNA sponge for miR-223 and inhibits its activity [132, 240]. It targets the abundantly expressed heart protein ARC (apoptosis repressor with CARD domain). Therefore, promotes cardiac hypertrophy and heart failure by directly targeting this anti-apoptotic protein [241, 242]. The wide spectrum of non-coding RNAs is utilized for the development of ncRNA based therapeutic strategies. The non-coding RNAs such as the miRNA, lncRNAs can serve as the efficient targets for the treatment of cardiovascular diseases

[243–246]. The siRNA based RNA interference is also used as a general tool for targeting mRNA and results in protein encoding gene silencing [247]. The rapid evolution of non-coding RNAs highlights their importance for human health [50, 248]. However, very little part of the genome has been investigated for the cardiovascular therapeutics [247].

8 miRNA as Therapeutic Target in Cardiovascular Diseases

The miRNAs have the remarkable ability to maintain expression of the several genes of different signaling pathways and makes them striking therapeutic targets. The different studies have been conducted in preclinical models to evaluate the therapeutic potential of miRNA in cardiovascular diseases. The miRNAs have the diverse range of targets because of the multiple target sites in different genes. This feature of the miRNA makes them superior over the other therapeutic strategies, as miRNA can potentially regulate complex signaling cascades [249]. Moreover, as miRNAs mostly target the different components in the signaling of the biological process, this may control the desensitization of a drug [156]. However, the limitations of the miRNA therapeutics include the way of delivery, off-target effects and stimulatory effects. All these are the major challenges for using the miRNA in clinical practice.

The miRNA therapeutic approaches are of two types.

- The inhibition of miRNA to lower the expression of pathological miRNAs.
- The miRNA replacement strategy to enhance the expression of beneficial miRNAs or the ones which are repressed in cardiac stress.

To attain these approaches, different strategies have been designed including the antisense oligonucleotides which are chemically modified and also the miRNA mimics.

8.1 Role in Acute Myocardial Infarction

The miRNAs are involved in the regulation of cardiac remodeling in variety of ways. In response to ischemia the miRNA-15 family is regulated and it modulates the hypoxia induced cardiomyocyte cell death [156]. The obstruction of miRNA-15 family members enhances postnatal cardiac regeneration [250]. With regard to mechanism, the key player of the mitochondrial function, Pyruvate dehydrogenase lipoamide kinase isozyme 4 and checkpoint kinase 1 have been recognized as the targets of miRNA-15 family members [156, 250]. In addition to ischemia, aging can also induce the expression of miRNA-34 family members and trigger the debilitate DNA damage control, cardiomyocyte cell death and promote telomere degradation, paving for their role as key regulators of cardiomyocytes repair [251–253]. Mechanistically, the cardiomyocyte cell death due to aging is directly related with the miRNA-34a regulated reduction of the target gene "protein phosphatase 1 nuclear-targeting subunit"(PNUTS). PNUTS regulates the DNA damage response and cardiomyocytes cell death, ultimately resulting in the recovery after acute myocardial infarction in mice. The expression of MiR-92 is elevated in ischemic tissues, but contrary to it exhibits the anti-angiogenicity by decreasing the Sirtuin 1 and resulting in the inhibition of ischemia-induced angiogenesis [254–256]. In addition miR-24 also targets Sirtuin 1 and acts as a key modulator of angiogenesis and endothelial cell death [149].

8.2 Role in Fibrosis

Several miRNAs control important processes which are involved in cardiac fibrosis by targeting cardiomyocytes death or by angiogenesis that contribute post-infarction injury and later remodeling responses [145]. The examples of miRNA which are directly hindering the fibrotic response are miRNA-29 and miRNA-21. The miRNA-29 targets different matrix proteins and reduces the fibrosis [257]. The miR-21 inhibits the Spry1 (sprout homologue 1), thus increase the ERK-MAP kinase associated fibrotic pathway. The expression of miRNA-21 is increased in fibroblasts in transverse aortic constriction or acute myocardial infarction [258]. The inhibition of ERK-MAP kinase signaling regulates the release of growth factor and also controls the survival of fibroblasts thus ultimately it regulates the hypertrophy and fibrosis. The role of miRNA-21 in cardiac fibrosis was firstly investigated in the mice model [259]. However, the studies in other models have also affirmed that inhibition of miR-21 reduces cardiac hypertrophy and fibrosis [260–263].

Another important miRNA which targets the collagen type-1 A1 is miRNA-133, its levels were found to be downregulated in case of hypertension and cardiac fibrosis. Due to the decreased levels of miRNA-133, there is the depression in collagen levels which confirms the role of miRNA-133 in promoting the extent of fibrosis [264]. However, another study has shown the role of miRNA-133 and miRNA-30 in regulation of the expression of connective tissue growth factor in both human and animal cardiac tissues [174].

Pan et al. elucidated the role of miRNA-101 in fibrosis. The levels of miRNA-101a and miRNA-101b were found to be downregulated in the infarct area after coronary artery ligation [265]. However, in-vitro studies have shown the decreased expression of miRNA-101a and b due to angiotensin II in the cardiac fibroblasts of the rats. In cardiac fibroblasts the overexpression of the miRNA-101a and miRNA-101b nullify the collagen production and proliferation. The co-transfection of miRNA-101a and b inhibitors along with the overexpression of miRNA-101a/b has abrogated the effects. The bioinformatic tools and luciferase gene reporter assays have shown the c-fos as a target of miRNA-101a. The angiotensin II treatment to the cardiac fibroblasts resulted in the significantly enhanced expression of c-fos and TGF-β1. Further experimental studies have elucidated the role of miRNA-101 by increasing the expression of c-fos, which resulted in the elevated expression of TGF-β1 and collagen, whereas by the use of miRNA-101 mimic the levels were diminished. The miRNA-101 also targets the several autophagy genes such as the Stathmin 1 and Rab-5A [266]. The miRNA-101 levels were reduced in the patients of stenosis and cardiomyopathy [144]. In previous studies the decreased levels of miRNA-101 have been reported in the case of rheumatic heart disease. Moreover, the cardiac stress is associated with the downregulation of miRNA-101, therefore the strategies to enhance the levels of miRNA-101 may serve as a therapeutic approach for cardiac fibrosis [267].

The members of the c-Jun family form the transcription factor activator protein 1 (AP-1). Different cytokines which are involved in the cellular differentiation and proliferation induces the expression of AP-1 [268]. The cell-cycle regulatory genes also mediate the expression of AP-1. The expression of the cardiac fibrosis related miRNA, the miRNA-21 is regulated by the AP-1. Moreover, the promoter region of the miRNA-29 also contains several putative binding sites for the AP-1 [269]. The binding of AP-1 to the promoter of miRNA-29 results in the reduction of fibrosis. The role of AP-1 in the ischemia/reperfusion was also investigated by Roy et al., it has been found that oxygen induces the expression of the TGFβ isoforms by the activation of AP-1 [270]. Specifically, the fos related AP-1 is essential in the regulation of TGF expression.

Interestingly, the miRNA-21 also contributes to the cardiac fibrosis by the restoration of the endothelial to mesenchymal transition (EMT). The TGFβ induces EMT in endothelial cells by the elevated levels of miRNA-21 [271]. The miRNA-101 also enhances the cardiac fibrosis by regulating the c-fos and c-fos related miRNAs. The activation of AP-1 activates the profibrotic pathways such as the activation of the miRNA-21. The miRNA-101 directly interferes with the expression of miRNA-21 and the expression of AP-1. However, the direct effect of miRNA-101 on the different miRNAs and the family members of c-Jun family is still explorable [272]. The in-vitro studies have shown no effect of miRNA-101 on cardiomyocytes apoptosis and suggest that miRNA-101 might have antiapoptotic effects in-vivo by the improvement in the cardiac function. In contrast, the miRNA-101 mimics have shown the positive effects on cardiac function and hemodynamic in myocardial infarcted rats. The underlie mechanism of miRNA-101 is yet need to be investigated for the enrichment of miRNA mimics by the viral based delivery approaches.

8.3 Role of miRNA in Cardiac Hypertrophy and Failure

The miR-133, miR-212/132, miRNA-208, miRNA-499, miRNA-208 and miRNA-25 are the major examples of miRNAs which are involved in cardiac hypertrophy and failure [173]. MiRNA also control the intracellular calcium homeostasis, which is deregulated in heart failure. Modification of the intracellular calcium levels improves the cardiomyocyte contractility, might serve as a promising therapy against cardiac failure. The inhibition of miR-25 represses the calcium uptake pump sarco/endoplasmic reticulum Ca^{+2} ATPase 2a, therefore it improves the calcium handling and restores cardiac function [273]. The decrease expression of miRNA-1 and miRNA-133 has been reported in mouse and human models of cardiac hypertrophy [274]. The invitro enhanced expression of the miRNA-133 and miRNA-1 has resulted in the inhibition of hypertrophy whereas; the inhibition of miRNA-133 by using antagomiRs has caused the substantial and sustained cardiac hypertrophy. The miRNA-133 targets the Rho A, Nelf-A/WHSC2 (a nuclear factor) and Cdc 42 which are involved in cardiac hypertrophy [173]. The miRNA-133 and miRNA-1 also regulate the cardiac muscle repolarization [275]. In contrary to miRNA133/1, the miRNA-212 and miRNA-132 expressions are increased by stimuli and maintain the growth of cardiomyocytes by directly regulating the FoxO3 (Forkhead box protein O3). The expression of Foxo3 is negatively correlated with the hypertrophy [161]. In response to hypothyroidism and stress the miRNA-208 is expressed by an intron of the *αMHC*. MiRNA-208 is known to play role in fibrosis, hypertrophy and in maintaining the level of βMHC (myosin heavy chain-β) [154].

8.4 Role of miRNA in Atherosclerosis and Remodeling

Atherosclerosis is an inflammatory reaction of the arterial wall, underlying the coronary artery disease. It is characterized by the dysfunctional responses of endothelial cells with dysregulated flow of immune cells [276]. It has been previously reported that diverse range of miRNAs has been emerged in atherosclerotic mouse model, which can provide a platform for designing potential therapeutic strategies using anti-miRNA or miRNA mimics [276]. The miRNa-92a, miRNA-126, miRNA-146 and miRNA-181 are involved in atherosclerosis [277]. In addition to these miRNAs, the miRNA-10a and 23b have shown the atheroprotective effects [278, 279]. The balloon injury in the vascular walls has shown the expression of miRNA-21 as a main regulator of cell proliferation, apoptosis and neointima formation [280]. Moreover, the analysis has also shown the role of miRNA-21 in cellular apoptosis by targeting PTEN and Bcl-2.

The miR-29 is age regulated and targets the collagen and other extracellular matrix proteins ultimately sensitizes the aorta for formation of aneurysms in later age [281, 282]. In disease conditions the levels of miRNA-29 is increased, causing the inhibition of its collagen target genes. The inhibition of miRNA-29 protects the vessel from rupturing by abrogating aortic dilation. Moreover, the intronic miRNAs such as the miRNA-33a and miRNA-33b are co-expressed with SREBF (sterol regulatory element-binding transcription factor) 1 and SREBF2, regulate lipid homeostasis thus, deletion at gene level was shown to increase circulating high density lipid cholesterol levels [283]. The endothelial miRNA-126 suppresses the expression of Notch1 inhibitor Dlk1 and thereby prevents atherosclerotic lesion formation. The few miRNAs also exhibit the anti-inflammatory potential such as the miRNA-146a and 181b, by inhibiting the 3′-untranslated region of TRAF6 and Importin alpha 3, ultimately inhibiting the activity of NF-kB [284, 285]. The altered level of miRNA-10a also plays role in maintaining the proinflammatory phenotypes that may affect the progression of atherosclerosis [286].

There are various miRNAs which are involved in the cardiovascular system regulation, accent their potential as worthy targets for the therapeutic intervention for different cardiovascular diseases.

8.5 miRNA as a Therapeutic Approach for CVDs

The miRNAs are playing diverse range of roles in regulation of different cardiac pathologies such as post-infarction angiogenesis, remodeling, cardiac fibrosis, hypertrophy, and atherosclerosis [145, 154, 258, 271, 287]. The role of miRNAs was mostly investigated either by viral vectors, RNA therapeutics or by using transgenic mice to overexpress or inhibit specific miRNAs. The antisense oligonucleotides or siRNAs are mainly used to inhibit the miRNA. The phosphorothioate backbones are chemically added to the antisense oligonucleotides or siRNA to increase their stability against RNases.

The cholesterol is also conjugated with certain RNAs to reduce the chances of initiating the immune response and to decrease the probability of off-target effects, thus ameliorating the pharmacodynamics by boosting cellular uptake. The antisense molecules base pairs with the given mRNA targets in complementary fashion and thereby block the inhibitory function of miRNA. The miRNA inhibitors known as antimiRs can also serve as the therapeutic strategy. The antimiRs are categorized into different groups on the basis of their chemical modifications.

9 miRNA Modification

The strategy to use miRNA as the therapeutic target is by using the miRNA inhibitor and miRNA sponge. The miRNA inhibitor should have the high affinity for the target mRNA sequence and high specificity. It should also display the nuclease resistance, less toxicity and low-cost for synthesis.

9.1 Antisense Oligonucleotides

The most eminent groups of antimiRs are the antagomiRs and locked nucleic acids. The antogomiRs are chemically modified by the conjugation of 3′cholesterol, 2′-O-methyl, 2′O-fluoro or 2′O-methoxymethyl oligonucleotides. The antagomiRs are complementary to the specific miRNA's mature sequence with the linkages of the phosphorothioate backbone that replaces non-bridging oxygen atom of the phosphate group with the Sulfur [288]. The phosphorothioate backbone supports the binding with the plasma protein in addition to the nuclease resistance, thus ultimately improves the pharmacokinetics [289]. Due to the addition of 2′-O-methyl, 2′-fluoro or 2′-methoxymethyl to the antagomiRs results in efficient binding and it also decreases the chances of off-targets effects, whereas the addition of cholesterol improves the cellular uptake of the antagomiRs [288]. The advancement of locked nucleic acids modified antimiRs has augmented the area of oligonucleotide chemistry.

The locked nucleic acids (LNAs) are chemically modified in such a way that a bridge locks the LNAs by connecting the 2′-oxygen and 4′-carbon in a ribonucleotide, thus mimics the C3′-endo conformation. The use of specific deoxyribonucleotide and locked ribonucleotide have exhibited the promising results in various *in-vivo* models [290]. The LNA-based antimiRs are 15-16nts in length whereas the shorter LNA-based antimiRs are also developed known as tiny LNAs or 8-mer LNA based AntimiR [291]. The 8-mer LNA based AntimiR binds to the seed region of the miRNA; therefore, we can target the complete miRNA family with coinciding functional activities which may potentiate the positive effect in certain pathological conditions. One of the examples of tiny LNA is for the miR-15 family members; it targets the seed region of all members including miRNA-15a, 15b, 16 to 1, 195, 16 to 2 and 497. It depresses the downstream targets more efficiently as compared to the previously used LNA- based antimir targeting only particular miRNA [156]. In case of cardiac tissues, the uptake of LNAs is not affected by the length of the LNAs. However, in some cases the efficiency of tiny LNAs is less as compared to longer LNAs, such as miR-21 targeted by antagomir treatment markedly reduce the cardiac hypertrophy and fibrosis whereas the tiny LNAs designed against miRNA-21 did not exhibit any restorative effects.

The functionality of LNA antimiRs has also been improved by the use of the two strategies that have been developed to ameliorate the actions of LNA antimiRs. The selenomethylene LNAs have shown the greater affinity and improved ability for miRNA-21 inhibition in cancerous cell lines. The other is known as small RNA zipper [292]. The small RNA zippers are designed on the basis of the LNA; inhibit the miRNA-221 and miRNA-17 in breast cancer [292]. However, to date there is no report of the potential application of these strategies for the therapeutics of cardiovascular diseases. The other class is the peptide nucleic acids; antisense oligonucleotides in which the backbone is replaced by the repetitive units of N-(2-aminomethyl) glycine to which the nitrogenous bases are linked through a methyl carbonyl linker. The peptide nucleic acids were successfully used against miRNA-155 in the B-cells of mice [293].

9.2 siRNAs

siRNAs are used to inhibit the miRNAs, these are the chemically modified RNA duplexes which improves the stability and cellular uptake [294]. The siRNas have been reported to downregulate the expression of miR-181a and leads to the reduced arrhythmogenicity of skeletal myoblasts replacement in rats having myocardial infarction [295]. The miRNAs are also targeted by using the miRNA target site blocker. They get attach to the miRNA target site of mRNA and ultimately prevents the miRNA binding to its target site [296]. In this way the certain targets of miRNA can be protected instead of targeting all in parallel. For example, Messina et al. (2016) has reported the use of blockers exhibited selective disability of miRNA-155 to target the CCAAT/enhancer binding protein- β in the juvenile hypothalamus. The function of miRNA can be modified by the use of miRNA sponges which are constructed from the transgene within the cells. The sponge RNAs have 4 to 10 complementary binding sites to the miRNA of interest introduced in 3′UTR of the RNA. The binding site can be any specific sequence of the miRNA or it can be the seed sequence of the mRNA [297]. The viral vectors are suitable for the delivery of miRNA sponges construct to the tissues of the living animals. The adenoviral eGFP (enhanced green fluorescence protein) sponge was used to target the miRNA-133 in cardiomyocytes of the cardiac hypertrophic mouse model. However, the limitation of this strategy is that as there is an excessive concentration of the endogenous miRNA within the cell so there should be the high concentration of sponges to bind. Various studies highlight the role of antimiRs in inhibition of miRNA function especially in cardiovascular research.

9.3 Restoration of miRNA Levels

Over the past few years the research has also been carried out to reintroduce the reduced miRNA into the effected cells. The levels of miRNA can be restored by either using the miRNA mimics or using the adeno-associated viruses (AAVs). miRNA mimics are the double stranded synthetic oligonucleotide sequences which are designed as a single strand for targeting the genes. The miRNA mimics are chemically modified in the similar manner as the antisense oligonucleotides technology. Montgomery et al. (2014) developed the functional miRNA -29 mimic for the treatment of cardiac fibrosis. They had conjugated the miRNA mimic with the cholesterol to increase the cellular uptake and it also had the mismatches to avoid it to act as the inhibitor [298]. Successful application of miRNA mimic in clinical trials has been reported [299, 300]. Inspite of the recent progress in this field to date still the delivery of miRNA mimics is a matter of debate, due to their short half-life. The efficient delivery system is required for better stability and cellular uptake of miRNA mimics. However, the issues regarding the dosage regimen and safety must need to be addressed too [301].

9.4 Therapeutic Potential of AntagomiRs

The antagomiRs have the wide range of therapeutic applications. The antagomir against miR-21 has been reported to reduce the extent of cardiac fibrosis and hypertrophy after TAC in mice [258]. The antagomiR which targets the miRNA-92a has displayed the increased neovascularization after ischemia and salubrious effects on myocardial infarction. A single injection of antagomir-92a intercepted the endothelial dysfunction and atherosclerosis [302, 303]. The seed sequence of the miRNA-25 is similar to the miRNA-92a, it is upregulated in heart failure and targeting it by the antagomiR results in ameliorative effects in mouse model [273]. The substantial studies have confirmed the protective effects of the antagomir-25 but another study showed that antagomir against the miRNA-25 injected intraperitoneally at a concentration of 80 mg/kg resulted in the spontaneous cardiac dysfunction [274]. However, it is still needed to investigate whether it is due to the difference in formulations or concentrations. The antagomiR-320 also showed the improved heart function after ischemia. In addition to these, the anatagomiR-212/132 rescued the cardiac heart failure after TAC in mice [161].

9.5 Therapeutic Potential of LNA AntimiRs

The LNA antimiRs have shown the promising effects as the inhibitors of miRNA in several disease models. The LNA based antimir which targets the miRNA-29 decreases the aneurysm development by enhancing the matrix formation and maintaining the structural integrity of the wall [281, 282]. The inhibition of miRNA-208 via the LNA antimir has manifested the improved heart function and survival after cardiac failure [304]. Moreover, the therapeutic targeting of the whole miRNA-34 family [253] or specifically miRNA-34a decreases apoptosis and cardiac fibrosis [251, 252]. A study has compared the therapeutic potential of both antagomiR and LNA-based antagomir-34a in the experimental mouse model, both the strategies showed the restorative effects from myocardial infarction [252]. The analeptic effects of the antagomir based targeting of miRNA-92a was also confirmed by using LNA antimiRs in ischemic model [254].

9.6 Challenges for AntimiR

There are wide range of therapeutic applications of miRNA inhibition in different experimental models, but still targeting the miRNA in cardiac tissue is more challenging than in any other organ. The administration of antimiRs can be done subcutaneously, intraperitoneally and intravenously. It manifests the long-term inhibition for many weeks. Mostly 0.5 to 25 mg/kg body weight dose of antimiRs are administered in either single or repetitive manner. However, the higher dose concentrations are required for the antagomiRs nearly 8 to 80 mg/kg body weight to effectively reduce miRNA in cardiovascular system. The optimum dose depends on the target chemistry and also on the target sequence. The miRNA-92a can be inhibited by the use of low dose (0.5 mg/kg) of LNA based antimiR-92a and also by the 8 mg/kg dose of antagomiR-92a [254]. However, for targeting the miRNA-34a the higher concentration was required although the target tissue was same as that for the miRNA-92a [252, 282].

10 miRNAs as Biomarker

With the recent advances in the research, the miRNAs are gaining more insight as the diagnostic and prognostic biomarkers for cardiovascular diseases. The different means of transportation and protection from RNAses adopted by the miRNA make them stable as compared to the mRNA. The miRNAs are enclosed in exosomes.

The miRNA form complexes with the RNA-binding proteins and are also transported in the high-density lipoprotein [305–307]. The expression pattern for the miRNA enclosed in exosomes reflects the expression pattern of those in whole blood [308].

The miRNAs serve as the useful clinical biomarkers as they can be easily accessible from the different body fluids which help in diagnosis. The use of miRNAs as biomarkers will play the key role in different clinical applications such as the diagnosis therapeutics and prognostics. In comparison to the tissue specific miRNAs the circulating miRNAs are the better option as a biomarker for CVD. The miRNAs are mostly conserved across the species, are resistant to RNase, harsh conditions, differential expression in disease condition and can easily be determined by various methods and all these features make them the promising candidate to serve as a biomarker [309, 310].

10.1 miRNA as Biomarker in Atherosclerosis

One of the major example of atherosclerotic biomarker is the miRNA-1, that is known to exhibit role in coronary artery disease. The pre-clinical trials exhibited that the miRNA-1 targets the ion channels which are the important players in cardiac physiology. One of the targets is the connexin 43; the gap junction channel which controls the intracellular conductance of ions in the ventricle while the second target is kir2.1; the K+ ion channel which maintains the resting membrane potential. The elevated expression of miRNA-1 is correlated with the repression in Kir2.1 ultimately leading to coronary artery disease [216].

miR-1 along with other heart-specific miRNAs might become a promising, specific and sensitive diagnostic biomarkers for AMI, because of their expected release into the circulation from injured cardiomyocytes. Presently, cardiac troponin (cTnT) is used for the diagnosis of Acute myocardial infarction but still there is a dire need for new biomarkers with enhanced specificity [311, 312].

The miRNA-1 levels are also positively corelated with the infarct size [313]. The miRNA-1 can serve as the biomarker for the acute coronary artery syndrome too. The miRNA-1, miRNA-133a and miRNA 208b were found to be significantly increased in case of acute myocardial infarction [314]. However, the differential levels of these miRNAs may serve as the better diagnostic marker to differentiate between myocardial infarction and unstable angina [314].

The mortality is also co-related with the levels of miRNA-133a and mIRNA-208b after acute coronary artery syndrome. These miRNAs did not give any prognostic information when they were adjusted with the troponin levels. Another related study has shown the very reduced levels of cardiac specific miRNAs in the plasma of the healthy subjects. The levels of miRNA-1, 133a and 208b were found to be increased in AMI patients but no significant variation was observed in case of any other cardiovascular disease patients. The pharmacological treatment to the patients reduced the plasma levels of miRNA-208a [307].

All the above findings suggest these miRNAs as a promising biomarker for the diagnosis of acute myocardial infarction. In comparison to the other miRNAs, the miRNA-208a is a better choice because the miRNA-1133 and 499 are also expressed in the skeletal muscles, so the injury to these may also increase the plasma levels of these miRNAs, whereas the miRNA-208a is specifically expressed in cardiac tissues.

The circulating levels of miRNA-133 and miRNA-208 were increased in coronary artery disease patients as compared to healthy subjects. In contrary to these miRNAs, the level of miRNA-126 (vascular miRNA), miRNA-17, inflammation related miRNA-155 and VSMC related miRNA-145 were significantly downregulated [315]. An appreciable elevated expression of miRNA-134, 370 and 198 was observed in unstable angina patients as compared to stable. They has been predicted as a clinical biomarkers for coronary artery disease especially in acute coronary events [316].

The human atherosclerosis and hypertension functions are associated with the renin-angiotensin-aldosterone system. The expression analysis of miRNA in the mononuclear cells treated with the renin antagonist (Aliskiren) exhibited more plaque progression in Aliskiren treated subjects. Among the 734 miRNAs, only three (miRNA-18b, miRNA-106b, miRNA-27a-3p) were downregulated and rest remained unaltered. The miRNA-18b and miRNA-106b are more specifically related to the progression of plaque, therefore could serve as the prognostic biomarkers for the atherosclerotic patients [317].

The miRNAs also play key roles in the pathophysiology of cardiovascular diseases via regulation of sarcoplasmic reticulum calcium ATPase (SERCA2a). It regulates the intracellular calcium level by pumping calcium from cytosol to the lumen of sarcoplasmic reticulum, thus replenish the calcium ions through ryanodine receptor channel at the time of contraction. The levels of SERCA2a are downregulated in case of cardiac failure and acute myocardial infarction [318]. The SERCA2a is the target of miRNA-574 which is found to be upregulated in case of infarcted heart tissues [319].

The use of miRNA as a therapeutic approach can facilitate the distinctive diagnosis of acute myocardial infarction patients. The myocardial infarction can be classified as the ST-elevation myocardial infarction (STEMI) and non-ST-elevation MI (NSTEMI). There is a unique expression pattern of circulating miRNA in both cases. The expression of miRNA-221 and miRNA-483 were found to be significantly increased in platelets and plasma of the NSTEMI patients only. However, the expression of miRNA-30d was upregulated in both NSTEMI and STEMI patients [320]. Similarly, the miRNA-499 may also serve as the promising biomarker for NSTEMI, as its level was found to be significantly upregulated in NSTEMI patients as compared to healthy subjects [321]. The use of miRNA-499 can be more reliable as compared to previously used markers, because those are unable to differentiate between NSTEMI and other cardiac disorders due to atypical symptoms of NSTEMI.

The therapeutic potential of miRNA-26 in atherosclerosis represents it as a better target for the treatment of acute myocardial infarction. Its level was found to be upregulated in case of acute coronary artery syndrome patients and mouse model [322]. The miRNA-26 inhibits the endothelial cells proliferation and their pro-angiogenic function via Smad1 signaling. The use of intravenous miRNA-26 inhibitor leads to the myocardial angiogenesis and reduction in infarct size in mice.

10.2 miRNAs as Biomarker in Ischemic Stroke

Stroke is a prime cause of death worldwide. The various miRNAs have been indicated in the development of stroke [323]. Currently, the tissue plasminogen is used as the treatment for the stroke [324]. Due the involvement of multiple signaling cascades in the stroke, the currently used endovascular strategies remained unsuccessful in clinical trials [325]. The miRNAs can serve as the solution to this problem, as they are the early responders to the ischemic stroke and also regulate the multiple signaling pathways [326].

The transient cerebral artery occlusion in experimental rat model has shown the dysregulation of 20 miRNAs among which 11 of these miRNAs were early responders just in 3 h after ischemic reperfusion. The targets of these miRNAs were mostly the gene promoters, which strongly strengthens their role in gene expression regulation. The further targets of these miRNAs are the genes which are involved in inflammation, ionic homeostasis and receptor function [327].

A recent study has shown that most of the altered miRNAs in ischemic patients have been involved in endothelial function, inflammation and hypoxia related process. The different types of ischemic strokes have shown the differential expression of miRNA profiles and this makes the miRNAs as promising diagnostic and prognostic biomarkers for ischemic stroke [328].

The miRNAs are being used as the successful predictors for ischemic stroke; the miRNA-21 and miRNA-221 are also used as the biomarkers for stroke [329]. The most important miRNAs which are up regulated in ischemic conditions are the miRNA-125b, miRNA-27a, miRNA-422a, miRNA-488 and miRNA-627, whereas the 32 miRNAs are differentially expressed based on the cause of stroke [193].

The emerging approach for the stroke treatment is the bone-marrow derived mesenchymal cells (BSMSCs) transplantation [330]. The beneficial attributes of this therapy are due to the release of exosomes. The miRNA-133 is translocated from the mesenchymal cells to the neuronal cells and thus promotes plasticity of the neurons [331]. The miRNA-210 and miRNA-107 are known to regulate the cell death [249]. The positive aspect in using the BMSCs as the therapeutic strategy is that they can be easily cultured as compared to embryonic stem cells.

Moreover, the BSMCs can also bypass the immune system of the body. After transplantation the BSMCs can migrate to the boundary zone of the ischemic stroke [332]. The BSCMs generated exosomes can also be used as therapeutic strategy for the ischemic stroke. According to Xin et al. (2013) the intravenous administration of multipotent mesenchymal stromal cells derived exosomes has resulted in significantly ameliorated effects. It has led to the neurovascular remodeling. The specific exosomes can be used for the treatment of stroke, consisting of the specific miRNAs or antimiRs against the detrimental miRNAs [333].

10.3 miRNAs as Biomarker in Hypertension

Hypertension is a major prognosticator of mortality for a wide range of cardiovascular disorders such as acute myocardial infarction, cardiac hypertrophy, ischemic stroke and heart failure [334]. Several genetic components may also play role in hypertension while the association of single nucleotide polymorphism with the hypertension still needs to be investigated [335, 336]. The single nucleotide polymorphism in the miRNAs binding sites of some RAAS genes effects the arterial blood pressure level and also acts as a risk for acute myocardial infarction. The higher level of angiotensin II receptor is associated with the cardiovascular disorder and they can be targeted for the treatment of hypertension. Different studies have demonstrated a link of 1166C allele of angiotensin II receptor gene with hypertension, hypertrophy and acute myocardial infarction [337]. The SNP at this locus annul the binding of miRNA-155 to the 3′UTR of the gene. The miRNA-155 and angiotensin II receptor (ATR1) are co-expressed in the kidney and thus regulate the blood pressure of the body [334]. The level of ATR1 is negatively correlated with miRNA-155 expression and positively with the blood pressure [338]. Therefore, the miRNA-155 plays role in the regulation of ATR1 expression. The reduced expression of miRNA-132 and miRNA-122 in the internal mammary arteries of the ATR1 blocker treated patients have been observed, whereas in case of the patients treated with β-blockers the levels of miRNA were not reduced [339]. This research unravels that all blood pressure reducing agents do not downregulate the miRNA-132 and miRNA-212. It suggests that miRNA-132 and miRNA-212 cluster in human beings might be due to the angiotensin II. Similar results have been reported by the study of angiotensin II induced hypertension rat model.

The miRNA-765 and miRNA-571 targets the T-allele of thromboxane A2 receptor by decreasing the arterial blood pressure [340]. The SNP is located in the putative seed recognition site thus may serve as a therapeutic target for hypertension. The miRNAs can serve as the prognostic biomarkers for hypertension. The level of miRNA-9 and 126 were found to be lowered in hypertension patients as compared to the healthy subjects [341]. The 24 h mean pulse is an establish prognosticator for the organ damage. The level of miRNA- 9 and miRNA-126 were observed to be positively correlated with the 24 h mean pulse [342] while the levels of miRNA-143 and 145 were found to be negatively correlated with the pulse rate. The miRNA-143 and 145 target the angiotensin converting enzyme, a key player in hypertension. Both miRNAs are also regulated by the myocardin.

The analysis of regulatory mechanism by which miRNA-9, miRNA-126 and miRNA-145 are playing role in pathophysiology of hypertension accentuate their practicality as the putative biomarkers for hypertension related cardiac damage and different cardiovascular complications.

10.4 miRNAs as Biomarker in Hypertrophy and Heart Failure

The cardiac hypertrophy is linked with wide range of cardiac complications such as hypertension, aortic stenosis and cardiomyopathies. The pathological hypertrophy may leads to the heart failure or sudden cardiac death [274]. Several studies have shown the differential expression of miRNAs in the case of heart failure as compared to the normal subjects [343]. The expression of miRNA-24, miRNA-125b, miRNA-195, miRNA-199a and miRNA-214 were found to be overexpressed in heart failure. The expression pattern of the miRNA in human heart is in consistent with rat model which suggests that differential expression of miRNA may serve as prognostic marker for cardiac remodeling. It has been reported that the increased expression of the miRNA-195 is sufficient to cause hypertrophy [344].

The expression pattern of miRNAs is specific depending upon the type of the cardiovascular disorder [344]. There is a differential pattern of miRNA expression in ischemic and cardiomyopathic conditions. As the expression of miRNA-382 is increased and miRNA-10b and 139 decreased only in cardiomyopathic conditions [345] while the miRNA-222 is found to be downregulated only in the case of ischemia. However, the few miRNAs which are expressed in both the conditions of heart failure are miRNA-100 and miRNA-195, are found to be upregulated in both cases whereas the miRNA-133a, 150, 221 are found to be downregulated. Moreover, the expression of cardiac specific miRNAs, miRNA-1 and miRNA-133 are found to be downregulated in cardiac hypertrophy and myopathic patients [173].

The studies of the mouse model have also confirmed that inhibition of miRNA-133 by the administration of antimir-133 has resulted in the induction of cardiac hypertrophy and by the upregulation of miRNA-133, the hypertrophy can be prevented. The inhibition of miRNA-100 has also shown preventive effects [173, 345]. The activation of different fetal genes is the hallmark of heart failure and specifically cardiac hypertrophy.

The wide ranges of miRNAs are being used as the diagnostic biomarkers for heart failure. The miRNA-423 specifically affects the left ventricle in case of heart failure [346]. The level of miRNA-423 can get increased in heart failure patients and is currently used as a biomarker for heart failure [347].

11 The Role of Long Non-coding RNA in Cardiovascular System

The lncRNAs play crucial role in the development of different organ systems. The recent studies have characterized the lncRNAs role in the hematopoietic lineage commitment and cardiac development. The lncRNAs are necessary for the lineage commitment of embryonic stem cells as Braveheart (*Bvht*). The Braveheart is a cardiac specific lncRNA [50] and plays vital role the in-vitro differentiation of cardiomyocytes and embryonic stem cells lineage commitment. The Bvht activates the mesoderm posterior 1 (Mesp 1), which regulates the expression of several downstream modulators that are involved in cardiac development. The transcription factors activated by Mesp1 are NKX2.5, GATA6, GATA1 and HAND1. The Bvht physically interact with the SUZ12, a main component of the poly comb repressive complex 2 (PRC 2). By this interaction the Bvht inhibits the trimethylation of histone lysine H3K27. The depletion of Bvht in neonatal mice cardiomyocytes reduces the maintenance of cardiac cell [50]. The murine lncRNA Fendrr is expressed in the mesoderm and is a critical regulator of cardiac wall development. The knockout of the *Fendrr* resulted in embryonic lethality and also the defects in pulmonary and gastrointestinal tract [199]. However, in another study instead of embryonic lethality, the homozygous mutant pups died perinatally [348]. Despite of the same genetic background the effects were different because the studies have used different approaches for *Fendrr* deletion. Grote et al. (2013) has used the replacement strategy, they replaced the first exon with stop codon whereas the Sauvageau et al. [348] inserted the lacZ cassette in place of lncRNA gene, however further studies are still required to elucidate the underlying mechanism [199, 348]. Like the Bvht, the *Fendrr* also interact with the PRC2 complex and it can bind with the promoters of the different transcriptional factors of cell cycle for example, Foxf1 and Pitx2. In this way the *Fendrr* acts as a guide for lncRNA that harbor the PRC2 to its target sites. Strikingly, the *Fendrr* also activates the chromatin mark by interaction with the HMT complex trithorax (TrxG/MLL) and catalyzes the trimethylation of H3K4 [349]. During mesoderm differentiation, the *Fendrr* is required for the methylation of H3K4 and H3K27 to regulate the gene programs ([350].

In another study Ounzain et al. (2015) compared the murine ESCs with the cardiac precursor cells and annotated the 2608 lncRNAs which were not annotated before. Several of these newly annotated lncRNAs were differentially expressed during differentiation [351]. The enhancer lncRNAs were also identified by the use of integrated chip-seq; as lncRNAs were overlapping the active enhancer elements with the H3K4 methylation and H3K27 acetylation. This study is also in accordance with the previous findings that the regulatory lncRNAs are also essential for the activity of the enhancer elements [352]. Moreover, this also exhibits the role of enhancer lncRNAs in regulation of cardiac regulatory proteins, involved in cardiac pathophysiology [353]. The *Carmen* (cardiac mesoderm enhancer-asscociated noncoding RNA) is a lncRNA which regulate the cardiac lineage specification and its continuation [351]. Interestingly, the silencing of Carmen results in the inhibition of Bvht expression which shows the role of Carmen in regulation of Bvht and cardiac specification. The miRNAs such as miRNA-143 and miRNA-154 are transcribed from the same locus but independent of the Carmen, as the decrease in Carmen expression has no effect on the expression of these miRNAs which are important in the cardiac development [354, 355].

The role of lncRNA in various developmental activities is achieved by the stage specific expression of lncRNAs. The expression pattern of lncRNA differs at different developmental stages. Under homeostatic conditions, the expression of lncRNA in human fetal and adult hearts was significantly different [356]. With the emerging advances in the field of RNAseq, nearly 5000 lncRNAs were investigated which expressed in both fetal and adult hearts, among these 277 were differentially expressed, 164 were upregulated and 113 were down regulated in the fetal heart. The difference in expression pattern is due to the epigenetic regulation with specific chromatin states. The structural analyses of the lncRNAs has revealed the shorter transcripts in fetal heart and increase number of sense lncRNAs in adult [356].

According to Matkovich et al. (2014) larger number of lncRNAs are expressed in tissue and in stage specific manner but these studies were unable to explain the link of these changes with cardiogenesis [357]. By the rapid increase in the sequencing data, the comparative analysis can be done which may serve as an evolving research area especially in the case of lncRNA biology.

Another study has used the RNA seq to investigate the lncRNAs which are involved in the cardiac development and also in the differentiation of ESC into the vascular endothelial cells. Among the several lncRNAs, the three lncRNA are characterized as the developmental stage specific. *TERMINATOR*, specifically expressed in pluripotent stem cells and plays role in maintaining the identity of the stem cells. The *ALIEN* is expressed in the vascular progenitor cells and is essential for cardiovascular development. The *PUNISHER* is specifically expressed in the mature endothelial cells and maintain the endothelial cell function [358].

The data of genome wide RNA sequencing has provided the substantial evidence that single nucleotide polymorphism in 3′UTR may have functional effects on the expression of long noncoding RNA. The expression of long noncoding RNA manifests the critical role in cardiovascular system. The expression of long non-coding RNAs is more anticipative as compared to the miRNA or mRNA in cardiac failure. The altered expression of lncRNAs in disease conditions, makes them an important target in cardiovascular therapeutics [359].

11.1 Role of lncRNA in Myocardial Infarction

The lncRNA "MIAT" (myocardial infarction-associated transcript) expressed by chromosome 22q.12.1 was analyzed as a risk factor for myocardial infarction [298]. However, the function of MIAT is yet need to be elucidated. It has been found that the MIAT acts a as a sponge for miR-150, targets the fibrosis related genes furin, TGF-β1 and also miRNA-24 [360]. The MIAT plays role in angiogenesis, migration and cellular proliferation, it serves an endogenous RNA to form a feedback loop with VEGF. The MIAT also form a feedback loop with the miR-150-5p to modulate endothelial cell function [251]. Several lncRNAs such as cardiac apoptosis-related lncRNA, autophagy promoting factor and mitochondrial dynamic related lncRNA target the specific miRNAs and thus regulate the cardiomyocytes apoptosis and play salubrious role in myocardial infarction.

11.2 Role of lncRNA in Cardiac Fibrosis and Hypertrophy

The lncRNA cardiac hypertrophy related factor (CHRF) serves as an miRNA sponge directly targets the miRNA-489 and regulate MyD88 expression in cardiac hypertrophy [361]. The genome wide transcript analysis showed the deregulation of several lncRNAs in cardiac hypertrophy [189] The pro-hypertrophic lncRNA "Chast" (Cardiac hypertrophy associated transcript) was found to be upregulated in cardiomyocytes after TAC induced cardiac hypertrophy. The NFAT transcriptionally target the Chast, while the overexpression of Chast can induce cardiac hypertrophy both in-vivo and in-vitro. However, its inhibition has shown the salubrious effects in TAC model. This suggests the lncRNA targeted therapy of cardiac hypertrophy. The human homologue of Chast was found to be increased in both ESC-cardiomyocytes and aortic stenotic patients. The Chast also regulates the expression of *Plekhm*, which is the regulator of autophagy and is present cis to Chast at opposite. It negatively regulates the PH domain containing family M member 1 and constrain the hypertrophy [189]. Likewise, Chast another lncRNA is "Chaer" which epigenetically regulates the cardiac hypertrophy by interacting with the PRC2 complex and thus inhibits the generation of transcriptionally silent chromatin.

Another study by the Han et al. (2014) has reported the cardiac specific cluster of the lncRNAs which expressed at the murine myosin heavy chain 7 (Myh7) locus. It is also known as the Mhrt (myosin heavy chain-associated RNA transcript). During the pressure-overload cardiac hypertrophy the Mhrt is repressed and imparts the cardioprotective effects [59]. The transgenic mice with overexpression of Mhrt exhibit the salubrious effects from heart failure and cardiac hypertrophy. It also regulates the Myh6, 7 and osteopontin by interfering with the chromatin remodeling factor Brg1. The Brg1 is the component of chromatin repressor complex, the binding of the Mhrt with the Brg1 prevents the epigenetic inhibition of Brg1 targets [59]. However, under the cardiac stress conditions, the levels of Brg1 increases and thus the cell fails to maintain the balance between the Mhrt and Brg1. The free Brg1 can easily repress the target gene Myh6 and Mhrt, ultimately resulting in cardiac failure. Piccoli et al. (2017) has reported the role of lncRNA Meg3 in fibrosis as its inhibition downregulates the matrix-metalloproteinase-2 in cardiac fibroblasts [362].

11.3 Role of lncRNA in Atherosclerosis and Angiogenesis

The chromosome 9p21 locus encodes for the major lncRNAs which are involved in carotid artery plaque, aneurysms, heart failure and cardiovascular mortality. The differential expression of ANRIL in the INK4 as well as the protein-coding genes at the INK/ARF locus was identified [363]. The ANRIL expresses in various cell types which are key players in atherogenesis. It plays role in different cellular processes such as cellular viability, adhesion and apoptosis. The ANRIL epigenetically regulates the target gene expression by binding to the polycomb family [363]. The differential expression of H19 located at chromosome 11p15.5 is related with coronary artery heart disease [364]. In normal physiological conditions the heart and skeletal muscle tissues have shown the downregulation of H19 (Boon et al. 2016). However, the expression is increased in case of vascular injury and atherosclerotic plaques. Mechanistically the H19 acts as a sponge for let-7, preventing its inhibitory effects on target genes in case of skeletal muscle differentiation [130].

The long intergenic non-coding RNA (lincRNA)-p21 plays major role in cellular proliferation and death in atherosclerosis, as it is directly targeted by p53. The p53 binds to its promoter and upregulates its expression. Whereas the expression of p53 is also regulated by the lincRNA-p21 by the positive feedback loop and thus results in the differential expression of several p53 target genes [244]. The expression of lincRNA-p21 was found to be downregulated in patients with coronary artery disease and also in the atherosclerotic plaques of mice.

Another long non-coding RNA which regulates the endothelial cell function and vessel growth is the Malat-1 (metastasis-associated lung adenocarcinoma transcript 1), is triggered by the hypoxia. Its expression is appreciably increased in case of diabetic conditions causing the endothelial dysfunction [191, 365].

In endothelial cells, the hypoxia induces the expression of the two more long non-coding RNAs, linc00323-003 and MIR503HG which play role in angiogenesis. They control cell proliferation by inhibiting the expression of the endothelial transcription factor GATA-binding protein 2 (GATA-2) [366]. Another lncRNA "SENCR" (smooth muscle and endothelial cell-enriched migration) is an inhibitor of smooth muscle cell migration [367]. The increased expression of lncRNA SENCR results in the increased mesoderm endothelial commitment and also increases the angiogenesis in the umbilical cord. However, the knock out model for SENCR has shown the decline in the smooth cell migration. The patients of premature coronary artery disease have shown the decreased levels of SENCR. The SENCR is localized in the cytoplasm which underlie the similar cell processes like the differentiation and tissue specific lineage commitment are also governed by the different lncRNAs at multiple levels [367].

The above examples showed that long non-coding RNAs play key roles in the regulation of cardiovascular system and thus may serve as a promising agents for the development of new therapeutic strategies.

12 Targeting lncRNA for the Treatment of Cardiovascular Diseases

The targeting of lncRNA by the antisense-based strategies, such as the siRNAs and antisense oligonucleotides which can target the cytoplasmic lncRNAs and the gapmers that pass into the nucleus and target the lncRNAs [368]. Most of the lncRNAs are located in the nucleus therefore the gapmers are most widely used for the inhibition of lncRNA. The chimeric gapmers are stabilized by the 2′-O modified ribonucleotides and also by the phosphothorotioate for the therapeutics.

The several gapmers are being used for the targeting of lncRNAs. PCSK9 is in the phase 1 of the clinical trials; however, it is facing the challenges due to the off-target effects which might cause hepatotoxicity [368].

Another studied gapmer against HIF-1α has not shown any concerns during the early observations [369, 370]. Several studies have shown the effective inhibition of lncRNAs in cardiovascular system. As the inhibition of Malat-1 and Chast by the gapmer reduces the endothelial cell proliferation and cardiac hypertrophy respectively. The gapmers against the Meg 3 can reduce cardiac fibrosis. Therefore, the use of gapmers and the antisense oligonucleotide targeting can serve as the potential therapeutic strategies against cardiac remodeling [362].

The siRNAs can also be used to target the lncRNAs as the lincRNA-p21 is known as the key player in cellular proliferation and atherosclerosis. The inhibition of lincRNA-p21 by the lentiviral based siRNA results in neointima hyperplasia in carotid artery disease model [244]. The siRNA inhibits the lncRNA APF to regulate the cell death by reducing the ischemia/reperfusion in mice [361].

12.1 Restoration of lncRNA by Overexpression

The viral vectors and synthetically modified RNAs are used as the therapeutic strategy to restore the function of lncRNA by its overexpression. However, the cis-regulatory lncRNAs can not be targeted in this way because they directly interferes the expression of adjacent genes. The appropriate localization of cis-regulatory lncRNAs may not be attained by using the vector based overexpression approach. The use of CRISPR/cas9 based RNA-guided gene activation may bypass the problem but it needs further investigation. Although it has shown promising effects in case of bacteria and human cells but still the trial in living cells needs more research [371]. The expression of lncRNA is in the form of different transcript variant and they may undergo the post translational modifications by methylation or editing. More specifically, the Alu sequence is mostly edited which is abundantly found in lncRNAs [372]. Large number of studies has reported the successful overexpression of the lncRNAs and their potential role in therapeutics. In cardiomyocytes the adenoviral transfection of the MDRL (mitochondrial dynamic-related lnRNA) overexpresses the lncRNA and inhibits the mitochondrial fission and apoptosis. Whereas, the transfection of MDRL siRNA has shown the increased mitochondrial fission and apoptosis [361]. The in-vivo studies exhibited the decreased myocardial infarction after the delivery of adenovirus-expressed MDRL in ischemic mice model. The lncRNA CARL also reduces the mitochondrial fission and cell death by targeting miR-539 and prohibitin 2 (PHB2), and the lncRNA CHRF regulates cardiac hypertrophy [361]. However, further studies are still required to check the tolerance for overexpression of lncRNA overexpression in living organisms.

12.2 Circulating LnRNA as Biomarkers for Cardiovascular Diseases

The lncRNA can serve as the biomarkers for cardiovascular dieases. The expression analysis of the mouse plasma and white blood cells has revealed the upregulation of 518 and downregulation of 908 lncRNA in case of acute heart failure [373]. However, the expression was more significantly altered in case of heart tissues in comparison to plasma or whole blood. The MIAT and LIPCAR are the lncRNA which are involved in myocardial infarction and heart failure. The ANRIL and CDKN2A/B are reported to be involved in atherosclerosis ([196, 374, 375].

12.3 Challenges for lncRNA Therapeutics

The repeated administration of siRNA is required for the efficient inhibition of lncRNA in-vivo. Depending upon the chemical nature of the inhibitor, the dose dependent toxicities are better to be considered during the preclinical trials.

Another challenge for the lncRNA therapeutics is its non-conservative nature among different species. As the animal models are being used for the investigation of the mode of action of interested lncRNA, still the toxicity profiling should be cautiously done before going into clinical trials. The designing of human specific sequence for the toxicology model is a better option then the endogenously expressed sequences. However, in this case only the hybridization independent toxicology can be evaluated.

The use of humanized model may serve as the better platform for the investigation of the action of the human-specific lncRNAs. This will underlie the importance of lncRNA role in the development of lncRNA as the therapeutic approach, because without understanding the exact mechanism the unwanted targets may lead to different hurdles.

Acknowledgments Higher Education Commission of Pakistan Grant to Murtaza I (6165/Federal/NRPU/R&D/HEC/2016) and the URF, QAU funds to Murtaza I.

Competing Financial Interests The authors declare no competing financial interests.

References

1. Bartel DP. MicroRNAs: target recognition and regulatory functions. Cell. 2009;136(2):215–33.
2. Carninci P, Kasukawa T, Katayama S, Gough J, Frith M, Maeda N, Oyama R, Ravasi T, Lenhard B, Wells C. The transcriptional landscape of the mammalian genome. Science. 2005;309(5740):1559–63.
3. Katayama S, Tomaru Y, Kasukawa T, Waki K, Nakanishi M, Nakamura M, Nishida H, Yap C, Suzuki M, Kawai J. Antisense transcription in the mammalian transcriptome. Science. 2005;309(5740):1564–6.
4. Hangauer MJ, Vaughn IW, McManus MT. Pervasive transcription of the human genome produces thousands of previously unidentified long intergenic noncoding RNAs. PLoS Genet. 2013;9(6):e1003569.
5. Taft RJ, Pheasant M, Mattick JS. The relationship between non-protein-coding DNA and eukaryotic complexity. BioEssays. 2007;29(3):288–99.
6. Melton C, Reuter JA, Spacek DV, Snyder M. Recurrent somatic mutations in regulatory regions of human cancer genomes. Nat Genet. 2015;47(7):710.
7. Wong C-M, Tsang FH-C, Ng IO-L. Non-coding RNAs in hepatocellular carcinoma: molecular functions and pathological implications. Nat Rev Gastroenterol Hepatol. 2018;15(3):137.
8. Viereck J, Thum T. Circulating noncoding RNAs as biomarkers of cardiovascular disease and injury. Circ Res. 2017;120(2):381–99.
9. Ingolia NT, Brar GA, Stern-Ginossar N, Harris MS, Talhouarne GJ, Jackson SE, Wills MR, Weissman JS. Ribosome profiling reveals pervasive translation outside of annotated protein-coding genes. Cell Rep. 2014;8(5):1365–79.
10. Anderson DM, Anderson KM, Chang C-L, Makarewich CA, Nelson BR, McAnally JR, Kasaragod P, Shelton JM, Liou J, Bassel-Duby R. A micropeptide encoded by a putative long noncoding RNA regulates muscle performance. Cell. 2015;160(4):595–606.
11. Crick FH. On protein synthesis. Symp Soc Exp Biol. 1958;1958:8.
12. Mirsky A, Ris H. The desoxyribonucleic acid content of animal cells and its evolutionary significance. J Gen Physiol. 1951;34(4):451.
13. Thomas CA Jr. The genetic organization of chromosomes. Annu Rev Genet. 1971;5(1):237–56.
14. Gall JG. Chromosome structure and the C-value paradox. J Cell Biol. 1981;91(3):3s–14s.
15. Ohno S. So much 'junk' DNA in our genome. In: Evolution of genetic systems, Brookhaven symposia in biology. New York: Gordon and Breach; 1972. p. 366–70.
16. John B, Miklos GLG. Functional aspects of satellite DNA and heterochromatin. Int Rev Cytol. 1979;58:1–114.
17. Lewin R. Repeated DNA still in search of a function. Science. 1982;217(4560):621–3.
18. Orgel LE, Crick FH. Selfish DNA: the ultimate parasite. Nature. 1980;284(5757):604.
19. Yunis JJ, Yasmineh WG. Heterochromatin, satellite DNA, and cell function. Science. 1971;174(4015):1200–9.
20. Holmes DS, Mayfield JE, Sander G, Bonner J. Chromosomal RNA: its properties. Science. 1972;177(4043):72–4.
21. Jarmolowski A, Zagorski J, Li H, Fournier M. Identification of essential elements in U14 RNA of Saccharomyces cerevisiae. EMBO J. 1990;9(13):4503–9.
22. Kiss T, Solymosy F. Sequence homologies between a viroid and a small nuclear RNA (snRNA) species of mammalian origin. FEBS Lett. 1982;144(2):318–20.
23. Bertone P, Stolc V, Royce TE, Rozowsky JS, Urban AE, Zhu X, Rinn JL, Tongprasit W, Samanta M, Weissman S. Global identification of human transcribed sequences with genome tiling arrays. Science. 2004;306(5705):2242–6.
24. Iyer MK, Niknafs YS, Malik R, Singhal U, Sahu A, Hosono Y, Barrette TR, Prensner JR, Evans JR, Zhao S. The landscape of long noncoding RNAs in the human transcriptome. Nat Genet. 2015;47(3):199.
25. Brannan CI, Dees EC, Ingram RS, Tilghman SM. The product of the H19 gene may function as an RNA. Mol Cell Biol. 1990;10(1):28–36.
26. Brockdorff N, Ashworth A, Kay GF, McCabe VM, Norris DP, Cooper PJ, Swift S, Rastan S. The product of the mouse Xist gene is a 15 kb inactive X-specific transcript containing no conserved ORF and located in the nucleus. Cell. 1992;71(3):515–26.
27. Brown CJ, Hendrich BD, Rupert JL, Lafrenière RG, Xing Y, Lawrence J, Willard HF. The human XIST gene: analysis of a 17 kb inactive X-specific RNA that contains conserved repeats and is highly localized within the nucleus. Cell. 1992;71(3):527–42.

28. Khorshidi A, Dhaliwal P, Yang BB. Noncoding RNAs in tumor angiogenesis. In: The long and short non-coding RNAs in cancer biology. Singapore: Springer; 2016. p. 217–41.
29. Winter J, Jung S, Keller S, Gregory RI, Diederichs S. Many roads to maturity: microRNA biogenesis pathways and their regulation. Nat Cell Biol. 2009;11(3):228.
30. Kim VN, Han J, Siomi MC. Biogenesis of small RNAs in animals. Nat Rev Mol Cell Biol. 2009;10(2):126.
31. Ha M, Kim VN. Regulation of microRNA biogenesis. Nat Rev Mol Cell Biol. 2014;15(8):509.
32. Siomi MC, Sato K, Pezic D, Aravin AA. PIWI-interacting small RNAs: the vanguard of genome defence. Nat Rev Mol Cell Biol. 2011;12(4):246.
33. Bartel DP. Metazoan MicroRNAs. Cell. 2018;173(1):20–51.
34. Mattick JS, Rinn JL. Discovery and annotation of long noncoding RNAs. Nat Struct Mol Biol. 2015;22(1):5.
35. Lee Y, Kim M, Han J, Yeom KH, Lee S, Baek SH, Kim VN. MicroRNA genes are transcribed by RNA polymerase II. EMBO J. 2004;23(20):4051–60.
36. Gregory RI, K-p Y, Amuthan G, Chendrimada T, Doratotaj B, Cooch N, Shiekhattar R. The Microprocessor complex mediates the genesis of microRNAs. Nature. 2004;432(7014):235.
37. Mercer TR, Mattick JS. Structure and function of long noncoding RNAs in epigenetic regulation. Nat Struct Mol Biol. 2013;20(3):300.
38. Wilusz JE, Sunwoo H, Spector DL. Long noncoding RNAs: functional surprises from the RNA world. Genes Dev. 2009;23(13):1494–504.
39. Batista PJ, Chang HY. Long noncoding RNAs: cellular address codes in development and disease. Cell. 2013;152(6):1298–307.
40. Laurent GS, Wahlestedt C, Kapranov P. The landscape of long noncoding RNA classification. Trends Genet. 2015;31(5):239–51.
41. Kapranov P, Cheng J, Dike S, Nix DA, Duttagupta R, Willingham AT, Stadler PF, Hertel J, Hackermüller J, Hofacker IL. RNA maps reveal new RNA classes and a possible function for pervasive transcription. Science. 2007;316(5830):1484–8.
42. Faghihi MA, Zhang M, Huang J, Modarresi F, Van der Brug MP, Nalls MA, Cookson MR, St-Laurent G, Wahlestedt C. Evidence for natural antisense transcript-mediated inhibition of microRNA function. Genome Biol. 2010;11(5):R56.
43. Cole SL, Vassar R. Linking vascular disorders and Alzheimer's disease: potential involvement of BACE1. Neurobiol Aging. 2009;30(10):1535–44.
44. Panda AC, Grammatikakis I, Munk R, Gorospe M, Abdelmohsen K. Emerging roles and context of circular RNAs. Wiley Interdiscip Rev: RNA. 2017;8(2):e1386.
45. Salzman J. Circular RNA expression: its potential regulation and function. Trends Genet. 2016;32(5):309–16.
46. Thum T, Condorelli G. Long noncoding RNAs and microRNAs in cardiovascular pathophysiology. Circ Res. 2015;116(4):751–62.
47. Uchida S, Dimmeler S. Long noncoding RNAs in cardiovascular diseases. Circ Res. 2015;116(4):737–50.
48. Holdt LM, Teupser D. From genotype to phenotype in human atherosclerosis-recent findings. Curr Opin Lipidol. 2013;24(5):410.
49. Li W, Notani D, Ma Q, Tanasa B, Nunez E, Chen AY, Merkurjev D, Zhang J, Ohgi K, Song X. Functional roles of enhancer RNAs for oestrogen-dependent transcriptional activation. Nature. 2013;498(7455):516.
50. Klattenhoff CA, Scheuermann JC, Surface LE, Bradley RK, Fields PA, Steinhauser ML, Ding H, Butty VL, Torrey L, Haas S. Braveheart, a long noncoding RNA required for cardiovascular lineage commitment. Cell. 2013;152(3):570–83.
51. Gong C, Maquat LE. lncRNAs transactivate STAU1-mediated mRNA decay by duplexing with 3′ UTRs via Alu elements. Nature. 2011;470(7333):284.
52. Yoon J-H, Abdelmohsen K, Srikantan S, Yang X, Martindale JL, De S, Huarte M, Zhan M, Becker KG, Gorospe M. LincRNA-p21 suppresses target mRNA translation. Mol Cell. 2012;47(4):648–55.
53. Yoon J-H, Abdelmohsen K, Gorospe M. Posttranscriptional gene regulation by long noncoding RNA. J Mol Biol. 2013;425(19):3723–30.
54. Cesana M, Cacchiarelli D, Legnini I, Santini T, Sthandier O, Chinappi M, Tramontano A, Bozzoni I. A long noncoding RNA controls muscle differentiation by functioning as a competing endogenous RNA. Cell. 2011;147(2):358–69.
55. Rinn JL, Chang HY. Genome regulation by long noncoding RNAs. Annu Rev Biochem. 2012;81:145–66.
56. Wang Z, Wang Y. Dawn of the Epi-LncRNAs: new path from Myheart. Circ Res. 2015;116(2):235–6.
57. Spitale RC, Tsai M-C, Chang HY. RNA templating the epigenome: long noncoding RNAs as molecular scaffolds. Epigenetics. 2011;6(5):539–43.
58. Monnier P, Martinet C, Pontis J, Stancheva I, Ait-Si-Ali S, Dandolo L. H19 lncRNA controls gene expression of the Imprinted Gene Network by recruiting MBD1. Proc Natl Acad Sci. 2013;110(51):20693–8.
59. Han P, Li W, Lin C-H, Yang J, Shang C, Nurnberg ST, Jin KK, Xu W, Lin C-Y, Lin C-J. A long noncoding RNA protects the heart from pathological hypertrophy. Nature. 2014;514(7520):102.
60. Djebali S, Davis CA, Merkel A, Dobin A, Lassmann T, Mortazavi A, Tanzer A, Lagarde J, Lin W, Schlesinger F. Landscape of transcription in human cells. Nature. 2012;489(7414):101.
61. de Hoon M, Shin JW, Carninci P. Paradigm shifts in genomics through the FANTOM projects. Mamm Genome. 2015;26(9–10):391–402.
62. Guttman M, Amit I, Garber M, French C, Lin MF, Feldser D, Huarte M, Zuk O, Carey BW, Cassady JP. Chromatin signature reveals over a thousand highly conserved large non-coding RNAs in mammals. Nature. 2009;458(7235):223.

63. Milligan MJ, Lipovich L. Pseudogene-derived lncRNAs: emerging regulators of gene expression. Front Genet. 2015;5:476.
64. Chen J, Sun M, Kent WJ, Huang X, Xie H, Wang W, Zhou G, Shi RZ, Rowley JD. Over 20% of human transcripts might form sense–antisense pairs. Nucleic Acids Res. 2004;32(16):4812–20.
65. Pandey RR, Mondal T, Mohammad F, Enroth S, Redrup L, Komorowski J, Nagano T, Mancini-DiNardo D, Kanduri C. Kcnq1ot1 antisense noncoding RNA mediates lineage-specific transcriptional silencing through chromatin-level regulation. Mol Cell. 2008;32(2):232–46.
66. Pastori C, Peschansky VJ, Barbouth D, Mehta A, Silva JP, Wahlestedt C. Comprehensive analysis of the transcriptional landscape of the human FMR1 gene reveals two new long noncoding RNAs differentially expressed in Fragile X syndrome and Fragile X-associated tremor/ataxia syndrome. Hum Genet. 2014;133(1):59–67.
67. Salzman J, Gawad C, Wang PL, Lacayo N, Brown PO. Circular RNAs are the predominant transcript isoform from hundreds of human genes in diverse cell types. PLoS One. 2012;7(2):e30733.
68. Mattick JS, Makunin IV. Non-coding RNA. Hum Mol Genet. 2006;15(suppl_1):R17–29.
69. Ozsolak F, Platt AR, Jones DR, Reifenberger JG, Sass LE, McInerney P, Thompson JF, Bowers J, Jarosz M, Milos PM. Direct RNA sequencing. Nature. 2009;461(7265):814.
70. Wei Y, Peng S, Wu M, Sachidanandam R, Tu Z, Zhang S, Falce C, Sobie EA, Lebeche D, Zhao Y. Multifaceted roles of miR-1s in repressing the fetal gene program in the heart. Cell Res. 2014;24(3):278.
71. Takahashi H, Kato S, Murata M, Carninci P. CAGE (cap analysis of gene expression): a protocol for the detection of promoter and transcriptional networks. In: Gene regulatory networks. New York: Springer; 2012. p. 181–200.
72. Z-k Z, Pang C, Yang Y, Duan Q, Zhang J, W-c L. Serum long noncoding RNA urothelial carcinoma-associated 1: a novel biomarker for diagnosis and prognosis of hepatocellular carcinoma. J Int Med Res. 2018;46(1):348–56.
73. Gardini A. Global run-on sequencing (GRO-Seq). In: Enhancer RNAs. New York: Springer; 2017. p. 111–20.
74. Shi Y, Shang J. Long noncoding RNA expression profiling using Arraystar LncRNA microarrays. In: Long non-coding RNAs. New York: Springer; 2016. p. 43–61.
75. Chen C, Li Z, Yang Y, Xiang T, Song W, Liu S. Microarray expression profiling of dysregulated long non-coding RNAs in triple-negative breast cancer. Cancer Biol Ther. 2015;16(6):856–65.
76. Zhu D, Fang C, Li X, Geng Y, Li R, Wu C, Jiang J, Wu C. Predictive analysis of long non-coding RNA expression profiles in diffuse large B-cell lymphoma. Oncotarget. 2017;8(14):23228.
77. Huang W, Thomas B, Flynn RA, Gavzy SJ, Wu L, Kim SV, Hall JA, Miraldi ER, Ng CP, Rigo F. DDX5 and its associated lncRNA Rmrp modulate T H 17 cell effector functions. Nature. 2015;528(7583):517.
78. Kashi K, Henderson L, Bonetti A, Carninci P. Discovery and functional analysis of lncRNAs: methodologies to investigate an uncharacterized transcriptome. Biochimica et Biophysica Acta (BBA)-Gene Regulatory Mechanisms. 2016;1859(1):3–15.
79. Guil S, Soler M, Portela A, Carrère J, Fonalleras E, Gómez A, Villanueva A, Esteller M. Intronic RNAs mediate EZH2 regulation of epigenetic targets. Nat Struct Mol Biol. 2012;19(7):664.
80. Cabili MN, Trapnell C, Goff L, Koziol M, Tazon-Vega B, Regev A, Rinn JL. Integrative annotation of human large intergenic noncoding RNAs reveals global properties and specific subclasses. Genes Dev. 2011;25(18):1915–27.
81. Conesa A, Madrigal P, Tarazona S, Gomez-Cabrero D, Cervera A, McPherson A, Szcześniak MW, Gaffney DJ, Elo LL, Zhang X. A survey of best practices for RNA-seq data analysis. Genome Biol. 2016;17(1):13.
82. Cheng J, Kapranov P, Drenkow J, Dike S, Brubaker S, Patel S, Long J, Stern D, Tammana H, Helt G. Transcriptional maps of 10 human chromosomes at 5-nucleotide resolution. Science. 2005;308(5725):1149–54.
83. Derrien T, Johnson R, Bussotti G, Tanzer A, Djebali S, Tilgner H, Guernec G, Martin D, Merkel A, Knowles DG. The GENCODE v7 catalog of human long noncoding RNAs: analysis of their gene structure, evolution, and expression. Genome Res. 2012;22(9):1775–89.
84. Galupa R, Heard E. X-chromosome inactivation: new insights into cis and trans regulation. Curr Opin Genet Dev. 2015;31:57–66.
85. Wutz A. Gene silencing in X-chromosome inactivation: advances in understanding facultative heterochromatin formation. Nat Rev Genet. 2011;12(8):542.
86. Brown CJ, Ballabio A, Rupert JL, Lafreniere RG, Grompe M, Tonlorenzi R, Willard HF. A gene from the region of the human X inactivation centre is expressed. Nature. 1991;349:3.
87. Chu C, Zhang QC, Da Rocha ST, Flynn RA, Bharadwaj M, Calabrese JM, Magnuson T, Heard E, Chang HY. Systematic discovery of Xist RNA binding proteins. Cell. 2015;161(2):404–16.
88. da Rocha ST, Heard E. Novel players in X inactivation: insights into Xist-mediated gene silencing and chromosome conformation. Nat Struct Mol Biol. 2017;24(3):197.
89. Shi Y, Downes M, Xie W, Kao H-Y, Ordentlich P, Tsai C-C, Hon M, Evans RM. Sharp, an inducible cofactor that integrates nuclear receptor repression and activation. Genes Dev. 2001;15(9):1140–51.
90. Schoeftner S, Sengupta AK, Kubicek S, Mechtler K, Spahn L, Koseki H, Jenuwein T, Wutz A. Recruitment of PRC1 function at the initiation of

X inactivation independent of PRC2 and silencing. EMBO J. 2006;25(13):3110–22.
91. Beltran M, Puig I, Peña C, García JM, Álvarez AB, Peña R, Bonilla F, de Herreros AG. A natural antisense transcript regulates Zeb2/Sip1 gene expression during Snail1-induced epithelial–mesenchymal transition. Genes Dev. 2008;22(6):756–69.
92. Szcześniak MW, Makałowska I. lncRNA-RNA interactions across the human transcriptome. PLoS One. 2016;11(3):e0150353.
93. Faghihi MA, Modarresi F, Khalil AM, Wood DE, Sahagan BG, Morgan TE, Finch CE, Laurent GS III, Kenny PJ, Wahlestedt C. Expression of a noncoding RNA is elevated in Alzheimer's disease and drives rapid feed-forward regulation of β-secretase. Nat Med. 2008;14(7):723.
94. Ma X, Shao C, Jin Y, Wang H, Meng Y. Long noncoding RNAs: a novel endogenous source for the generation of Dicer-like 1-dependent small RNAs in Arabidopsis thaliana. RNA Biol. 2014;11(4):373–90.
95. Cai X, Cullen BR. The imprinted H19 noncoding RNA is a primary microRNA precursor. RNA. 2007;13(3):313–6.
96. Ebert MS, Neilson JR, Sharp PA. MicroRNA sponges: competitive inhibitors of small RNAs in mammalian cells. Nat Methods. 2007;4(9):721.
97. Park E, Maquat LE. Staufen-mediated mRNA decay. Wiley Interdiscip Rev: RNA. 2013;4(4):423–35.
98. Kim YK, Furic L, DesGroseillers L, Maquat LE. Mammalian Staufen1 recruits Upf1 to specific mRNA 3′ UTRs so as to elicit mRNA decay. Cell. 2005;120(2):195–208.
99. Kretz M, Siprashvili Z, Chu C, Webster DE, Zehnder A, Qu K, Lee CS, Flockhart RJ, Groff AF, Chow J. Control of somatic tissue differentiation by the long non-coding RNA TINCR. Nature. 2013;493(7431):231.
100. Ong C-T, Corces VG. Enhancer function: new insights into the regulation of tissue-specific gene expression. Nat Rev Genet. 2011;12(4):283.
101. Papanayotou C, Benhaddou A, Camus A, Perea-Gomez A, Jouneau A, Mezger V, Langa F, Ott S, Sabéran-Djoneidi D, Collignon J. A novel nodal enhancer dependent on pluripotency factors and smad2/3 signaling conditions a regulatory switch during epiblast maturation. PLoS Biol. 2014;12(6):e1001890.
102. Kim T-K, Hemberg M, Gray JM, Costa AM, Bear DM, Wu J, Harmin DA, Laptewicz M, Barbara-Haley K, Kuersten S. Widespread transcription at neuronal activity-regulated enhancers. Nature. 2010;465(7295):182.
103. Andersson R, Gebhard C, Miguel-Escalada I, Hoof I, Bornholdt J, Boyd M, Chen Y, Zhao X, Schmidl C, Suzuki T. An atlas of active enhancers across human cell types and tissues. Nature. 2014;507(7493):455.
104. Lam MT, Cho H, Lesch HP, Gosselin D, Heinz S, Tanaka-Oishi Y, Benner C, Kaikkonen MU, Kim AS, Kosaka M. Rev-Erbs repress macrophage gene expression by inhibiting enhancer-directed transcription. Nature. 2013;498(7455):511.
105. Ørom UA, Derrien T, Beringer M, Gumireddy K, Gardini A, Bussotti G, Lai F, Zytnicki M, Notredame C, Huang Q. Long noncoding RNAs with enhancer-like function in human cells. Cell. 2010;143(1):46–58.
106. Lai F, Orom UA, Cesaroni M, Beringer M, Taatjes DJ, Blobel GA, Shiekhattar R. Activating RNAs associate with Mediator to enhance chromatin architecture and transcription. Nature. 2013;494(7438):497.
107. Zeng Y. Principles of micro-RNA production and maturation. Oncogene. 2006;25(46):6156.
108. Saini HK, Griffiths-Jones S, Enright AJ. Genomic analysis of human microRNA transcripts. Proc Natl Acad Sci. 2007;104(45):17719–24.
109. Calin GA, Dumitru CD, Shimizu M, Bichi R, Zupo S, Noch E, Aldler H, Rattan S, Keating M, Rai K. Frequent deletions and down-regulation of micro-RNA genes miR15 and miR16 at 13q14 in chronic lymphocytic leukemia. Proc Natl Acad Sci. 2002;99(24):15524–9.
110. Lerner M, Harada M, Lovén J, Castro J, Davis Z, Oscier D, Henriksson M, Sangfelt O, Grandér D, Corcoran MM. DLEU2, frequently deleted in malignancy, functions as a critical host gene of the cell cycle inhibitory microRNAs miR-15a and miR-16-1. Exp Cell Res. 2009;315(17):2941–52.
111. Kasar S, Underbayev C, Yuan Y, Hanlon M, Aly S, Khan H, Chang V, Batish M, Gavrilova T, Badiane F. Therapeutic implications of activation of the host gene (Dleu2) promoter for miR-15a/16-1 in chronic lymphocytic leukemia. Oncogene. 2014;33(25):3307.
112. Morenos L, Chatterton Z, Ng JL, Halemba MS, Parkinson-Bates M, Mechinaud F, Elwood N, Saffery R, Wong NC. Hypermethylation and down-regulation of DLEU2 in paediatric acute myeloid leukaemia independent of embedded tumour suppressor miR-15a/16-1. Mol Cancer. 2014;13(1):123.
113. Slezak-Prochazka I, Kluiver J, de Jong D, Kortman G, Halsema N, Poppema S, Kroesen B-J, van den Berg A. Cellular localization and processing of primary transcripts of exonic microRNAs. PLoS One. 2013;8(9):e76647.
114. Tam W. Identification and characterization of human BIC, a gene on chromosome 21 that encodes a noncoding RNA. Gene. 2001;274(1–2):157–67.
115. Elton TS, Selemon H, Elton SM, Parinandi NL. Regulation of the MIR155 host gene in physiological and pathological processes. Gene. 2013;532(1):1–12.
116. de Pontual L, Yao E, Callier P, Faivre L, Drouin V, Cariou S, Van Haeringen A, Geneviève D, Goldenberg A, Oufadem M. Germline deletion of the miR-17∼ 92 cluster causes skeletal and growth defects in humans. Nat Genet. 2011;43(10):1026.
117. Keniry A, Oxley D, Monnier P, Kyba M, Dandolo L, Smits G, Reik W. The H19 lincRNA is a develop-

mental reservoir of miR-675 that suppresses growth and Igf1r. Nat Cell Biol. 2012;14(7):659.
118. Thomas M, Lieberman J, Lal A. Desperately seeking microRNA targets. Nat Struct Mol Biol. 2010;17(10):1169.
119. Seitz H. Redefining microRNA targets. Curr Biol. 2009;19(10):870–3.
120. Salmena L, Poliseno L, Tay Y, Kats L, Pandolfi PP. A ceRNA hypothesis: the Rosetta Stone of a hidden RNA language? Cell. 2011;146(3):353–8.
121. Wang Y, Xu Z, Jiang J, Xu C, Kang J, Xiao L, Wu M, Xiong J, Guo X, Liu H. Endogenous miRNA sponge lincRNA-RoR regulates Oct4, Nanog, and Sox2 in human embryonic stem cell self-renewal. Dev Cell. 2013;25(1):69–80.
122. Kumar SM, Liu S, Lu H, Zhang H, Zhang PJ, Gimotty PA, Guerra M, Guo W, Xu X. Acquired cancer stem cell phenotypes through Oct4-mediated dedifferentiation. Oncogene. 2012;31(47):4898.
123. Wang L, Guo Z-Y, Zhang R, Xin B, Chen R, Zhao J, Wang T, Wen W-H, Jia L-T, Yao L-B. Pseudogene OCT4-pg4 functions as a natural micro RNA sponge to regulate OCT4 expression by competing for miR-145 in hepatocellular carcinoma. Carcinogenesis. 2013;34(8):1773–81.
124. An Y, Furber KL, Ji S. Pseudogenes regulate parental gene expression via ce RNA network. J Cell Mol Med. 2017;21(1):185–92.
125. Poliseno L, Salmena L, Zhang J, Carver B, Haveman WJ, Pandolfi PP. A coding-independent function of gene and pseudogene mRNAs regulates tumour biology. Nature. 2010;465(7301):1033.
126. Thomson DW, Dinger ME. Endogenous microRNA sponges: evidence and controversy. Nat Rev Genet. 2016;17(5):272.
127. Rutnam ZJ, Du WW, Yang W, Yang X, Yang BB. The pseudogene TUSC2P promotes TUSC2 function by binding multiple microRNAs. Nat Commun. 2014;5:2914.
128. Yang J, Li T, Gao C, Lv X, Liu K, Song H, Xing Y, Xi T. FOXO1 3′ UTR functions as a ceRNA in repressing the metastases of breast cancer cells via regulating miRNA activity. FEBS Lett. 2014;588(17):3218–24.
129. Mercer TR, Wilhelm D, Dinger ME, Solda G, Korbie DJ, Glazov EA, Truong V, Schwenke M, Simons C, Matthaei KI. Expression of distinct RNAs from 3′ untranslated regions. Nucleic Acids Res. 2010;39(6):2393–403.
130. Kallen AN, Zhou X-B, Xu J, Qiao C, Ma J, Yan L, Lu L, Liu C, Yi J-S, Zhang H. The imprinted H19 lncRNA antagonizes let-7 microRNAs. Mol Cell. 2013;52(1):101–12.
131. Imig J, Brunschweiger A, Brümmer A, Guennewig B, Mittal N, Kishore S, Tsikrika P, Gerber AP, Zavolan M, Hall J. miR-CLIP capture of a miRNA targetome uncovers a lincRNA H19–miR-106a interaction. Nat Chem Biol. 2015;11(2):107.
132. Hansen TB, Jensen TI, Clausen BH, Bramsen JB, Finsen B, Damgaard CK, Kjems J. Natural RNA circles function as efficient microRNA sponges. Nature. 2013;495(7441):384.
133. Hansen TB, Wiklund ED, Bramsen JB, Villadsen SB, Statham AL, Clark SJ, Kjems J. miRNA-dependent gene silencing involving Ago2-mediated cleavage of a circular antisense RNA. EMBO J. 2011;30(21):4414–22.
134. Memczak S, Jens M, Elefsinioti A, Torti F, Krueger J, Rybak A, Maier L, Mackowiak SD, Gregersen LH, Munschauer M. Circular RNAs are a large class of animal RNAs with regulatory potency. Nature. 2013;495(7441):333.
135. Li Z, Huang C, Bao C, Chen L, Lin M, Wang X, Zhong G, Yu B, Hu W, Dai L. Exon-intron circular RNAs regulate transcription in the nucleus. Nat Struct Mol Biol. 2015;22(3):256.
136. Lee JT, Bartolomei MS. X-inactivation, imprinting, and long noncoding RNAs in health and disease. Cell. 2013;152(6):1308–23.
137. Geisler S, Coller J. RNA in unexpected places: long non-coding RNA functions in diverse cellular contexts. Nat Rev Mol Cell Biol. 2013;14(11):699.
138. Nagano T, Fraser P. No-nonsense functions for long noncoding RNAs. Cell. 2011;145(2):178–81.
139. Beermann J, Piccoli M-T, Viereck J, Thum T. Non-coding RNAs in development and disease: background, mechanisms, and therapeutic approaches. Physiol Rev. 2016;96(4):1297–325.
140. Dinger ME, Amaral PP, Mercer TR, Pang KC, Bruce SJ, Gardiner BB, Askarian-Amiri ME, Ru K, Soldà G, Simons C. Long noncoding RNAs in mouse embryonic stem cell pluripotency and differentiation. Genome Res. 2008;18(9):1433–45.
141. Feng J, Bi C, Clark BS, Mady R, Shah P, Kohtz JD. The Evf-2 noncoding RNA is transcribed from the Dlx-5/6 ultraconserved region and functions as a Dlx-2 transcriptional coactivator. Genes Dev. 2006;20(11):1470–84.
142. Ng S-Y, Bogu GK, Soh BS, Stanton LW. The long noncoding RNA RMST interacts with SOX2 to regulate neurogenesis. Mol Cell. 2013;51(3):349–59.
143. Tripathi V, Ellis JD, Shen Z, Song DY, Pan Q, Watt AT, Freier SM, Bennett CF, Sharma A, Bubulya PA. The nuclear-retained noncoding RNA MALAT1 regulates alternative splicing by modulating SR splicing factor phosphorylation. Mol Cell. 2010;39(6):925–38.
144. Ikeda S, Kong SW, Lu J, Bisping E, Zhang H, Allen PD, Golub TR, Pieske B, Pu WT. Altered microRNA expression in human heart disease. Physiol Genomics. 2008;31:367–73.
145. Boon RA, Dimmeler S. MicroRNAs in myocardial infarction. Nat Rev Cardiol. 2015;12(3):135.
146. Chen J-F, Murchison EP, Tang R, Callis TE, Tatsuguchi M, Deng Z, Rojas M, Hammond SM, Schneider MD, Selzman CH. Targeted deletion of Dicer in the heart leads to dilated cardiomyopathy and heart failure. Proc Natl Acad Sci. 2008;105(6):2111–6.

147. da Costa Martins PA, Bourajjaj M, Gladka M, Kortland M, van Oort RJ, Pinto YM, Molkentin JD, De Windt LJ. Clinical perspective. Circulation. 2008;118(15):1567–76.
148. Suárez Y, Fernández-Hernando C, Pober JS, Sessa WC. Dicer dependent microRNAs regulate gene expression and functions in human endothelial cells. Circ Res. 2007;100(8):1164–73.
149. Fiedler J, Jazbutyte V, Kirchmaier BC, Gupta SK, Lorenzen J, Hartmann D, Galuppo P, Kneitz S, Pena JT, Sohn-Lee C. MicroRNA-24 regulates vascularity after myocardial infarction. Circulation. 2011;124(6):720–30.
150. Kumar S, Kim CW, Simmons RD, Jo H. Role of flow-sensitive microRNAs in endothelial dysfunction and atherosclerosis: mechanosensitive athero-miRs. Arterioscler Thromb Vasc Biol. 2014;34(10):2206–16.
151. Wang S, Aurora AB, Johnson BA, Qi X, McAnally J, Hill JA, Richardson JA, Bassel-Duby R, Olson EN. The endothelial-specific microRNA miR-126 governs vascular integrity and angiogenesis. Dev Cell. 2008;15(2):261–71.
152. Boštjančič E, Zidar N, Štajer D, Glavač D. MicroRNAs miR-1, miR-133a, miR-133b and miR-208 are dysregulated in human myocardial infarction. Cardiology. 2010;115(3):163–9.
153. Satoh M, Minami Y, Takahashi Y, Tabuchi T, Nakamura M. Expression of microRNA-208 is associated with adverse clinical outcomes in human dilated cardiomyopathy. J Card Fail. 2010;16(5):404–10.
154. van Rooij E, Sutherland LB, Qi X, Richardson JA, Hill J, Olson EN. Control of stress-dependent cardiac growth and gene expression by a microRNA. Science. 2007;316(5824):575–9.
155. Callis TE, Pandya K, Seok HY, Tang R-H, Tatsuguchi M, Huang Z-P, Chen J-F, Deng Z, Gunn B, Shumate J. MicroRNA-208a is a regulator of cardiac hypertrophy and conduction in mice. J Clin Invest. 2009;119(9):2772–86.
156. Hullinger TG, Montgomery RL, Seto AG, Dickinson BA, Semus HM, Lynch JM, Dalby CM, Robinson K, Stack C, Latimer PA. Inhibition of miR-15 protects against cardiac ischemic injury. Circ Res. 2012;110(1):71–81.
157. Zidar N, Boštjančič E, Glavač D, Štajer D. MicroRNAs, innate immunity and ventricular rupture in human myocardial infarction. Dis Markers. 2011;31(5):259–65.
158. Wu T, Wu D, Wu Q, Zou B, Huang X, Cheng X, Wu Y, Hong K, Li P, Yang R. Knockdown of long non-coding RNA-ZFAS1 protects cardiomyocytes against acute myocardial infarction via anti-apoptosis by regulating miR-150/CRP. J Cell Biochem. 2017;118(10):3281–9.
159. Devaux Y, Vausort M, McCann GP, Zangrando J, Kelly D, Razvi N, Zhang L, Ng LL, Wagner DR, Squire IB. MicroRNA-150: a novel marker of left ventricular remodeling after acute myocardial infarction. Circ Cardiovasc Genet. 2013;6(3):290–8.
160. Thum T, Galuppo P, Wolf C, Fiedler J, Kneitz S, van Laake LW, Doevendans PA, Mummery CL, Borlak J, Haverich A. MicroRNAs in the human heart. Circulation. 2007;116(3):258–67.
161. Ucar A, Gupta SK, Fiedler J, Erikci E, Kardasinski M, Batkai S, Dangwal S, Kumarswamy R, Bang C, Holzmann A. The miRNA-212/132 family regulates both cardiac hypertrophy and cardiomyocyte autophagy. Nat Commun. 2012;3:1078.
162. Cheng Y, Zhang C. MicroRNA-21 in cardiovascular disease. J Cardiovasc Transl Res. 2010;3(3):251–5.
163. Liang H, Zhang C, Ban T, Liu Y, Mei L, Piao X, Zhao D, Lu Y, Chu W, Yang B. A novel reciprocal loop between microRNA-21 and TGFβRIII is involved in cardiac fibrosis. Int J Biochem Cell Biol. 2012;44(12):2152–60.
164. Roy S, Khanna S, Hussain S-RA, Biswas S, Azad A, Rink C, Gnyawali S, Shilo S, Nuovo GJ, Sen CK. MicroRNA expression in response to murine myocardial infarction: miR-21 regulates fibroblast metalloprotease-2 via phosphatase and tensin homologue. Cardiovasc Res. 2009;82(1):21–9.
165. Bang C, Batkai S, Dangwal S, Gupta SK, Foinquinos A, Holzmann A, Just A, Remke J, Zimmer K, Zeug A. Cardiac fibroblast–derived microRNA passenger strand-enriched exosomes mediate cardiomyocyte hypertrophy. J Clin Invest. 2014;124(5):2136–46.
166. Jayawardena TM, Egemnazarov B, Finch EA, Zhang L, Payne JA, Pandya K, Zhang Z, Rosenberg P, Mirotsou M, Dzau VJ. MicroRNA-mediated in vitro and in vivo direct reprogramming of cardiac fibroblasts to cardiomyocytes. Circ Res. 2012;110(11):1465–73.
167. Ikeda S, He A, Kong SW, Lu J, Bejar R, Bodyak N, Lee K-H, Ma Q, Kang PM, Golub TR. MicroRNA-1 negatively regulates expression of the hypertrophy-associated calmodulin and Mef2a genes. Mol Cell Biol. 2009;29(8):2193–204.
168. Rau F, Freyermuth F, Fugier C, Villemin J-P, Fischer M-C, Jost B, Dembele D, Gourdon G, Nicole A, Duboc D. Misregulation of miR-1 processing is associated with heart defects in myotonic dystrophy. Nat Struct Mol Biol. 2011;18(7):840.
169. Karakikes I, Chaanine AH, Kang S, Mukete BN, Jeong D, Zhang S, Hajjar RJ, Lebeche D. Therapeutic cardiac-targeted delivery of miR-1 reverses pressure overload–induced cardiac hypertrophy and attenuates pathological remodeling. J Am Heart Assoc. 2013;2(2):e000078.
170. Bagnall RD, Tsoutsman T, Shephard RE, Ritchie W, Semsarian C. Global microRNA profiling of the mouse ventricles during development of severe hypertrophic cardiomyopathy and heart failure. PLoS One. 2012;7(9):e44744.
171. Lagos-Quintana M, Rauhut R, Yalcin A, Meyer J, Lendeckel W, Tuschl T. Identification of tissue-specific microRNAs from mouse. Curr Biol. 2002;12(9):735–9.

172. Chen J-F, Mandel EM, Thomson JM, Wu Q, Callis TE, Hammond SM, Conlon FL, Wang D-Z. The role of microRNA-1 and microRNA-133 in skeletal muscle proliferation and differentiation. Nat Genet. 2006;38(2):228.
173. Care A, Catalucci D, Felicetti F, Bonci D, Addario A, Gallo P, Bang M-L, Segnalini P, Gu Y, Dalton ND. MicroRNA-133 controls cardiac hypertrophy. Nat Med. 2007;13(5):613.
174. Duisters RF, Tijsen AJ, Schroen B, Leenders JJ, Lentink V, van der Made I, Herias V, van Leeuwen RE, Schellings MW, Barenbrug P. miR-133 and miR-30 regulate connective tissue growth factor: implications for a role of microRNAs in myocardial matrix remodeling. Circ Res. 2009;104(2):170–8.
175. Castaldi A, Zaglia T, Di Mauro V, Carullo P, Viggiani G, Borile G, Di Stefano B, Schiattarella GG, Gualazzi MG, Elia L. MicroRNA-133 modulates the β1-adrenergic receptor transduction cascade. Circ Res. 2014;115(2):273–83.
176. Ali T, Mushtaq I, Maryam S, Farhan A, Saba K, Jan MI, Sultan A, Anees M, Duygu B, Hamera S. Interplay of N acetyl cysteine and melatonin in regulating oxidative stress-induced cardiac hypertrophic factors and microRNAs. Arch Biochem Biophys. 2019;661:56–65.
177. Liu F, Li N, Long B, Fan Y, Liu C, Zhou Q, Murtaza I, Wang K, Li P. Cardiac hypertrophy is negatively regulated by miR-541. Cell Death Dis. 2014;5(4):e1171.
178. Lin Z, Murtaza I, Wang K, Jiao J, Gao J, Li P-F. miR-23a functions downstream of NFATc3 to regulate cardiac hypertrophy. Proc Natl Acad Sci. 2009;106(29):12103–8.
179. Jan MI, Khan RA, Ali T, Bilal M, Bo L, Sajid A, Malik A, Urehman N, Waseem N, Nawab J. Interplay of mitochondria apoptosis regulatory factors and microRNAs in valvular heart disease. Arch Biochem Biophys. 2017;633:50–7.
180. Long B, Wang K, Li N, Murtaza I, Xiao J-Y, Fan Y-Y, Liu C-Y, Li W-H, Cheng Z, Li P. miR-761 regulates the mitochondrial network by targeting mitochondrial fission factor. Free Radic Biol Med. 2013;65:371–9.
181. Wang J-X, Gao J, Ding S-L, Wang K, Jiao J-Q, Wang Y, Sun T, Zhou L-Y, Long B, Zhang X-J. Oxidative modification of miR-184 enables it to target Bcl-xL and Bcl-w. Mol Cell. 2015;59(1):50–61.
182. Ong S-B, Subrayan S, Lim SY, Yellon DM, Davidson SM, Hausenloy DJ. Inhibiting mitochondrial fission protects the heart against ischemia/reperfusion injury. Circulation. 2010;121(18):2012.
183. Frank S, Gaume B, Bergmann-Leitner ES, Leitner WW, Robert EG, Catez F, Smith CL, Youle RJ. The role of dynamin-related protein 1, a mediator of mitochondrial fission, in apoptosis. Dev Cell. 2001;1(4):515–25.
184. Dagda RK, Cherra SJ, Kulich SM, Tandon A, Park D, Chu CT. Loss of PINK1 function promotes mitophagy through effects on oxidative stress and mitochondrial fission. J Biol Chem. 2009;284(20):13843–55.
185. Wang K, Zhou L-Y, Wang J-X, Wang Y, Sun T, Zhao B, Yang Y-J, An T, Long B, Li N. E2F1-dependent miR-421 regulates mitochondrial fragmentation and myocardial infarction by targeting Pink1. Nat Commun. 2015;6:7619.
186. Li J, Zhou J, Li Y, Qin D, Li P. Mitochondrial fission controls DNA fragmentation by regulating endonuclease G. Free Radic Biol Med. 2010;49(4):622–31.
187. Li J, Li Y, Jiao J, Wang J, Li Y, Qin D, Li P. Mitofusin 1 is negatively regulated by microRNA 140 in cardiomyocyte apoptosis. Mol Cell Biol. 2014;34(10):1788–99.
188. Yang K-C, Yamada KA, Patel AY, Topkara VK, George I, Cheema FH, Ewald GA, Mann DL, Nerbonne JM. Deep RNA sequencing reveals dynamic regulation of myocardial noncoding RNAs in failing human heart and remodeling with mechanical circulatory support. Circulation. 2014;129(9):1009–21.
189. Viereck J, Kumarswamy R, Foinquinos A, Xiao K, Avramopoulos P, Kunz M, Dittrich M, Maetzig T, Zimmer K, Remke J. Long noncoding RNA Chast promotes cardiac remodeling. Sci Transl Med. 2016;8(326):326ra322.
190. Michalik KM, You X, Manavski Y, Doddaballapur A, Zörnig M, Braun T, John D, Ponomareva Y, Chen W, Uchida S. Long noncoding RNA MALAT1 regulates endothelial cell function and vessel growth. Circ Res. 2014;114(9):1389–97.
191. Liu J, Yao J, Li X, Song Y, Wang X, Li Y, Yan B, Jiang Q. Pathogenic role of lncRNA-MALAT1 in endothelial cell dysfunction in diabetes mellitus. Cell Death Dis. 2014;5(10):e1506.
192. Wang Y-N-Z, Shan K, Yao M-D, Yao J, Wang J-J, Li X, Liu B, Zhang Y-Y, Ji Y, Jiang Q. Long noncoding RNA-GAS5: a novel regulator of hypertension-induced vascular remodeling. Hypertension. 2016;68(3):736–48.
193. Sepramaniam S, Tan J-R, Tan K-S, DeSilva D, Tavintharan S, Woon F-P, Wang C-W, Yong F-L, Karolina D-S, Kaur P. Circulating microRNAs as biomarkers of acute stroke. Int J Mol Sci. 2014;15(1):1418–32.
194. Ounzain S, Micheletti R, Beckmann T, Schroen B, Alexanian M, Pezzuto I, Crippa S, Nemir M, Sarre A, Johnson R. Genome-wide profiling of the cardiac transcriptome after myocardial infarction identifies novel heart-specific long non-coding RNAs. Eur Heart J. 2014;36(6):353–68.
195. Wang K, Long B, Zhou L-Y, Liu F, Zhou Q-Y, Liu C-Y, Fan Y-Y, Li P-F. CARL lncRNA inhibits anoxia-induced mitochondrial fission and apoptosis in cardiomyocytes by impairing miR-539-dependent PHB2 downregulation. Nat Commun. 2014;5:3596.
196. Ishii N, Ozaki K, Sato H, Mizuno H, Saito S, Takahashi A, Miyamoto Y, Ikegawa S, Kamatani N, Hori M. Identification of a novel non-coding RNA,

MIAT, that confers risk of myocardial infarction. J Hum Genet. 2006;51(12):1087.
197. Eicher JD, Chami N, Kacprowski T, Nomura A, Chen M-H, Yanek LR, Tajuddin SM, Schick UM, Slater AJ, Pankratz N. Platelet-related variants identified by exomechip meta-analysis in 157,293 individuals. Am J Hum Genet. 2016;99(1):40–55.
198. Frade AF, Laugier L, Ferreira LRP, Baron MA, Benvenuti LA, Teixeira PC, Navarro IC, Cabantous S, Ferreira FM, da Silva Cândido D. Myocardial infarction–associated transcript, a long noncoding RNA, is overexpressed during dilated cardiomyopathy due to chronic chagas disease. J Infect Dis. 2016;214(1):161–5.
199. Grote P, Wittler L, Hendrix D, Koch F, Währisch S, Beisaw A, Macura K, Bläss G, Kellis M, Werber M. The tissue-specific lncRNA Fendrr is an essential regulator of heart and body wall development in the mouse. Dev Cell. 2013;24(2):206–14.
200. Caretti G, Schiltz RL, Dilworth FJ, Di Padova M, Zhao P, Ogryzko V, Fuller-Pace FV, Hoffman EP, Tapscott SJ, Sartorelli V. The RNA helicases p68/p72 and the noncoding RNA SRA are coregulators of MyoD and skeletal muscle differentiation. Dev Cell. 2006;11(4):547–60.
201. Hube F, Velasco G, Rollin J, Furling D, Francastel C. Steroid receptor RNA activator protein binds to and counteracts SRA RNA-mediated activation of MyoD and muscle differentiation. Nucleic Acids Res. 2010;39(2):513–25.
202. Finnemore A, Groves A. Physiology of the fetal and transitional circulation. In: Seminars in fetal and neonatal medicine: 2015. New York: Elsevier; 2015. p. 210–6.
203. Touma M, Kang X, Zhao Y, Cass AA, Gao F, Biniwale R, Coppola G, Xiao X, Reemtsen B, Wang Y. Decoding the long noncoding RNA during cardiac maturation: a roadmap for functional discovery. Circ Cardiovasc Genet. 2016;9(5):395–407.
204. de Boer BA, van den Berg G, de Boer PA, Moorman AF, Ruijter JM. Growth of the developing mouse heart: an interactive qualitative and quantitative 3D atlas. Dev Biol. 2012;368(2):203–13.
205. Sun L, Zhang Y, Zhang Y, Gu Y, Xuan L, Liu S, Zhao X, Wang N, Huang L, Huang Y. Expression profile of long non-coding RNAs in a mouse model of cardiac hypertrophy. Int J Cardiol. 2014;177(1):73–5.
206. Kadar A, Glasz T. Development of atherosclerosis and plaque biology. Cardiovasc Surg. 2001;9(2):109–21.
207. Kroemer G, Galluzzi L, Vandenabeele P, Abrams J, Alnemri ES, Baehrecke E, Blagosklonny M, El-Deiry W, Golstein P, Green D. Classification of cell death: recommendations of the Nomenclature Committee on Cell Death 2009. Cell Death Differ. 2009;16(1):3.
208. Bergsbaken T, Fink SL, Cookson BT. Pyroptosis: host cell death and inflammation. Nat Rev Microbiol. 2009;7(2):99.
209. Orogo AM, Gustafsson ÅB. Cell death in the myocardium: my heart won't go on. IUBMB Life. 2013;65(8):651–6.
210. Skommer J, Rana I, Marques F, Zhu W, Du Z, Charchar F. Small molecules, big effects: the role of microRNAs in regulation of cardiomyocyte death. Cell Death Dis. 2014;5(7):e1325.
211. Gao CF, Ren S, Zhang L, Nakajima T, Ichinose S, Hara T, Koike K, Tsuchida N. Caspase-dependent cytosolic release of cytochrome c and membrane translocation of Bax in p53-induced apoptosis. Exp Cell Res. 2001;265(1):145–51.
212. Jiang X, Wang X. Cytochrome c promotes caspase-9 activation by inducing nucleotide binding to Apaf-1. J Biol Chem. 2000;275(40):31199–203.
213. Clerk A, Cullingford TE, Fuller SJ, Giraldo A, Markou T, Pikkarainen S, Sugden PH. Signaling pathways mediating cardiac myocyte gene expression in physiological and stress responses. J Cell Physiol. 2007;212(2):311–22.
214. Boštjančič E, Zidar N, Glavač D. MicroRNA microarray expression profiling in human myocardial infarction. Dis Markers. 2009;27(6):255–68.
215. Tang Y, Zheng J, Sun Y, Wu Z, Liu Z, Huang G. MicroRNA-1 regulates cardiomyocyte apoptosis by targeting Bcl-2. Int Heart J. 2009;50(3):377–87.
216. Yang B, Lin H, Xiao J, Lu Y, Luo X, Li B, Zhang Y, Xu C, Bai Y, Wang H. The muscle-specific microRNA miR-1 regulates cardiac arrhythmogenic potential by targeting GJA1 and KCNJ2. Nat Med. 2007;13(4):486.
217. Xu C, Lu Y, Pan Z, Chu W, Luo X, Lin H, Xiao J, Shan H, Wang Z, Yang B. The muscle-specific microRNAs miR-1 and miR-133 produce opposing effects on apoptosis by targeting HSP60, HSP70 and caspase-9 in cardiomyocytes. J Cell Sci. 2007;120(17):3045–52.
218. Matkovich SJ, Wang W, Tu Y, Eschenbacher WH, Dorn LE, Condorelli G, Diwan A, Nerbonne JM, Dorn GW. MicroRNA-133a protects against myocardial fibrosis and modulates electrical repolarization without affecting hypertrophy in pressure-overloaded adult hearts. Circ Res. 2010;106(1):166–75.
219. Wang H, Li J, Chi H, Zhang F, Zhu X, Cai J, Yang X. Micro RNA-181c targets Bcl-2 and regulates mitochondrial morphology in myocardial cells. J Cell Mol Med. 2015;19(9):2084–97.
220. Cheng Y, Liu X, Zhang S, Lin Y, Yang J, Zhang C. MicroRNA-21 protects against the H2O2-induced injury on cardiac myocytes via its target gene PDCD4. J Mol Cell Cardiol. 2009;47(1):5–14.
221. Li J, Donath S, Li Y, Qin D, Prabhakar BS, Li P. miR-30 regulates mitochondrial fission through targeting p53 and the dynamin-related protein-1 pathway. PLoS Genet. 2010;6(1):e1000795.
222. Rane S, He M, Sayed D, Vashistha H, Malhotra A, Sadoshima J, Vatner DE, Vatner SF, Abdellatif M. Downregulation of miR-199a derepresses hypoxia-inducible factor-1a and Sirtuin 1 and reca-

pitulates hypoxia preconditioning in cardiac myocytes. Circ Res. 2009;104(7):879–86.
223. Ren X-P, Wu J, Wang X, Sartor MA, Qian J, Jones K, Nicolaou P, Pritchard TJ, Fan G-C. Clinical perspective. Circulation. 2009;119(17):2357–66.
224. Murtaza I, Wang H-X, Mushtaq S, Javed Q, Li P-F. Interplay of phosphorylated apoptosis repressor with CARD, casein kinase-2 and reactive oxygen species in regulating endothelin-1–induced cardiomyocyte hypertrophy. Iran J Basic Med Sci. 2013;16(8):928.
225. Cassidy-Stone A, Chipuk JE, Ingerman E, Song C, Yoo C, Kuwana T, Kurth MJ, Shaw JT, Hinshaw JE, Green DR. Chemical inhibition of the mitochondrial division dynamin reveals its role in Bax/Bak-dependent mitochondrial outer membrane permeabilization. Dev Cell. 2008;14(2):193–204.
226. Li P. MicroRNAs in cardiac apoptosis. J Cardiovasc Transl Res. 2010;3(3):219–24.
227. Wang J-X, Jiao J-Q, Li Q, Long B, Wang K, Liu J-P, Li Y-R, Li P-F. miR-499 regulates mitochondrial dynamics by targeting calcineurin and dynamin-related protein-1. Nat Med. 2011;17(1):71.
228. Wang K, Zhang D, Long B, An T, Zhang J, Zhou L, Liu C, Li P. NFAT4-dependent miR-324-5p regulates mitochondrial morphology and cardiomyocyte cell death by targeting Mtfr1. Cell Death Dis. 2015;6(12):e2007.
229. Singal PK, Iliskovic N. Doxorubicin-induced cardiomyopathy. N Engl J Med. 1998;339(13):900–5.
230. Octavia Y, Tocchetti CG, Gabrielson KL, Janssens S, Crijns HJ, Moens AL. Doxorubicin-induced cardiomyopathy: from molecular mechanisms to therapeutic strategies. J Mol Cell Cardiol. 2012;52(6):1213–25.
231. Tony H, Yu K, Qiutang Z. MicroRNA-208a silencing attenuates doxorubicin induced myocyte apoptosis and cardiac dysfunction. Oxidative Med Cell Longev. 2015;2015:1–6.
232. Wang J, Zhang X, Feng C, Sun T, Wang K, Wang Y, Zhou L, Li P. MicroRNA-532-3p regulates mitochondrial fission through targeting apoptosis repressor with caspase recruitment domain in doxorubicin cardiotoxicity. Cell Death Dis. 2015;6(3):e1677.
233. Tong Z, Jiang B, Wu Y, Liu Y, Li Y, Gao M, Jiang Y, Lv Q, Xiao X. MiR-21 protected cardiomyocytes against doxorubicin-induced apoptosis by targeting BTG2. Int J Mol Sci. 2015;16(7):14511–25.
234. Roca-Alonso L, Castellano L, Mills A, Dabrowska A, Sikkel M, Pellegrino L, Jacob J, Frampton A, Krell J, Coombes R. Myocardial MiR-30 downregulation triggered by doxorubicin drives alterations in β-adrenergic signaling and enhances apoptosis. Cell Death Dis. 2015;6(5):e1754.
235. Papait R, Kunderfranco P, Stirparo GG, Latronico MV, Condorelli G. Long noncoding RNA: a new player of heart failure? J Cardiovasc Transl Res. 2013;6(6):876–83.
236. Wang KC, Chang HY. Molecular mechanisms of long noncoding RNAs. Mol Cell. 2011;43(6):904–14.
237. Piccoli M-T, Gupta SK, Thum T. Noncoding RNAs as regulators of cardiomyocyte proliferation and death. J Mol Cell Cardiol. 2015;89:59–67.
238. Ginger MR, Shore AN, Contreras A, Rijnkels M, Miller J, Gonzalez-Rimbau MF, Rosen JM. A noncoding RNA is a potential marker of cell fate during mammary gland development. Proc Natl Acad Sci. 2006;103(15):5781–6.
239. Kanduri C. Kcnq1ot1: a chromatin regulatory RNA. In: Seminars in cell & developmental biology: 2011. New York: Elsevier; 2011. p. 343–50.
240. Wang K, Long B, Liu F, Wang J-X, Liu C-Y, Zhao B, Zhou L-Y, Sun T, Wang M, Yu T. A circular RNA protects the heart from pathological hypertrophy and heart failure by targeting miR-223. Eur Heart J. 2016;37(33):2602–11.
241. Koseki T, Inohara N, Chen S, Núñez G. ARC, an inhibitor of apoptosis expressed in skeletal muscle and heart that interacts selectively with caspases. Proc Natl Acad Sci. 1998;95(9):5156–60.
242. Li Y-Z, Lu D-Y, Tan W-Q, Wang J-X, Li P-F. p53 initiates apoptosis by transcriptionally targeting the antiapoptotic protein ARC. Mol Cell Biol. 2008;28(2):564–74.
243. Haussecker D, Kay MA. Drugging RNAi. Science. 2015;347(6226):1069–70.
244. Wu SY, Lopez-Berestein G, Calin GA, Sood AK. RNAi therapies: drugging the undruggable. Sci Transl Med. 2014;6(240):240ps247.
245. Maheshwari R, Tekade M, A Sharma P, Kumar Tekade R. Nanocarriers assisted siRNA gene therapy for the management of cardiovascular disorders. Curr Pharm Des. 2015;21(30):4427–40.
246. Fire A, Xu S, Montgomery MK, Kostas SA, Driver SE, Mello CC. Potent and specific genetic interference by double-stranded RNA in Caenorhabditis elegans. Nature. 1998;391(6669):806.
247. Poller W, Dimmeler S, Heymans S, Zeller T, Haas J, Karakas M, Leistner D-M, Jakob P, Nakagawa S, Blankenberg S. Non-coding RNAs in cardiovascular diseases: diagnostic and therapeutic perspectives. Eur Heart J. 2017;39(29):2704–16.
248. Necsulea A, Soumillon M, Warnefors M, Liechti A, Daish T, Zeller U, Baker JC, Grützner F, Kaessmann H. The evolution of lncRNA repertoires and expression patterns in tetrapods. Nature. 2014;505(7485):635.
249. Olson EN. MicroRNAs as therapeutic targets and biomarkers of cardiovascular disease. Sci Transl Med. 2014;6(239):239ps233.
250. Porrello ER, Mahmoud AI, Simpson E, Johnson BA, Grinsfelder D, Canseco D, Mammen PP, Rothermel BA, Olson EN, Sadek HA. Regulation of neonatal and adult mammalian heart regeneration by the miR-15 family. Proc Natl Acad Sci. 2013;110(1):187–92.
251. Yang Y, Cheng H-W, Qiu Y, Dupee D, Noonan M, Lin Y-D, Fisch S, Unno K, Sereti K-I, Liao R. MicroRNA-34a plays a key role in cardiac repair and regeneration following myocardial infarction. Circ Res. 2015;117(5):450–9.

252. Boon RA, Iekushi K, Lechner S, Seeger T, Fischer A, Heydt S, Kaluza D, Tréguer K, Carmona G, Bonauer A. MicroRNA-34a regulates cardiac ageing and function. Nature. 2013;495(7439):107.
253. Bernardo BC, Gao X-M, Winbanks CE, Boey EJ, Tham YK, Kiriazis H, Gregorevic P, Obad S, Kauppinen S, Du X-J. Therapeutic inhibition of the miR-34 family attenuates pathological cardiac remodeling and improves heart function. Proc Natl Acad Sci. 2012;109(43):17615–20.
254. Hinkel R, Penzkofer D, Zühlke S, Fischer A, Husada W, Xu Q-F, Baloch E, van Rooij E, Zeiher AM, Kupatt C. Inhibition of microRNA-92a protects against ischemia/reperfusion injury in a large-animal model. Circulation. 2013;128(10):1066–75.
255. Bellera N, Barba I, Rodriguez-Sinovas A, Ferret E, Asín MA, Gonzalez-Alujas MT, Pérez-Rodon J, Esteves M, Fonseca C, Toran N. Single intracoronary injection of encapsulated antagomir-92a promotes angiogenesis and prevents adverse infarct remodeling. J Am Heart Assoc. 2014;3(5):e000946.
256. Bonauer A, A Boon R, Dimmeler S. Vascular micrornas. Curr Drug Targets. 2010;11(8):943–9.
257. Van Rooij E, Sutherland LB, Thatcher JE, DiMaio JM, Naseem RH, Marshall WS, Hill JA, Olson EN. Dysregulation of microRNAs after myocardial infarction reveals a role of miR-29 in cardiac fibrosis. Proc Natl Acad Sci. 2008;105(35):13027–32.
258. Thum T, Gross C, Fiedler J, Fischer T, Kissler S, Bussen M, Galuppo P, Just S, Rottbauer W, Frantz S. MicroRNA-21 contributes to myocardial disease by stimulating MAP kinase signalling in fibroblasts. Nature. 2008;456(7224):980.
259. Patrick DM, Montgomery RL, Qi X, Obad S, Kauppinen S, Hill JA, van Rooij E, Olson EN. Stress-dependent cardiac remodeling occurs in the absence of microRNA-21 in mice. J Clin Invest. 2010;120(11):3912–6.
260. Gupta SK, Itagaki R, Zheng X, Batkai S, Thum S, Ahmad F, Van Aelst LN, Sharma A, Piccoli M-T, Weinberger F. miR-21 promotes fibrosis in an acute cardiac allograft transplantation model. Cardiovasc Res. 2016;110(2):215–26.
261. Lee DI, Zhu G, Sasaki T, Cho G-S, Hamdani N, Holewinski R, Jo S-H, Danner T, Zhang M, Rainer PP. Phosphodiesterase 9A controls nitric-oxide-independent cGMP and hypertrophic heart disease. Nature. 2015;519(7544):472.
262. Liu G, Friggeri A, Yang Y, Milosevic J, Ding Q, Thannickal VJ, Kaminski N, Abraham E. miR-21 mediates fibrogenic activation of pulmonary fibroblasts and lung fibrosis. J Exp Med. 2010;207(8):1589–97.
263. Thum T, Chau N, Bhat B, Gupta SK, Linsley PS, Bauersachs J, Engelhardt S. Comparison of different miR-21 inhibitor chemistries in a cardiac disease model. J Clin Invest. 2011;121(2):461–2.
264. Castoldi G, Di Gioia CR, Bombardi C, Catalucci D, Corradi B, Gualazzi MG, Leopizzi M, Mancini M, Zerbini G, Condorelli G. MiR-133a regulates collagen 1A1: potential role of miR-133a in myocardial fibrosis in angiotensin II-dependent hypertension. J Cell Physiol. 2012;227(2):850–6.
265. Pan Z, Sun X, Shan H, Wang N, Wang J, Ren J, Feng S, Xie L, Lu C, Yuan Y. MicroRNA-101 inhibited postinfarct cardiac fibrosis and improved left ventricular compliance via the FBJ osteosarcoma oncogene/transforming growth factor-β1 pathway. Circulation. 2012;126(7):840–50.
266. Frankel LB, Wen J, Lees M, Høyer-Hansen M, Farkas T, Krogh A, Jäättelä M, Lund AH. microRNA-101 is a potent inhibitor of autophagy. EMBO J. 2011;30(22):4628–41.
267. Lu Y, Zhang Y, Wang N, Pan Z, Gao X, Zhang F, Zhang Y, Shan H, Luo X, Bai Y. MicroRNA-328 contributes to adverse electrical remodeling in atrial fibrillation. Circulation. 2010;122(23):2378–87.
268. Hess J, Angel P, Schorpp-Kistner M. AP-1 subunits: quarrel and harmony among siblings. J Cell Sci. 2004;117(25):5965–73.
269. Noetel A, Kwiecinski M, Elfimova N, Huang J, Odenthal M. microRNA are central players in anti- and profibrotic gene regulation during liver fibrosis. Front Physiol. 2012;3:49.
270. Roy S, Khanna S, Azad A, Schnitt R, He G, Weigert C, Ichijo H, Sen CK. Fra-2 mediates oxygen-sensitive induction of transforming growth factor β in cardiac fibroblasts. Cardiovasc Res. 2010;87(4):647–55.
271. Thum T. MicroRNA therapeutics in cardiovascular medicine. EMBO Mol Med. 2012;4(1):3–14.
272. Su H, Yang J-R, Xu T, Huang J, Xu L, Yuan Y, Zhuang S-M. MicroRNA-101, down-regulated in hepatocellular carcinoma, promotes apoptosis and suppresses tumorigenicity. Cancer Res. 2009;69(3):1135–42.
273. Wahlquist C, Jeong D, Rojas-Muñoz A, Kho C, Lee A, Mitsuyama S, van Mil A, Park WJ, Sluijter JP, Doevendans PA. Inhibition of miR-25 improves cardiac contractility in the failing heart. Nature. 2014;508(7497):531.
274. Dirkx E, da Costa Martins PA, De Windt LJ. Regulation of fetal gene expression in heart failure. Biochimica et Biophysica Acta (BBA)-Molecular Basis of Disease. 2013;1832(12):2414–24.
275. Besser J, Malan D, Wystub K, Bachmann A, Wietelmann A, Sasse P, Fleischmann BK, Braun T, Boettger T. MiRNA-1/133a clusters regulate adrenergic control of cardiac repolarization. PLoS One. 2014;9(11):e113449.
276. Schober A, Nazari-Jahantigh M, Weber C. MicroRNA-mediated mechanisms of the cellular stress response in atherosclerosis. Nat Rev Cardiol. 2015;12(6):361.
277. Boon RA, Hergenreider E, Dimmeler S. Atheroprotective mechanisms of shear stress-regulated microRNAs. Thromb Haemost. 2012;108(10):616–20.
278. Qin X, Wang X, Wang Y, Tang Z, Cui Q, Xi J, Li Y-SJ, Chien S, Wang N. MicroRNA-19a mediates the suppressive effect of laminar flow on cyclin

D1 expression in human umbilical vein endothelial cells. Proc Natl Acad Sci. 2010;107(7):3240–4.
279. Wang K-C, Garmire LX, Young A, Nguyen P, Trinh A, Subramaniam S, Wang N, Shyy JY, Li Y-S, Chien S. Role of microRNA-23b in flow-regulation of Rb phosphorylation and endothelial cell growth. Proc Natl Acad Sci. 2010;107(7):3234–9.
280. Ji R, Cheng Y, Yue J, Yang J, Liu X, Chen H, Dean DB, Zhang C. MicroRNA expression signature and antisense-mediated depletion reveal an essential role of MicroRNA in vascular neointimal lesion formation. Circ Res. 2007;100(11):1579–88.
281. Maegdefessel L, Azuma J, Toh R, Merk DR, Deng A, Chin JT, Raaz U, Schoelmerich AM, Raiesdana A, Leeper NJ. Inhibition of microRNA-29b reduces murine abdominal aortic aneurysm development. J Clin Invest. 2012;122(2):497–506.
282. Boon RA, Seeger T, Heydt S, Fischer A, Hergenreider E, Horrevoets AJ, Vinciguerra M, Rosenthal N, Sciacca S, Pilato M. MicroRNA-29 in aortic dilation: implications for aneurysm formation. Circ Res. 2011;109(10):1115–9.
283. Schober A, Nazari-Jahantigh M, Wei Y, Bidzhekov K, Gremse F, Grommes J, Megens RT, Heyll K, Noels H, Hristov M. MicroRNA-126-5p promotes endothelial proliferation and limits atherosclerosis by suppressing Dlk1. Nat Med. 2014;20(4):368.
284. Li K, Ching D, Luk FS, Raffai RL. Apolipoprotein E enhances microRNA-146a in monocytes and macrophages to suppress nuclear factor-κB–driven inflammation and atherosclerosis. Circ Res. 2015;117(1):e1–e11.
285. Sun X, He S, Wara A, Icli B, Shvartz E, Tesmenitsky Y, Belkin N, Li D, Blackwell TS, Sukhova GK. Systemic delivery of microRNA-181b inhibits nuclear factor-κb activation, vascular inflammation, and atherosclerosis in apolipoprotein E–deficient mice. Circ Res. 2014;114(1):32–40.
286. Fang Y, Shi C, Manduchi E, Civelek M, Davies PF. MicroRNA-10a regulation of proinflammatory phenotype in athero-susceptible endothelium in vivo and in vitro. Proc Natl Acad Sci. 2010;107(30):13450–5.
287. Van Rooij E, Kauppinen S. Development of microRNA therapeutics is coming of age. EMBO Mol Med. 2014;6(7):851–64.
288. Krützfeldt J, Rajewsky N, Braich R, Rajeev KG, Tuschl T, Manoharan M, Stoffel M. Silencing of microRNAs in vivo with 'antagomirs'. Nature. 2005;438(7068):685.
289. Lennox KA, Behlke MA. A direct comparison of anti-microRNA oligonucleotide potency. Pharm Res. 2010;27(9):1788–99.
290. Elmén J, Lindow M, Schütz S, Lawrence M, Petri A, Obad S, Lindholm M, Hedtjärn M, Hansen HF, Berger U. LNA-mediated microRNA silencing in non-human primates. Nature. 2008;452(7189):896.
291. Obad S, dos Santos CO, Petri A, Heidenblad M, Broom O, Ruse C, Fu C, Lindow M, Stenvang J, Straarup EM. Silencing of microRNA families by seed-targeting tiny LNAs. Nat Genet. 2011;43(4):371.
292. Meng L, Liu C, Lü J, Zhao Q, Deng S, Wang G, Qiao J, Zhang C, Zhen L, Lu Y. Small RNA zippers lock miRNA molecules and block miRNA function in mammalian cells. Nat Commun. 2017;8:13964.
293. Fabani MM, Abreu-Goodger C, Williams D, Lyons PA, Torres AG, Smith KG, Enright AJ, Gait MJ, Vigorito E. Efficient inhibition of miR-155 function in vivo by peptide nucleic acids. Nucleic Acids Res. 2010;38(13):4466–75.
294. Behlke MA. Chemical modification of siRNAs for in vivo use. Oligonucleotides. 2008;18(4):305–20.
295. Li Y-G, Zhang P-P, Jiao K-L, Zou Y-Z. Knockdown of microRNA-181 by lentivirus mediated siRNA expression vector decreases the arrhythmogenic effect of skeletal myoblast transplantation in rat with myocardial infarction. Microvasc Res. 2009;78(3):393–404.
296. Choi W-Y, Giraldez AJ, Schier AF. Target protectors reveal dampening and balancing of Nodal agonist and antagonist by miR-430. Science. 2007;318(5848):271–4.
297. Messina A, Langlet F, Chachlaki K, Roa J, Rasika S, Jouy N, Gallet S, Gaytan F, Parkash J, Tena-Sempere M. A microRNA switch regulates the rise in hypothalamic GnRH production before puberty. Nat Neurosci. 2016;19(6):835.
298. Montgomery RL, Yu G, Latimer PA, Stack C, Robinson K, Dalby CM, Kaminski N, van Rooij E. MicroRNA mimicry blocks pulmonary fibrosis. EMBO Mol Med. 2014;6(10):1347–56.
299. Lin R, Van Zandwijk N, Reid G. MicroRNA therapeutics—back in vogue. J Investig Genomics. 2014;1(2):57–8.
300. Bader AG. miR-34–a microRNA replacement therapy is headed to the clinic. Front Genet. 2012;3:120.
301. Kwekkeboom RF, Lei Z, Doevendans PA, Musters RJ, Sluijter JP. Targeted delivery of miRNA therapeutics for cardiovascular diseases: opportunities and challenges. Clin Sci. 2014;127(6):351–65.
302. Iaconetti C, Polimeni A, Sorrentino S, Sabatino J, Pironti G, Esposito G, Curcio A, Indolfi C. Inhibition of miR-92a increases endothelial proliferation and migration in vitro as well as reduces neointimal proliferation in vivo after vascular injury. Basic Res Cardiol. 2012;107(5):296.
303. Loyer X, Potteaux S, Vion A-C, Guérin CL, Boulkroun S, Rautou P-E, Ramkhelawon B, Esposito B, Dalloz M, Paul J-L. Inhibition of microRNA-92a prevents endothelial dysfunction and atherosclerosis in mice. Circ Res. 2014;114(3):434–43.
304. Montgomery RL, Hullinger TG, Semus HM, Dickinson BA, Seto AG, Lynch JM, Stack C, Latimer PA, Olson EN, van Rooij E. Therapeutic inhibition of miR-208a improves cardiac function and survival during heart failure. Circulation. 2011;124(14):1537–47.
305. Norata GD, Sala F, Catapano AL, Fernández-Hernando C. MicroRNAs and lipoproteins: a con-

nection beyond atherosclerosis? Atherosclerosis. 2013;227(2):209–15.
306. Arroyo JD, Chevillet JR, Kroh EM, Ruf IK, Pritchard CC, Gibson DF, Mitchell PS, Bennett CF, Pogosova-Agadjanyan EL, Stirewalt DL. Argonaute2 complexes carry a population of circulating microRNAs independent of vesicles in human plasma. Proc Natl Acad Sci. 2011;108(12):5003–8.
307. Wang G-K, Zhu J-Q, Zhang J-T, Li Q, Li Y, He J, Qin Y-W, Jing Q. Circulating microRNA: a novel potential biomarker for early diagnosis of acute myocardial infarction in humans. Eur Heart J. 2010;31(6):659–66.
308. Karolina DS, Tavintharan S, Armugam A, Sepramaniam S, Pek SLT, Wong MT, Lim SC, Sum CF, Jeyaseelan K. Circulating miRNA profiles in patients with metabolic syndrome. J Clin Endocrinol Metabol. 2012;97(12):E2271–6.
309. Corsten MF, Dennert R, Jochems S, Kuznetsova T, Devaux Y, Hofstra L, Wagner DR, Staessen JA, Heymans S, Schroen B. Circulating MicroRNA-208b and MicroRNA-499 reflect myocardial damage in cardiovascular disease. Circ Cardiovasc Genet. 2010;3(6):499–506.
310. Huang F, Zhu X, Hu X-Q, Fang Z-F, Tang L, Lu X-L, Zhou S-H. Mesenchymal stem cells modified with miR-126 release angiogenic factors and activate Notch ligand Delta-like-4, enhancing ischemic angiogenesis and cell survival. Int J Mol Med. 2013;31(2):484–92.
311. Sharma S, Jackson P, Makan J. Cardiac troponins. London: BMJ Publishing Group; 2004.
312. Thygesen K, Alpert JS, White HD, Jaffe AS, Apple FS, Galvani M, Katus HA, Newby LK, Ravkilde J, Chaitman B. Universal definition of myocardial infarction: Kristian Thygesen, Joseph S. Alpert and Harvey D. White on behalf of the Joint ESC/ACCF/AHA/WHF Task Force for the Redefinition of Myocardial Infarction. Eur Heart J. 2007;28(20):2525–38.
313. Holland R, Brooks H. The QRS complex during myocardial ischemia. An experimental analysis in the porcine heart. J Clin Invest. 1976;57(3):541–50.
314. Widera C, Gupta SK, Lorenzen JM, Bang C, Bauersachs J, Bethmann K, Kempf T, Wollert KC, Thum T. Diagnostic and prognostic impact of six circulating microRNAs in acute coronary syndrome. J Mol Cell Cardiol. 2011;51(5):872–5.
315. Fichtlscherer S, De Rosa S, Fox H, Schwietz T, Fischer A, Liebetrau C, Weber M, Hamm CW, Röxe T, Müller-Ardogan M. Circulating microRNAs in patients with coronary artery disease. Circ Res. 2010;107(5):677–84.
316. C-f X, Yu C-h, Li Y-m. Regulation of hepatic microRNA expression in response to ischemic preconditioning following ischemia/reperfusion injury in mice. OMICS J Integr Biol. 2009;13(6):513–20.
317. Wronska A, Kurkowska-Jastrzebska I, Santulli G. Application of micro RNA s in diagnosis and treatment of cardiovascular disease. Acta Physiol. 2015;213(1):60–83.
318. Periasamy M, Bhupathy P, Babu GJ. Regulation of sarcoplasmic reticulum Ca2+ ATPase pump expression and its relevance to cardiac muscle physiology and pathology. Cardiovasc Res. 2007;77(2):265–73.
319. Boštjančič E, Zidar N, Glavač D. MicroRNAs and cardiac sarcoplasmic reticulum calcium ATPase-2 in human myocardial infarction: expression and bioinformatic analysis. BMC Genomics. 2012;13(1):552.
320. Ward JA, Esa N, Pidikiti R, Freedman JE, Keaney JF, Tanriverdi K, Vitseva O, Ambros V, Lee R, McManus DD. Circulating cell and plasma microRNA profiles differ between non-ST-segment and ST-segment-elevation myocardial infarction. Fam Med Med Sci Res. 2013;2(2):108.
321. Olivieri F, Antonicelli R, Lorenzi M, D'Alessandra Y, Lazzarini R, Santini G, Spazzafumo L, Lisa R, La Sala L, Galeazzi R. Diagnostic potential of circulating miR-499-5p in elderly patients with acute non ST-elevation myocardial infarction. Int J Cardiol. 2013;167(2):531–6.
322. Icli B, Dorbala P, Feinberg MW. An emerging role for the miR-26 family in cardiovascular disease. Trends Cardiovasc Med. 2014;24(6):241–8.
323. Rink C, Khanna S (2010) MicroRNA in ischemic stroke etiology and pathology. Am J Physiol Heart Circ Physiol
324. Sandercock PA, Soane T. Corticosteroids for acute ischaemic stroke. Cochrane Database Syst Rev. 2011;9:CD000064.
325. Ouyang Y-B, Giffard RG. MicroRNAs regulate the chaperone network in cerebral ischemia. Transl Stroke Res. 2013;4(6):693–703.
326. Stary CM, Giffard RG. Advances in astrocyte-targeted approaches for stroke therapy: an emerging role for mitochondria and microRNAS. Neurochem Res. 2015;40(2):301–7.
327. Dharap A, Bowen K, Place R, Li L-C, Vemuganti R. Transient focal ischemia induces extensive temporal changes in rat cerebral microRNAome. J Cereb Blood Flow Metab. 2009;29(4):675–87.
328. Tan J, Tan K, Koo Y, Yong F, Wang C, Armugam A, Jeyaseelan K. Blood microRNAs in low or no risk ischemic stroke patients. Int J Mol Sci. 2013;14(1):2072–84.
329. Tsai P-C, Liao Y-C, Wang Y-S, Lin H-F, Lin R-T, Juo S-HH. Serum microRNA-21 and microRNA-221 as potential biomarkers for cerebrovascular disease. J Vasc Res. 2013;50(4):346–54.
330. Chen J, Li Y, Wang L, Zhang Z, Lu D, Lu M, Chopp M. Therapeutic benefit of intravenous administration of bone marrow stromal cells after cerebral ischemia in rats. Stroke. 2001;32(4):1005–11.
331. Xin H, Li Y, Cui Y, Yang JJ, Zhang ZG, Chopp M. Systemic administration of exosomes released from mesenchymal stromal cells promote functional recovery and neurovascular plasticity after stroke in rats. J Cereb Blood Flow Metab. 2013;33(11):1711–5.

332. Li K, Zhang T, Fan H, Li Q, Ito W, Torzewski J, Guo J, Liu Z. The analysis of microRNA expression profiling for coronary artery disease. Cardiology. 2014;127(1):62–9.
333. Xin M, Olson EN, Bassel-Duby R. Mending broken hearts: cardiac development as a basis for adult heart regeneration and repair. Nat Rev Mol Cell Biol. 2013;14(8):529.
334. Santulli G, Cipolletta E, Sorriento D, Del Giudice C, Anastasio A, Monaco S, Maione AS, Condorelli G, Puca A, Trimarco B. CaMK4 gene deletion induces hypertension. J Am Heart Assoc. 2012;1(4):e001081.
335. Kumar R, Kohli S, Mishra A, Garg R, Alam P, Stobdan T, Nejatizadeh A, Gupta M, Tyagi S, Pasha MQ. Interactions between the genes of vasodilatation pathways influence blood pressure and nitric oxide level in hypertension. Am J Hypertens. 2014;28(2):239–47.
336. Santulli G, Trimarco B, Iaccarino G. G-protein-coupled receptor kinase 2 and hypertension. High Blood Press Cardiovas Prevent. 2013;20(1):5–12.
337. Hindorff LA, Heckbert SR, Tracy R, Tang Z, Psaty BM, Edwards KL, Siscovick DS, Kronmal RA, Nazar-Stewart V. Angiotensin II type 1 receptor polymorphisms in the cardiovascular health study: relation to blood pressure, ethnicity, and cardiovascular events. Am J Hypertens. 2002;15(12):1050–6.
338. Ceolotto G, Papparella I, Bortoluzzi A, Strapazzon G, Ragazzo F, Bratti P, Fabricio AS, Squarcina E, Gion M, Palatini P. Interplay between miR-155, AT1R A1166C polymorphism, and AT1R expression in young untreated hypertensives. Am J Hypertens. 2011;24(2):241–6.
339. Eskildsen T, Jeppesen P, Schneider M, Nossent A, Sandberg M, Hansen P, Jensen C, Hansen M, Marcussen N, Rasmussen L. Angiotensin II regulates microRNA-132/-212 in hypertensive rats and humans. Int J Mol Sci. 2013;14(6):11190–207.
340. Nossent AY, Hansen JL, Doggen C, Quax PH, Sheikh SP, Rosendaal FR. SNPs in microRNA binding sites in 3′-UTRs of RAAS genes influence arterial blood pressure and risk of myocardial infarction. Am J Hypertens. 2011;24(9):999–1006.
341. Kontaraki J, Marketou M, Zacharis E, Parthenakis F, Vardas P. Differential expression of vascular smooth muscle-modulating microRNAs in human peripheral blood mononuclear cells: novel targets in essential hypertension. J Hum Hypertens. 2014;28(8):510.
342. Carpinella G, Pagano G, Buono F, Petitto M, Guarino G, Orefice G, Rengo G, Trimarco B, Morisco C. Prognostic value of combined target-organ damage in patients with essential hypertension. Am J Hypertens. 2014;28(1):127–34.
343. Latronico MV, Condorelli G. microRNAs in hypertrophy and heart failure. Exp Biol Med. 2011;236(2):125–31.
344. Van Wagoner DR, Nerbonne JM. Molecular basis of electrical remodeling in atrial fibrillation. J Mol Cell Cardiol. 2000;32(6):1101–17.
345. Sucharov C, Bristow MR, Port JD. miRNA expression in the failing human heart: functional correlates. J Mol Cell Cardiol. 2008;45(2):185–92.
346. Tijsen AJ, Pinto YM, Creemers EE. Circulating microRNAs as diagnostic biomarkers for cardiovascular diseases. Am J Phys Heart Circ Phys. 2012;303:H1085.
347. Ellis KL, Cameron VA, Troughton RW, Frampton CM, Ellmers LJ, Richards AM. Circulating microRNAs as candidate markers to distinguish heart failure in breathless patients. Eur J Heart Fail. 2013;15(10):1138–47.
348. Sauvageau M, Goff LA, Lodato S, Bonev B, Groff AF, Gerhardinger C, Sanchez-Gomez DB, Hacisuleyman E, Li E, Spence M. Multiple knockout mouse models reveal lincRNAs are required for life and brain development. elife. 2013;2:e01749.
349. Schuettengruber B, Martinez A-M, Iovino N, Cavalli G. Trithorax group proteins: switching genes on and keeping them active. Nat Rev Mol Cell Biol. 2011;12(12):799.
350. Rizki G, Boyer LA. Lnc ing epigenetic control of transcription to cardiovascular development and disease. Circ Res. 2015;117(2):192–206.
351. Ounzain S, Micheletti R, Arnan C, Plaisance I, Cecchi D, Schroen B, Reverter F, Alexanian M, Gonzales C, Ng SY. CARMEN, a human super enhancer-associated long noncoding RNA controlling cardiac specification, differentiation and homeostasis. J Mol Cell Cardiol. 2015;89:98–112.
352. Kowalczyk MS, Hughes JR, Garrick D, Lynch MD, Sharpe JA, Sloane-Stanley JA, McGowan SJ, De Gobbi M, Hosseini M, Vernimmen D. Intragenic enhancers act as alternative promoters. Mol Cell. 2012;45(4):447–58.
353. Ounzain S, Pezzuto I, Micheletti R, Burdet F, Sheta R, Nemir M, Gonzales C, Sarre A, Alexanian M, Blow MJ. Functional importance of cardiac enhancer-associated noncoding RNAs in heart development and disease. J Mol Cell Cardiol. 2014;76:55–70.
354. Boucher JM, Peterson SM, Urs S, Zhang C, Liaw L. The miR-143/145 cluster is a novel transcriptional target of Jagged-1/Notch signaling in vascular smooth muscle cells. J Biol Chem. 2011;286(32):28312–21.
355. Cordes KR, Sheehy NT, White MP, Berry EC, Morton SU, Muth AN, Lee T-H, Miano JM, Ivey KN, Srivastava D. miR-145 and miR-143 regulate smooth muscle cell fate and plasticity. Nature. 2009;460(7256):705.
356. He C, Hu H, Wilson KD, Wu H, Feng J, Xia S, Churko J, Qu K, Chang HY, Wu JC. Systematic characterization of long noncoding RNAs reveals the contrasting coordination of cis-and trans-molecular regulation in human fetal and adult hearts. Circ Cardiovasc Genet. 2016;9(2):110–8.
357. Matkovich SJ, Edwards JR, Grossenheider TC, de Guzman Strong C, Dorn GW. Epigenetic coordination of embryonic heart transcription by dynamically

regulated long noncoding RNAs. Proc Natl Acad Sci. 2014;111(33):12264–9.
358. Kurian L, Aguirre A, Sancho-Martinez I, Benner C, Hishida T, Nguyen TB, Reddy P, Nivet E, Krause MN, Nelles DA. Identification of novel long noncoding RNAs underlying vertebrate cardiovascular development. Circulation. 2015;131(14):1278–90.
359. Yang X, Gao L, Guo X, Shi X, Wu H, Song F, Wang B. A network based method for analysis of lncRNA-disease associations and prediction of lncRNAs implicated in diseases. PLoS One. 2014;9(1):e87797.
360. Qu X, Du Y, Shu Y, Gao M, Sun F, Luo S, et al. MIAT is a pro-fibrotic long non-coding RNA governing cardiac fibrosis in post-infarct myocardium. Sci Rep. 2017;7:42657.
361. Wang K, Liu F, Zhou L-Y, Long B, Yuan S-M, Wang Y, Liu C-Y, Sun T, Zhang X-J, Li P-F. The long noncoding RNA CHRF regulates cardiac hypertrophy by targeting miR-489. Circ Res. 2014;114(9):1377–88.
362. Piccoli M-T, Gupta SK, Viereck J, Foinquinos A, Samolovac S, Kramer FL, Garg A, Remke J, Zimmer K, Batkai S. Inhibition of the cardiac fibroblast–enriched lncRNA Meg3 prevents cardiac fibrosis and diastolic dysfunction. Circ Res. 2017;121(5):575–83.
363. Holdt LM, Hoffmann S, Sass K, Langenberger D, Scholz M, Krohn K, Finstermeier K, Stahringer A, Wilfert W, Beutner F. Alu elements in ANRIL noncoding RNA at chromosome 9p21 modulate atherogenic cell functions through trans-regulation of gene networks. PLoS Genet. 2013;9(7):e1003588.
364. Gao W, Zhu M, Wang H, Zhao S, Zhao D, Yang Y, Wang Z-M, Wang F, Yang Z-J, Lu X. Association of polymorphisms in long non-coding RNA H19 with coronary artery disease risk in a Chinese population. Mutat Res/Fundam Mol Mech Mutagen. 2015;772:15–22.
365. Ali T, Waheed H, Shaheen F, Mahmud M, Javed Q, Murtaza I. Increased endogenous serotonin level in diabetic conditions may lead to cardiac valvulopathy via reactive oxygen species regulation. Biologia. 2015;70(2):273–8.
366. Fiedler J, Breckwoldt K, Remmele CW, Hartmann D, Dittrich M, Pfanne A, Just A, Xiao K, Kunz M, Müller T. Development of long noncoding RNA-based strategies to modulate tissue vascularization. J Am Coll Cardiol. 2015;66(18):2005–15.
367. Bell RD, Long X, Lin M, Bergmann JH, Nanda V, Cowan SL, Zhou Q, Han Y, Spector DL, Zheng D. Identification and initial functional characterization of a human vascular cell–enriched long noncoding RNA. Arterioscler Thromb Vasc Biol. 2014;34(6):1249–59.
368. Burel SA, Hart CE, Cauntay P, Hsiao J, Machemer T, Katz M, Watt A, Bui H-h, Younis H, Sabripour M. Hepatotoxicity of high affinity gapmer antisense oligonucleotides is mediated by RNase H1 dependent promiscuous reduction of very long pre-mRNA transcripts. Nucleic Acids Res. 2015;44(5):2093–109.
369. Lucas T, Dimmeler S. RNA therapeutics for treatment of cardiovascular diseases: promises and challenges. Circ Res. 2016;119(7):794–7.
370. Kasuya T, Hori S-i, Watanabe A, Nakajima M, Gahara Y, Rokushima M, Yanagimoto T, Kugimiya A. Ribonuclease H1-dependent hepatotoxicity caused by locked nucleic acid-modified gapmer antisense oligonucleotides. Sci Rep. 2016;6:30377.
371. Maeder ML, Linder SJ, Cascio VM, Fu Y, Ho QH, Joung JK. CRISPR RNA–guided activation of endogenous human genes. Nat Methods. 2013;10(10):977.
372. Batzer MA, Deininger PL. Alu repeats and human genomic diversity. Nat Rev Genet. 2002;3(5):370.
373. Li D, Chen G, Yang J, Fan X, Gong Y, Xu G, Cui Q, Geng B. Transcriptome analysis reveals distinct patterns of long noncoding RNAs in heart and plasma of mice with heart failure. PLoS One. 2013;8(10):e77938.
374. Congrains A, Kamide K, Oguro R, Yasuda O, Miyata K, Yamamoto E, Kawai T, Kusunoki H, Yamamoto H, Takeya Y. Genetic variants at the 9p21 locus contribute to atherosclerosis through modulation of ANRIL and CDKN2A/B. Atherosclerosis. 2012;220(2):449–55.
375. Kumarswamy R, Bauters C, Volkmann I, Maury F, Fetisch J, Holzmann A, Lemesle G, de Groote P, Pinet F, Thum T. Circulating long noncoding RNA, LIPCAR, predicts survival in patients with heart failure. Circ Res. 2014;114(10):1569–75.

Part II

Bioinformatics and Interactions

Bioinformatics Research Methodology of Non-coding RNAs in Cardiovascular Diseases

2

Marina C. Costa, André F. Gabriel, and Francisco J. Enguita

Abstract

The transcriptional complexity generated by the human genomic output is within the core of cell and organ physiology, but also could be in the origin of pathologies. In cardiovascular diseases, the role of specific families of RNA transcripts belonging to the group of the non-coding RNAs started to be unveiled in the last two decades. The knowledge of the functional rules and roles of non-coding RNAs in the context of cardiovascular diseases is an important factor to derive new diagnostic methods, but also to design targeted therapeutic strategies. The characterization and analysis of ncRNA function requires a deep knowledge of the regulatory mechanism of these RNA species that often relies on intricated interaction networks. The use of specific bioinformatic tools to interrogate biological data and to derive functional implications is particularly relevant and needs to be extended to the general practice of translational researchers. This chapter briefly summarizes the bioinformatic tools and strategies that could be used for the characterization and functional analysis of non-coding RNAs, with special emphasis in their applications to the cardiovascular field.

Keywords

Non-coding RNAs · Bioinformatics · miRNAs · circRNAs · lncRNAs · Cardiovascular diseases · Analytical methods · Quantification · Databases

1 Introduction

Pervasive transcription of the human genome is one of the pivotal factors that contributes to the diversity of the transcriptome. Among all the transcriptome components, the non-coding RNAs (ncRNAs) are essential regulatory players that control the flow of information from the genome and are involved in many physiological processes including the proper development and homeostasis of the cardiovascular system. Non-proliferative organs as the heart are specially dependent on the presence and balanced function of all the ncRNA regulators, and in consequence, many cardiovascular diseases can be characterized by a specific misregulation patter of those molecular species [1–3].

Molecular biology techniques devoted to the characterization and functional analysis of

M. C. Costa · A. F. Gabriel · F. J. Enguita (✉)
Instituto de Medicina Molecular João Lobo Antunes, Faculdade de Medicina, Universidade de Lisboa, Lisbon, Portugal

Cardiomics Unit, Centro de Cardiologia da Universidade de Lisboa (CCUL), Faculdade de Medicina, Universidade de Lisboa, Lisbon, Portugal
e-mail: fenguita@medicina.ulisboa.pt

J. Xiao (ed.), *Non-coding RNAs in Cardiovascular Diseases*, Advances in Experimental Medicine and Biology 1229, https://doi.org/10.1007/978-981-15-1671-9_2

ncRNA function are becoming widely applied in the context of cardiovascular diseases. Since the discovery of the first specific ncRNAs generated by the myocardium, the community of cardiovascular researchers integrating clinicians and fundamental scientists, developed a deep interest for this field as a source of explanations for observed pathologies but also as a potential intervention target for therapy. Precision medicine initiatives and projects have empowered the characterization of new relevant ncRNA species and their functions related with the onset, development, diagnosis, prognosis and therapeutic response in cardiovascular diseases [4, 5]. The analytical methods used for molecular biology should be accompanied by the development of specific bioinformatic tools that could help in the positioning of ncRNA molecules in the context of cardiovascular diseases.

Here we present a practical compendium of the more relevant topics related with the application of bioinformatic methods and protocols for the functional characterization of ncRNAs in cardiovascular diseases, with specific focus on the considerations to be taken in the experimental obtention of RNA samples, data processing and analysis, and functional *in silico* characterization of three of the principal ncRNA families: microRNAs (miRNAs), long non-coding RNAs (lncRNAs) and circular RNAs (circRNAs).

2 Wet-Lab Methodological Considerations

The study of cardiovascular diseases in humans is a complex scientific enterprise when analysed from the point of view of the ncRNA biology. This fact is due to the intrinsic difficulties subjacent to the manipulation of human biological samples, the low abundance of some ncRNA families, and connected with the establishment of experimental models which are often not reliable for the mimicking of the human condition.

2.1 Sample Preparation

The study of ncRNAs in biological samples is always dependent on the obtention of a good starting material for analysis. Cardiac tissue is always a difficult sample to handle for RNA obtention, due to the fibrous nature of the myocardium which often prevents an optimal RNA extraction. Cardiac biopsies must be rapidly collected from human patients or animal models and preserved frozen at −80 °C until use in appropriate buffers. Typically, non-phenolic lysis buffers containing guanidinium salts for RNA extraction are not good enough and may be supplemented with reducing agents such as beta-mercaptoethanol at a concentration between 1–2% to abolish RNAse activity [6]. Prior do RNA extraction, the homogenization of the tissue is also a critical factor, that needs to be performed carefully. For this purpose, the use bead-beater or mechanical homogenizers is advisable before RNA extraction. NcRNAs present in homogenized samples can be extracted by several methods, including phenol-chloroform extraction and precipitation and anion-exchange purification under hydrophobic conditions. Depending on the myocardial origin of the biopsies, the standard protocols must be modified, such in the case of the extraction of RNA from heart valves or other more fibrous heart locations [7]. In all the considered cases, researchers need to consider that the final quality of the RNA samples obtained from heart biopsies is not too high, when compared with other softer tissues such as liver, brain or kidney. As a quality check, typical RNA Integrity Numbers (RIN) observed in RNA preparations from myocardium range between 7 and 9, being perfectly suitable for analysis by quantification methods such as microarrays, qPCR or next-generation sequencing.

Moreover, cardiovascular diseases are a wide range of conditions that often need to be studied from the systemic point of view. Biomarker research has become a hot topic in cardiovascular diseases within the frame of personalized medicine. Considering that cells are able to secrete ncRNAs and that these molecular species can be detected in circulating biofluids, ncRNAs belonging to diverse families (mainly miRNAs and circRNAs) have been proposed to be used as biomarkers for prognosis and therapeutic response in several cardiovascular diseases [8]. Extraction of ncRNA from biofluids is a relative standard protocol when considering serum or plasma [9], that can be modified and adapted to other biofluids such as urine or saliva [10]. Biofluid sample collection and preservation must follow protocols to maximize the RNA stability and extraction yield. For circulating ncRNAs in blood samples, the use of plasma is widely extended. Laboratory technicians from the clinical field engaged in research projects involving these samples must be aware of the quantification methods to be further used before sample collection. Plasma samples devoted for ncRNA extraction and quantification must be collected in heparin-free tubes since the polymeric nature of heparin would interfere with the analytical procedures, namely qPCR quantification and library preparation for next-generation sequencing experiments [11]. For normalization purposes, RNA samples extracted from biofluids need to be spiked with synthetic RNA molecules to ensure a proper quality check before and after RNA extraction [12].

2.2 Non-coding RNA Quantification

Protocols applied for the quantification of ncRNAs in the context of the study of cardiovascular diseases are dependent on the source of the analysed biological sample and on the family of ncRNAs to be analysed. In general, we can distinguish two main families of methods by their ability to perform just a quantification of a selected ncRNA or to screen a group of different ncRNAs (Table 2.1). Classical quantification methods as Northern blot can be only applied to specific experimental setup where it is possible to obtain a high amount of total RNA from a biological sample and perform with a low sensitivity [1]. In general, modern molecular biology labs prefer to use quantitative PCR methods to analyse ncRNAs in the context of cardiovascular diseases, since they require a smaller amount of RNA and show increased sensitivity and specificity when compared with Northern blot.

Screening methods for the quantification of ncRNAs are generally used for the simultaneous quantification of a group of ncRNAs. The hybridization-based methods as the classical microarrays were widely used before the appearance of next-generation sequencing techniques mainly for the quantification of miRNAs. Nowadays they are less used, but still employed for the screening and quantification of specific groups of ncRNAs such as circRNAs [13, 14]. Hybridization methods are robust and reliable, but for the quantification of small ncRNAs such as miRNAs they suffer from a lack of specificity and a high background noise that allows only to be applied for highly represented ncRNA species. Among the screening methods, qPCR low-density arrays are the most reliable tools for parallel quantitative analysis of gene expression signatures of a focused panel of genes in a medium throughput approach. For miRNA expression profile they are available from several manufacturers in 96-well and 384-well, which can be adapted to most qPCR systems. The detection chemistry used in qPCR arrays is either DNA binding dyes (mainly SYBR® Green) or optimized probe-based primer sets (mainly TaqMan® probes or LNA® probes). They can be used for a genomic-wide screening of expressed ncRNA or sub-panels, e.g. pathway- or disease-focused gene families or customized to contain a panel of genes tailored to your specific research interests [15, 16]. Low-density arrays typically showed a sensitivity down to 1 ng per reaction setup or 1 μg of total RNA and replicate correlation coefficients of $r > 0.99$, indicates that experimental samples can be reliably compared across array plates and within multiple runs. These qPCR panels are especially reliable for low abundance ncRNA species, and poor-quality RNA samples, allowing to be used for quantification of ncRNAs in biofluids. Recently, some new technologies for the quantification of RNA molecules have been emerged in the cardiovascular field, such as the Nanostring® nCounter system, which is based on a targeted capture of RNA molecules

Table 2.1 Methods for the detection and quantification of ncRNAs

Method	Advantages	Drawbacks	Application	Reference
Northern blot	Cheap	Tedious. Low sensitivity. High amount of RNA required.	Quantification	[1]
Hybridization microarrays	Cheap Easy Robust	Low specificity. High background noise. Not adequate for low-expressed ncRNAs.	Screening Quantification	[13, 14]
qPCR-low density arrays	Easy Sensitive Robust Specific	Expensive. Closed panels with a limited number of ncRNAs.	Screening Quantification	[15, 16]
qPCR	Easy Sensitive Robust Specific	Individual study.	Quantification	[53, 55, 80]
Nanostring®	Sensitive Specific Not dependent on PCR amplification.	Expensive. Propietary technology design. Limited number of transcripts analyzed.	Screening Quantification	[17, 18]
Next generation sequencing	High-yield and throughtput method. Useful for low-expressed ncRNAs.	Expensive. Specific data processing and analysis protocols.	Discovery Screening Quantification	[81–83]

and a quantitative analysis by fluorescent barcoded primers. This system offers the possibility of custom-made screening primers for the quantification of up to 800 different transcripts without previous sample amplification, and has been applied for the characterization of ncRNAs in cardiovascular diseases [17, 18].

Despite their different sensitivities and specificities, none of the already described methods allow a discovery approach for the detection and quantification of novel ncRNAs, since they are strictly dependent on a previous knowledge of the sequence of the selected ncRNAs for the design of specific detection probes or amplification primers. The discovery approach is particularly interesting in those ncRNA families, such as circRNAs, which biogenesis is dependent on processes that are not totally understood, and very important in the context of pathological processes such as cardiovascular diseases. Next-generation sequencing (NGS) techniques combine the possibility of using a small amount of starting RNA sample together with a myriad of possible applications, including the discovery of new and functionally relevant ncRNA species. Their limitations are more associated with post-processing events, including the bioinformatics approach for data analysis and the high amount of generated data. More specific applications of NGS in the context of cardiovascular diseases and related with every group of ncRNA will be further discussed along the chapter.

2.3 Data Processing from Quantification Methods

The advantages and disadvantages of all the available quantification methods for ncRNAs have been already discussed. At this point it will be important to analyse the data processing strategies for each quantification method.

Hybridization methods as microarrays are a solid option for ncRNA quantification, and typically affordable in economic terms. Microarray data processing is a very well standardized protocol for all the available microarrays. Despite of the availability of proprietary software for each microarray manufacturer, there are some good freeware alternatives such as AltAnalyze [19] or TM4 [20], that could be applicable to any type of microarrays. Microarray data processing software often provides a user-friendly interface integrating several normalization methods and strategies and data representation options. An excellent integrated option is NetworkAnalyst 3.0 which provides an online interface for data processing and functional analysis in a graphical environment [21].

Quantitative PCR methods (qPCR) are other of the quantification options for ncRNAs in the context of cardiovascular diseases. All of them rely on fluorescent probes that are selective bound to the double-stranded DNA during PCR amplification. There are two main methods for processing such data: The Delta-Ct and the standard curve methods. The Delta-Ct method is an indirect method of quantification that requires the presence of an internal normalizer and a reference group, and the results will be expressed in the form of fold change units of the experimental group in reference to the control. This strategy can be widely applied for any kind of ncRNA quantification including qPCR low-density arrays and individual determinations even when the amount of starting material is very low as in the case of circulating RNAs in biofluids. The selection of the internal normalizer is the most critical point in the Delta-Ct method, since it needs to show a constant expression among all the experimental conditions. For tissue or cells, internal normalizers need to be chosen accordingly to the size of the ncRNA that needs to be quantified; for miRNAs, typically a tRNA or a small rRNA is preferred, whereas for bigger ncRNAs such as lncRNAs, a snoRNA could be an appropriate choice. In the case of biofluids, there is a still not solved experimental controversy about the selection of the internal normalizers. In our experience, the use of other circulating ncRNAs is not recommended, since their levels can vary dramatically among different experimental conditions. For this reason, we typically used synthetic RNAs that are used to spike-in the biofluid samples prior to RNA extraction, serving as normalizers but also as internal control to determine the extraction yields [22]. It is frequent that manufacturers sell proprietary software for qPCR data processing and analysis with detection equipment. However, there are also free alternatives for analysis such as DataAssist software from Thermo Fisher Scientific® or LinRegPCR [23] that can be used for low-density array analysis and individual determinations.

Next generation sequencing (NGS) protocols for ncRNA analysis have become widely used in translational and personalized medicine focused on cardiovascular diseases [4]. Detailed protocols for transcriptomic analysis by NGS are out of the scope of this chapter and have been reviewed elsewhere [2]. In a brief summary, transcriptomic data obtained from NGS consist of a series of short DNA reads in a number that depends on the redundancy of the applied protocol, but typically range from 10 to 100 million. The relative abundance of these short reads is related with the quantity of the specific RNA transcript. Data collection protocols from NGS needs to be carefully designed to cover all the selected ncRNA families. In general, for human miRNAs, an output of 10–20 million reads per sample are enough to cover all the miRNA species. For lncRNAs, which are typically low-abundance species, an increase redundancy would be required, and the minimum reads to be collected for sample are around 50 million. Besides of transcriptomic quantification, the studies involving lncRNAs can also be source of other functional information such as the splicing pattern. Collection of data for lncRNA splicing studies require to employ the paired-end strategy, whereas the quantification of other ncRNAs as miRNAs could be performed by using the single-end strategy [24]. Obtained reads will then need to be aligned to the reference genome and the corresponding transcripts assembled and annotated within the genomic context. The alignment protocol and software used are critical steps in NGS data analysis, and have been extensively reviewed in other publications [25].

NGS data processing is often performed in a terminal-based way, using software applications that could be non-intuitive for an inexperienced computer user. For specific groups of ncRNAs such as miRNAs, several laboratories have developed user-friendly interfaces that can be accessible in a web-based manner. Oasis2, is a web-server that performs all the steps in miRNA quantification from NGS data starting from the genomic alignment of the reads from raw data, the annotation of miRNAs and the final differential expression from sample groups [26]. Oasis2 also performs a functional target analysis using the differentially expressed miRNAs between sample groups. SRNAbench and sRNAtoolbox 2019 is also an intuitive web suite of tools for for expression profiling and subsequent downstream analysis of miRNA-seq analysis [27]. In the last years, a considerable effort has been also made to develop user-friendly applications for the analysis of NGS data at the whole transcriptomic level that could be widely applicable for any family of RNA transcripts. We can cite the interesting examples of deepTools2 [28], a NGS analysis system based on the Galaxy platform, and the recently developed Maser [29], a full suite of analysis tools that can integrate NGS data and produce a complete range of functional analysis with quality graphic output.

Among all the ncRNA groups, the methods for the quantification of circRNAs from NGS data are specifically different due to their intrinsic characteristics. Specialized software as Uroborus [30], CircExplorer [31] or CIRI2 [32] have been developed to analyze these ncRNA species. All the cited software is designed to identify back-spliced junction reads and to filter false positives derived from repetitive sequences and mapping errors. Detailed protocols for circRNAs analysis and quantification from NGS data have been also reviewed elsewhere [33, 34].

3 Analysis of ncRNA Functions by Computational Methods

3.1 *In Silico* Analysis of miRNAs Function

Since their discovery and functional characterization in *Caenorhabditis elegans* in 1993 by Gary Ruvkun and Victor Ambros research teams, microRNAs (miRNAs) have been described as central players in cell biology and human disease [35, 36]. MiRNAs are small ncRNAs (19–23 nucleotides) generated by the processing of specialized transcription units, able to act as negative post-transcriptional regulators of gene expression and can be considered as molecular buffers that regulate the protein levels generated from mRNA transcripts. The miRNA mechanism of action involves a base-pairing event of its mature form to the target mRNA transcript, typically involving the 3′-UTR end. The role of miRNAs in cardiac physiology is well known since the discovery of miR-1 as a key player in heart development and function [3].

In humans and other higher eukaryotes, miRNAs are only partially complementary to their mRNA targets which allow a high degree of promiscuity in their regulatory effects. Physiological redundancy of this regulatory effect often involves several miRNA-mRNA interactions in the control of a specific metabolic process. The knowledge of the complete sequence of the human genome and the governing rules of miRNA-mRNA interactions allow to predict the putative regulatory effects of a miRNA over their cognate targets, and vice versa, the possible regulating miRNAs acting over a selected mRNA transcript. For this purpose, many bioinformatic target prediction algorithms have been developed in the last two decades. In general, target prediction algorithms are fundamentally based in the rule of the Watson-Crick base complementarity between the miRNA and its target, however the partial base complementarity between both RNAs and the small size of the mature miRNAs often produce false positive results. In order to reduce the output noise of the methods, specific approaches have been included in different target prediction algorithms to improve their success rate (Table 2.2). Classical target prediction algorithms as RNA22 [37], MiRanda [38] or Targetscan [39] combine the base pairing rules between miRNAs and their cognate targets with the binding energy of the hybrid. Some other applications as PITA introduce additional factors to improve the prediction, namely the secondary structure and target accessibility of the mRNA [40]. Complex target binding algorithms as miSTAR [41] or PicTar [42] with improved performance also used advanced mathematical models as random forest and logistic regressions, that

Table 2.2 Computer algorithms and applications for miRNA target prediction

Algorithm	Parameters contributing to the final score	Description	Assesment	Reference
miRanda	Complementarity and free energy	Algorithm for finding genomic targets for miRNAs. It is useful when working with non-model genomes.	**PROS**: Good for prediction of sites with imperfect binding within the seed region. There is a standalone version of the software.	[38]
			CONS: Low precision, too many false positives.	
miRWalk	Complementarity, seed match, and pairing probability	MirWalk is an integrated miRNA portal which includes its own target prediction algorithm, but also cross-talk with other algorithms.	**PROS**: Excellent interface and good performance. Very customizable interface for advanced target prediction using different criteria.	[84]
			CONS: Tendency to overestimate the number of targets when appeared in the same mRNA.	
miSTAR	Complementary, pairing probability and genomic content	miSTAR uses a logistic regression and random forest models to predict miRNA targets.	**PROS**: Good and easy to use interface. Uses the influence of binding site genomic context to increase accuracy.	[41]
			CONS: Obtained results are very accurate, but some non-canonical targets are missing.	
PicTar	Binding energy, complementarity of the seed and conservation among species	Classical algorithm for the predcition of mIRNA targets in several organisms. It can be searched locally but all the data can be also downloaded by local use.	**PROS**: miRNAs with high species conservation are more favorable to give good targeting scores.	[42]
			CONS: It does not predict non-canonical sites.	
TargetScan	Seed match, 3′ complementarity, local AU content and position contribution	Prediction of miRNA targets for mammal genomes, fish, fly and *C. elegans*. It can be searched by gene symbol or by miRNA ID. It gives information about the conservation of different miRNA families in all the scanned genomes.	**PROS**: Many parameters are included in the targeting score which is typically correlated with the protein downregulation in wet-lab experiments.	[39]
			CONS: Sites with poor seed pairing are often omitted.	
TargetScanS	Seed match type	Focused on the search of miRNA targets within ORFs of vertebrate genomes.	**PROS**: Simple tool for search conserved sites with strong seed pairing.	[85]
			CONS: It usually underestimates miRNAs with multiple target sites.	

(continued)

Table 2.2 (continued)

Algorithm	Parameters contributing to the final score	Description	Assesment	Reference
Diana	Free binding energy and complementarity	It is a integrated portal for miRNA target prediction and analysis. The prediction module is based on artificial neural networks. It may be used to search for target genes of annotated or user defined miRNA sequences.	**PROS**: It gives a score probability for each target site. Great interface. **CONS**: Some miRNAs with multiple target sites in the same 3′-UTR may be omitted.	[86]
PITA	Target site accessibility and binding energy	Target prediction tool that takes into consideration the secondary structure of the target mRNA. The interface is easily customizable and can be used to search for miRNA, genes and also for UTR sequences.	**PROS**: The secondary structure of the target mRNA is considered for the predictions. **CONS**: Low efficiency in comparison with other algorithms.	[40]
RNA22	Pattern recognition and folding energy of the miRNA-mRNA hybrid	Algorithm for miRNA target prediction that uses input sequences for miRNA and UTR. Whole genomic predictions are available for download and browsing.	**PROS**: Allows to identify sites targeted by new miRNAs. **CONS**: Low efficiency in comparison with other algorithms.	[37]

could be also combined with the genomic content and conservation of targets among species.

Despite of the differences in methodology showed by all the miRNA target prediction algorithms, all of them are based on the complementarity between the miRNA and its mRNA target and could potentially result in false positive determinations. In order to circumvent this problem, it would be advisable to simultaneously use several target prediction algorithms and combine their results. For this purpose, recent web-based applications can interrogate different target predictors and show a combined result (Table 2.3). The targets predicted by more applications would have more realistic probability to be true and could be selected for further biological or functional validations [43].

Moreover, the accumulation of biological evidences of the regulatory role of miRNAs in general biological processes in the last two decades allowed the construction and development of databases containing validated miRNA targets. These databases could be a complementary source of information in miRNA studies together with the computer predictions. MiRTarBase currently in its 7.0 version, contains more than 400,000 curated miRNA-mRNA interactions validated by biological means along 23 different species including humans [44]. Tarbase v.8 is also an experimentally validated database for miRNA targets, comprising more than one million of biological interactions classified by species, cell types and tissues [45].

The availability of functional data about miRNAs and their roles in human disease allowed to develop specialized databases that link the role of these ncRNAs in the context of several human conditions (Table 2.4). Mir2Disease [46] and miRGator3 [47] databases are manually curated databases spanning the role of miRNAs in a wide range of human diseases including heart and cardiovascular ones. Specially interesting is the HDncRNA database, a compendium of functional implication of two families of ncRNAs, miRNAs and lncRNAs, in the onset, development and progression of cardiovascular diseases [48]. This database offers a friendly user interface and contains associations between miRNAs and lncRNAs with cardiovascular conditions. Interestingly, the HDncRNA database compiles information in 6 species including human, mouse, rat, pig, calf and dog, allowing the comparison of ncRNA regula-

Table 2.3 Multiple miRNA target predictors

Application	Comments	Species	Reference
miRecords	Resource for animal miRNA-target interactions. miRecords consists of two components: a database of validated targets and a combined resource which simultaneously uses eleven applications for miRNA target prediction, and multiple species.	Human, mouse, rat, fly and zebrafish	[87]
miRWalk2	A comprehensive database that provides information on miRNA from human, mouse and rat on their predicted as well as validated binding sites on their target genes combining eight different applications for target prediction.	Human, mouse and rat	[88]
miRSystem	miRSystem is a database which integrates seven well known miRNA target gene prediction programs: DIANA, miRanda, miRBridge, PicTar, PITA, rna22, and TargetScan.	Human and mouse	[89]
MIRDIP	MIRDIP integrates twelve microRNA prediction datasets from six microRNA prediction databases, allowing users to customize their microRNA target searches. Combining microRNA predictions allows users to obtain more robust target predictions, giving you more confidence in your microRNA targets.	Human, mouse and rat	[90]

Table 2.4 Specialized miRNA databases related with human diseases

Database	Comments	Reference
miR2Disease	Manually curated database designed as a comprehensive resource for the study of miRNA influence in several human diseases.	[46]
miRGator3	Aims to be the microRNA (miRNA) portal encompassing microRNA diversity, expression profiles, target relationships, and various supporting tools. Include 73 deep sequencing datasets on human samples from GEO, SRA, and TCGA archives, which amounts to 4.1 billion short reads and 2.5 billion aligned reads, and curated into 38 diseases and 71 anatomic categories.	[47]
PhenomiR	Provides information about differentially regulated miRNA expression in diseases and other biological processes. The content of PhenomiR is completely generated by manual curation of experienced annotators.	[91]
HMDD	The human microRNA disease database which contains miRNA names, disease names, dysfunction evidences, and the literature PubMed ID.	[92, 93]
miRCancer	Comprehensive collection of microRNA expression profiles in various human cancers which are automatically extracted from published literature in PubMed.	[94]
PROGmiR	A prognostic database for cancers based on their miRNA expression signature.	[95]
HDncRNA	Heart Disease-related Non-coding RNAs Database (HDncRNA), is a manually curated database that compiles ncRNA and cardiovascular diseases. Include functional associations for miRNAs and lncRNAs with cardiovascular diseases. Currently, the database contains 2304 associations for 133 conditions in 6 species including human, mouse, rat, pig, calf and dog.	[48]

tory effects in several widely used laboratory models for the study of cardiovascular diseases.

3.2 *In Silico* Analysis of lncRNAs Function

LncRNAs (Long Non-Coding RNAs) are a rich family of non-coding genes able to generate long transcripts >200 bases in length. Structurally, lncRNAs are very similar to protein coding genes but they harbour a reduced coding potential. They are typically controlled by specific promoters and contain exons and introns, having the potential of produce diverse isoforms by alternative splicing. The last version of NONCODE database [49] annotated around 96,000 lncRNA genes producing more than 170,000 different transcripts in the human genome. Other more conservative annotation resources as GENCODE, quantified the number of lncRNAs genes in the human genome by 16,000 and the number of generated transcripts around 30,000 [50]. LncRNAs are versatile and heterogeneous molecules in their function that usually involve different molecular players and can be compartmentalized either in the nucleus or the cytoplasm, and have the tendency to be species-specific [51]. An interesting fact is related with the dual nature of lncRNAs, which can be illustrated by the presence of sequence and structural information. LncRNAs have been widely considered as scaffold molecules that can help to the formation of macromolecular complexes and target these complexes to their specific place of action, acting as functional guides [52]. They have been involved in the control of gene expression at the chromatin level by interacting with chromatin remodelling complexes [53], in regulatory events controlling translation in the cytoplasm by controlling mRNA stability [54], and as sponges of other ncRNAs as central players of the so called complementary endogenous RNAs (ceRNAs) [55]. Since their discovery, lncRNAs have been studied on the context of cardiovascular diseases, and their roles have been extensively reviewed [56–58].

Braveheart lncRNA was one of the first characterized examples of the functional role of these family of ncRNAs in cardiovascular physiology. In mouse, Braveheart is strictly required for a proper recruitment of the lineage of cardiovascular precursor cells and to form a functional heart [17]. Other lncRNAs such as PFL or H19 have been involved in cardiac fibrosis or ischemic and reperfusion injury [55, 59]. Recently, an interesting example of the pivotal role of these ncRNAs have been characterized for the case of CPR lncRNA, which is a natural negative regulator of cardiomyocyte proliferation that could be putatively used as a pharmacological target. The silencing of CPR lncRNA significantly increased the cardiomyocyte proliferation, improved cardiac contractility and reduced the scar formation after an infarction episode [60].

Inferring molecular functions of lncRNAs by pure computational methods is a difficult task, since there ncRNAs have no clear sequence or structure patterns that could allow to predict their molecular functions. Prediction of lncRNA function often involves a combined approach, where experimental data and bioinformatic analysis are combined. The "guilty-by-association" protocol is based on the analysis of the expression of coding mRNA transcripts and lncRNAs in a biological process [61]. The correlation expression patterns found between mRNAs and lncRNAs, and the further functional classification of the coding transcripts could act as an association factor for the prediction of the function of lncRNAs. Some computer applications such as decodeRNA integrate information derived from the guilty-by-association method to predict the function of lncRNAs in the context of cancer [62]. Among other tools that contain functional correlations between lncRNAs and coding transcripts, lncRNA2Function is a database that contains correlation data between mRNAs and lncRNAs in healthy human tissues, that can be searched by gene ontology terms and biological pathways [63]. The lncRNA2disease web portal integrate around 3000 lncRNA-disease associations and it is manually curated by text mining, and includes information about cardiovascular diseases [64]. Unfortunately, with the exception of HDncRNA which is a general ncRNA resource [48], there is not any specific tool for lncRNA function in the context of cardiovascular disease, but the existing ones often harbour useful information that can be applied for cardiovascular studies. Other relevant tools devoted for lncRNA classification, function and analysis are compiled on Table 2.5.

A particularly interesting functional role of lncRNAs is related with their inclusion in the ceRNA networks, acting as sponges of other ncRNAs mainly represented by miRNAs. The importance of this sequestering process in cardiovascular biology has been described mainly in the myocardium, being characterized as an essential regulatory process to control cardiomyocyte function. The sequestering activity of MALAT1 lncRNA over miR-200a has been involved in the negative regulation of cardiomyocyte proliferation and cell cycle in mouse models [65]. Other lncRNAs such as PFL were

Table 2.5 lncRNA databases useful in cardiovascular research

Database	Comments	Reference
NONCODE	Reference resource containing sequences of 527,336 lncRNAs in 16 different species. For human and mouse, the lncRNA numbers are 167,150 and 130,558, respectively. Available information includes conservation annotation, the relationships between lncRNAs and diseases and an interface to choose datasets through predicted scores, literature support and sequencing method support.	[49]
LNCipedia	LNCipedia is a public manually curated database for long non-coding RNA (lncRNA) sequence and annotation. The current release contains 127,802 transcripts and 56,946 genes. Contains data of species conservation and integrates genomic visualization tools.	[96]
DIANA-LncBase	Database containing in silico predicted miRNA Recognition Elements (MREs) on lncRNAs. The database includes more than 70,000 low and high-throughput miRNA-lncRNA experimentally supported interactions, derived from manually curated publications and the analysis of 153 AGO CLIP-Seq libraries.	[68]
LncReg	Database collecting regulatory relationships of the lncRNAs with 1081 validated lncRNA-associated regulatory entries, including 258 non-redundant lncRNAs and 571 non-redundant genes. It provides overall perspectives of regulatory networks of lncRNAs which is useful for understanding the functional roles of lncRNAs.	[97]
lncRNA2Function	Database with expression correlations between lncRNAs and protein-coding genes across 19 human normal tissues, associated with functional gene ontology and human biological pathways collected from 12 pathway databases. It enables browsing the lncRNAs associated with a specific functional term, the functional terms associated with a specific lncRNA, or to assign functional terms to a set of human lncRNA genes, such as a cluster of co-expressed lncRNAs.	[63]
LncRNADisease	LncRNADisease is a database for collection of experimental supported lncRNA-disease associations. It provides the transcriptional regulatory relationships among lncRNA, mRNA and miRNA, providing a confidence score for each lncRNA-disease association and integrating experimentally supported RNA disease associations.	[64]
lncRNAtor	Database for functional investigation of lncRNAs that encompasses annotation, sequence analysis, gene expression, protein binding and phylogenetic conservation, integrating lncRNAs from six species (human, mouse, zebrafish, fruit fly, worm and yeast) from ENSEMBL, HGNC, MGI and lncRNAdb.	[98]
Linc2go	A web resource that aims to provide comprehensive functional annotations for human lincRNA. MicroRNA-mRNA and microRNA-lincRNA interaction data were integrated to generate lincRNA functional annotations based on the 'competing endogenous RNA hypothesis'.	[67]

also characterized as a fibrotic factor by a mechanism that involves the capture of let-7d miRNA [55]. In the context of cardiovascular diseases, the case of MEG3 lncRNAs is very relevant, as a regulatory factor but also as a potential therapeutic target. MEG3 was initially characterized as overexpressed in many human cancers, whereas is also involved in the development of cardiac hypertrophy by induction of cardiomyocyte cell growth via a selective blocking of miR-361-5p [66]. The intrinsic nature of the ceRNA networks allowed the development of specific bioinformatic tools that could predict the potential sponging ability of a selected lncRNA over a group of miRNAs (Table 2.5). For instance, Linc2GO is a web resource that aims to provide comprehensive functional annotations for human lincRNAs, considering miRNA-mRNA and miRNA-lincRNA interaction data that were integrated to infer lincRNA functional associations based on the ceRNA hypothesis [67]. Diana-lncBase is another useful tool for dissecting lncRNA-centered ceRNA networks, since it integrates more than 70,000 miRNA-lncRNA experimentally supported interactions, derived from manually curated publications and the analysis of 153 AGO CLIP-Seq libraries [68].

3.3 *In Silico* Analysis of circRNAs Function

Circular RNAs (circRNAs) were initially considered as bystander products of transcription and splicing of genomic loci producing coding or non-coding RNA transcripts. However, the advent of next-generation sequencing techniques showed that the global pattern of circRNAs expression was dependent on the physiological state of the cell, suggesting a putative functional role of these biochemical species. CircRNAs are generate by a non-canonical splicing evet, generically called as "back-splicing", where the 5′ and 3′ ends of a splicing product (containing either exons or introns, or a combination of them) are ligated in a circular manner, being more stable to degradation by RNAses than the linear RNA molecules.

CircRNAs sequences and genomic localization are compiled in the circBase database [69]. Comparing with other central resources such the miRbase database for miRNAs [70], there is an unmet and urgent need for the standardization of the circRNAs nomenclature. It is very frequent to find divergent annotations of these ncRNAs either following manufacturers specific designations or other non-conventional annotations outside of circBase. The standard annotation is particularly needed in the field of circRNAs due to their heterogeneity in origins, considering the parental gene and the splicing pattern observed [71, 72].

The functional roles of circRNAs characterized from experimental evidences, suggested that these ncRNAs act as scavengers of other biomolecules, namely RNAs or proteins. The participation of circRNAs in regulatory networks involving complementary-endogenous RNA (ceRNA) interactions by sequestering miRNAs has been recently characterized in cardiovascular pathologies. The role of some of the characterized circRNAs-miRNAs interactions appeared to have a protective function for the development of cardiovascular diseases. This is particularly evident for processes related with cardiomyocyte death [73] or myocardium hypertrophy [74]. However, some recent working evidences described the pivotal role of circRNAs within complex RNA-regulatory networks to the establishment of chronic cardiovascular conditions such as atrial fibrillation [75].

In cardiovascular research, some general-purpose computer resources can be applied for the functional study of RNA regulatory networks mediated by circRNAs. For experimentally validated associations, the starBase platform is an essential database that systematically compile experimental data to identify RNA-RNA and RNA-protein interaction networks from PAR-CLIP, HITS-CLIP, iCLIP and CLASH experiments [76]. The last version of starBase (2.0) contains approximately 9000 miRNA-circRNA interaction pairs obtained from 37 independent studies. CircInteractome is also an interesting web-based tool that performs an in silico prediction of the putative protein or miRNA interacting partners of a given circRNA [77, 78]. For experimental design of specific primers and for the determination of sponging activity of circRNAs, circPrimer is a standalone software based on the Windows® environment with a user-friendly interface that combines the information from circBase together with miRNA target prediction algorithms as MiRanda [79].

4 Conclusions and Further Perspectives

Cardiovascular research field is probably the clinical discipline where the importance of ncRNAs has been earlier recognized either by clinicians or by translational researchers. Development of personalized medicine concepts and methods had a considerable benefit over the global knowledge of the roles of ncRNAs in cardiovascular conditions. Management of big data generated from the new techniques of genome analysis, namely next generation sequencing and its applications for transcriptome analysis, has prompted to the develop of a myriad of bioinformatic tools that can be easily applied in the cardiovascular research on ncRNAs.

As stated in this chapter, the development of user-friendly interfaces and computer applications for the analysis of ncRNA function has been essential for the engagement of the medical community within the field. It is no longer required to have a deep knowledge about computer programming or operating systems to interact, use, and apply bioinformatic software and algorithms to any field of research, including the medical one.

The different roles of ncRNAs in the context of cardiovascular diseases requires a multidisciplinary research approach to characterize their functions. Particularly interesting is the recently characterized RNA regulatory networks involving the interactions between several ncRNA molecules. Entangled functional interactions are very relevant for the synchronicity of the myocardium, but also for the essential homeostasis of the whole cardiovascular system. The characterization of these RNA regulatory networks by using the point of view of the systems biology will be in the core of further research in the cardiovascular field.

Bioinformatic tools applied to the ncRNA field have extensively evolved in the last decade, and nowadays benefit from the new computer processors and algorithms based on new methods such as the artificial intelligence. The commitment of the cardiovascular medical community in the translational research has pointed out the intrinsic importance of ncRNAs as essential tools for understanding the basis of many cardiovascular diseases, but it will need a specific training in the use and application of bioinformatic methods for an integrative analysis of ncRNA function. It is still a long road to drive, but we are getting closer to the medical application of ncRNAs for diagnosis and therapeutics of cardiovascular diseases, and their integration in the general practical medical guidelines for cardiovascular medicine.

References

1. van Rooij E, Sutherland LB, Liu N, Williams AH, McAnally J, Gerard RD, Richardson JA, Olson EN. A signature pattern of stress-responsive microRNAs that can evoke cardiac hypertrophy and heart failure. Proc Natl Acad Sci U S A. 2006;103(48):18255–60.
2. Wirka RC, Pjanic M, Quertermous T. Advances in transcriptomics: investigating cardiovascular disease at unprecedented resolution. Circ Res. 2018;122(9):1200–20.
3. Zhao Y, Ransom JF, Li A, Vedantham V, von Drehle M, Muth AN, Tsuchihashi T, McManus MT, Schwartz RJ, Srivastava D. Dysregulation of cardiogenesis, cardiac conduction, and cell cycle in mice lacking miRNA-1-2. Cell. 2007;129(2):303–17.
4. Gullapalli RR, Lyons-Weiler M, Petrosko P, Dhir R, Becich MJ, LaFramboise WA. Clinical integration of next-generation sequencing technology. Clin Lab Med. 2012;32(4):585–99.
5. Gandhi S, Ruehle F, Stoll M. Evolutionary patterns of non-coding RNA in cardiovascular biology. Noncoding RNA. 2019;5(1)
6. Asp M, Salmen F, Stahl PL, Vickovic S, Felldin U, Lofling M, Fernandez Navarro J, Maaskola J, Eriksson MJ, Persson B, Corbascio M, Persson H, Linde C, Lundeberg J. Spatial detection of fetal marker genes expressed at low level in adult human heart tissue. Sci Rep. 2017;7(1):12941.
7. Cecilia Valadares A, Gorki H, Liebold A, Hoenicka M. Extraction of total RNA from calcified human heart valves for gene expression analysis. J Heart Valve Dis. 2017;26(2):185–92.
8. Stepien E, Costa MC, Kurc S, Drozdz A, Cortez-Dias N, Enguita FJ. The circulating non-coding RNA landscape for biomarker research: lessons and prospects from cardiovascular diseases. Acta Pharmacol Sin. 2018;39(7):1085–99.
9. Bergallo M, Gambarino S, Martino S, Montin D, Montanari P, Galliano I, Tovo PA. Comparison of two available RNA extraction protocols for microRNA amplification in serum samples. J Clin Lab Anal. 2016;30(4):277–83.
10. Martinez-Fernandez M, Paramio JM, Duenas M. RNA detection in urine: from RNA extraction to good normalizer molecules. J Mol Diagn. 2016;18(1):15–22.
11. Plieskatt JL, Feng Y, Rinaldi G, Mulvenna JP, Bethony JM, Brindley PJ. Circumventing qPCR inhibition to amplify miRNAs in plasma. Biomark Res. 2014;2:13.
12. Marabita F, de Candia P, Torri A, Tegner J, Abrignani S, Rossi RL. Normalization of circulating microRNA expression data obtained by quantitative real-time RT-PCR. Brief Bioinform. 2016;17(2):204–12.
13. Zhang S, Zeng X, Ding T, Guo L, Li Y, Ou S, Yuan H. Microarray profile of circular RNAs identifies hsa_circ_0014130 as a new circular RNA biomarker in non-small cell lung cancer. Sci Rep. 2018;8(1):2878.
14. Tan WL, Lim BT, Anene-Nzelu CG, Ackers-Johnson M, Dashi A, See K, Tiang Z, Lee DP, Chua WW, Luu TD, Li PY, Richards AM, Foo RS. A landscape of circular RNA expression in the human heart. Cardiovasc Res. 2017;113(3):298–309.
15. Gevaert AB, Witvrouwen I, Vrints CJ, Heidbuchel H, Van Craenenbroeck EM, Van Laere SJ, Van Craenenbroeck AH. MicroRNA profiling in plasma samples using qPCR arrays: recommendations for correct analysis and interpretation. PLoS One. 2018;13(2):e0193173.

16. Chen Y, Gelfond JA, McManus LM, Shireman PK. Reproducibility of quantitative RT-PCR array in miRNA expression profiling and comparison with microarray analysis. BMC Genomics. 2009;10:407.
17. Klattenhoff CA, Scheuermann JC, Surface LE, Bradley RK, Fields PA, Steinhauser ML, Ding H, Butty VL, Torrey L, Haas S, Abo R, Tabebordbar M, Lee RT, Burge CB, Boyer LA. Braveheart, a long non-coding RNA required for cardiovascular lineage commitment. Cell. 2013;152(3):570–83.
18. Schonrock N, Harvey RP, Mattick JS. Long noncoding RNAs in cardiac development and pathophysiology. Circ Res. 2012;111(10):1349–62.
19. Emig D, Salomonis N, Baumbach J, Lengauer T, Conklin BR, Albrecht M. AltAnalyze and DomainGraph: analyzing and visualizing exon expression data. Nucleic Acids Res. 2010;38(Web Server issue):W755–62.
20. Saeed AI, Bhagabati NK, Braisted JC, Liang W, Sharov V, Howe EA, Li J, Thiagarajan M, White JA, Quackenbush J. TM4 microarray software suite. Methods Enzymol. 2006;411:134–93.
21. Zhou G, Soufan O, Ewald J, Hancock REW, Basu N, Xia J. NetworkAnalyst 3.0: a visual analytics platform for comprehensive gene expression profiling and meta-analysis. Nucleic Acids Res. 2019;47:W234–41.
22. Costa MC, Leitao AL, Enguita FJ. MicroRNA profiling in plasma or serum using quantitative RT-PCR. Methods Mol Biol. 2014;1182:121–9.
23. Brunet-Vega A, Pericay C, Quilez ME, Ramirez-Lazaro MJ, Calvet X, Lario S. Variability in microRNA recovery from plasma: comparison of five commercial kits. Anal Biochem. 2015;488:28–35.
24. Lizio M, Abugessaisa I, Noguchi S, Kondo A, Hasegawa A, Hon CC, de Hoon M, Severin J, Oki S, Hayashizaki Y, Carninci P, Kasukawa T, Kawaji H. Update of the FANTOM web resource: expansion to provide additional transcriptome atlases. Nucleic Acids Res. 2019;47(D1):D752–8.
25. Mielczarek M, Szyda J. Review of alignment and SNP calling algorithms for next-generation sequencing data. J Appl Physiol. 2016;57(1):71–9.
26. Rahman RU, Gautam A, Bethune J, Sattar A, Fiosins M, Magruder DS, Capece V, Shomroni O, Bonn S. Oasis 2: improved online analysis of small RNA-seq data. BMC Bioinformatics. 2018;19(1):54.
27. Aparicio-Puerta E, Lebron R, Rueda A, Gomez-Martin C, Giannoukakos S, Jaspez D, Medina JM, Zubkovic A, Jurak I, Fromm B, Marchal JA, Oliver J, Hackenberg M. sRNAbench and sRNAtoolbox 2019: intuitive fast small RNA profiling and differential expression. Nucleic Acids Res. 2019;47:W530–5.
28. Ramirez F, Ryan DP, Gruning B, Bhardwaj V, Kilpert F, Richter AS, Heyne S, Dundar F, Manke T. deepTools2: a next generation web server for deep-sequencing data analysis. Nucleic Acids Res. 2016;44(W1):W160–5.
29. Kinjo S, Monma N, Misu S, Kitamura N, Imoto J, Yoshitake K, Gojobori T, Ikeo K. Maser: one-stop platform for NGS big data from analysis to visualization. Database (Oxford). 2018;2018
30. Song X, Zhang N, Han P, Moon BS, Lai RK, Wang K, Lu W. Circular RNA profile in gliomas revealed by identification tool UROBORUS. Nucleic Acids Res. 2016;44(9):e87.
31. Dong R, Ma XK, Chen LL, Yang L. Genome-wide annotation of circRNAs and their alternative back-splicing/splicing with CIRCexplorer pipeline. Methods Mol Biol. 2019;1870:137–49.
32. Gao Y, Zhang J, Zhao F. Circular RNA identification based on multiple seed matching. Brief Bioinform. 2018;19(5):803–10.
33. Zheng Y, Zhao F. Detection and reconstruction of circular RNAs from transcriptomic data. Methods Mol Biol. 2018;1724:1–8.
34. Zeng X, Lin W, Guo M, Zou Q. A comprehensive overview and evaluation of circular RNA detection tools. PLoS Comput Biol. 2017;13(6):e1005420.
35. Lee RC, Feinbaum RL, Ambros V. The C. elegans heterochronic gene lin-4 encodes small RNAs with antisense complementarity to lin-14. Cell. 1993;75(5):843–54.
36. Wightman B, Ha I, Ruvkun G. Posttranscriptional regulation of the heterochronic gene lin-14 by lin-4 mediates temporal pattern formation in C. elegans. Cell. 1993;75(5):855–62.
37. Loher P, Rigoutsos I. Interactive exploration of RNA22 microRNA target predictions. Bioinformatics. 2012;28(24):3322–3.
38. Enright AJ, John B, Gaul U, Tuschl T, Sander C, Marks DS. MicroRNA targets in Drosophila. Genome Biol. 2003;5(1):R1.
39. Agarwal V, Bell GW, Nam JW, Bartel DP. Predicting effective microRNA target sites in mammalian mRNAs. Elife. 2015;4
40. Kertesz M, Iovino N, Unnerstall U, Gaul U, Segal E. The role of site accessibility in microRNA target recognition. Nat Genet. 2007;39(10):1278–84.
41. Van Peer G, De Paepe A, Stock M, Anckaert J, Volders PJ, Vandesompele J, De Baets B, Waegeman W. miSTAR: miRNA target prediction through modeling quantitative and qualitative miRNA binding site information in a stacked model structure. Nucleic Acids Res. 2017;45(7):e51.
42. Krek A, Grun D, Poy MN, Wolf R, Rosenberg L, Epstein EJ, MacMenamin P, da Piedade I, Gunsalus KC, Stoffel M, Rajewsky N. Combinatorial microRNA target predictions. Nat Genet. 2005;37(5):495–500.
43. Leitao AL, Costa MC, Enguita FJ. A guide for miRNA target prediction and analysis using web-based applications. Methods Mol Biol. 2014;1182:265–77.
44. Chou CH, Chang NW, Shrestha S, Hsu SD, Lin YL, Lee WH, Yang CD, Hong HC, Wei TY, Tu SJ, Tsai TR, Ho SY, Jian TY, Wu HY, Chen PR, Lin NC, Huang HT, Yang TL, Pai CY, Tai CS, Chen WL, Huang CY, Liu CC, Weng SL, Liao KW, Hsu WL, Huang HD. miRTarBase 2016: updates to the experimentally validated miRNA-target interactions database. Nucleic Acids Res. 2016;44(D1):D239–47.

45. Paraskevopoulou MD, Vlachos IS, Hatzigeorgiou AG. DIANA-TarBase and DIANA suite tools: studying experimentally supported microRNA targets. Curr Protoc Bioinformatics. 2016;55:12.14.11–8.
46. Jiang Q, Wang Y, Hao Y, Juan L, Teng M, Zhang X, Li M, Wang G, Liu Y. miR2Disease: a manually curated database for microRNA deregulation in human disease. Nucleic Acids Res. 2009;37(Database):D98–104.
47. Cho S, Jang I, Jun Y, Yoon S, Ko M, Kwon Y, Choi I, Chang H, Ryu D, Lee B, Kim VN, Kim W, Lee S. MiRGator v3.0: a microRNA portal for deep sequencing, expression profiling and mRNA targeting. Nucleic Acids Res. 2013;41(Database issue):D252–7.
48. Wang WJ, Wang YM, Hu Y, Lin Q, Chen R, Liu H, Cao WZ, Zhu HF, Tong C, Li L, Peng LY. HDncRNA: a comprehensive database of non-coding RNAs associated with heart diseases. Database (Oxford). 2018:2018.
49. Zhao Y, Li H, Fang S, Kang Y, Wu W, Hao Y, Li Z, Bu D, Sun N, Zhang MQ, Chen R. NONCODE 2016: an informative and valuable data source of long non-coding RNAs. Nucleic Acids Res. 2016;44(D1):D203–8.
50. Frankish A, Diekhans M, Ferreira AM, Johnson R, Jungreis I, Loveland J, Mudge JM, Sisu C, Wright J, Armstrong J, Barnes I, Berry A, Bignell A, Carbonell Sala S, Chrast J, Cunningham F, Di Domenico T, Donaldson S, Fiddes IT, Garcia Giron C, Gonzalez JM, Grego T, Hardy M, Hourlier T, Hunt T, Izuogu OG, Lagarde J, Martin FJ, Martinez L, Mohanan S, Muir P, Navarro FCP, Parker A, Pei B, Pozo F, Ruffier M, Schmitt BM, Stapleton E, Suner MM, Sycheva I, Uszczynska-Ratajczak B, Xu J, Yates A, Zerbino D, Zhang Y, Aken B, Choudhary JS, Gerstein M, Guigo R, Hubbard TJP, Kellis M, Paten B, Reymond A, Tress ML, Flicek P. GENCODE reference annotation for the human and mouse genomes. Nucleic Acids Res. 2019;47(D1):D766–73.
51. Marchese FP, Raimondi I, Huarte M. The multidimensional mechanisms of long noncoding RNA function. Genome Biol. 2017;18(1):206.
52. Aguilo F, Di Cecilia S, Walsh MJ. Long non-coding RNA ANRIL and polycomb in human cancers and cardiovascular disease. Curr Top Microbiol Immunol. 2016;394:29–39.
53. Grote P, Wittler L, Hendrix D, Koch F, Wahrisch S, Beisaw A, Macura K, Blass G, Kellis M, Werber M, Herrmann BG. The tissue-specific lncRNA Fendrr is an essential regulator of heart and body wall development in the mouse. Dev Cell. 2013;24(2):206–14.
54. Rashid F, Shah A, Shan G. Long non-coding RNAs in the cytoplasm. Genomics Proteomics Bioinformatics. 2016;14(2):73–80.
55. Liang H, Pan Z, Zhao X, Liu L, Sun J, Su X, Xu C, Zhou Y, Zhao D, Xu B, Li X, Yang B, Lu Y, Shan H. LncRNA PFL contributes to cardiac fibrosis by acting as a competing endogenous RNA of let-7d. Theranostics. 2018;8(4):1180–94.
56. Sallam T, Sandhu J, Tontonoz P. Long noncoding RNA discovery in cardiovascular disease: decoding form to function. Circ Res. 2018;122(1):155–66.
57. Garg A, Gupta SK, Thum T. Long non-coding RNAs: a crucial part of the vasculature puzzle. Vasc Pharmacol. 2019;114:131–8.
58. Hobuss L, Bar C, Thum T. Long non-coding RNAs: at the heart of cardiac dysfunction? Front Physiol. 2019;10:30.
59. Luo H, Wang J, Liu D, Zang S, Ma N, Zhao L, Zhang L, Zhang X, Qiao C. The lncRNA H19/miR-675 axis regulates myocardial ischemic and reperfusion injury by targeting PPARalpha. Mol Immunol. 2019;105:46–54.
60. Ponnusamy M, Liu F, Zhang YH, Li RB, Zhai M, Zhou LY, Liu CY, Yan KW, Dong YH, Wang M, Qian LL, Shan C, Xu S, Wang Q, Li PF, Zhang J, Wang K. The long non-coding RNA CPR regulates cardiomyocyte proliferation and cardiac repair. Circulation. 2019;20:336–40.
61. Li Y, Xu J, Shao T, Zhang Y, Chen H, Li X. RNA function prediction. Methods Mol Biol. 2017;1654:17–28.
62. Lefever S, Anckaert J, Volders PJ, Luypaert M, Vandesompele J, Mestdagh P. decodeRNA- predicting non-coding RNA functions using guilt-by-association. Database (Oxford). 2017;2017
63. Jiang Q, Ma R, Wang J, Wu X, Jin S, Peng J, Tan R, Zhang T, Li Y, Wang Y. LncRNA2Function: a comprehensive resource for functional investigation of human lncRNAs based on RNA-seq data. BMC Genomics. 2015;16(Suppl 3):S2.
64. Bao Z, Yang Z, Huang Z, Zhou Y, Cui Q, Dong D. LncRNADisease 2.0: an updated database of long non-coding RNA-associated diseases. Nucleic Acids Res. 2019;47(D1):D1034–7.
65. Sun R, Zhang L. Long non-coding RNA MALAT1 regulates cardiomyocytes apoptosis after hypoxia/reperfusion injury via modulating miR-200a-3p/PDCD4 axis. Biomed Pharmacother. 2019;111:1036–45.
66. Zhang J, Liang Y, Huang X, Guo X, Liu Y, Zhong J, Yuan J. STAT3-induced upregulation of lncRNA MEG3 regulates the growth of cardiac hypertrophy through miR-361-5p/HDAC9 axis. Sci Rep. 2019;9(1):460.
67. Liu K, Yan Z, Li Y, Sun Z. Linc2GO: a human LincRNA function annotation resource based on ceRNA hypothesis. Bioinformatics. 2013;29(17):2221–2.
68. Paraskevopoulou MD, Vlachos IS, Karagkouni D, Georgakilas G, Kanellos I, Vergoulis T, Zagganas K, Tsanakas P, Floros E, Dalamagas T, Hatzigeorgiou AG. DIANA-LncBase v2: indexing microRNA targets on non-coding transcripts. Nucleic Acids Res. 2016;44(D1):D231–8.
69. Glazar P, Papavasileiou P, Rajewsky N. circBase: a database for circular RNAs. RNA. 2014;20(11):1666–70.
70. Kozomara A, Birgaoanu M, Griffiths-Jones S. miRBase: from microRNA sequences to function. Nucleic Acids Res. 2019;47(D1):D155–62.

71. Chen LL, Yang L. Regulation of circRNA biogenesis. RNA Biol. 2015;12(4):381–8.
72. Huang C, Shan G. What happens at or after transcription: insights into circRNA biogenesis and function. Transcription. 2015;6(4):61–4.
73. Wang K, Gan TY, Li N, Liu CY, Zhou LY, Gao JN, Chen C, Yan KW, Ponnusamy M, Zhang YH, Li PF. Circular RNA mediates cardiomyocyte death via miRNA-dependent upregulation of MTP18 expression. Cell Death Differ. 2017;24(6):1111–20.
74. Wang K, Long B, Liu F, Wang JX, Liu CY, Zhao B, Zhou LY, Sun T, Wang M, Yu T, Gong Y, Liu J, Dong YH, Li N, Li PF. A circular RNA protects the heart from pathological hypertrophy and heart failure by targeting miR-223. Eur Heart J. 2016;37(33):2602–11.
75. Costa MC, Cortez-Dias N, Gabriel A, de Sousa J, Fiuza M, Gallego J, Nobre A, Pinto FJ, Enguita FJ. circRNA-miRNA cross-talk in the transition from paroxysmal to permanent atrial fibrillation. Int J Cardiol. 2019;290:134–7.
76. Li JH, Liu S, Zhou H, Qu LH, Yang JH. starBase v2.0: decoding miRNA-ceRNA, miRNA-ncRNA and protein-RNA interaction networks from large-scale CLIP-Seq data. Nucleic Acids Res. 2014;42(Database issue):D92–7.
77. Panda AC, Dudekula DB, Abdelmohsen K, Gorospe M. Analysis of circular RNAs using the web tool circinteractome. Methods Mol Biol. 2018;1724:43–56.
78. Dudekula DB, Panda AC, Grammatikakis I, De S, Abdelmohsen K, Gorospe M. CircInteractome: a web tool for exploring circular RNAs and their interacting proteins and microRNAs. RNA Biol. 2016;13(1):34–42.
79. Zhong S, Wang J, Zhang Q, Xu H, Feng J. CircPrimer: a software for annotating circRNAs and determining the specificity of circRNA primers. BMC Bioinformatics. 2018;19(1):292.
80. Jiang XY, Ning QL. Expression profiling of long noncoding RNAs and the dynamic changes of lncRNA-NR024118 and Cdkn1c in angiotensin II-treated cardiac fibroblasts. Int J Clin Exp Pathol. 2014;7(4):1325–36.
81. Pawlak M, Niescierowicz K, Winata CL. Decoding the heart through next generation sequencing approaches. Genes (Basel). 2018;9(6):289.
82. Yang KC, Yamada KA, Patel AY, Topkara VK, George I, Cheema FH, Ewald GA, Mann DL, Nerbonne JM. Deep RNA sequencing reveals dynamic regulation of myocardial noncoding RNAs in failing human heart and remodeling with mechanical circulatory support. Circulation. 2014;129(9):1009–21.
83. Morini E, Sangiuolo F, Caporossi D, Novelli G, Amati F. Application of next generation sequencing for personalized medicine for sudden cardiac death. Front Genet. 2015;6:55.
84. Dweep H, Gretz N, Sticht C. miRWalk database for miRNA-target interactions. Methods Mol Biol. 2014;1182:289–305.
85. Lewis BP, Burge CB, Bartel DP. Conserved seed pairing, often flanked by adenosines, indicates that thousands of human genes are microRNA targets. Cell. 2005;120(1):15–20.
86. Paraskevopoulou MD, Georgakilas G, Kostoulas N, Vlachos IS, Vergoulis T, Reczko M, Filippidis C, Dalamagas T, Hatzigeorgiou AG. DIANA-microT web server v5.0: service integration into miRNA functional analysis workflows. 2013;41(Web Server issue):W169–73.
87. Xiao F, Zuo Z, Cai G, Kang S, Gao X, Li T. miRecords: an integrated resource for microRNA-target interactions. Nucleic Acids Res. 2009;37(Database):D105–10.
88. Dweep H, Gretz N. miRWalk2.0: a comprehensive atlas of microRNA-target interactions. Nat Methods. 2015;12(8):697.
89. Lu TP, Lee CY, Tsai MH, Chiu YC, Hsiao CK, Lai LC, Chuang EY. miRSystem: an integrated system for characterizing enriched functions and pathways of microRNA targets. PLoS One. 2012;7(8):e42390.
90. Shirdel EA, Xie W, Mak TW, Jurisica I. NAViGaTing the micronome – using multiple microRNA prediction databases to identify signalling pathway-associated microRNAs. PLoS One. 2011;6(2):e17429.
91. Ruepp A, Kowarsch A, Theis F. PhenomiR: microRNAs in human diseases and biological processes. Methods Mol Biol. 2012;822:249–60.
92. Li Y, Qiu C, Tu J, Geng B, Yang J, Jiang T, Cui Q. HMDD v2.0: a database for experimentally supported human microRNA and disease associations. Nucleic Acids Res. 2014;42(Database issue):D1070–4.
93. Huang Z, Shi J, Gao Y, Cui C, Zhang S, Li J, Zhou Y, Cui Q. HMDD v3.0: a database for experimentally supported human microRNA-disease associations. Nucleic Acids Res. 2019;47(D1):D1013–7.
94. Xie B, Ding Q, Han H, Wu D. miRCancer: a microRNA-cancer association database constructed by text mining on literature. Bioinformatics. 2013;29(5):638–44.
95. Goswami CP, Nakshatri H. PROGmiR: a tool for identifying prognostic miRNA biomarkers in multiple cancers using publicly available data. J Clin Bioinforma. 2012;2(1):23.
96. Volders PJ, Anckaert J, Verheggen K, Nuytens J, Martens L, Mestdagh P, Vandesompele J. LNCipedia 5: towards a reference set of human long non-coding RNAs. Nucleic Acids Res. 2019;47(D1):D135–9.
97. Zhou Z, Shen Y, Khan MR, Li A. LncReg: a reference resource for lncRNA-associated regulatory networks. Database (Oxford). 2015;2015
98. Park C, Yu N, Choi I, Kim W, Lee S. lncRNAtor: a comprehensive resource for functional investigation of long non-coding RNAs. Bioinformatics. 2014;30(17):2480–5.

Online Databases and Non-coding RNAs in Cardiovascular Diseases

3

Rui Chen, Chao Shi, Jianhua Yao, and Wei Chen

Abstract

Cardiovascular disease is characterized by its highest morbidity and mortality. One of the main pathological basis of this disease is the dysregulation of gene expression. Non-coding RNA (ncRNA) is a kind of functional RNA, which is transcript from DNA but not translated into proteins. More and more studies have established the important roles of ncRNAs, including transcription, RNA maturation, translation, protein degradation, and their involvement in the pathogenesis of diseases such as cancer and cardiovascular diseases. This chapter will focus on the biological functions of ncRNAs and their advances in cardiovascular disease. With the development of sequencing and computer technology, more and more databases can be easily obtained on the internet. In another part of this chapter, we will summarize some commonly used non-coding RNA databases, which can be easily and quickly used for relevant research.

Keywords

Cardiovascular disease · Non-coding RNA · Online database

1 Introduction

Cardiovascular disease was one of the diseases with the highest morbidity and mortality in the world. However, the basic research on cardiovascular disease was still limited [1, 2]. In-depth basic research could provide a guiding direction for new methods in treating cardiovascular diseases [3]. Therefore, exploring the molecular and cellular mechanisms in the pathogenesis of cardiovascular disease could help us understand the disease process, discover new biomarkers, and find new therapeutic targets [4, 5]. Over the past decade, the development of high-throughput sequencing technologies given us an opportunity to expand our understanding of human transcriptomes [6, 7]. Previous studies have suggested that proteins are the main regulators of cardiovascular

R. Chen
Shanghai Applied Radiation Institute, School of Environmental and Chemical Engineering, Shanghai University, Shanghai, China

C. Shi
Cardiac Regeneration and Ageing Lab, Institute of Cardiovascular Sciences, School of Life Science, Shanghai University, Shanghai, China

J. Yao (✉)
Department of Cardiology, Shanghai Tenth People's Hospital, Tongji University School of Medicine, Shanghai, China
e-mail: yaojianhua@tongji.edu.cn

W. Chen (✉)
Emergency Department, Shanghai Tongji Hospital, Tongji University School of Medicine, Shanghai, China

J. Xiao (ed.), *Non-coding RNAs in Cardiovascular Diseases*, Advances in Experimental Medicine and Biology 1229, https://doi.org/10.1007/978-981-15-1671-9_3

disease [8, 9]. However, with the understanding of the complexity human transcriptomes, it was revealed that most human genomes can transcribe RNA, of which more than 98% were untranslated proteins [10]. The number of non-coding RNAs was far exceeds the amount of mRNA encoding proteins [11, 12].

Although the expression level of ncRNAs were generally low and did not encode proteins, they could show strong tissue specificity and express abnormalities in various human diseases and biological processes such as organ development, internal and external environmental stimulation and disease occurrence [13, 14, 15]. So far, more and more studies have shown the important regulatory functions of ncRNAs in participate in biosynthetic steps such as transcription [16], RNA maturation [17], translation [18], protein degradation [19], and found ncRNAs play an important role in pathological processes such as tumors and cardiovascular diseases [20]. Based on their size, these non-coding RNAs were classified into microRNAs (miRNAs, <200 nucleotides), and long non-coding RNAs (lncRNAs, >200 nucleotides), in which lncRNAs can also exhibit a circular shape called circular RNAs (circRNAs). In this section, we will illuminate the important role of non-coding RNAs in the development of cardiovascular diseases through their special biological function. The main classification of non-coding RNA and its formation in the cell is shown in Fig. 3.1.

2 miRNAs in Cardiovascular Diseases

A miRNA was an endogenous non-coding RNA, typically 18–25 nucleotides, which regulated the expression of a target gene by binding to the 3′UTR of the mRNA and inhibiting its translation. The precursor of the miRNA first existed in the nucleus. Then after the transcription and subsequently matured by several enzymatic reactions, mRNAs transferred to the cytoplasm to exert their biological functions. miRNAs exerted their regulatory functions by recruiting specific silencing proteins to form an RNA-induced silencing complex (RISC). It was speculated that about 60% of mRNA will be target by miRNA, while a miRNA may target more than 100 mRNAs in human. Specific miRNAs have significantly different expression levels in cardiac tissue and cardiovascular, and played as regulators of cardiovascular function, including cardiovascular cell differentiation, growth, proliferation and apoptosis, angiogenesis and cell contractility regulation. Meanwhile, the pathological changes in the cardiovascular system always accompanied with some specific miRNAs changes. These miRNAs changes have been confirmed to be associated with cardiovascular diseases such as arrhythmia, cardiac hypertrophy, fibrosis, myocardial infarction and heart failure. Recent studies indicated that miRNAs with specific changes in the progression of heart valve disease play key role in the processes of disease progression, such as fibrosis, calcification, matrix degradation remodeling, and inflammation. In addition, some miRNAs could also regulate extracellular body through exosomes and participate in circulation in the exocrine [21–23]. Further studies revealed that these miRNAs can be used as biomarkers for cardiovascular diseases for clinical diagnosis and personalized medicine.

3 lncRNAs in Cardiovascular Diseases

lncRNAs were the heterogeneous RNA transcripts, which contain more than200 nucleotides in length. lncRNAs could be classified into sense, antisense, intron, genomic and divergent lncRNAs based on their relative genomic location. lncRNAs were involved in many biological processes, such as chromatin structural changes, transcription, post-transcriptional processing, intracellular trafficking, and regulation of enzyme activity.

lncRNA could also regulate other endogenous ncRNAs, particularly miRNAs, through competitive binding. Compared to miRNAs, lncRNAs were less conserved, suggesting that these RNA

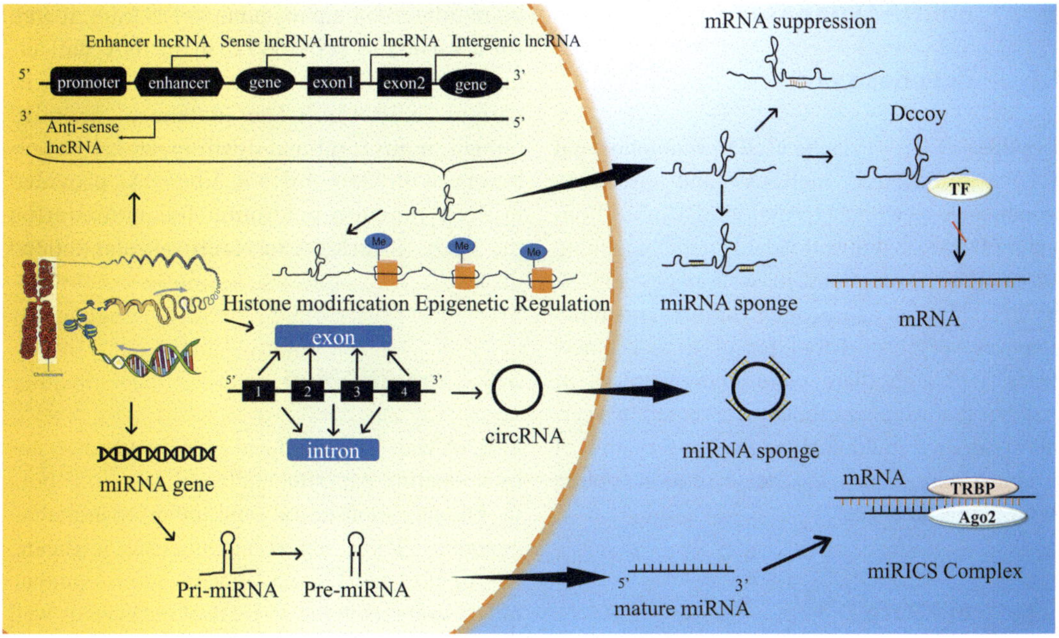

Fig. 3.1 The main classification of non-coding RNA and its formation in the cell

molecules have a species-specific effect. Although the dysregulation of lncRNAs was associated with various human diseases, their mechanism of action still remained unclear. To date, it has been reported that lncRNAs dysregulation was detected in many cardiovascular diseases such as myocardial infarction, myocardial fibrosis, cardiac hypertrophy and heart failure.

4 circRNAs in Cardiovascular Diseases

Circular RNAs (circRNAs) transcripts were first identified in the early 1990s, but knowledge of these species has remained limited, due to their difficult study through traditional methods of RNA analysis. circRNAs were a peculiar group of RNAs, consisting of at least a few hundred nucleotides and relatively stable in their circular state. circRNAs were involved in a wide range of biological processes, that expression disorder of circRNAs might lead to abnormal cellular functions and disease. However, the regulation of circRNAs in cardiovascular diseases remains largely unexplored. As the develop of RNA-Seq studies, large number of different circRNAs were detected to be expressed in cardiac tissues from human and rodents.

As the roles of non-coding RNAs in cardiovascular diseases were gradually unearthed, a large amount of data was reported every year, including non-coding RNA sites, regulatory mechanisms, etc. Document summarization and data induction became a daunting task when summarizing the rules and guiding the direction of the next step. With the development of electronic computer hardware and software such as artificial intelligence and cloud computing, many non-coding RNAs databases have been established. These databases summarized the existing research data of miRNAs and lncRNAs with the combination of bioinformatics analysis. These gave us a way to generalize the functions reported by miRNAs and lncRNAs and predict other possible sites of their effects. The rational use of these databases could significantly improve the efficiency of our researchers. Below we will introduce some of the more mature online databases.

5 miRNA Database

5.1 deepBase v1.0

deepBase v1.0 [24] can be used to annotation and discovery miRNAs, lncRNAs and circRNAs sequencing, view the expression of various non-coding RNAs, and downloadable data. Searching for miRNA expressions in web pages can be retrieved by gene names and symbols. This function was very useful tool for us to select new genes. Although there were many choices of lncRNA that were specifically expressed in a certain tissue, we could analyze the conservation of a non-coding RNA in the evolution option through this database.

5.2 miRBase

miRBase [25] was an online miRNA database, which was developed by researchers at the University of Chester. The database contained more than 200 species and close to 40,000 miRNAs. It was the most comprehensive miRNA database in which we can do species specific particular miRNA search and browses, such as the numbering of the precursor miRNA, the relative expression, the starting position of the miRNA precursor on the chromosome, and gives confidence to judge. miRbase also assigned names to newly discovered miRNAs, which provided a convenient and fast communication platform for researchers.

5.3 microRNA.org

microRNA.org [26] was a comprehensive database of miRNA target prediction and expression. The target predictions provided by the website were implemented by the MiRanda algorithm, which combined current research reports on miRNAs and provided data from a large number of mammalian tissue synthesis sequencing projects. Through the latest algorithms, users could search for genes that may be regulated by a particular miRNA, or search for a variety of miRNAs that regulate the certain gene, as well as the expression profiles of various miRNAs. The database included human, mouse, rat and other species, by combining with 250 miRNA libraries, provided miRNA function prediction functions during the study of miRNA in cardiovascular-related diseases.

5.4 miRNAMap

miRNAMap [27] validated miRNA target genes by collecting experimentally validated miRNAs in human, mouse, rat and other mammalian genomes. Three algorithms include miRanda, RNAhybrid and TargetScan were used to validate miRNA targets in the 3′-UTR of the gene as well as known miRNA targets. By using filtration of multiple algorithms to speculate the target site of the miRNA in order to reduce the probability of predicting false positives in the miRNA target site prediction.

5.5 Cupid

Cupid [28] was an online database that validated the high-throughput validation analysis in breast cancer cell lines by simultaneously predicting miRNA-target interactions and their mediated endogenous RNA interactions. The database publisher verified the accuracy of the interaction of 500 miRNAs with the target to make sure the accuracy of this database.

5.6 TargetScan

TargetScan [29] was a website for predicting miRNA target genes, which contained human, orangutan, macaque, mouse, rat and other species. The website could display the prediction after inputting the gene name or the ENST label. This website also predicted target genes' possible role through miRNAs.

5.7 miRTarBase

miRTarBase [30] was a manually collected, experimentally validated miRNA target gene database, which provided a variety way to search, such as miRNA ID, target genes, KEGG pathways, validated methods, or diseases. The database was incubated with a unique miRNA-target interactions (MTS) number for each miRNA target gene. miRTarBase not only provided highly reliable miRNA target gene information, but also provided information on miRNA and diseases that were reported in the literature.

5.8 Diana-microT-CDS

Diana-microT-CDS [31] was an online database, which provided computer simulations of miRNA-mRNA interactions with a good user interface. This database provided sufficient information on predicting miRNA target genes, such as global scores of interactions and visualized results. microT-CDS was the only miRNA target prediction algorithm available online that was specifically designed to identify miRNA targets in the 3′UTR and CDS regions. The database contained miRNA target information in the mRNA sequences of human, mus musculus, drosophila melanogaster and C. elegans, which contained a wealth of tooltips and convenient menu options that were easy to use. In addition, the new system that combined advanced workflows also supported massive data analysis from Next Generation Sequencing (NGS).

5.9 miRecords

miRecords [32] was an online database that provided animal miRNA-target gene prediction. The database consisted of two parts, one was a proven large, high-quality database, which also includeed artificially screened miRNA targets. The other one was an online target gene prediction algorithm, which the algorithm provided by the database emphasized experimental data support of miRNA targets.

5.10 PicTar

PicTar [33] database used a certain algorithm to identify the target of a microRNA. The searchable website provided detailed predictions of microRNA targets from the following species, including: vertebrate, seven drosophila species, three nematode species, and human non-conserved but co-expressed microRNA targets (e.g.: Express microRNA and mRNA in the same tissue).

5.11 TarBase

TarBase [34] was a database of miRNA target genes prediction website that was supported by experimental data. After 10 years of data compilation, the database provided information on miRNA target genes in various species such as humans and mice. For each target gene data, such as the relevant literature, organization type, and test method were given. In TarBase, each experimental evidence was divided into two categories, low and high. Low represented the traditional experimental method. Compared with the high-throughput sequencing analysis, the reliability of the result was higher. We can filter the miRNA target supported through the low method in order to obtain a high-quality miRNA target gene data set.

5.12 miRWalk

miRWalk [35] was a comprehensive miRNA target gene database containing miRNA target gene information from human, mouse and other species. It was an integrated database that integrated information from miRDB, TargetScan, miRTarBase and other databases. The regulation network between the miRNAs and the target genes visualized the function of graph and gene set enrichment, supported the enrichment analysis and the analysis of reactive pathway, KEGG pathway, and gene ontology. The miRNA databases URLs and related information listed above are shown in Table 3.1.

Table 3.1 microRNA databases

Name	Weblink	Data content
deepBase	http://biocenter.sysu.edu.cn/deepBase/	A platform containing evolution and expression patterns of diverse ncRNAs across 19 species from 5 clades.
miRBase	http://www.mirbase.org/	A searchable database of published miRNA sequences and annotation.
microRNA	http://www.microrna.org/	Predict microRNA targets & target downregulation scores. Experimentally observed expression patterns.
miRNAMap	http://mirnamap.mbc.nctu.edu.tw/	Collect experimental verified microRNAs and their target genes in human, mouse, rat, and other metazoan genomes.
Cupid	http://cupidtool.sourceforge.net/	A method for simultaneous prediction of miRNA-target interactions and their mediated competitive endogenous RNA interactions.
TargetScan	http://www.targetscan.org/vert_72/	Predict biological targets of miRNAs by searching for the presence of conserved 8mer, 7mer, and 6mer sites that match the seed region of each miRNA.
miRTarBase	http://mirtarbase.mbc.nctu.edu.tw/php/index.php	Accumulated more than 360,000 miRNA-target interactions (MTIs).
Diana-microT-CDS	http://diana.imis.athena-innovation.gr/	Specifically trained on a positive and a negative set of miRNA Recognition Elements (MREs) located in both the 3′-UTR and CDS regions.
miRecords	http://c1.accurascience.com/miRecords/	Hosts 2705 records of interactions between 644 miRNAs and 1901 target genes in 9 animal species.
PicTar	https://pictar.mdc-berlin.de/	An algorithm for the identification of microRNA targets.
TarBase	http://carolina.imis.athena-innovation.gr	Containing more than 1,000,000 miRNA-gene interactions.
miRWalk	http://mirwalk.umm.uni-heidelberg.de/	Stores predicted data obtained with a machine learning algorithm including experimentally verified miRNA-target interactions.

6 lncRNA Databases

6.1 LNCipedia

LNCipedia [36–38] was a comprehensive human lncRNA database that integrated lncRNA records from multiple databases and articles and gave them a uniform ID or named new reported lncRNA. The database summarizes lncRNAdb, Broad Institute, Ensembl, Gencode, Refseq, NONCODE, FANTOM and other lncRNA databases.

6.2 lncRNAdb

lncRNAdb [39, 40] was available at the website http://www.lncrnadb.org/. In order to make it easy for the users to compile and update the information of lncRNAs, researchers established this database containing comprehensive lncRNAs and their biological functions. lncRNAdb provided users with plenty information of lncRNAs, including lncRNA sequences, struction, genomic context and so on. Users could search for the published lncRNA names and sequences species, associated protein-coding genes. Also, this database was linked to the UCSC Genome Browser and Noncoding RNA Expression Database, making various sources of lncRNAs. With 4 years development, there existed version 2.0 lncRNAdb. This new version contained 287 eukaryotic lncRNAs, and a more accessible interface for users to search the sequence information and expression data. There were some new features of the version 2.0, including the nucleotide sequence information and an easier way for users to export the information they searched. With deeper study of lncRNAs, there will be more lncRNAs adding to this database and make it better for the future research.

6.3 LncRNAWiki

LncRNAWiki [41] database integrateed the sequences and annotation information of human lncRNAs in GENCODE, NONCODE, and LNCipedia databases. It now has 105,255 non-redundant lncRNAs, of which 103 have full annotation and biological function tests. The database was also an editable public platform that not only allowed users to annotate, update, and organize existing lncRNAs, but also open a permission for all user to share their new detected lncRNAs. This database was an open platform for human lncRNA information.

6.4 MONOCLdb

MONOCLdb [42] fully called the Mouse Non-Code Lung interactive database, which was available at https://www.monocldb.org/. The lncRNAs from this database were based on the mice infected by influenza and SARS-CoV viruses.5329 of 20,728 mouse lncRNAs genes showed differently expressed after infected by these two viruses. In this database, developers annotated the difference of the expression by two computational methods, module-based and rank-based, so that users can retrieve the annotations, expression profiles and the functional enrichment of lncRNAs. Also, via MONOCLdb, users could generate the expression heatmaps and the functional enrichment results on-the-fly. This database provided users with association scores between lncRNAs and pathogenicity variables MONOCLdb was an integrative and interactive database containing abundant lncRNAs in order to make convenience for the researchers to learn more about their role during the viruses infection.

6.5 NONCODE

NONCODE [43, 44], located at the web server http://www.bioinfo.org/noncode/, was a database which showed complete collection of the lncRNAs. Based on the third-generation sequencing method, developers could get plenty correct annotations and establish this database. NONCODE contained 527,336 lncRNAs from 16 different species, including 167,150 human lncRNAs and 130,558 mouse lncRNAs. Compared with other database, NONCODE really had a large number of lncRNAs. Except the large number, NONCODE contained three unique features, including a conservation annotation of the lncRNAs, a relationship annotation between lncRNAs and diseases, and a platform for users to choose the high-quality datasets. This database decided to show the relationship between the lncRNAs and diseases to make a systematic network about the noncoding regions and the diseases. Also, it made more convenient for the disease study users to get their interested information. Although there still existed some uncleared things in the development of this database, the developers will attempt to solve the problem and make NONCODE a better database for the users.

6.6 lncRNome

lncRNome [45] was a comprehensive database that integrated lots of significant annotations for lncRNAs, and now became one of the largest database of lncRNAs in the world. It was available at the website http://genome.igib.res.in/lncRNome/. In lncRNome, each lncRNA has its own page including the information about the annotation sets. Through the links on this page, users could easily get other information of this lncRNA including the sequence, structure, interactions, variations and so on. There existed 937 quadruplex and 40 hairpins motifs, 3716 miRNA binding sites and more than 10,000 binding sites for proteins on the lncRNA in lncRNome. Also, lncRNome provided 345,351 genomic variations associated with lncRNAs and 11,790 epigenetic marks in the promoters of lncRNAs. Furthermore, this database has multiple options for users to search for the lncRNAs, such as thename or known targets. In addition, the representative of the available associated genomic annotations was also one of the features of this database.

6.7 C-It-Loci

C-It-Loci [46] was an database that allowed users to browse the transcripts specific in tissue from human, mouse and zebrafish. It was an available and free web server, which was established in 2015. User can used through the website http://c-it-loci.uni-frankfurt.de/. C-It-Loci made it easier for users to identify ncRNAs and protein-coding genes from various tissues. Not only normal lncRNAs, but also the housekeeping genes and its housekeep lncRNAs were contained in this database. To make convenience for the users with limited knowledge, C-It-Loci allowed users to see the different types of transcripts C-It-Loci had a quick search function on the page, which made it easy for users to compare the difference of two transcripts. C-It-Loci also offered a diagram for the users to analyze the conserved regions and explore the detailed information of the lncRNA they searched. Compared with other databases, C-It-Loci had the latest human genomic assembly, and defined lncRNAs with three organisms. Furthermore, C-It-Loci was the only database that has both protein-coding genes and lncRNAs transcripts. There would be a great prospect to study on lncRNAs through this database.

6.8 MiTranscriptome

MiTranscriptome [47] was a database about genome-wide lncRNA expression, constructed by Matthew K Iyer and his colleagues in 2015. The web server of this database is http://www.mitranscriptome.org/. In order to build this database, they curated 7256 RNA-seq from tumors, normal tissues and cell lines, which was comprising from 25 independent studies. Finally, they got a transcriptome of 91,013 expressed gene, 68% was lncRNAs. Interestingly, 79% of them were unannotated in previous study. Then they used non-parametric differential expression test to filtrate and finally got 7942 lncRNAs that were associated with disease or cancer. These lncRNA could be valuable for the further study of cancer and the development of biomarker. Therefore, MiTranscriptome provided a foundation for lncRNA genomics, biomarker development and the delineation of cancer.

6.9 slncky Evolution Browser

slncky Evolution Browser [48] was developed in 2016. The website of this database was https://scripts.mit.edu/~jjenny/. slncky was a tool for searching conserved lncRNAs through a sensitive noncoding aligning method. This database could be efficiently used to produce high quality lncRNAs from RNA-sequencing data. It could separateed lncRNAs accurately from coding genes, pseudogenes, assembly artifacts, and also identify novel proteins including small peptides. On the basis of this tool, they develop the database called slncky Evolution Browser. Through this database, they list 233 constrained lncRNAs out of the currently annotated transcripts. With the powerful tool like slncky, this database would contain more valuable lncRNAs which will do a lot to the research of cancer and relative diseases. The lncRNA databases URLs and related information listed above are shown in Table 3.2.

7 circRNA Databases

7.1 starBase

starBase [49, 50] (http://starbase.sysu.edu.cn/) was established for the researchers to identify the interaction networks of RNAs systematically. The data of the circRNAs in starBase came from 108 CLIP-Seq datasets in 37 studies. Totally 9000 miRNA-circRNAs, 16,000 miRNAs pseudogene and 285,000 protein-RNA relationships wereidentified in this database. With the updated version, starBase V2.0 began to provide users with miRNA-mRNA and miRNA-lncRNA interaction networks. In this new version, developers also identified 10,000 ceRNA pairs and developed miRNA and ceRNA Functions, which made it easier for users to predict the function of the RNAs, which drafted the first interaction maps between miRNAs and circRNAs. Through this

Table 3.2 Long non-coding RNA databases

Name	Weblink	Data content
LNCipedia	https://lncipedia.org/	A public database for long non-coding RNA (lncRNA) sequence and annotation, contains 127,802 transcripts and 56,946 genes.
lncRNAdb	http://lncrnadb.com/	Database that provides comprehensive annotations of eukaryotic long non-coding RNAs.
LncRNAWiki	http://lncrna.big.ac.cn/index.php	Contains 106,063 human long non-coding RNAs.
MONOCLdb	https://www.monocldb.org/	20,728 mouse lncRNA genes.
NONCODE	http://www.noncode.org/	An integrated knowledge database of non-coding RNAs from 17 species.
lncRNome	http://genome.igib.res.in/lncRNome/	Over 17,000 long non-coding RNAs in human.
C-It-Loci	http://c-it-loci.uni-frankfurt.de/	Including the expression profiles of yet-to-be-characterized long non-coding RNAs (lncRNAs).
MiTranscriptome	http://mitranscriptome.org/	Contains over 91,000 genes.
slncky Evolution Browser	https://scripts.mit.edu/~jjenny/	Contains alignments and evolutionary metrics of conserved lncRNAs.

database, users could get more information about the interaction between miRNAs and circRNAs. With the development of technology, the starBase continued to update their data service for searching. Furthermore, this database will to add RNA data about cancer to improve the understanding the network of circRNAs and miRNAs.

7.2 circBase

circBase [51], a database that you can browse and download the datasets of circRNAs and their expression supporting evidence, also it provided users with the sequencing data of uncovered and novel circRNAs. The available website for this database was http://www.circbase.org/. Before construct this database, developers put forward some expectation on this database, for example, it should provide the genomic context and the available expression of the circRNAs,should summarize the existence and expression for each circRNA. To achieve this goal, they putted together all the datasets from other different laboratories. For the current version of circBase, it contained the simple search interface, various methods of data retrieval and unifying, merging and annotating published datasets. There were three main ways to search for the circRNAs in circBase, including the simple search, list search and table browser. Through these three methods, users could extend their information of circRNAs from this database. However, circBase doesn't support users to submit the new circRNA data by themselves right now. With the update of circBase, it will be more useful to the researchers in the study of circRNAs.

7.3 CircNet

CircNet [52] was constructed by 464 RNA-seq samples using transcriptome sequencing, which could be available on http://circnet.mbc.nctu.edu.tw/. This database was established by the purpose of extending the catalog of reported circRNAs. CircNet provided lots of information of the circRNAs, including novel circRNAs, integrated miRNA targets, expression profiles of circRNAs etc. When clicked on any of the circRNAs, it will display the complete information of the entire circRNA, including its position on the chromosome, length and sequence information. CireNet was the first database that provided circRNA expression profiles specific in tissue and circRNA-miRNA-gene regulatory networks. CircNet not only contained the latest circRNAs, but also provided a comprehensive analysis between the reported circRNAs and the novel RNAs. Meanwhile, it made a regulatory network that illustrates the regulation between circRNAs, miRNAs and genes. All in all, this database was a convenient tool for the users to get the information they need easily.

7.4 Circ2Traits

Circ2Traits [53] was a database of circRNAs, which was available on http://gyanxet-beta.com/circdb/. This database was the first comprehensive database containing with the circRNAs of diseased human, which classified the circRNAs by their potential association with diseases. By analyzing the interaction of circRNAs with diseases associated miRNAs they established the association between circRNAs and the diseases. Till now the Circ2Traits contains 1951 human circRNAs with the association of 105 human diseases. What's more, this database contained the complete miRNA-circRNA-mRNA-lncRNA interaction network, in order to help users see the interaction table of each disease clearly. Meanwhile, the ceRNA regulatory network of circRNA was also constructed in this database to further analyze circRNA regulatory pathways. According to the searched circRNA, you could not only get the normal information of that circRNA, but also know its interaction sites SNPs.

7.5 CircBank

CircBank [51] database contained more than 140,000 annotated human circRNAs from many different source, which was a comprehensive database of human circRNA. The available website for this database iwas http://www.circbank.cn/. This database was publicly available with a lot of service, including circRNA modification, circRNA conservation etc. Despite the simple information, there were many new features in this database, including the predicted binding miRNA, circRNA mutation and circRNA methylation. Furthermore, CircBank also put forward a new nomenclature system based on the host gene name, start position and end position, so that researchers will not be bothered with the ID of circRNA right now. With CircBank, it could be easier for researchers to get enough information of circRNAs they need.

7.6 exoRBase

exoRBase [54], containing circRNA, lncRNA and mRNA, which were derived from RNA-seq data analyses of human blood exosomes. It was established by Prof. Li from Fudan University, who aimed to collect and demonstrate all long RNA species in human blood exosomes. Researchers can visit this database through the website http://www.exoRBase.org/. The first version of this database contained 58,330 circRNAs, 15,501 lncRNAs and 18,333 mRNAs, based on the RNA-seq data from normal samples and disease patients. This database also provided researchers with the annotation, expression level and possible original tissues of the circRNAs. What's more, there were 77 experimental validations from the published articles included in exoRBase. Through the website, users could conveniently browse and download the information of the circRNAs. Different from other database, exoRBase allowed researchers to submit new profiles of the RNAs in human blood exosomes, which will help researchers identify new exosome biomarkers and find their influence on human diseases.

7.7 circRNADb

circRNADb [55] was a diversified-source circRNA database, which built for further study of the circRNAs and its related functions. It contained 32,194 human exonic circRNAs. It was free for the researchers to search the circRNAs they need by the web server at http://reprod.njmu.edu.cn/circrnadb. They could get various kinds of detailed information of the circRNAs, including genomic information, exon splicing, genome sequence, internal ribosome entry site and open reading frame. The raw circRNAs dataset were collected from related literatures, and only included the circRNA which was supported more than twice. Now there were 16,328 annotated circRNAs with a longer than 100 amino acids open reading frame, and 7170 of them had internal ribosome entry site elements. CircRNADb was designed to be a comprehensive and interactive database, providing advanced search, resource download and many other functions for the users. It could do a lot to the circRNA studies by providing users with the detailed genomic and protein-coding information of each circRNA. Furthermore, developers will update the newly identified circRNAs with their detailed information to the database, in order to build circRNADb a powerful information platform for circRNAs.

7.8 CSCD

CSCD [56] (Cancer-specific circRNA database) was a cancer circRNAs specific database, which was developed by the researchers from Wuhan University. It provided genomic coordinates and gene annotation for each file of cancer-specific circRNA. The available website for this database was http://gb.whu.edu.cn/CSCD/. This database now contained total 272,152 circRNAs, which were identified from both cancer and normal cell lines. There are 950,962 circRNAs recognized from normal samples and 179,909 from both normal and tumor samples. What's more, they identified many circRNAs only in CSCD, which contained many different samples including cancer samples. This database also contained the prediction of the microRNA response element sites and RNA binding protein sites for each circRNA, which could be better used for the researchers to understand the functional effects of circRNAs. The developers also predicted each splicing event in linear transcripts of the circRNAs in order to comprehend the association between the linear splicing and the back-splicing. As the first comprehensive cancer-specific circRNA database, CSCD provided potential open reading frames in cancer-specific circRNAs, which could significantly contribute to the circRNAs research in cancer.

7.9 circAtlas

circAtlas [57] was a database newly established by Ji et al. in 2019, which was the most abundant and comprehensive circRNAs database from normal samples. They provided many aspects of circRNAs on their circRNA Atlas web server, including their expression patterns, genomic features, conservations and functional annotations. This database was available at http://circatlas.biols.ac.cn/. Researchers could browse, visualize and prioritize the circRNAs they need and get the related information from this database. This database enlarged our knowledge of circRNAs by exploring the landscape of circRNAs in human, macaque and mouse, elucidating their diversities in various tissues. The developers also invented a new method to prioritize disease related circRNAs, which ranked the circRNAs by considering both circAtlas networks and circRNA conservation. As a starting point to investigate the biological importance of circRNAs, cireAtlas will provide a powerful foundation for circRNA studies, and help the circRNA community to annotate and prioritize circRNAs. The circRNA database URLs and related information listed above are shown in Table 3.3.

8 Conclusion

This chapter reviewed the role of ncRNAs in cardiac pathology, which abnormally elevated or decreased expression could lead cardiovascular disease. Although there are a lot of reports on these ncRNAs, but how to quickly find the information you need from tons data was an important issue that needs to be addressed. Therefore, we summarized some online databases that were currently available. These databases have powerful functions, such as predicting ncRNA targets, viewing ncRNA basic information, etc.. In addition, the biological function of the currently

Table 3.3 circRNA databases

Name	Weblink	Data content
starBase	http://starbase.sysu.edu.cn/starbase2/mirCircRNA.php	View the predicted miRNA-circRNA interactions by scanning circRNA sequences overlapping with CLIP-Seq peaks for potential microRNA targets and then output the detailed information.
circBase	http://circrna.org/	Contains thousands of recently showed circular RNAs (circRNAs) that expressed in eukaryotic cells.
CircNet	http://syslab5.nchu.edu.tw/CircNet/	Provides tissue-specific circRNA expression profiles and circRNA-miRNA-gene regulatory networks.
Circ2Traits	http://gyanxet-beta.com/circdb/	A comprehensive knowledge base on potential association of circular RNAs with diseases in human.
CircBank	http://www.circbank.cn/	A comprehensive database of human circRNAs which included more than 140,000 annotated circRNAs from different source.
exoRBase	http://www.exorbase.org/	A repository of circular RNA, long non-coding RNA (lncRNA) and messenger RNA (mRNA) derived from human blood exosomes RNA-seq data analyses.
circRNADb	http://reprod.njmu.edu.cn/circrnadb/circRNADb.php	A comprehensive database of circular RNA molecules in humans, which contains 32,914 annotated exonic circRNAs,
CSCD	http://gb.whu.edu.cn/CSCD/#	A database developed for cancer-specific circRNAs, which contains 272,152 cancer-specific circRNAs.
circAtlas	http://circatlas.biols.ac.cn	circAtlas 2.0 integrates millions of circRNAs across 7 species (human, macaca, mouse, rat, pig, chicken, dog) and a variety of tissues.

known ncRNA was only the tip of the iceberg, and there were still many unknown functions needed to be perfected. Therefore, based on the summarized existing research data, new ncRNA targets can be discovered by design algorithm.

Acknowledgements This chapter was supported by the Fundamental Research Funds for the Central Universities (22120180384 to Jianhua Yao).

References

1. Sabatine MS, Giugliano RP, Keech AC, Honarpour N, Wiviott SD, Murphy SA, Kuder JF, Wang H, Liu T, Wasserman SM. Evolocumab and clinical outcomes in patients with cardiovascular disease. N Engl J Med. 2017;376(18):1713–22.
2. Fitzgibbons TP, Czech MP. Epicardial and perivascular adipose tissues and their influence on cardiovascular disease: basic mechanisms and clinical associations. J Am Heart Assoc. 2014;3(2):e000582.
3. Liu C-L, Guo J, Zhang X, Sukhova GK, Libby P, Shi G-P. Cysteine protease cathepsins in cardiovascular disease: from basic research to clinical trials. Nat Rev Cardiol. 2018;1
4. Shah MS, Brownlee M. Molecular and cellular mechanisms of cardiovascular disorders in diabetes. Circ Res. 2016;118(11):1808–29.
5. Olson EN. MicroRNAs as therapeutic targets and biomarkers of cardiovascular disease. Sci Transl Med. 2014;6(239):239ps233.
6. Reuter JA, Spacek DV, Snyder MP. High-throughput sequencing technologies. Mol Cell. 2015;58(4):586–97.
7. Kukurba KR, Montgomery SB. RNA sequencing and analysis. Cold Spring Harbor Protoc. 2015;2015(11):pdb.top084970.
8. Sharma S, Garg I, Ashraf MZ. TLR signalling and association of TLR polymorphism with cardiovascular diseases. Vasc Pharmacol. 2016;87:30–7.
9. Castro EA, Peinado AB, Benito PJ, Galindo M, Gonzalez-Gross M, Cupeiro R, Group PS. What is the most effective exercise protocol to improve cardiovascular fitness in overweight and obese subjects? J Sport Health Sci. 2017;6(4):454–61.
10. Mattick JS, Makunin IV. Non-coding RNA. Hum Mol Genet. 2006;15(suppl_1):R17–29.
11. Esteller M. Non-coding RNAs in human disease. Nat Rev Genet. 2011;12(12):861.
12. Palazzo AF, Lee ES. Non-coding RNA: what is functional and what is junk? Front Genet. 2015;6:2.
13. Matsui M, Corey DR. Non-coding RNAs as drug targets. Nat Rev Drug Discov. 2017;16(3):167.
14. Beermann J, Piccoli M-T, Viereck J, Thum T. Non-coding RNAs in development and disease: back-

ground, mechanisms, and therapeutic approaches. Physiol Rev. 2016;96(4):1297–325.
15. Li Y, Liang Y, Zhu Y, Zhang Y, Bei Y. Noncoding RNAs in cardiac hypertrophy. J Cardiovasc Transl Res. 2018;11(6):439–49.
16. Li W, Notani D, Rosenfeld MG. Enhancers as non-coding RNA transcription units: recent insights and future perspectives. Nat Rev Genet. 2016;17(4):207.
17. Holdt LM, Stahringer A, Sass K, Pichler G, Kulak NA, Wilfert W, Kohlmaier A, Herbst A, Northoff BH, Nicolaou A. Circular non-coding RNA ANRIL modulates ribosomal RNA maturation and atherosclerosis in humans. Nat Commun. 2016;7:12429.
18. Gong C, Li Z, Ramanujan K, Clay I, Zhang Y, Lemire-Brachat S, Glass DJ. A long non-coding RNA, LncMyoD, regulates skeletal muscle differentiation by blocking IMP2-mediated mRNA translation. Dev Cell. 2015;34(2):181–91.
19. Sengupta S. Noncoding RNAs in protein clearance pathways: implications in neurodegenerative diseases. J Genet. 2017;96(1):203–10.
20. Anastasiadou E, Jacob LS, Slack FJ. Non-coding RNA networks in cancer. Nat Rev Cancer. 2018;18(1):5.
21. Goldberg L, Tirosh-Wagner T, Vardi A, Abbas H, Pillar N, Shomron N, Nevo-Caspi Y, Paret G. Circulating microRNAs: a potential biomarker for cardiac damage, inflammatory response, and left ventricular function recovery in pediatric viral myocarditis. J Cardiovasc Transl Res. 2018;11(4):319–28.
22. Wang L, Lv Y, Li G, Xiao J. MicroRNAs in heart and circulation during physical exercise. J Sport Health Sci. 2018;7(4):433–41.
23. Batacan RB Jr, Duncan MJ, Dalbo VJ, Buitrago GL, Fenning AS. Effect of different intensities of physical activity on cardiometabolic markers and vascular and cardiac function in adult rats fed with a high-fat high-carbohydrate diet. J Sport Health Sci. 2018;7(1):109–19.
24. Yang J-H, Shao P, Zhou H, Chen Y-Q, Qu L-H. deepBase: a database for deeply annotating and mining deep sequencing data. Nucleic Acids Res. 2009;38(suppl_1):D123–30.
25. Kozomara A, Griffiths-Jones S. miRBase: annotating high confidence microRNAs using deep sequencing data. Nucleic Acids Res. 2013;42(D1):D68–73.
26. Betel D, Wilson M, Gabow A, Marks DS, Sander C. The microRNA. org resource: targets and expression. Nucleic Acids Res. 2008;36(suppl_1):D149–53.
27. Hsu S-D, Chu C-H, Tsou A-P, Chen S-J, Chen H-C, Hsu PW-C, Wong Y-H, Chen Y-H, Chen G-H, Huang H-D. miRNAMap 2.0: genomic maps of microRNAs in metazoan genomes. Nucl Acids Res. 2007;36(suppl_1):D165–9.
28. Chiu H-S, Llobet-Navas D, Yang X, Chung W-J, Ambesi-Impiombato A, Iyer A, Kim HR, Seviour EG, Luo Z, Sehgal V. Cupid: simultaneous reconstruction of microRNA-target and ceRNA networks. Genome Res. 2015;25(2):257–67.
29. Lewis BP, Burge CB, Bartel DP. Conserved seed pairing, often flanked by adenosines, indicates that thousands of human genes are microRNA targets. Cell. 2005;120(1):15–20.
30. Chou C-H, Shrestha S, Yang C-D, Chang N-W, Lin Y-L, Liao K-W, Huang W-C, Sun T-H, Tu S-J, Lee W-H. miRTarBase update 2018: a resource for experimentally validated microRNA-target interactions. Nucleic Acids Res. 2017;46(D1):D296–302.
31. Paraskevopoulou MD, Georgakilas G, Kostoulas N, Vlachos IS, Vergoulis T, Reczko M, Filippidis C, Dalamagas T, Hatzigeorgiou AG. DIANA-microT web server v5.0: service integration into miRNA functional analysis workflows. Nucleic Acids Res. 2013;41(Web Server issue):W169–73.
32. Xiao F, Zuo Z, Cai G, Kang S, Gao X, Li T. miRecords: an integrated resource for microRNA–target interactions. Nucl Acids Res. 2008;37(suppl_1):D105–10.
33. Krek A, Grün D, Poy MN, Wolf R, Rosenberg L, Epstein EJ, MacMenamin P, Da Piedade I, Gunsalus KC, Stoffel M. Combinatorial microRNA target predictions. Nat Genet. 2005;37(5):495.
34. Karagkouni D, Paraskevopoulou MD, Chatzopoulos S, Vlachos IS, Tastsoglou S, Kanellos I, Papadimitriou D, Kavakiotis I, Maniou S, Skoufos G. DIANA-TarBase v8: a decade-long collection of experimentally supported miRNA–gene interactions. Nucleic Acids Res. 2017;46(D1):D239–45.
35. Dweep H, Sticht C, Pandey P, Gretz N. miRWalk–database: prediction of possible miRNA binding sites by "walking" the genes of three genomes. J Biomed Inform. 2011;44(5):839–47.
36. Volders P-J, Helsens K, Wang X, Menten B, Martens L, Gevaert K, Vandesompele J, Mestdagh P. LNCipedia: a database for annotated human lncRNA transcript sequences and structures. Nucleic Acids Res. 2012;41(D1):D246–51.
37. Volders P-J, Verheggen K, Menschaert G, Vandepoele K, Martens L, Vandesompele J, Mestdagh P. An update on LNCipedia: a database for annotated human lncRNA sequences. Nucleic Acids Res. 2014;43(D1):D174–80.
38. Volders P-J, Anckaert J, Verheggen K, Nuytens J, Martens L, Mestdagh P, Vandesompele J. LNCipedia 5: towards a reference set of human long non-coding RNAs. Nucleic Acids Res. 2018;47(D1):D135–9.
39. Amaral PP, Clark MB, Gascoigne DK, Dinger ME, Mattick JS. lncRNAdb: a reference database for long noncoding RNAs. Nucleic Acids Res. 2010;39(suppl_1):D146–51.
40. Quek XC, Thomson DW, Maag JL, Bartonicek N, Signal B, Clark MB, Gloss BS, Dinger ME. lncRNAdb v2.0: expanding the reference database for functional long noncoding RNAs. Nucleic Acids Res. 2014;43(D1):D168–73.
41. Ma L, Li A, Zou D, Xu X, Xia L, Yu J, Bajic VB, Zhang Z. LncRNAWiki: harnessing community knowledge in collaborative curation of human long non-coding RNAs. Nucleic Acids Res. 2014;43(D1):D187–92.
42. Josset L, Tchitchek N, Gralinski LE, Ferris MT, Eisfeld AJ, Green RR, Thomas MJ, Tisoncik-Go J, Schroth GP, Kawaoka Y. Annotation of long non-

coding RNAs expressed in collaborative cross founder mice in response to respiratory virus infection reveals a new class of interferon-stimulated transcripts. RNA Biol. 2014;11(7):875–90.
43. Liu C, Bai B, Skogerbø G, Cai L, Deng W, Zhang Y, Bu D, Zhao Y, Chen R. NONCODE: an integrated knowledge database of non-coding RNAs. Nucleic Acids Res. 2005;33(suppl_1):D112–5.
44. Zhao Y, Li H, Fang S, Kang Y, Wu W, Hao Y, Li Z, Bu D, Sun N, Zhang MQ. NONCODE 2016: an informative and valuable data source of long non-coding RNAs. Nucleic Acids Res. 2015;44(D1):D203–8.
45. Bhartiya D, Pal K, Ghosh S, Kapoor S, Jalali S, Panwar B, Jain S, Sati S, Sengupta S, Sachidanandan C. lncRNome: a comprehensive knowledgebase of human long noncoding RNAs. Database. 2013;2013
46. Weirick T, John D, Dimmeler S, Uchida S. C-It-Loci: a knowledge database for tissue-enriched loci. Bioinformatics. 2015;31(21):3537–43.
47. Iyer MK, Niknafs YS, Malik R, Singhal U, Sahu A, Hosono Y, Barrette TR, Prensner JR, Evans JR, Zhao S. The landscape of long noncoding RNAs in the human transcriptome. Nat Genet. 2015;47(3):199.
48. Chen J, Shishkin AA, Zhu X, Kadri S, Maza I, Guttman M, Hanna JH, Regev A, Garber M. Evolutionary analysis across mammals reveals distinct classes of long non-coding RNAs. Genome Biol. 2016;17(1):19.
49. Yang J-H, Li J-H, Shao P, Zhou H, Chen Y-Q, Qu L-H. starBase: a database for exploring microRNA–mRNA interaction maps from Argonaute CLIP-Seq and Degradome-Seq data. Nucleic Acids Res. 2010;39(suppl_1):D202–9.
50. Li J-H, Liu S, Zhou H, Qu L-H, Yang J-H. starBase v2.0: decoding miRNA-ceRNA, miRNA-ncRNA and protein–RNA interaction networks from large-scale CLIP-Seq data. Nucleic Acids Res. 2013;42(D1):D92–7.
51. Glažar P, Papavasileiou P, Rajewsky N. circBase: a database for circular RNAs. RNA. 2014;20(11):1666–70.
52. Liu Y-C, Li J-R, Sun C-H, Andrews E, Chao R-F, Lin F-M, Weng S-L, Hsu S-D, Huang C-C, Cheng C. CircNet: a database of circular RNAs derived from transcriptome sequencing data. Nucleic Acids Res. 2015;44(D1):D209–15.
53. Ghosal S, Das S, Sen R, Basak P, Chakrabarti J. Circ2Traits: a comprehensive database for circular RNA potentially associated with disease and traits. Front Genet. 2013;4:283.
54. Li S, Li Y, Chen B, Zhao J, Yu S, Tang Y, Zheng Q, Li Y, Wang P, He X. exoRBase: a database of circRNA, lncRNA and mRNA in human blood exosomes. Nucleic Acids Res. 2017;46(D1):D106–12.
55. Chen X, Han P, Zhou T, Guo X, Song X, Li Y. circRNADb: a comprehensive database for human circular RNAs with protein-coding annotations. Sci Rep. 2016;6:34985.
56. Xia S, Feng J, Chen K, Ma Y, Gong J, Cai F, Jin Y, Gao Y, Xia L, Chang H. CSCD: a database for cancer-specific circular RNAs. Nucleic Acids Res. 2017;46(D1):D925–9.
57. Ji P, Wu W, Chen S, Zheng Y, Zhou L, Zhang J, Cheng H, Yan J, Zhang S, Yang P. Expanded expression landscape and prioritization of circular RNAs in mammals. Cell Rep. 2019;26(12):3444–3460.e5.

Interactions Among Regulatory Non-coding RNAs Involved in Cardiovascular Diseases

4

André F. Gabriel, Marina C. Costa, and Francisco J. Enguita

Abstract

Non-coding RNAs (ncRNAs) are important regulatory players in human cells that have been shown to modulate different cellular processes and biological functions through controlling gene expression, being also involved in pathological conditions such as cardiovascular diseases. Among them, long non-coding RNAs (lncRNAs) and circular (circRNAs) could act as competing endogenous RNAs (ceRNAs) sequestering other ncRNAs. This entangled network of interactions has been reported to trigger the decay of the targeted ncRNAs having important roles in gene regulation. Growing evidences have been demonstrated that the regulatory mechanism underlying the crosstalk between different ncRNA species, namely lncRNAs, circRNAs and miRNAs has also an important role in the pathophysiological processes of cardiovascular diseases. In this chapter, the main regulatory relationship among lncRNAs, circRNAs and miRNAs were summarized and their role in the control and development of cardiovascular diseases was highlighted.

Keywords

Long noncoding RNA · Circular RNA · microRNA · Interaction and cardiovascular disease · RNA-regulatory networks · Competing endogenous RNA

1 Introduction

Cardiovascular diseases (CVDs) are important causes of mortality and morbidity worldwide. Following a stress stimulus, the development of hypertrophy, autophagy, necrosis and apoptosis of cardiomyocytes, proliferation and differentiation of cardiac fibroblasts, endothelial cells (ECs) and vascular smooth muscle cells (VSMCs), contribute to the emergence and progression of CVDs. However, the molecular mechanisms underlying these processes are not completely understood. Therefore, investigating the key molecules involved in CVDs are key steps to explore effective prevention strategies and treatment methods.

The development of high-throughput deep sequencing techniques has enabled genomic and transcriptomic sequencing with higher sensitivity and accuracy. More than 98% of the human genome comprises non-coding regions, which are actively transcribed following a pervasive

A. F. Gabriel · M. C. Costa · F. J. Enguita (✉)
Instituto de Medicina Molecular João Lobo Antunes, Faculdade de Medicina, Universidade de Lisboa, Lisbon, Portugal

Cardiomics Unit, Centro de Cardiologia da Universidade de Lisboa (CCUL), Faculdade de Medicina, Universidade de Lisboa, Lisbon, Portugal
e-mail: fenguita@medicina.ulisboa.pt

J. Xiao (ed.), *Non-coding RNAs in Cardiovascular Diseases*, Advances in Experimental Medicine and Biology 1229, https://doi.org/10.1007/978-981-15-1671-9_4

transcription mechanism, generating thousands of non-coding RNA species with functional relevance [1, 2]. Transcriptomic studies driven by next-generation sequencing techniques allowed to characterize the dynamic profiles of all the functional RNA species (coding and non-coding), and to establish functional relationships in the context of cell physiology and human disease.

In recent years, several studies have revealed the important role of ncRNAs in the development of various CVDs by their involvement in the regulation of cell differentiation [3], proliferation [4], autophagy [5], necrosis [6] and apoptosis [7]. Adding to the numerous evidences showing that ncRNAs have an important role in the genomic functional output, growing data also indicates that different ncRNAs species can interact with each other constituting complex RNA-regulatory networks [8–10].

In this chapter, we describe the leading research on the interaction between long non-coding RNAs (lncRNAs), circular RNAs (circRNAs) and micro-RNAs (miRNAs), illustrating their significance in the understanding of cardiovascular pathophysiology.

2 Biogenesis of ncRNAs and Functional Interactions

The discovery of the phenomenon of pervasive transcription and the existence of ncRNAs has altered our perception of the dynamics of the human genome [11]. Generally, researchers have classified ncRNAs into three main groups based on their length: short-sized ncRNAs, including microRNAs (miRNAs) [19–25 nucleotides], short interfering RNAs (siRNAs) [~21 nucleotides] and Piwi-interacting RNAs (piRNAS) [26–31 nucleotides]; medium-sized ncRNAs including stable non-coding RNAs, as small nucleolar RNAs (snoRNAs) [60–300 nucleotides]; long-sized ncRNAs, including long intergenic ncRNAs (lincRNAs), circular RNAs (circRNAs) and other long ncRNAs (lncRNAs) [>200 nucleotides].

2.1 Biogenesis of microRNAs (miRNAs)

MiRNAs are small non-coding RNAs of approximately 19–25 nucleotides in length, found both in animals and plants and involved post-transcriptional silencing of specific messenger RNA (mRNA) targets. According to the general repository miRBase (current version 22.1; www.mirbase.org), the catalogue of human miRNAs comprises 2693 sequences of mature miRNAs, while only 2013 mature miRNAs are annotated in the mouse genome. In their biogenesis, miRNAs are synthesized by RNA polymerase II that transcribes miRNA genes into pri-miRNAs (long primary transcripts). Then, the microprocessor complex, composed by RNase-III Drosha and its co-factor DGCR8, cleaves the pri-miRNAs into pre-miRNAs (~70 nt-long precursor molecules). Pre-miRNAs are then transported to the cytosol by the nuclear exporting protein Exportin-5 [12]. In the cytosol, the RNase-III Dicer and the RNA binding cofactor trans-activation response RNA binding protein (TRBP) complex cleaves pre-miRNAs to form 19–25 nt long double-stranded miRNA molecules [12]. Subsequently, miRNAs go through the RNA-induced silencing complex (RISC) undergoing a strand-selection process which will select the mature single-stranded miRNA. The main components of RISC complex are Argonaute proteins, such as Ago2, which is responsible for the negative regulatory effect of miRNAs over coding mRNA transcripts. Several other enzymes take part into processes of decapping, deadenylation and subsequent degradation of mRNA target. It is proposed that miRNAs could modulate over 30% of the human protein coding genes, having an important role in the regulation of biological processes by the establishment of intricated networks involving multiple miRNA-mRNA interactions [13].

2.2 Biogenesis of Long Non-coding RNAs (lncRNAs)

LncRNAs are a heterogeneous group of RNA transcripts longer than 200 nucleotides that account for a large proportion of the non-coding transcriptome [11]. According to NONCODE database (www.noncode.org), there are currently 172,216 and 131,697 lncRNA genes for human and mouse, respectively. Unlike small ncRNAs, such as miRNAs, which are highly conserved and involved in transcriptional and post-transcriptional gene silencing, lncRNAs are poorly conserved and can regulate gene expression by various mechanisms, not yet fully understood [14]. The lncRNA biogenesis is largely similar to mRNAs, as its transcription is mediated by RNA polymerase II, and typically controlled by specific lncRNA promoters. Also, lncRNAs can be or not polyadenylated, can have alternative polyadenylation, and can undergo alternative splicing [15]. Alternative splicing contributes to the fact that lncRNAs display reduced sequence conservation compared to coding sequences, but emerging evidences have been reported that lncRNAs have essential and multiple functions in several biological processes regardless of their limited expression levels. LncRNAs can be classified into five groups as sense, antisense, bidirectional, intergenic and intronic lncRNAs, according to their position on the genome or their relationships to the neighbouring coding genes [15]. Functionally, lncRNAs are involved in regulating gene expression at transcriptional, post-transcriptional and epigenetic levels or could directly control protein activity [16].

2.3 Biogenesis of Circular RNAs (circRNAs)

Circular RNAs (circRNAs) are a ubiquitous group of circular covalently closed molecules generated by non-canonical back-splicing of coding and non-coding transcriptional units [17, 18]. Circular RNA molecules were first discovered as plant-infecting viroids in 1976 [19] and later on, were also discovered in eukaryotes, however these molecules were initially considered as a result of splicing defects [20]. Today it is known that circRNAs are mostly generated from protein coding genes and are mainly composed by exons [21]. The presence of circRNAs has been reported in practically every tissue and organ, being, in some situations, tissue-enriched [17, 22].

Jeck and colleagues proposed the term back-splicing to describe the pre-mRNA process of circularization and covalent joining of the 5′- to 3′-end via phosphodiester bonds [21]. Inverted repeat elements, such as Alu repeats, are *cis*-factors that participate in back-splicing. These sequences are found in exon-bordering introns and can bind each other by base pair complementarity, which causes the splice sites to close in a circular structure [21, 23]. RNA binding proteins (RBPs) were also shown to be involved in back-splicing events. For instance, Muscleblind protein (MBL) and Quaking protein (QKI) are two *trans*-acting factors that regulate circRNA synthesis. These RBPs are able to bridge the two exon-bordering introns together, leading to RNA circularization [24, 25]. CircRNAs may also be a product of "alternative circularization", by which the same locus is able to produce several circRNA isoforms [26]. Once the circular structure is formed, circRNAs become highly resistant to nuclease action, such as RNAse R [27, 28], which means that their half-life is usually higher than other linear RNA molecules [29]. Some circRNAs contain intronic elements and are originated from intronic lariats and exon-containing lariats by exon skipping [30].

CircRNAs are classified in three different groups: exonic circRNA (ecircRNA), intronic circRNA (ciRNA) and exon and intron-containing circRNA (EIciRNA) [21]; these two last circRNAs are mainly found in the nucleus and are responsible for transcription events, being present in the spliceosome and even taking part in alternative splicing [31, 32]. Among other functions, ecircRNAs were shown to participate in regulation of gene expression by interacting with RBPs [24, 25] and also with other non-coding RNAs, such as miRNAs [18, 28, 33].

2.4 Functional Interactions Among ncRNAs

In general, four main types of regulatory interactions between ncRNAs have been proposed: lncRNAs and circRNAs as miRNA sponges, lncRNAs and miRNAs co-expression, reciprocal repression of lncRNAs and miRNAs, and miRNAs negative regulation of lncRNAs.

The most prevalent interaction between ncRNAs, namely lncRNAs and circRNAs, and miRNAs involves a "sponge-effect", consisting on the ability of ncRNAs to sequestrate miRNAs molecules by the competing endogenous RNA (ceRNA) mechanism (Fig. 4.1). This effect occurs through binding to the miRNA response elements (MREs), thus down-regulating them. In order to act as a ceRNA, the MRE does not require complete complementarity to bind to miRNA. So, the interactions between ncRNAs and miRNAs do not usually trigger decay of the interacting RNAs or trigger only slow decays [34].

Interactions between ncRNAs are described to control different cellular processes, in particular in CVDs (Tables 4.1 and 4.2), establishing intertwined and complex regulatory networks (Fig. 4.2), described below.

3 lncRNA–miRNA Interactions in Cardiovascular Diseases

3.1 Cardiac Hypertrophy

Cardiac hypertrophy is a physiological adaptive reaction of the heart mainly characterized by enlarged cardiomyocyte size and sustained cardiac increased volume that can lead to heart failure and even sudden death [35]. Recent studies have showed that dysregulation of lncRNAs can induce cardiac hypertrophy [36, 37]. Several ncRNAs have been described as relevant players in this pathology, including also functional RNA-RNA interactions.

The lncRNA H19, a 2.3 kb lncRNA transcribed from the H19 gene, is highly expressed in

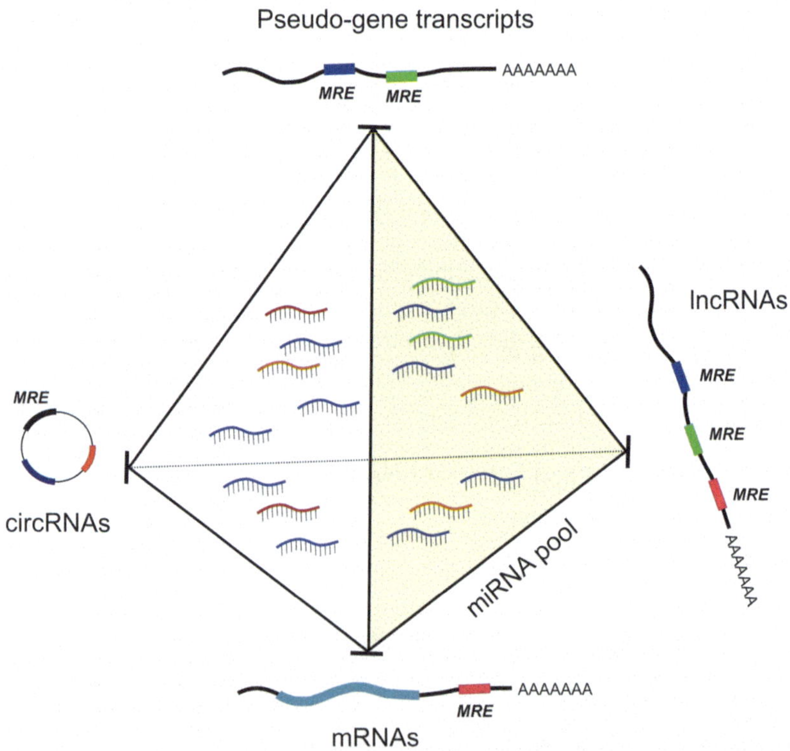

Fig. 4.1 The ncRNA interactions according to complementary endogenous (ceRNA) hypothesis. MiRNAs are the focal point of the ceRNA hypothesis by interacting with other RNA molecules through their miRNA response elements (MREs). MiRNAs act as negative regulators of gene expression by targeting mRNAs, but their levels could be regulated by other RNAs. LncRNAs and circRNAs harbouring specific MREs can act as molecular sponges of miRNAs by sequence complementarity, decreasing their available levels within the cell. Pseudo-gene are also described to act as miRNA decoys

Table 4.1 LncRNA and miRNA interactions in cardiovascular diseases

lncRNA	miRNA	mRNA target	Function	References
Cardiac hypertrophy				
H19	miR-675	CaMKIId	Inhibits cardiac hypertrophy	[41]
		USP10	Protects CPCc senescence	[43]
CHRF	miR-489	Myd88	Promotes cardiac hypertrophy and dysfunction	[44]
MIAT	miR-150		Promotes cardiac hypertrophy	[50]
	miR-93	TLR4	Promotes cardiac hypertrophy	[51]
ROR	miR-133		Promotes hypertrophy	[36]
Plscr4	miR-214	Mfn2	Inhibits hypertrophy	[55]
HOTAIR	miR-19	PTEN	Inhibits hypertrophy	[57]
CASC15	miR-432-5p	VDR	Promotes hypertrophy	[59]
XIST	miR-330-3p	S100B	Promotes hypertrophy	[64]
	miR-101	TLR2	Promotes hypertrophy	[66]
Myocardial infarction				
MIAT	miR-24	Furin, TGF-β1	Increases cardiac interstitial fibrosis	[68]
APF	miR-188-3p	ATG7	Suppress I/R injury and protect cardiac function when down-regulated	[69]
MALAT1	miR-320	PTEN	Promotes cardiomyocite apoptosis	[71]
	miR-125	JMJD6	Promotes CPC proliferation	[143]
H19	miR-139	Sox8	Suppresses hypoxia-induced cell injury	[72]
MEG3	miR-183	p27	Promoted hypoxia-induced cell injury	[73]
Galont	miR-338	ATG5	Promotes anoxia/reoxygenation-induced autophagy and cell death in cardiomyocytes	[74]
ZFAS1	miR-150	CRP	Prevented cardiomyocytes apoptosis	[75]
CRRL	miR-199a-3p	Hopx	Promotes post-MI remodeling and inhibit cardiac function	[76]
Heart failure				
CARL	miR-539	PHB2	Inhibited mitochondrial fission, apoptosis and reduced I/R injury	[78]
MDRL	miR-361		Suppressed I/R injury and protected cardiac function	[80]
H19	miR-19b	Sox6	Inhibited proliferation and promoted apoptosis in cardiomyocytes	[40]
	miR-103/107	FADD	Prevented I/R injury and protected cardiac function	[6]
NFR	miR-873	RIPK1/RIPK3	Induced I/R injury and cardiac dysfunction	[81]
FTX	miR-29b-1-5p	Bcl2l27	Inhibited cardiomyocyte apoptosis	[82]
SNHG1	miR-195	Bcl2l27	Inhibited cardiomyocyte apoptosis	[83]
AZIN2-sv	miR-214	PTEN	Inhibited endogenous cardiac regeneration	[84]
Atrial fibrillation				
TCONS_00075467	miR-328	CACNA1C	Reduced atrial effective refractory; induced AF as it was knockdown	[85]
Cardiac fibrosis				
GAS5	miR-21	PTEN	Inhibited CFs growth	[87]
H19	miR-455	CTGF	Promotes fibrosis-associated protein synthesis	[88]
PFL	Let-7d		Promotes fibrogenesis	[89]

(continued)

Table 4.1 (continued)

lncRNA	miRNA	mRNA target	Function	References
n379519	miR-30		Inhibited MI induced cardiac fibrosis an cardiac dysfunction	[90]
SRA1	miR-148b		Reduces cardiac fibrosis	[91]
Atherosclerosis				
Ang 262	miR-221/-222		Promoted proliferation of VSMCs	[92]
MALAT1	miR-22-3p	CXCR2	Prevented ECs apoptosis	[93]
RP5-833A20.1	miR-382-5p	NFIA	Induced atherosclerosis	[94]
RNCR3	miR-185	KLF2	Prevented proliferation of ECs	[95]
DIGIT	miR-134		Inhibited growth, migration and tube formation of ECs	[96]
Diabetic cardiomyopathy				
MIAT	miR-22-3p	DAPK2	Inhibited cardiomyocyte apoptosis and improve left ventricular function in diabetic rats when knockdown	[98]
Kcnq1ot1	miR-214-3p	Caspase-1	Inhibited pyroptosis	[99]
Aortic valve disease				
MALAT1	miR-204	Smad4	Promoted osteogenic differentiation of VICs	[100]

Table 4.2 CircRNAs and miRNA interactions in cardiovascular diseases

circRNA	circRNA locus	miRNA	miRNA target	No. MREs	Phenotypes up-regulated circRNA	References
Cardiac hypertrophy and heart failure						
HRCR	Pwwp2a	miR-223	ARC	6	HRCR protects the heart from pathological hypertrophy by inhibiting cardiomyocyte apoptosis	[102]
Myocardial infarction						
cdr1as	CDR1	miR-7a	PARP, SP1	63	Apoptotic cardiomyocytes and worsening of MI symptoms	[101]
MFACR	Smyd4	miR-652-3p	MTP18	15	Cardiomyocyte mitochondrial fission and apoptosis	[7]
circNCX1	ncx1	miR-133a-3p	Cdip1	8	Apoptotic cardiomyocytes	[111]
circRNA_081881	NA	miR-548	PPARγ	7	Decreased foam cell formation	[114]
MICRA	ZNF609	miR-150	ADRB1, CRP	N/A	Decreased LV dysfunction risk	[116, 122]
Cardiac fibrosis in diabetic cardiomyopathy						
circRNA_000203	Myo9a	miR-26b-5p	Col1a2, CTGF	2	Arrhythmia and heart failure due to fibrotic tissue	[103]
circRNA_010567	NA	miR-141	TGF-β1	N/A	Arrhythmia and heart failure due to fibrotic tissue	[125]
Hypoxic angiogenesis and endothelial disorders						
circZNF609	ZNF609	miR-615	MEF2A	1	Worsening of endothelial damage	[128]
hsa_circ_000595	BTBD7	miR-19a	NF-κB, COX-2	N/A	Aortic smooth muscle cell apoptosis. Aortic aneurism	[130]

(continued)

Table 4.2 (continued)

circRNA	circRNA locus	miRNA	miRNA target	No. MREs	Phenotypes up-regulated circRNA	References
hsa_circ_0010729	HSPG2	miR-186	HIF-1α	N/A	Angiogenesis proliferation and apoptosis suppression	[131]
Stroke						
circDLGAP4	DLGAP4	miR-143	HECTD1	1	Decreased neural deficits, decreased infarction area and mitigation of BBB damage	[135]
circHECTD1	HECTD1	miR-142	TIPARP	1	Astrocyte activation and brain infarction	[136]
Atherosclerosis						
hsa_circ_0000284	HIPK3	miR-221	$p27^{Kip1}$	1	Carotid plaque rupture and eventually stroke	[115]
Coronary artery disease						
hsa_circ_0089378	VAV2	miR-130a-3p	TRPM3	N/A	CAD typical phenotype	[140]
hsa_circ_0083357	CTSB	miR-130a-3p	TRPM3	N/A	CAD typical phenotype	[140]
hsa_circ_0082824	CUL1	miR-130a-3p	TRPM3	N/A	CAD typical phenotype	[140]
hsa_circ_0068942	ADD1	miR-130a-3p	TRPM3	N/A	CAD typical phenotype	[140]
hsa_circ_0057576	HECW2	miR-130a-3p	TRPM3	N/A	CAD typical phenotype	[140]
hsa_circ_0054537	PSME4	miR-130a-3p	TRPM3	N/A	CAD typical phenotype	[140]
hsa_circ_0051172	AXL	miR-130a-3p	TRPM3	N/A	CAD typical phenotype	[140]
hsa_circ_0032970	TC2N	miR-130a-3p	TRPM3	N/A	CAD typical phenotype	[140]
hsa_circ_0006323	DPYD	miR-130a-3p	TRPM3	N/A	CAD typical phenotype	[140]

several tissues of the foetus, but its transcriptional levels are significantly reduced after birth [38]. So far, there is increasing evidence that lncRNA H19 can regulate several cellular functions by targeting different miRNAs acting via either as a sponge of miRNAs, including miR-103/107 [39] and miR-19b [40], or as miRNA precursor involved in the regulation of cardiomyocyte hypertrophy. The miR-675 precursor is located in the first exon of H19 gene, and in the hypertrophic heart, both H19 lncRNA and miR-675 were up-regulated [41]. The H19 overexpression was correlated with the miR-675 up-regulation and therefore reduced the levels of several cardiomyocyte foetal genes; whereas H19 down-regulation would overturn those effects. The Ca^{2+}/calmodulin-dependent protein kinase IId (CaMKIId) was identified as a target gene of miR-675. Down-regulation of CaMKIId gene transcript by miR-675 partly reverted the hypertrophic phenotype caused by H19 down-regulation. H19 can inhibit the hypertrophy of cardiomyocytes both by modulating of miR-675-CaMKIId axis and by suppressing the expression of CaMKIId [42].

Also, H19 and its encoded miR-675 have been reported playing a key role in the regulating of cellular senescence. Under stress conditions, cardiac progenitor cells (CPCs) lose capacity of proliferation and differentiation due to the contribution of senescence to cell aging which would lead to cardiac dysfunction. Besides, both H19 and miR-675 were inhibited in H_2O_2-treated CPCs. Inhibition of H19 or miR-675 would result

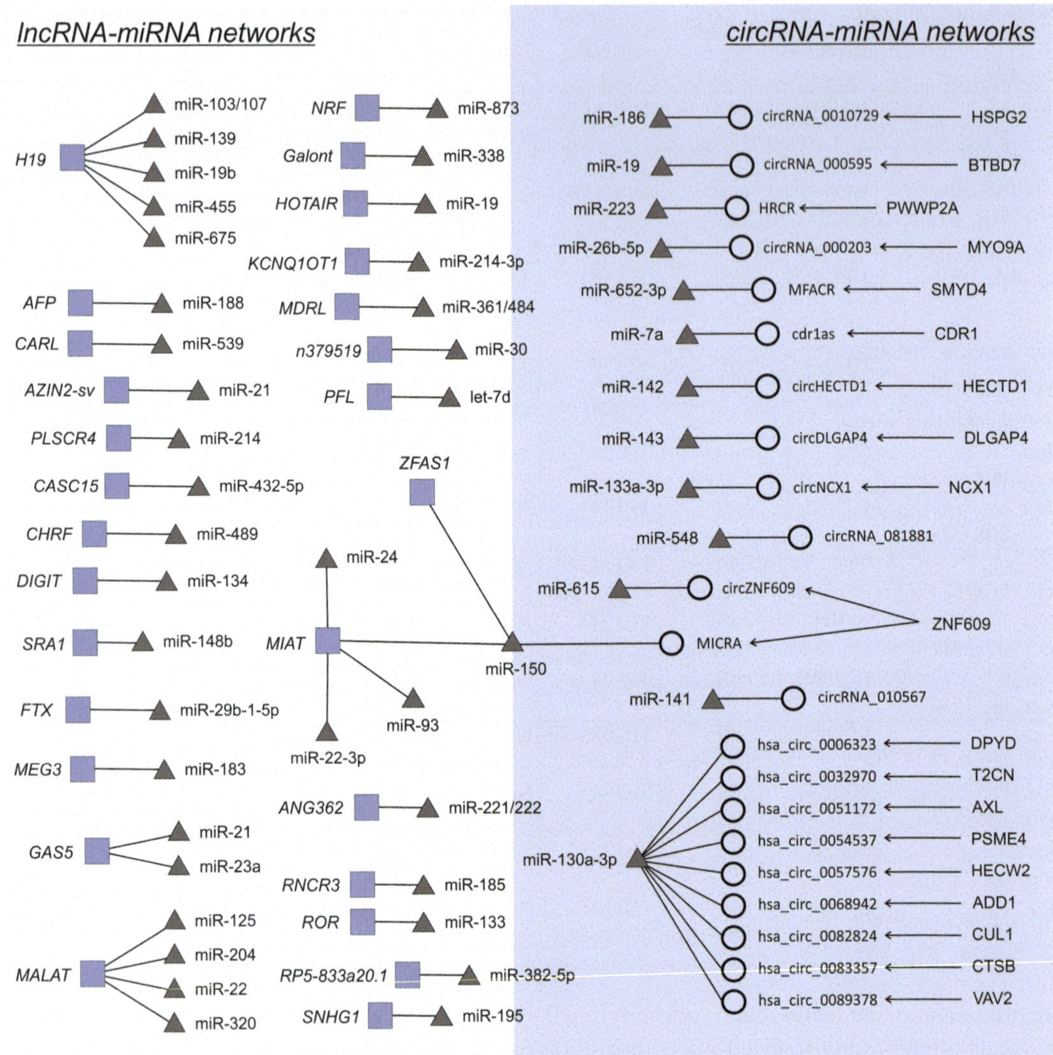

Fig. 4.2 Regulatory networks in the lncRNA/miRNA/mRNA and circRNA/miRNA/mRNA axis in cardiovascular diseases. miRNAs are depicted as triangles, circRNAs as open circles and lncRNAs as squares. Functional RNA-RNA interactions are represented by lines, whereas the genes leading to the production of specific circRNAs by back-splicing are connected by arrows with the corresponding circRNA designation

in the loss of protection of CPCs ageing caused by melatonin through a ubiquitin-specific protease 10 (USP10) suppression mechanism [43].

In 2014, Wang and colleagues showed that lncRNA AK048451, named as cardiac hypertrophy related factor (CHRF) could function as miR-489 endogenous sponge that directly sequester this miRNA in a sequence-specific manner and decreases its regulatory activity. This sponging-activity was demonstrated through bioinformatics, luciferase and RNA pull-down assays [44]. CHRF overexpression would promote cardiac hypertrophy, while CHRF inhibition could attenuate angiotensin II (AngII)-induced cardiac hypertrophic effects. These observations suggested that CHRF can serve as an upstream regulator of the miR-489/Myd88 axis after hypertrophic stress [44].

LncRNA myocardial infarction-associated transcript (MIAT) is mostly expressed in heart and foetal brain tissues and it has been demonstrated that deregulated expression of MIAT is associated with cell proliferation, apoptosis, and migration in various diseases, including myocardial infarction [45–49]. Early reports showed that MIAT was significantly up-regulated in AngII-induced cardiac hypertrophy and could enhance the pathology by partly sponging miR-150 [50]. In rat isolated cardiomyocytes, Li et al. proposed that MIAT could also act as a ceRNA for miR-93 [51]. In their recent study, the authors showed that MIAT was up-regulated and miR-93 was down-regulated in AngII-treated cardiomyocytes and validated MIAT as a molecular sponge of miR-93 in cardiomyocytes. Also, TLR4 was identified as a target of miR-93 and MIAT promoted TLR4 expression by sponging miR-93. Additionally, enforced expression of TLR4 partially reversed the protective effect of miR-93 overexpression on AngII-induced cardiac hypertrophy [51].

The lncRNA ROR is also known to act as sponge of miRNAs, including miR-145, miR-205 and the let-7 family, and to be involved in the control of embryonic stem cells differentiation [9], and cancer cells proliferation, migration and invasion [52, 53]. In hypertrophic cardiomyocytes, a reciprocal repression mechanism between ROR and miR-133 was first described by Jiang and co-workers, demonstrated by a reciprocal-correlation between ROR and miR-133 levels [36]. The down-regulation of ROR transcript was negatively correlated with the expression of miR-133, and miR-133 mimics reduced the expression of ROR [36].

Mitochondrial physiology is important for healthy heart function as cardiomyocytes are dependent on mitochondrial oxidative phosphorylation to generate ATP for cardiac contraction [54]. In a recent study, Lv and colleagues found the lncRNA Plscr4 to be a negative regulator of cardiac hypertrophy in vivo and in vitro by regulating the miR-214-Mfn2 axis [55]. Mitofusin 2 (Mfn2) is a protein located at the mitochondrial outer membrane and with a key role in the maintenance of mitochondrial homeostasis [56]. The authors verified that Plscr4 was up-regulated in hypertrophic mice hearts and in AngII-treated cardiomyocytes. When inhibited, Plscr4 induced a hypertrophic response in cardiomyocytes. Conversely, the overexpression of Plscr4 attenuated cardiac hypertrophy in vitro and in vivo models. The authors proposed that Plscr4 acted as an endogenous sponge of miR-214 since an overexpression of Plscr4 was able to down-regulate miR-214 expression promoting Mfn2 and reducing the hypertrophic phenotype. In contrast, knockdown of Plscr4 led to up-regulation of miR-214 and induced cardiomyocyte hypertrophy [55].

HOTAIR was one of the first lncRNAs identified as a key regulator of the progression of cancers, and recently proposed as member of a ceRNA-centered regulatory network in CVDs [57, 58]. In mice, Lai et al. detected the down-regulation of HOTAIR expression in pathological cardiac hypertrophy and in AngII-stimulated hypertrophic cultured cardiomyocytes [57]. Later, following bioinformatics analysis, induced overexpression and luciferase reporter assays the authors were able to demonstrate that HOTAIR could sponge miR-19. In addition, the levels of the phosphatase and tensin homologue gene (PTEN, a miR-19 target) in hypertrophic mouse hearts was reported to be positively correlated with HOTAIR. These results indicate that HOTAIR function as a negative regulator of cardiac hypertrophy via facilitating the expression of PTEN by competitively binding to miR-19 [57].

Recent findings show that the lncRNA CASC15 can also facilitate cardiac hypertrophy by interacting with miR-432-5p [59]. Li and colleagues demonstrated that CASC15 was up-regulated in hypertrophic cardiomyocytes in vivo and stimulated hypertrophic responses in cardiomyocytes treated with angiotensin II. In this study, the transcription factor VDR appeared to up-regulate CASC15 expression to facilitate cardiac hypertrophy. Furthermore, it was demonstrated that the expression of CASC15 correlated negatively with the expression of miR-432-5p in a cardiac hypertrophy model. Luciferase assays validated the inhibitory function of miR-432-5p by CASC15. In conclusion, these results suggest that the up-regulation of CASC15 induced by VDR facilitates cardiac hypertrophy by modulating miR-432-5p [59].

X-inactive specific transcript (XIST) RNA is a 17-kb lncRNA that regulates X-chromosome inactivation [60]. Recently, XIST was found to target miRNAs to regulate pathological process of several diseases including myocardial infarction [61–63]. A recent study revealed that XIST was up-regulated in hypertrophic cardiac animal model and phenylephrine (PE)-treated cardiomyocytes [64]. Silencing XIST induced a hypertrophic response of cardiomyocyte; in contrast overexpression of XIST attenuated cardiomyocyte hypertrophy induced by PE. Additionally, using bioinformatic tools and functional assays, the authors demonstrated that XIST regulated the hypertrophic response through directly binding to miR-330-3p. Also, miR-330-3p was found to target S100B, a Ca^{2+}-binding protein that impacts on cardiac pathology [65]. The authors observed that XIST modulated S100B expression by sponging miR-330-3p, leading to a decrease in the hypertrophic response [64].

In another study, new evidences associate XIST expression with the regulation of cardiac hypertrophy by targeting a different miRNA [66]. I was reported the up-regulation of XIST, and down-regulation of miR-101, in hypertrophic mouse hearts and PE-treated cardiomyocytes [66]. The knockdown of XIST led to a reduction in PE-induced cardiomyocyte hypertrophy. On the other hand, overexpression of XIST aggravated cardiac hypertrophy in the animal model. With the use of Luciferase reporter and RNA-binding protein immunoprecipitation (RIP) assays, the authors demonstrated that XIST could regulate cardiac hypertrophy by targeting miR-101. Furthermore, rescue assays confirmed that XIST supported the progression of cardiac hypertrophy by binding with miR-101 leading to an increase of the expression of TLR2, also a target of miR-101 [66].

3.2 Myocardial Infarction

Myocardial infarction (MI) occurs when the supply of blood to the heart is diminished (ischemia) for a long time. Heart ischemia is the main cause of hypoxia and can lead to serious tissue damage and functional complications [67].

The lncRNA MIAT was identified as risk factor for the development and progression of myocardial infarction, through a large scale case-control association study [45]. Recently, Qu and colleagues investigated the role of MIAT interaction with miR-24 in the regulation of cardiac fibrosis, in consequence of a MI event [68]. In a mouse model of MI, MIAT was abnormally up-regulated and accompanied by cardiac interstitial fibrosis. MIAT up-regulation was also accompanied by a deregulation of fibrosis-related modulators, namely down-regulation of miR-24 and up-regulation of Furin and TGF-β1. When the authors performed the knockdown of endogenous MIAT by siRNA it reduced cardiac fibrosis and improved cardiac function, also restoring the deregulated expression of the fibrosis-related regulators. In cardiac fibroblasts treated with serum or angiotensin II, similar up-regulation of MIAT and down-regulation of miR-24 were observed [68].

In 2015, Wang et al., reported that one lncRNA, named autophagy promoting factor (APF), could regulate autophagic cell death by targeting miR-188-3p and ATG7 (autophagy associated gene), an enzyme of the autophagy system with a critical role in membrane elongation [69]. In this report, the authors showed that miR-188-3p contributed to the regulation of ATG7 expression, and inhibited autophagy and cell death in vitro and in vivo. Luciferase reporter assays revealed that APF was able to directly bind to miR-188-3p and regulate its activity.

The lncRNA metastasis-associated lung adenocarcinoma transcript 1 (MALAT1) has been associated with the development of acute myocardial infarction (AMI), specifically as a predictor of left ventricular dysfunction [47]. Genome-wide miRNA profiles and transcriptional analysis by microarrays showed that miR-320 was down-regulated in AMI patients [70]. Additionally, bioinformatics analyses revealed that MALAT1 and PTEN shared the same regulatory sites for miR-320. Based in these evidences, Hu and colleagues proposed that MALAT1 could function as ceRNA to control PTEN expression through sponging miR-320, thus playing an important role in the progression of AMI [71]. To test this hypothesis, the expression levels of MALAT1, miR-320 and PTEN in a mouse model of AMI and sham-operated mice were determined by quantitative PCR and western blotting, respectively. MALAT1 and PTEN were highly expressed, while miR-320 expression was reduced in AMI group. By luciferase reporter assay, the authors confirmed that MALAT1 functioned as a ceRNA of miR-320 to regulate PTEN in mouse cardiomyocytes. MALAT1 and PTEN expressions were up-regulated with time dependent hypoxia treatment and miR-320 expression was reduced. Also, hypoxia stimulated the apoptosis of mouse cardiomyocytes. Additionally, the overexpression of miR-320 or the down-regulation of PTEN partly reversed the pro-apoptotic effect induced by MALAT1 overexpression. These data suggested that MALAT1 could target miR-320 to promote the apoptosis of mouse cardiomyocytes through up-regulation of PTEN [71].

Other evidences show that MALAT1 may contribute to the development of MI, by interacting with other miRNAs. Recently, Li et al. showed that the expression of MALAT1 was markedly up-regulated in a $CoCl_2$-induced hypoxia cardiac progenitor cells (CPCs) model [71]. CPCs play a key role in heart muscle regeneration in patients after myocardial infarction and MALAT1 down-regulation reduced CPC proliferation under hypoxic conditions. Additionally, MALAT1 acted as a sponge for miR-125. Inhibition of miR-125 restored the proliferation potential of CPCs after a MALAT1 knockdown in hypoxia. Additional analyses demonstrated that JMJD6, a histone lysine demethylase, was a target of miR-125 and negatively regulated by this miRNA. Moreover, JMJD6 knockdown blocked miR-125 inhibitor's protective effect on CPC function in hypoxia [71].

In 2017, Gong and colleagues designed a study to assess the effects of lncRNA H19 on hypoxic rat H9c2 cells and mouse HL-1 cells [72]. In vitro, the authors verified the hypoxia-induced up-regulation of H19 as well as cell injury in H9c2 cells. Also, hypoxia-induced cell injury effect was exacerbated by knockdown of H19 but alleviated by overexpression of H19. When the miR-139 was suppressed they could reverse the effects of H19 knockdown. With the use of bioinformatics tools and functional experiments the authors showed that transcription factor Sox8 was negatively regulated by miR-139. Moreover, Sox8 overexpression mitigated hypoxia-induced cell injury of H9c2 cells. These data suggested that H19 controlled hypoxia-induced myocardial injury through miR-139-mediated up-regulation of Sox8 axis [72].

Later and using a similar methodological approach, the same research group studied the role of lncRNA maternally expressed gene 3 (MEG3) on hypoxic rat cardiomyocyte-derived H9c2 cells [73]. Their results depicted that hypoxia induced an increase of MEG3 expression and silencing MEG3 caused a decrease in hypoxia-induced injury in H9c2 cells. Additionally, the knockdown of MEG3 also increased miR-183 expression, which was identified as a target of MEG3. When silenced, the effects of MEG3 knockdown on the hypoxic cells were reversed. Next, the cyclin dependent kinase inhibitor p27 was identified as a target gene of miR-183, and its expression was negatively regulated by miR-183. Together, these findings proposed that knockdown of MEG3 diminished hypoxia-induced H9c2 cell injury by miR-183-mediated suppression of p27 [73].

The hypernomic autophagy is a cellular process associated with several cardiovascular diseases, including myocardial infarction. The GATA1 activated lncRNA (Galont) was found to promote anoxia/reoxygenation-induced autophagy and cell death in cardiomyocytes by targeting miR-338 [74]. In the Yin study, Galont interacted directly with miR-338 and promoted ATG5-mediated autophagic cell death in mouse cardiomyocytes. Galont was up-regulated by anoxia/reoxygenation (A/R) stimulus, and stimulated autophagy and cell death in cardiomyocytes exposed to A/R. Also, miR-338 suppressed autophagy and cell death. These findings illustrate that Galont could play an important role in regulating autophagy in cardiomyocytes through Galont/miR-338/ATG5 axis.

ZFAS1 is a cardiac-related lncRNA implicated in the molecular mechanism of cardiomyocyte apoptosis induced by MI by targeting miR-150 [75]. The relative expression of ZFAS1 was significantly up-regulated and miR-150 was significantly down-regulated in MI-induced rats. RNA pull-down assays indicated that ZFAS1 could interact directly with miR-150. C-reactive protein (CRP) was found to be regulated by ZFAS1/miR-150 axis and negatively targeted by miR-150. Also, knockdown of ZFAS1 or miR-150 overexpression effectively reduced induced myocardial infarction rats [75].

In an investigation of endogenous cardiomyocyte (CM) regeneration to improve cardiac function and cardiac remodelling after MI, a screening of human foetal and adult hearts RNA-seq data identified a novel lncRNA (NONHSAG007671), later named cardiomyocyte regeneration-related lncRNA (CRRL) [76]. It was observed that the loss of CRRL reduced post-MI remodelling and protected cardiac function in adult rats. Also, CRRL knockdown promoted neonatal rat CM proliferation both in vivo and in vitro. CRRL operated as a ceRNA by directly binding to miR-199a-3p and thereby increasing the expression of Hopx, a target gene of miR-199a-3p and a critical negative regulatory factor of CM proliferation.

3.3 Heart Failure

Heart failure is a widespread and complex clinical syndrome that arises from functional and/or structural heart disorders and impairs ventricular ejection of the blood to the systemic circulation. Cardiomyocyte apoptosis or necrosis is a major cause of heart failure, though the underlying mechanism remains unknown [77].

Mitochondrial fission and fusion are one of the biological processes which are related with cardiomyocyte apoptosis [78]. The lncRNA AK017121, named cardiac apoptosis-related lncRNA (CARL), was identified as a functional sponge of miR-539 [79]. CARL overexpression inhibited mitochondrial fission, apoptosis and ischaemia/reperfusion (I/R) injury by directly suppressing miR-539 expression and subsequently up-regulating its target gene prohibitin 2 (PHB2) [78].

The lncRNA AK009271, named mitochondrial dynamic related lncRNA (MDRL), is also involved in mitochondrial fission and fusion under stress condition. MDRL could directly interact with miR-361 suppressing the activity of miR-361, decreasing mitochondrial fission and apoptosis after anoxia/reoxygenation treatment. MiR-361 was found to base-paring with the primary transcript of miR-484, restricting the processing of pri-miR-484 in the nucleus. The effects of MDRL overexpression over the counteracting miRNA were reverted when MDRL expression was knocked down [80].

The lncRNA H19 appears to be a crucial regulator in this process as it was described to suppress miR-19b-Sox6 and miR-103/107-FADD (Fas-associated protein with death domain) cascades inhibiting proliferation, promoting apoptosis in P19CL6 cells and preventing cardiomyocyte necrosis. In 2016, Han et al. revealed that during the late stage of cardiac differentiation of P19CL6 cells, miR-19b was negatively regulated by H19, evidenced by luciferase assay and quantitative PCR. H19 overexpression would inhibit cell proliferation and benefit cell apoptosis by regulating miR-19b and its target gene Sox6, whereas down-regulation of H19 reversed these effects [40]. In another study, H19 was found to contain three potential miR-103/107 binding sites and was implicated in cardiomyocyte necrosis by inhibiting the expression levels of miR-103/107 and its target FADD, in response to H_2O_2 treatment [39]. Knockdown of miR-103/107 reduced necrosis in the cellular model and also MI in a mouse ischemia/reperfusion (I/R) model.

Another lncRNA, named necrosis-related factor (NRF), was associated to necrotic death of cardiomyocytes by sponging miR-873. Silencing of NRF resulted in an increase of miR-873 levels and a subsequent down-regulation of its cognate targets receptor-interacting serine/threonine protein kinase 1 (RIPK1) and RIPK3, leading to a severe reduction in myocardial necrosis [81].

Recently, new lncRNAs-miRNAs associations were proposed to be also playing a significant role in cardiomyocyte cell fate and development of heart failure. In 2018, a novel FTX/miR-29b-1-5p/Bcl2l27 axis was suggested in the regulation of cardiomyocyte apoptosis [82]. In the Long et al. study, authors found that FTX was significantly down-regulated upon ischemia/reperfusion injury and H_2O_2 treatment. When enhanced, the expression of FTX inhibited cardiomyocyte apoptosis. Also, miR-29b-1-5p was found to interact with FTX and regulate the expression of BCL2-Like Protein 2 (Bcl2l2). Furthermore, inhibition of miR-29b-1-5p attenuated cardiomyocyte apoptosis upon hydrogen peroxide treatment.

In another report, the lncRNA SNHG1 also seemed to regulate cardiomyocyte apoptosis by targeting miR-195 and modulating Bcl2l2 [83]. SNHG1 was found to limit cell apoptosis via regulating miR-195 and Bcl2l2 in human cardiomyocytes (HCMs). Overexpression of SNHG1 alleviated the effects of H_2O_2 on HCMs. Also, SNHG1 was found to sponge miR-195 in HCMs. The increase levels of miR-195 suppressed cell viability and induced apoptosis in HCMs, and miR-195 was found to negatively regulate the expression of Bcl2l2.

The high-throughput sequencing of foetal and adult human heart tissue was used to identify a novel lncRNA up-regulated in the adult heart and named splice variant of the AZIN2 gene (AZIN2-sv). The lncRNA AZIN2-sv inhibited endogenous cardiac regeneration in vivo and in vitro, while loss of AZIN2-sv attenuated adverse remodelling and improved cardiac function. It was found that AZIN2-sv mediated cardiac regeneration involved a ceRNA sponging activity over miR-214 which is on the basis of the modulation of the PTEN-Akt signalling pathway [84].

3.4 Atrial Fibrillation

Atrial fibrillation (AF) is a the most prevalent of heart arrythmia, characterized by abnormal electrical activities in the heart atrial tissues. The loss of electrical synchronization in the myocardium often contributes to cardiac remodelling, fibrosis and failure. The disease starts with an isolated fibrillation event that will evolve to a paroxysmal and later to a chronical and permanent condition. Underlying molecular mechanisms for the onset and transition to a permanent condition are still poorly understood.

The lncRNA expression profiles of right atria were investigated in AF and non-AF rabbit models by using RNA sequencing techniques and validated using quantitative PCR [85]. Bioinformatics analysis was conducted to predict the functions and interactions of the aberrantly expressed genes, and one lncRNA, TCONS_00075467, was selected to study its effects and mechanisms on electrical remodelling. Knock-down of TCONS_00075467 led to reduced atrial effective refractory period in vivo and diminished L-type calcium current and action potential duration in vitro. Also, the expression of miR-328 was negatively correlated with TCONS_00075467. Additionally, TCONS_00075467 could target miR-328 in vitro and in vivo to modulate CACNA1C, a calcium voltage-gated channel subunit alpha1 C protein. The expression of miR-328 was up-regulated and CACNA1C protein levels were reduced when TCONS_00075467 was silenced in vivo and in vitro, while miR-328 negatively modulates TCONS_00075467 [85].

3.5 Cardiac Fibrosis

Myocardial fibrosis represents an important health issue associated with almost all forms of heart disease. Cardiac fibroblasts are an essential cell type in the heart in charge of homeostasis of the extracellular matrix. However, after a stress stimuli or injury these cells can change to a myofibroblast phenotype and progress to cardiac fibrosis. This transformation involves physiopathological changes such as cardiomyocyte hypertrophy, chamber dilation and apoptosis, and eventually leads to the progression to heart failure [86]. In cardiac fibrosis, several ncRNAs, including lncRNAs and miRNAs, have been reported to play a pivotal role in the regulation of the fibrotic phenotype [4, 68].

A key mechanism in the development of fibrosis is the fibroblast activation. In TGF-β1-activated cardiac fibroblasts (CFs), the lncRNA GAS5 was shown to be down-regulated, while the level of miR-21 was increased [87]. However, overexpression of GAS5 prevented the growth of CFs and inhibited the expressions levels of type I collagen protein (Col1A1) and smooth muscle alpha-action protein (α-SMA) by negatively regulating miR-21 and its target PTEN. These data suggested that the regulation of miR-21/PTEN by GAS5 could have a significant role in the development of cardiac fibrosis.

Also, the lncRNA H19 has been implicated in the development of cardiac fibrosis by regulating miR-455 [88]. In a report by Huang and colleagues, after miRNA microarray analysis, miR-455 was found to be significantly down-regulated in diabetic mouse myocardium and in Ang II-induced CFs. Loss and gain-of-function assays showed that miR-455 expression levels were negatively correlated with collagen I and III expression in CFs. Also, bioinformatic analyses predicted that miR-455 targeted CTGF (connective tissue growth factor) and H19, which was validated by luciferase reporter assay. Furthermore, it was described that H19 knockdown could increase the antifibrotic role of miR-455 by diminishing CTGF expression and fibrosis-associated protein synthesis.

Recently a novel lncRNA designated as a pro-fibrotic lncRNA (PFL) was found to be up-regulated in fibrotic CFs and in the hearts of mice in response to myocardial infarction (MI) [89]. PFL knockdown attenuated cardiac interstitial fibrosis and improved ejection fraction (EF) and fractional shortening (FS) in MI mice. Also, forced expression of PFL promoted proliferation, fibroblast-to-myofibroblast transition and fibrogenesis in CFs by modulating let-7d, while inhibition of PFL reduced TGF-β1-induced myofibroblast generation and fibrogenesis. Furthermore, PFL acted as a ceRNA of let-7d, as overexpression of PFL reduced the level and activity of let-7d.

Another example of the modulation of cardiac fibrosis in post-infarcted myocardium by lncRNA-miRNA association was documented by Wang and colleagues [90]. These authors described the role of the lncRNA n379519-miR-30 axis as a negative regulator MI induced cardiac fibrosis and the associated cardiac dysfunction [90]. They observed that the expression of n379519 was up-regulated in the hearts of mice with MI and in the fibrotic CFs. Silencing of endogenous n379519 improved the heart function and reduced collagen deposition and the process of cardiac fibrosis. Also, they showed the opposite tendency of expression between n379519 and miR-30. Bioinformatics analysis and luciferase reporter assay indicated that n379519 could directly bind to miR-30. Moreover, miR-30 inhibitor abolished the collagen synthesis inhibition induced by n379519.

Recent data examine the role of lncRNA SRA1 in the activation of cardiac myofibroblasts in cardiac fibrosis. Results showed that SRA1 was up-regulated followed by cardiac fibrosis in an abdominal aortic banding-treated rat model. Angiotensin-II treatment amplified the SRA1 expression in cardiac myofibroblasts, while SRA1 silencing inhibited the proliferation, myofibroblast conversion and collagen production of cardiac myofibroblasts. Furthermore miR-148b was predicted to be a targeted microRNA of SRA1. Sequence alignment, luciferase activity, and MS2 RNA immunoprecipitation were conducted to detect the interaction between SRA1 and miR-148b and suggested that SRA1 negatively regulated miR-148b in cardiac myofibroblasts. Moreover, miR-148b knockdown stimulated cardiac myofibroblast activation, and miR-148b mediated promoting effect of SRA1 on cardiac myofibroblast activation [91].

3.6 Atherosclerosis

Atherosclerosis is a major cause of cardiovascular disease characterized by a chronic inflammatory response, with immune competent cells in lesions that produce mostly pro-inflammatory cytokines. Atherosclerosis is a very prevalent and important cardiac disease, involving the heart and brain.

Growing data has exposed the positive regulatory relationship between lncRNA and miRNA that modulate the proliferation and hypertrophy of vascular smooth muscle cells (VSMCs), contributing to the formation of atherosclerotic plaques. The lncRNA Ang362 was detected to be proximal to miR-221/222 gene and it was co-transcribed with miR-221/222 in VSMCs. The levels of Ang362 and miR-221/222 were increased upon AngII treatment in a time-dependent manner. Down-regulation of Ang362 reduced the expression of miR-221/222, as well as inhibited the proliferation of VSMCs. Evidences shown that lncRNA Ang362 exacerbated AngII-triggered vascular dysfunction via positive modulation of miR-221/222 [92].

In 2015, Tang and colleagues hypothesize that MALAT1 could regulate CXCR2 post-transcriptionally via ceRNA network in reaction to oxidized low-density lipoprotein (ox-LDL) induced endothelial dysfunction, that can lead to the development of atherosclerosis [93]. In patients with unstable angina MALAT1 was up-regulated and silencing of this lncRNA significantly down-regulated the expression of the gene CXCR2, a target for miR-22-3p, resulting in the increase of ox-LDL-induced endothelial injury. The authors proposed MALAT1 as a protector of the endothelium from ox-LDL-induced endothelial dysfunction by competing with miR-22-3p for endogenous RNA.

The lncRNA RP5-833A20.1 is located within intron 2 of the nuclear factor IA (NFIA) sequence, and its transcription direction is opposite to the host gene. NFIA expression was down-regulated in human acute monocytic leukemia macrophage-derived foam cells [94]. Also, it was demonstrated that RP5-833A20.1 could decrease NFIA expression by inducing miR-382-5p expression. The RP5-833A20.1/miR-382-5p/NFIA pathway was depicted as essential to the regulation of cholesterol homeostasis and inflammatory responses in human acute monocytic leukemia macrophages, although the gene relationship between RP5-833A20.1 and miR-382-5p remain barely explored and will need to be further investigated.

In 2016, miR-185-5p was identified as a negative regulator of the lncRNA retinal noncoding RNA3 (RNCR3) in the proliferation of endothelial cells (ECs) and vascular smooth muscle cells (VSMCs) [95]. The expression level of RNCR3 was found to be up-regulated in aortic atherosclerotic lesions and silencing of RNCR3 reduced the proliferation of ECs and VSMCs. When overexpressed, miR-185-5p decreased the levels of RNCR3, and knockdown of miR-185-5p increased the viability and proliferation of HUVECs, whilst this was partially reversed by RNCR3 silencing. The Krüppel-like factor 2 (KLF2) was detected as a target of miR-185-5p, regulated by RNCR3 as well. RNCR3 knockdown decreased the expression level of KLF2 and attenuated the viability and proliferation of HUVECs, while KLF2 overexpression compromised these effects.

The lncRNA DIGIT (divergent to GSC induced by TGF-β family signalling) was found to accelerate tube formation of vascular endothelial cells by targeting miR-134 [96]. The study by C. Miao, described that DIGIT silencing could significantly reduce cell viability, migration, tube-like structures formation and induced apoptosis in HMEC-1 cells. Also, DIGIT was demonstrated to be a sponge for miR-134, and the antigrowth, anti-migratory and anti-tube-formation functions of DIGIT silence on HMEC-1 cells were cancelled by miR-134 suppression.

3.7 Diabetic Cardiomyopathy

Diabetic cardiomyopathy (DCM) is a common complication of diabetes and can cause heart failure, arrhythmia, even sudden death. The pathogenesis of DCM includes altered metabolism, mitochondrial dysfunction, oxidative stress, inflammation, cardiac fibrosis, cell death and extracellular matrix remodelling [97].

In the research work by Zhou and colleagues, a rat model of DCM was established and the modulation by MIAT was characterized [98]. Later, they intended to determine the pathologic role of MIAT in the development of DCM. MIAT down-regulation was found to reduce cardiomyocyte apoptosis and improve left ventricular function in diabetic rats. The results of luciferase reporter and RNA immunoprecipitation assays revealed that MIAT targeted miR-22-3p. In addition, DAPK2 (death-associated protein kinase 2) a kinase involved in the regulation of cellular apoptosis, was characterized as a direct target of miR-22-3p. Also, MIAT overexpression counteracted the inhibitory effect of miR-22-3p on DAPK2. In addition, MIAT knockdown reduced DAPK2 expression and inhibit apoptosis in cardiomyocytes exposed to high glucose.

In a recent report, the lncRNA Kcnq1ot1 was documented to mediate a type of programmed cell death related to inflammation, pyroptosis in DCM [99]. The expression of Kcnq1ot1 was increased in patients with diabetes, high glucose-induced cardiomyocytes and diabetic mouse cardiac tissue. Knockdown of Kcnq1ot1 reduced pyroptosis by targeting miR-214-3p and caspase-1. In addition, inhibition of Kcnq1ot1 reduced cell death, cytoskeletal structure abnormalities and calcium overload in vitro and improved cardiac function and morphology in vivo.

3.8 Aortic Valve Disease

Aortic valve disease is a disorder caused by the malfunction of the valve between the left ventricle and aorta. Aortic valve disease may be a condition present at birth such as congenital heart disease, or it may result from other causes.

MALAT1, a highly abundant and conserved lncRNA, has been implicated in many cardiovascular diseases. Ectopic expression of MALAT1 was observed in calcific valves and after osteogenic induction in human aortic valve interstitial cells (VICs). In vitro experiments revealed that MALAT1 acted as a positive regulator of osteogenic differentiation by repressing miR-204 expression and activity and thereby promoting expression of osteoblast-specific markers, including alkaline phosphatase, mineralized bone matrix formation and osteocalcin. Smad4, protein involved in signal transduction, was identified as a direct target of miR-204. Data showed that MALAT1 could interact with miR-204 and overexpression of miR-204 reversed the up-regulation of Smad4 induced by MALAT1. Thus, MALAT1 positively regulated the expression of Smad4 through sponging miR-204, and promoted osteogenic differentiation of VICs [100].

4 circRNA–miRNA Interactions in Cardiovascular Diseases

Currently, circBase (www.circbase.org) registers 92,375 human circRNAs and 1903 mouse circRNAs. These molecules have been described to play relevant roles not only in the development of organisms, but also during pathological processes such as cardiovascular, neuronal diseases, cancer and other diseases [18, 101–105]. Their functional roles in specific biological contexts and their involvement in RNA-interaction networks are sources of further investigation.

4.1 Cardiac Hypertrophy and Heart Failure

The Heart-Related circRNA (HRCR) was discovered as the first circRNA that protects the heart from hypertrophy and heart failure. In fact HRCR was also the first circRNA whose association with pathological cardiac hypertrophy was observed [102]. This circRNA is transcribed from the Pwwp2a gene and is part of the HRCR/miR-223/ARC axis. Since HRCR has 6 binding sites for the miR-223, it down-regulates its activity. MiR-223 is a miRNA that down-regulates the expression of the Apoptosis Repressor with CARD Domain (ARC), as a negative inhibitor. Using a mouse model, Wang and colleagues, 2016, showed that the decreased levels of ARC in cardiomyocytes is responsible for hypertrophy and also found that HRCR has the ability to bind miR-223, repressing its function. The decreased availability of miR-223 is correlated with an increase in ARC protein production, which contributes to a lower number of apoptotic cardiomyocytes, therefore diminishing the effects of isoproterenol-induced cardiomyocyte hypertrophy and of pathological cardiac hypertrophy and heart failure [102].

4.2 Myocardial Infarction

Myocardial infarction (MI) is a major cause of morbidity and mortality worldwide, despite substantial improvements in diagnosis, prognosis and treatment over the past decades.

Among the relevant circRNAs involved in MI, Cdr1as was previously described as a miRNA sponge able to sequester miR-7 in neural cells by sequence complementarity [18, 33]. Geng et al. 2016, also verified that Cdr1as has a significant capacity to bind to miR-7a in mouse myocardial cells, thus regulating MI [101]. It was previously demonstrated that miR-7a protects the heart from MI in hypoxic cardiomyocytes, by negatively regulating the Poly (ADP-ribose) polymerase (PARP) and Sp1 transcription factor, thus suppressing ischemia/reperfusion-induced apoptosis [106]. PARP is a nuclear enzyme involved in many important cellular processes such as DNA damage repair and apoptosis, being the presence of cleaved PARP an indicator of apoptosis. During a cascade of apoptotic events, caspases 3/7 are activated and gain the ability to use PARP as substrate, thus proceeding to its cleavage and decreasing its ability to repair DNA errors [101, 106]. In ischemia/reperfusion (I/R) cardiomyocytes, this process is responsible for programmed cell death, which may lead to MI. Sp1 is a zinc-finger transcription factor that was also shown to play a major role in MI [101, 107]. Thus, miR-7a silencing is responsible for programmed cell death and the development of an MI typical phenotype [101].

Being a contractile and very dynamic organ, the heart requires a large amount of energy that is only produced if O_2 is profusely available. Myocardial mitochondria are very abundant, being major key players in the production of energy in the form of ATP by the electron transport chain [108]. Wang and colleagues found for the first time that circRNA molecules are also implied in the regulation of heart mitochondrial dynamics and consequent cardiomyocyte apoptosis. Recurring to anoxia-reoxygenation (A/R)-induced mouse cardiomyocytes and a model of ischemia-reperfusion (I/R)-induced MI mice, they have shown that the mitochondrial fission and apoptosis-related circRNA (MFACR) is responsible for mitochondrial fission. MFACR is expressed in oxygen deprivation and it originates from the exon 5 of the SET and MYND domain-containing 4 (Smyd4) gene. The mitochondrial protein 18 (MTP18) is overexpressed in cardiomyocytes under conditions of A/R. MTP18 actively participates in MI, activating mitochondrial fission and cardiomyocyte apoptosis [7, 109, 110]. MiR-652-3p has the ability to suppress apoptosis by binding to the 3′-UTR region of the mRNA generated by transcription of the MTP18 gene, inhibiting its expression and reducing the number of apoptotic cells [7]. The circRNA MFACR has 15 MREs for miR-652-3p and it is able to competitively down-regulate miR-652-3p [7]. In summary, MFACR is a pro-apoptotic circRNA that indirectly and positively regulates the expression of MTP18, which increases mitochondrial fission and cardiomyocyte apoptosis in ischemic hearts [7].

Moreover, Li and colleagues, 2018, recurring to in vitro methodologies, have demonstrated that circNCX1 is also associated with apoptosis in mouse cardiomyocytes. They have shown that an increase in the levels of circNCX1 in hydrogen peroxide-exposed stressed neonatal cardiomyocytes and H9c2 cells and in a MI mouse model, leads to a drastic increase in cardiomyocyte apoptotic rate [111]. This circRNA is generated from the second exon of the sodium/calcium exchanger 1 (ncx1) gene. This circRNA's up-regulation occurs as a result of exposure to reactive oxygen species (ROS) and was shown to worsen the myocardial I/R damage effects. Increased circNCX1 synthesis leads to decreased levels of miR-133a-3p, a miRNA that was previously shown to be linked to hypertrophic cardiomyopathy and heart failure [111, 112]. CircNCX1 harbors 8 putative binding-sites that exhibit imperfect complementarity to miR-133a-3p. MiR-133a-3p targets the cell death-inducing p53-target protein 1 (CDIP1), a transducer that mediates some major steps of apoptotic events [113]. Thus, low levels of miR-133a-3p lead to an increase in the number of apoptotic cardiomyocytes. Li's work was the first to demonstrate the relation of the circNCX1/miR-133a-3p/CDIP1 axis with myocardial injury [111].

NcRNAs can be found in various body fluids and may function as disease biomarkers [114–116]. Extracellular circRNA may be found encapsulated inside extracellular vesicles, like exosomes [117, 118]. The blood transcriptome is an excellent source of RNA biomarkers for many diseases: For instance circulating hsa_circ_0001785 can be used to detect breast cancer [105] and circulating hsa_circ_0124644 can be detected as a biomarker of coronary artery disease (CAD) [119]. As circRNAs are very abundant in peripheral blood and resistant to exoribonuclease action, these molecules may be used as non-invasive biomarkers of heart disease [21, 22, 115, 116, 119, 120]. For example Deng et al. demonstrated that circRNA_081881 is down-regulated in the plasma of Acute Myocardial Infarction (AMI) patients alongside with the Peroxisome proliferator-activated receptor gamma (PPARγ), a transcription factor. Knockdown of circRNA_081881 by siRNA had an impact on the decrease of PPARγ, which suggested that circRNA_081881 is directly related to PPARγ expression. Moreover, the group showed that this circRNA has 7 MREs for miR-548, being PPARγ one of its targets [114].

Additionally, the Myocardial Infarction-associated circular RNA (MICRA), a circRNA that is originated from the exon 1 of the zinc finger protein 609 (ZNF609) gene is down-regulated in the blood of MI patients. Salgado-Somoza et al. reported that MICRA, may be used to diagnose left ventricular (LV) dysfunction risk and differentiate its severity in three different groups in patients that undergo through AMI at reperfusion time [116]. It was shown in colon tissue that a similar circular transcript (circZNF609) derived from the same gene locus, regulates miR-150-5p [121]. As miR-150 is up-regulated in LV remodeling after AMI [122], it is predicted that MICRA is able to regulate miR-150 in MI [116].

4.3 Cardiac Fibrosis

Fibrosis is a condition characterized by myofibroblast activation and an increase of fibrotic protein synthesis. These proteins are actively secreted into the extracellular space, forming a collagen matrix that increases the myocardium stiffness. Cases of arrhythmia and heart failure may occur due to fibrosis in conditions such as diabetic cardio-myopathy (DCM) [103, 123, 124].

Tang et al. 2017, studied the effect of circRNA_000203 on the development of DCM in a diabetic mice model. This circRNA is transcribed from the Myo9a gene and it contains the exons 7–15 and respective flanking sequences of the introns 6 and 15. Two binding sites for miR-26b-5p, a miRNA involved in the suppression of Col1a2 and CTGF expression, were reported within circRNA_000203 [103]. Col1a2 is a peptide that can be found in type I collagen and CTGF is an extracellular growth factor protein responsible for the regeneration of damaged tissue that can be found in fibrotic tissues as well [103, 125]. The circRNA_000203/miR-26b-5p interaction results in an overexpression of Col1a2 and CTGF, which are the main cause for the appearance of a fibrotic phenotype in DCM. Moreover, higher levels of circRNA_000203 in mouse diabetic myocardium and in Ang-II-induced cardiac fibroblasts are responsible, not only for the Col1a2 and CTGF up-regulation but they are also accompanied by an increase in Col3a1 and α-SMA levels. Therefore, an increased cardiac rigidity, arrhythmias and decreased myocardial thickness may occur when circRNA_000203 is up-regulated [103].

In addition to circRNA_000203, circRNA_010567 has also been shown to be involved in diabetic cardiomyopathy in diabetic mouse myocardium and in Ang-II-induced cardiac fibroblasts (CFs) [125]. Zhou and colleagues, 2017, recurring to in silico techniques, found that circRNA_010567 has miR-141 binding sites in its structure. MiR-141 negatively regulates the expression of the pivotal fibrosis protein TGF-β1, as demonstrated by a validation performed by dual-luciferase assay [125]. Since

TGF-β1 is a fibrotic protein, its overexpression is responsible for the fibrotic phenotype that is characteristic in DCM hearts. The down-regulation of circRNA_010567 is able to ameliorate the fibrotic condition and is also accompanied by decreased expression of Col1a2, Col3a1 and α-SMA, all of them fibrosis-associated proteins [125]. A better understanding of regulatory events involving these pro-fibrotic circRNAs (circRNA_000203 and circRNA_010567) it would be of great importance to derive new treatments for DCM [103, 125].

4.4 Hypoxic Angiogenesis and Endothelial Disorders

ZNF609 locus may produce at least two different major circRNA isoforms: MICRA, which was discussed previously, and circZNF609 (Fig. 4.2). CircZNF609 was shown to be abundant in endothelial cells of individuals that suffered from diabetes mellitus, hypertension and coronary artery disease (CAD), thus causing pathological angiogenesis. CircZNF609 may act as a miRNA sponge by interacting with miR-615, which is a negative regulator of the Myocyte Enhancer Factor 2A (MEF2A), a protein that acts as a transcription factor and is intricately associated with CAD and MI [126]. In hypoxic and high glucose content conditions, circZNF609 is up-regulated and may cause tube formation, migration of endothelial cells and even trigger programmed cell death. The silencing of circZNF609 diminishes the effects of endothelial damage [127, 128]. Surprisingly, circZNF609 contains an small open reading frame in its sequence that could be translated, although further investigation is necessary to understand the physiological role of the encoded micro-peptide sequence [129].

Other putative "sponge-effects" involving circRNA molecules were also described in knock-down assays carried out on hypoxic conditions. For instance, hsa_circ_000595 can promote apoptosis in aortic smooth muscle cells. It was shown that the overexpression of this circRNA is accompanied by miR-19a down-regulation [130]. On the other hand, hsa_circ_0010729 was characterized as a vascular cell apoptosis suppressor by inhibiting the activity of miR-186. This miRNA acts as a pro-apoptotic factor that down-regulates the activity of the hypoxia inducible factor 1 alpha (HIF-1α), an anti-stress protein involved in angiogenesis during hypoxic conditions. It was verified that hsa_circ_0010729 diminishes the effects of hypoxia by regulating the vascular endothelial cell proliferation [131].

4.5 Stroke

Stroke occurs when the supply of O_2 that reaches the brain decreases dramatically, leading to serious tissue damage that worsens the normal function of the organ and can have severe consequences for patients. Most of the strokes are caused by ischemic events (ischemic stroke; IS), in which the blood flow decreases due to plaque formation. However with less frequency, vascular rupture may also occur leading to hemorrhagic stroke [132–134].

Recurring to miRNA pull down assays and FISH (fluorescent in situ hybridization), Bai and her group revealed that circDLGAP4 is down-regulated in IS patients and in a transient middle cerebral artery occlusion (tMCAO) mouse model. CircDLGAP4 is back-spliced from exons 8–10 of the DLGAP4 gene and has sponging activity over miR-143. High levels of miR-143 are responsible for a lower expression of tight junction proteins which leads to epithelial-mesenchymal transition. In fact miR-143 negatively regulates the homologous to the E6-AP C-terminus domain E3 ubiquitin protein ligase 1 (HECTD1), whose down-regulation is responsible for increasing neurological deficits, an increase in the damage induced in the blood-brain barrier and ultimately IS [135].

Additionally, it was found in tMCAO, in human glioblastoma A172 cell line treated with oxygen glucose deprivation-reperfusion and in IS patients' blood, that the same HECTD1 locus is able to produce a circRNA that down-regulates the expression of miR-142, called circHECTD1. CircHECTD1 contains the exons 23 and 24 of the HECTD1 gene. The effect of this interaction is responsible for astrocyte activation due to the expression of autophagic proteins, thus leading to cerebral infarction. TCDD-inducible poly (ADP-ribose) polymerase (TIPARP) is a target of miR-142 and participates in ischemic stroke. Down-regulation of circHECTD1 is responsible for lower levels of TIPARP, which reduces the risk for brain infarction [136].

4.6 Atherosclerosis

Atherosclerosis is a consequence of plaque deposition in arteries. In a worse case, atherosclerosis can lead to coronary artery disease (CAD), which is one of the major causes of cardiovascular diseases in the world [137]. Carotid artery disease occurs during plaque deposition in the walls of the arteries of the same name.

Bazan and colleagues studied the relative abundance of hsa_circ_0000284 (which they refer as circR-284) and miR-221 in the plasma of patients that suffered from recent carotid-related cerebrovascular ischemic event and a control group. MiR-221 is able to down-regulate the expression of the cyclin-dependent kinase p27^{Kip1} [138, 139]. This kinase blocks the cell cycle of vascular smooth muscle cells (VSMC). The down-regulation of this protein is able to promote carotid Intima-media thickness [138]. It was found that circR-284 levels were elevated in the patients that suffered carotid artery disease in the past 5 days, whilst miR-221 levels were down-regulated, in comparison with the control group. This suggested that circR-284 may inhibit miR-221 activity by sponging it. In fact, the same group reported one binding site in the circRNA molecule. Moreover, relative amounts of circR-284 and miR-221 constitute a biomarker to diagnose plaque rupture in the carotid artery, as in other arteries. Additionally, they claim that these molecules ratio can be considered as a prognostic biomarker for stroke risk [115].

4.7 Coronary Artery Disease

As already mentioned, CAD is a cardiovascular disease that presents high mortality and morbidity [137]. Several research groups have focused on the study of circRNA and miRNA co-expression in CAD patients in order to find molecular biomarkers for this disease [140, 141]. In one of these studies, 24 circRNAs were differentially expressed in the blood of individuals with CAD. Among these 24 circRNAs, 9 (hsa_circ_0089378, hsa_circ_0083357, hsa_circ_0082824, hsa_circ_0068942, hsa_circ_0057576, hsa_circ_0054537, hsa_circ_0051172, hsa_circ_0032970 and hsa_circ_0006323) were up-regulated, along with the Transient Receptor Potential Cation Channel Subfamily M Member 3 (TRPM3) [140]. TRPM3 is a channel protein able to regulate the calcium membrane gradient and it is responsible for the proliferation and contractility of vascular smooth muscle cells [142]. This channel protein is regulated by miR-130a-3p and it is not expressed in individuals with CAD. Using bioinformatics tools, Pan and his colleagues revealed that these 9 circRNAs have binding sites for miR-130a-3p. This study is merely prospective and requires validation of the in silico results by laboratorial methods [140].

5 Conclusion and Perspectives

Increasing evidence suggests that ncRNAs displays distinctive functions in the regulation of genomic output. Also, emerging data highlights the regulation of several molecular events under pathological circumstances through interactions between lncRNAs, circRNAs and miRNAs (Tables 4.1 and 4.2). These entangled networks of RNA regulatory and functional interactions appeared to be in the core of the delicate molecular balance that controls cell homeostasis. Understanding this RNA regulatory crosstalk may clarify the cell gene regulatory networks and can have new implications in the characterization of the molecular events that control cell physiology and disease.

In this chapter, we described that ncRNAs interactions can regulate multiple pathological processes in CVDs including myocardial hypertrophy, fibrosis, necrosis, apoptosis, autophagy as well as vascular cell apoptosis and proliferation. Additionally, the manipulation of ncRNAs expression levels by either inhibiting the up-regulated lncRNAs/circRNAs or increasing down-regulated lncRNAs/circRNAs illustrate future novel therapeutic strategies in cardiovascular diseases.

In the future, development of high-throughput sequencing and new interfering technologies may lead to further identification of ncRNAs involved in the pathophysiology of cardiovascular diseases, and more meaningful translational studies will be needed.

References

1. Carninci P, Kasukawa T, Katayama S, Gough J, Frith MC, Maeda N, Oyama R, Ravasi T, Lenhard B, Wells C, Kodzius R, Shimokawa K, Bajic VB, Brenner SE, Batalov S, Forrest AR, Zavolan M, Davis MJ, Wilming LG, Aidinis V, Allen JE, Ambesi-Impiombato A, Apweiler R, Aturaliya RN, Bailey TL, Bansal M, Baxter L, Beisel KW, Bersano T, Bono H, Chalk AM, Chiu KP, Choudhary V, Christoffels A, Clutterbuck DR, Crowe ML, Dalla E, Dalrymple BP, de Bono B, Della Gatta G, di Bernardo D, Down T, Engstrom P, Fagiolini M, Faulkner G, Fletcher CF, Fukushima T, Furuno M, Futaki S, Gariboldi M, Georgii-Hemming P, Gingeras TR, Gojobori T, Green RE, Gustincich S, Harbers M, Hayashi Y, Hensch TK, Hirokawa N, Hill D, Huminiecki L, Iacono M, Ikeo K, Iwama A, Ishikawa T, Jakt M, Kanapin A, Katoh M, Kawasawa Y, Kelso J, Kitamura H, Kitano H, Kollias G, Krishnan SP, Kruger A, Kummerfeld SK, Kurochkin IV, Lareau LF, Lazarevic D, Lipovich L, Liu J, Liuni S, McWilliam S, Madan Babu M, Madera M, Marchionni L, Matsuda H, Matsuzawa S, Miki H, Mignone F, Miyake S, Morris K, Mottagui-Tabar S, Mulder N, Nakano N, Nakauchi H, Ng P, Nilsson R, Nishiguchi S, Nishikawa S, Nori F, Ohara O, Okazaki Y, Orlando V, Pang KC, Pavan WJ, Pavesi G, Pesole G, Petrovsky N, Piazza S, Reed J, Reid JF, Ring BZ, Ringwald M, Rost B, Ruan Y, Salzberg SL, Sandelin A, Schneider C, Schonbach C, Sekiguchi K, Semple CA, Seno S, Sessa L, Sheng Y, Shibata Y, Shimada H, Shimada K, Silva D, Sinclair B, Sperling S, Stupka E, Sugiura K, Sultana R, Takenaka Y, Taki K, Tammoja K, Tan SL, Tang S, Taylor MS, Tegner J, Teichmann SA, Ueda HR, van Nimwegen E, Verardo R, Wei CL, Yagi K, Yamanishi H, Zabarovsky E, Zhu S, Zimmer A, Hide W, Bult C, Grimmond SM, Teasdale RD, Liu ET, Brusic V, Quackenbush J, Wahlestedt C, Mattick JS, Hume DA, Kai C, Sasaki D, Tomaru Y, Fukuda S, Kanamori-Katayama M, Suzuki M, Aoki J, Arakawa T, Iida J, Imamura K, Itoh M, Kato T, Kawaji H, Kawagashira N, Kawashima T, Kojima M, Kondo S, Konno H, Nakano K, Ninomiya N, Nishio T, Okada M, Plessy C, Shibata K, Shiraki T, Suzuki S, Tagami M, Waki K, Watahiki A, Okamura-Oho Y, Suzuki H, Kawai J, Hayashizaki Y, Consortium F, Group RGER, Genome Science G. The transcriptional landscape of the mammalian genome. Science. 2005;309(5740):1559–63.
2. Zhang XO, Fu Y, Mou H, Xue W, Weng Z. The temporal landscape of recursive splicing during Pol II transcription elongation in human cells. PLoS Genet. 2018;14(8):e1007579.
3. Klattenhoff CA, Scheuermann JC, Surface LE, Bradley RK, Fields PA, Steinhauser ML, Ding H, Butty VL, Torrey L, Haas S, Abo R, Tabebordbar M, Lee RT, Burge CB, Boyer LA. Braveheart, a long noncoding RNA required for cardiovascular lineage commitment. Cell. 2013;152(3):570–83.
4. Micheletti R, Plaisance I, Abraham BJ, Sarre A, Ting CC, Alexanian M, Maric D, Maison D, Nemir M, Young RA, Schroen B, Gonzalez A, Ounzain S, Pedrazzini T. The long noncoding RNA Wisper controls cardiac fibrosis and remodeling. Sci Transl Med. 2017;9(395):pii: eaai9118.
5. Gupta SK, Foinquinos A, Thum S, Remke J, Zimmer K, Bauters C, de Groote P, Boon RA, de Windt LJ, Preissl S, Hein L, Batkai S, Pinet F, Thum T. Preclinical development of a MicroRNA-based therapy for elderly patients with myocardial infarction. J Am Coll Cardiol. 2016;68(14):1557–71.
6. Wang K, An T, Zhou LY, Liu CY, Zhang XJ, Feng C, Li PF. E2F1-regulated miR-30b suppresses Cyclophilin D and protects heart from ischemia/reperfusion injury and necrotic cell death. Cell Death Differ. 2015;22(5):743–54.
7. Wang K, Gan TY, Li N, Liu CY, Zhou LY, Gao JN, Chen C, Yan KW, Ponnusamy M, Zhang YH, Li PF. Circular RNA mediates cardiomyocyte death via miRNA-dependent upregulation of MTP18 expression. Cell Death Differ. 2017;24:1111–20.
8. Kumar SM, Liu S, Lu H, Zhang H, Zhang PJ, Gimotty PA, Guerra M, Guo W, Xu X. Acquired cancer stem cell phenotypes through Oct4-mediated dedifferentiation. Oncogene. 2012;31(47):4898–911.
9. Wang Y, Xu Z, Jiang J, Xu C, Kang J, Xiao L, Wu M, Xiong J, Guo X, Liu H. Endogenous miRNA sponge lincRNA-RoR regulates Oct4, Nanog, and Sox2 in human embryonic stem cell self-renewal. Dev Cell. 2013;25(1):69–80.
10. Yang J, Li T, Gao C, Lv X, Liu K, Song H, Xing Y, Xi T. FOXO1 3′UTR functions as a ceRNA in repressing the metastases of breast cancer

cells via regulating miRNA activity. FEBS Lett. 2014;588(17):3218–24.
11. Esteller M. Non-coding RNAs in human disease. Nat Rev Genet. 2011;12(12):861–74.
12. Ha M, Kim VN. Regulation of microRNA biogenesis. Nat Rev Mol Cell Biol. 2014;15(8):509–24.
13. Huntzinger E, Izaurralde E. Gene silencing by microRNAs: contributions of translational repression and mRNA decay. Nat Rev Genet. 2011;12(2):99–110.
14. Whitehead J, Pandey GK, Kanduri C. Regulation of the mammalian epigenome by long noncoding RNAs. Biochim Biophys Acta. 2009;1790(9):936–47.
15. Quinn JJ, Chang HY. Unique features of long non-coding RNA biogenesis and function. Nat Rev Genet. 2016;17(1):47–62.
16. Marchese FP, Raimondi I, Huarte M. The multidimensional mechanisms of long noncoding RNA function. Genome Biol. 2017;18(1):206.
17. Salzman J, Gawad C, Wang PL, Lacayo N, Brown PO. Circular RNAs are the predominant transcript isoform from hundreds of human genes in diverse cell types. PLoS One. 2012;7(2):e30733.
18. Memczak S, Jens M, Elefsinioti A, Torti F, Krueger J, Rybak A, Maier L, Mackowiak SD, Gregersen LH, Munschauer M, Loewer A, Ziebold U, Landthaler M, Kocks C, le Noble F, Rajewsky N. Circular RNAs are a large class of animal RNAs with regulatory potency. Nature. 2013;495(7441):333–8.
19. Sanger HL, Klotz G, Riesner D, Gross HJ, Kleinschmidt AK. Viroids are single-stranded covalently closed circular RNA molecules existing as highly base-paired rod-like structures. Proc Natl Acad Sci U S A. 1976;73(11):3852–6.
20. Cocquerelle C, Mascrez B, Hetuin D, Bailleul B. Mis-splicing yields circular RNA molecules. FASEB J. 1993;7(1):155–60.
21. Jeck WR, Sorrentino JA, Wang K, Slevin MK, Burd CE, Liu J, Marzluff WF, Sharpless NE. Circular RNAs are abundant, conserved, and associated with ALU repeats. RNA. 2013;19(2):141–57.
22. Maass PG, Glazar P, Memczak S, Dittmar G, Hollfinger I, Schreyer L, Sauer AV, Toka O, Aiuti A, Luft FC, Rajewsky N. A map of human circular RNAs in clinically relevant tissues. J Mol Med. 2017;95(11):1179–89.
23. Liang D, Wilusz JE. Short intronic repeat sequences facilitate circular RNA production. Genes Dev. 2014;28(20):2233–47.
24. Ashwal-Fluss R, Meyer M, Pamudurti NR, Ivanov A, Bartok O, Hanan M, Evantal N, Memczak S, Rajewsky N, Kadener S. circRNA biogenesis competes with pre-mRNA splicing. Mol Cell. 2014;56(1):55–66.
25. Conn SJ, Pillman KA, Toubia J, Conn VM, Salmanidis M, Phillips CA, Roslan S, Schreiber AW, Gregory PA, Goodall GJ. The RNA binding protein quaking regulates formation of circRNAs. Cell. 2015;160(6):1125–34.
26. Zhang XO, Dong R, Zhang Y, Zhang JL, Luo Z, Zhang J, Chen LL, Yang L. Diverse alternative back-splicing and alternative splicing landscape of circular RNAs. Genome Res. 2016;26(9):1277–87.
27. Salzman J, Chen RE, Olsen MN, Wang PL, Brown PO. Cell-type specific features of circular RNA expression. PLoS Genet. 2013;9(9):e1003777.
28. Bachmayr-Heyda A, Reiner AT, Auer K, Sukhbaatar N, Aust S, Bachleitner-Hofmann T, Mesteri I, Grunt TW, Zeillinger R, Pils D. Correlation of circular RNA abundance with proliferation-exemplified with colorectal and ovarian cancer, idiopathic lung fibrosis, and normal human tissues. Sci Rep. 2015;5:8057.
29. Enuka Y, Lauriola M, Feldman ME, Sas-Chen A, Ulitsky I, Yarden Y. Circular RNAs are long-lived and display only minimal early alterations in response to a growth factor. Nucleic Acids Res. 2016;44(3):1370–83.
30. Ebbesen KK, Kjems J, Hansen TB. Circular RNAs: identification, biogenesis and function. Biochim Biophys Acta. 2016;1859(1):163–8.
31. Talhouarne GJ, Gall JG. Lariat intronic RNAs in the cytoplasm of Xenopus tropicalis oocytes. RNA. 2014;20(9):1476–87.
32. Li Z, Huang C, Bao C, Chen L, Lin M, Wang X, Zhong G, Yu B, Hu W, Dai L, Zhu P, Chang Z, Wu Q, Zhao Y, Jia Y, Xu P, Liu H, Shan G. Exon-intron circular RNAs regulate transcription in the nucleus. Nat Struct Mol Biol. 2015;22(3):256–64.
33. Hansen TB, Jensen TI, Clausen BH, Bramsen JB, Finsen B, Damgaard CK, Kjems J. Natural RNA circles function as efficient microRNA sponges. Nature. 2013;495(7441):384–8.
34. Salmena L, Poliseno L, Tay Y, Kats L, Pandolfi PP. A ceRNA hypothesis: the Rosetta Stone of a hidden RNA language? Cell. 2011;146(3):353–8.
35. Shimizu I, Minamino T. Physiological and pathological cardiac hypertrophy. J Mol Cell Cardiol. 2016;97:245–62.
36. Jiang F, Zhou X, Huang J. Long non-coding RNA-ROR mediates the reprogramming in cardiac hypertrophy. PLoS One. 2016;11(4):e0152767.
37. Salamon I, Saccani Jotti G, Condorelli G. The long noncoding RNA landscape in cardiovascular disease: a brief update. Curr Opin Cardiol. 2018;33(3):282–9.
38. Gabory A, Ripoche MA, Yoshimizu T, Dandolo L. The H19 gene: regulation and function of a non-coding RNA. Cytogenet Genome Res. 2006;113(1–4):188–93.
39. Wang JX, Zhang XJ, Li Q, Wang K, Wang Y, Jiao JQ, Feng C, Teng S, Zhou LY, Gong Y, Zhou ZX, Liu J, Wang JL, Li PF. MicroRNA-103/107 regulate programmed necrosis and myocardial ischemia/reperfusion injury through targeting FADD. Circ Res. 2015;117(4):352–63.
40. Han Y, Xu H, Cheng J, Zhang Y, Gao C, Fan T, Peng B, Li B, Liu L, Cheng Z. Downregulation of long non-coding RNA H19 promotes P19CL6 cells proliferation and inhibits apoptosis during late-stage

cardiac differentiation via miR-19b-modulated Sox6. Cell Biosci. 2016;6:58.
41. Keniry A, Oxley D, Monnier P, Kyba M, Dandolo L, Smits G, Reik W. The H19 lincRNA is a developmental reservoir of miR-675 that suppresses growth and Igf1r. Nat Cell Biol. 2012;14(7):659–65.
42. Liu L, An X, Li Z, Song Y, Li L, Zuo S, Liu N, Yang G, Wang H, Cheng X, Zhang Y, Yang X, Wang J. The H19 long noncoding RNA is a novel negative regulator of cardiomyocyte hypertrophy. Cardiovasc Res. 2016;111(1):56–65.
43. Cai B, Ma W, Bi C, Yang F, Zhang L, Han Z, Huang Q, Ding F, Li Y, Yan G, Pan Z, Yang B, Lu Y. Long noncoding RNA H19 mediates melatonin inhibition of premature senescence of c-kit(+) cardiac progenitor cells by promoting miR-675. J Pineal Res. 2016;61(1):82–95.
44. Wang K, Liu F, Zhou LY, Long B, Yuan SM, Wang Y, Liu CY, Sun T, Zhang XJ, Li PF. The long noncoding RNA CHRF regulates cardiac hypertrophy by targeting miR-489. Circ Res. 2014;114(9):1377–88.
45. Ishii N, Ozaki K, Sato H, Mizuno H, Saito S, Takahashi A, Miyamoto Y, Ikegawa S, Kamatani N, Hori M, Saito S, Nakamura Y, Tanaka T. Identification of a novel non-coding RNA, MIAT, that confers risk of myocardial infarction. J Hum Genet. 2006;51(12):1087–99.
46. Papait R, Kunderfranco P, Stirparo GG, Latronico MV, Condorelli G. Long noncoding RNA: a new player of heart failure? J Cardiovasc Transl Res. 2013;6(6):876–83.
47. Vausort M, Wagner DR, Devaux Y. Long noncoding RNAs in patients with acute myocardial infarction. Circ Res. 2014;115(7):668–77.
48. Yan B, Yao J, Liu JY, Li XM, Wang XQ, Li YJ, Tao ZF, Song YC, Chen Q, Jiang Q. lncRNA-MIAT regulates microvascular dysfunction by functioning as a competing endogenous RNA. Circ Res. 2015;116(7):1143–56.
49. Sun C, Huang L, Li Z, Leng K, Xu Y, Jiang X, Cui Y. Long non-coding RNA MIAT in development and disease: a new player in an old game. J Biomed Sci. 2018;25(1):23.
50. Zhu XH, Yuan YX, Rao SL, Wang P. LncRNA MIAT enhances cardiac hypertrophy partly through sponging miR-150. Eur Rev Med Pharmacol Sci. 2016;20(17):3653–60.
51. Li Y, Wang J, Sun L, Zhu S. LncRNA myocardial infarction-associated transcript (MIAT) contributed to cardiac hypertrophy by regulating TLR4 via miR-93. Eur J Pharmacol. 2018;818:508–17.
52. Hou P, Zhao Y, Li Z, Yao R, Ma M, Gao Y, Zhao L, Zhang Y, Huang B, Lu J. LincRNA-ROR induces epithelial-to-mesenchymal transition and contributes to breast cancer tumorigenesis and metastasis. Cell Death Dis. 2014;5:e1287.
53. Fu Z, Li G, Li Z, Wang Y, Zhao Y, Zheng S, Ye H, Luo Y, Zhao X, Wei L, Liu Y, Lin Q, Zhou Q, Chen R. Endogenous miRNA sponge LincRNA-ROR promotes proliferation, invasion and stem cell-like phenotype of pancreatic cancer cells. Cell Death Dis. 2017;3:17004.
54. Wang K, Xu Y, Sun Q, Long J, Liu J, Ding J. Mitochondria regulate cardiac contraction through ATP-dependent and independent mechanisms. Free Radic Res. 2018;52(11–12):1256–65.
55. Lv L, Li T, Li X, Xu C, Liu Q, Jiang H, Li Y, Liu Y, Yan H, Huang Q, Zhou Y, Zhang M, Shan H, Liang H. The lncRNA Plscr4 controls cardiac hypertrophy by regulating miR-214. Mol Ther Nucleic Acids. 2018;10:387–97.
56. Schrepfer E, Scorrano L. Mitofusins, from mitochondria to metabolism. Mol Cell. 2016;61(5):683–94.
57. Lai Y, He S, Ma L, Lin H, Ren B, Ma J, Zhu X, Zhuang S. HOTAIR functions as a competing endogenous RNA to regulate PTEN expression by inhibiting miR-19 in cardiac hypertrophy. Mol Cell Biochem. 2017;432(1–2):179–87.
58. Luan W, Li R, Liu L, Ni X, Shi Y, Xia Y, Wang J, Lu F, Xu B. Long non-coding RNA HOTAIR acts as a competing endogenous RNA to promote malignant melanoma progression by sponging miR-152-3p. Oncotarget. 2017;8(49):85401–14.
59. Li C, Zhou G, Feng J, Zhang J, Hou L, Cheng Z. Upregulation of lncRNA VDR/CASC15 induced by facilitates cardiac hypertrophy through modulating miR-432-5p/TLR4 axis. Biochem Biophys Res Commun. 2018;503(4):2407–14.
60. Minajigi A, Froberg J, Wei C, Sunwoo H, Kesner B, Colognori D, Lessing D, Payer B, Boukhali M, Haas W, Lee JT. Chromosomes A comprehensive Xist interactome reveals cohesin repulsion and an RNA-directed chromosome conformation. Science. 2015;349(6245)
61. Zhou T, Qin G, Yang L, Xiang D, Li S. LncRNA XIST regulates myocardial infarction by targeting miR-130a-3p. J Cell Physiol. 2017;234(6):8659–67.
62. Wang H, Shen Q, Zhang X, Yang C, Cui S, Sun Y, Wang L, Fan X, Xu S. The long non-coding RNA XIST controls non-small cell lung cancer proliferation and invasion by modulating miR-186-5p. Cell Physiol Biochem. 2017;41(6):2221–9.
63. Gu S, Xie R, Liu X, Shou J, Gu W, Che X. Long coding RNA XIST contributes to neuronal apoptosis through the downregulation of AKT phosphorylation and is negatively regulated by miR-494 in rat spinal cord injury. Int J Mol Sci. 2017;18(4):pii: E732.
64. Chen Y, Liu X, Chen L, Chen W, Zhang Y, Chen J, Wu X, Zhao Y, Wu X, Sun G. The long noncoding RNA XIST protects cardiomyocyte hypertrophy by targeting miR-330-3p. Biochem Biophys Res Commun. 2018;505(3):807–15.
65. Tsoporis JN, Mohammadzadeh F, Parker TG. S100B: a multifunctional role in cardiovascular pathophysiology. Amino Acids. 2011;41(4):843–7.
66. Xiao L, Gu Y, Sun Y, Chen J, Wang X, Zhang Y, Gao L, Li L. The long noncoding RNA XIST regulates cardiac hypertrophy by targeting miR-101. J Cell Physiol. 2019;234(8):13680–92.

67. Reed GW, Rossi JE, Cannon CP. Acute myocardial infarction. Lancet. 2017;389(10065):197–210.
68. Qu X, Du Y, Shu Y, Gao M, Sun F, Luo S, Yang T, Zhan L, Yuan Y, Chu W, Pan Z, Wang Z, Yang B, Lu Y. MIAT is a pro-fibrotic long non-coding RNA governing cardiac fibrosis in post-infarct myocardium. Sci Rep. 2017;7:42657.
69. Wang K, Liu CY, Zhou LY, Wang JX, Wang M, Zhao B, Zhao WK, Xu SJ, Fan LH, Zhang XJ, Feng C, Wang CQ, Zhao YF, Li PF. APF lncRNA regulates autophagy and myocardial infarction by targeting miR-188-3p. Nat Commun. 2015;6:6779.
70. Huang S, Chen M, Li L, He M, Hu D, Zhang X, Li J, Tanguay RM, Feng J, Cheng L, Zeng H, Dai X, Deng Q, Hu FB, Wu T. Circulating MicroRNAs and the occurrence of acute myocardial infarction in Chinese populations. Circ Cardiovasc Genet. 2014;7(2):189–98.
71. Hu H, Wu J, Li D, Zhou J, Yu H, Ma L. Knockdown of lncRNA MALAT1 attenuates acute myocardial infarction through miR-320-Pten axis. Biomed Pharmacother. 2018;106:738–46.
72. Gong LC, Xu HM, Guo GL, Zhang T, Shi JW, Chang C. Long non-coding RNA H19 protects H9c2 cells against hypoxia-induced injury by targeting microRNA-139. Cell Physiol Biochem. 2017;44(3):857–69.
73. Gong L, Xu H, Chang H, Tong Y, Zhang T, Guo G. Knockdown of long non-coding RNA MEG3 protects H9c2 cells from hypoxia-induced injury by targeting microRNA-183. J Cell Biochem. 2018;119(2):1429–40.
74. Yin G, Yang X, Li Q, Guo Z. GATA1 activated lncRNA (Galont) promotes anoxia/reoxygenation-induced autophagy and cell death in cardiomyocytes by sponging miR-338. J Cell Biochem. 2018;119(5):4161–9.
75. Wu T, Wu D, Wu Q, Zou B, Huang X, Cheng X, Wu Y, Hong K, Li P, Yang R, Li Y, Cheng Y. Knockdown of long non-coding RNA-ZFAS1 protects cardiomyocytes against acute myocardial infarction via anti-apoptosis by regulating miR-150/CRP. J Cell Biochem. 2017;118(10):3281–9.
76. Chen G, Li H, Li X, Li B, Zhong L, Huang S, Zheng H, Li M, Jin G, Liao W, Liao Y, Chen Y, Bin J. Loss of long non-coding RNA CRRL promotes cardiomyocyte regeneration and improves cardiac repair by functioning as a competing endogenous RNA. J Mol Cell Cardiol. 2018;122:152–64.
77. van Empel VP, Bertrand AT, Hofstra L, Crijns HJ, Doevendans PA, De Windt LJ. Myocyte apoptosis in heart failure. Cardiovasc Res. 2005;67(1):21–9.
78. Suen DF, Norris KL, Youle RJ. Mitochondrial dynamics and apoptosis. Genes Dev. 2008;22(12):1577–90.
79. Wang K, Long B, Zhou LY, Liu F, Zhou QY, Liu CY, Fan YY, Li PF. CARL lncRNA inhibits anoxia-induced mitochondrial fission and apoptosis in cardiomyocytes by impairing miR-539-dependent PHB2 downregulation. Nat Commun. 2014;5:3596.
80. Wang K, Sun T, Li N, Wang Y, Wang JX, Zhou LY, Long B, Liu CY, Liu F, Li PF. MDRL lncRNA regulates the processing of miR-484 primary transcript by targeting miR-361. PLoS Genet. 2014;10(7):e1004467.
81. Wang K, Liu F, Liu CY, An T, Zhang J, Zhou LY, Wang M, Dong YH, Li N, Gao JN, Zhao YF, Li PF. The long noncoding RNA NRF regulates programmed necrosis and myocardial injury during ischemia and reperfusion by targeting miR-873. Cell Death Differ. 2016;23(8):1394–405.
82. Long B, Li N, Xu XX, Li XX, Xu XJ, Guo D, Zhang D, Wu ZH, Zhang SY. Long noncoding RNA FTX regulates cardiomyocyte apoptosis by targeting miR-29b-1-5p and Bcl2l2. Biochem Biophys Res Commun. 2018;495(1):312–8.
83. Zhang N, Meng X, Mei L, Hu J, Zhao C, Chen W. The long non-coding RNA SNHG1 attenuates cell apoptosis by regulating miR-195 and BCL2-like protein 2 in human cardiomyocytes. Cell Physiol Biochem. 2018;50(3):1029–40.
84. Li X, He X, Wang H, Li M, Huang S, Chen G, Jing Y, Wang S, Chen Y, Liao W, Liao Y, Bin J. Loss of AZIN2 splice variant facilitates endogenous cardiac regeneration. Cardiovasc Res. 2018;114(12):1642–55.
85. Li Z, Wang X, Wang W, Du J, Wei J, Zhang Y, Wang J, Hou Y. Altered long non-coding RNA expression profile in rabbit atria with atrial fibrillation: TCONS_00075467 modulates atrial electrical remodeling by sponging miR-328 to regulate CACNA1C. J Mol Cell Cardiol. 2017;108:73–85.
86. Travers JG, Kamal FA, Robbins J, Yutzey KE, Blaxall BC. Cardiac fibrosis: the fibroblast awakens. Circ Res. 2016;118(6):1021–40.
87. Tao H, Zhang JG, Qin RH, Dai C, Shi P, Yang JJ, Deng ZY, Shi KH. LncRNA GAS5 controls cardiac fibroblast activation and fibrosis by targeting miR-21 via PTEN/MMP-2 signaling pathway. Toxicology. 2017;386:11–8.
88. Huang ZW, Tian LH, Yang B, Guo RM. Long noncoding RNA H19 acts as a competing endogenous RNA to mediate CTGF expression by sponging miR-455 in cardiac fibrosis. DNA Cell Biol. 2017;36(9):759–66.
89. Liang H, Pan Z, Zhao X, Liu L, Sun J, Su X, Xu C, Zhou Y, Zhao D, Xu B, Li X, Yang B, Lu Y, Shan H. LncRNA PFL contributes to cardiac fibrosis by acting as a competing endogenous RNA of let-7d. Theranostics. 2018;8(4):1180–94.
90. Wang X, Yong C, Yu K, Yu R, Zhang R, Yu L, Li S, Cai S. Long noncoding RNA (lncRNA) n379519 promotes cardiac fibrosis in post-infarct myocardium by targeting miR-30. Med Sci Monit. 2018;24:3958–65.
91. Zhang S, Gao S, Wang Y, Jin P, Lu F. lncRNA SRA1 promotes the activation of cardiac myofibroblasts through negative regulation of miR-148b. DNA Cell Biol. 2019;38(4):385–94.
92. Leung A, Trac C, Jin W, Lanting L, Akbany A, Saetrom P, Schones DE, Natarajan R. Novel long noncoding RNAs are regulated by angiotensin II in vascular smooth muscle cells. Circ Res. 2013;113(3):266–78.

93. Tang Y, Jin X, Xiang Y, Chen Y, Shen CX, Zhang YC, Li YG. The lncRNA MALAT1 protects the endothelium against ox-LDL-induced dysfunction via upregulating the expression of the miR-22-3p target genes CXCR2 and AKT. FEBS Lett. 2015;589(20 Pt B):3189–96.
94. Hu YW, Zhao JY, Li SF, Huang JL, Qiu YR, Ma X, Wu SG, Chen ZP, Hu YR, Yang JY, Wang YC, Gao JJ, Sha YH, Zheng L, Wang Q. RP5-833A20.1/miR-382-5p/NFIA-dependent signal transduction pathway contributes to the regulation of cholesterol homeostasis and inflammatory reaction. Arterioscler Thromb Vasc Biol. 2015;35(1):87–101.
95. Shan K, Jiang Q, Wang XQ, Wang YN, Yang H, Yao MD, Liu C, Li XM, Yao J, Liu B, Zhang YY, JY, Yan B. Role of long non-coding RNA-RNCR3 in atherosclerosis-related vascular dysfunction. Cell Death Dis. 2016;7(6):e2248.
96. Miao C, Cao H, Zhang Y, Guo X, Wang Z, Wang J. LncRNA DIGIT accelerates tube formation of vascular endothelial cells by sponging miR-134. Int Heart J. 2018;59(5):1086–95.
97. Hu X, Bai T, Xu Z, Liu Q, Zheng Y, Cai L. Pathophysiological fundamentals of diabetic cardiomyopathy. Compr Physiol. 2017;7(2):693–711.
98. Zhou X, Zhang W, Jin M, Chen J, Xu W, Kong X. lncRNA MIAT functions as a competing endogenous RNA to upregulate DAPK2 by sponging miR-22-3p in diabetic cardiomyopathy. Cell Death Dis. 2017;8(7):e2929.
99. Yang F, Qin Y, Wang Y, Li A, Lv J, Sun X, Che H, Han T, Meng S, Bai Y, Wang L. LncRNA KCNQ1OT1 mediates pyroptosis in diabetic cardiomyopathy. Cell Physiol Biochem. 2018;50(4):1230–44.
100. Xiao X, Zhou T, Guo S, Guo C, Zhang Q, Dong N, Wang Y. LncRNA MALAT1 sponges miR-204 to promote osteoblast differentiation of human aortic valve interstitial cells through up-regulating Smad4. Int J Cardiol. 2017;243:404–12.
101. Geng HH, Li R, Su YM, Xiao J, Pan M, Cai XX, Ji XP. The circular RNA Cdr1as promotes myocardial infarction by mediating the regulation of miR-7a on its target genes expression. PLoS One. 2016;11(3):e0151753.
102. Wang K, Long B, Liu F, Wang JX, Liu CY, Zhao B, Zhou LY, Sun T, Wang M, Yu T, Gong Y, Liu J, Dong YH, Li N, Li PF. A circular RNA protects the heart from pathological hypertrophy and heart failure by targeting miR-223. Eur Heart J. 2016;37(33):2602–11.
103. Tang CM, Zhang M, Huang L, Hu ZQ, Zhu JN, Xiao Z, Zhang Z, Lin QX, Zheng XL, Yang M, Wu SL, Cheng JD, Shan ZX. CircRNA_000203 enhances the expression of fibrosis-associated genes by derepressing targets of miR-26b-5p, Col1a2 and CTGF, in cardiac fibroblasts. Sci Rep. 2017;7:40342.
104. Yang Y, Gao X, Zhang M, Yan S, Sun C, Xiao F, Huang N, Yang X, Zhao K, Zhou H, Huang S, Xie B, Zhang N. Novel role of FBXW7 circular RNA in repressing glioma tumorigenesis. J Natl Cancer Inst. 2018;110(3):304–15.
105. Yin WB, Yan MG, Fang X, Guo JJ, Xiong W, Zhang RP. Circulating circular RNA hsa_circ_0001785 acts as a diagnostic biomarker for breast cancer detection. Clin Chim Acta. 2018;487:363–8.
106. Li B, Li R, Zhang C, Bian HJ, Wang F, Xiao J, Liu SW, Yi W, Zhang MX, Wang SX, Zhang Y, Su GH, Ji XP. MicroRNA-7a/b protects against cardiac myocyte injury in ischemia/reperfusion by targeting poly(ADP-ribose) polymerase. PLoS One. 2014;9(3):e90096.
107. Eltzschig HK, Kohler D, Eckle T, Kong T, Robson SC, Colgan SP. Central role of Sp1-regulated CD39 in hypoxia/ischemia protection. Blood. 2009;113(1):224–32.
108. Piquereau J, Caffin F, Novotova M, Lemaire C, Veksler V, Garnier A, Ventura-Clapier R, Joubert F. Mitochondrial dynamics in the adult cardiomyocytes: which roles for a highly specialized cell? Front Physiol. 2013;4:102.
109. Tondera D, Santel A, Schwarzer R, Dames S, Giese K, Klippel A, Kaufmann J. Knockdown of MTP18, a novel phosphatidylinositol 3-kinase-dependent protein, affects mitochondrial morphology and induces apoptosis. J Biol Chem. 2004;279(30):31544–55.
110. Tondera D, Czauderna F, Paulick K, Schwarzer R, Kaufmann J, Santel A. The mitochondrial protein MTP18 contributes to mitochondrial fission in mammalian cells. J Cell Sci. 2005;118(Pt 14):3049–59.
111. Li M, Ding W, Tariq MA, Chang W, Zhang X, Xu W, Hou L, Wang Y, Wang J. A circular transcript of ncx1 gene mediates ischemic myocardial injury by targeting miR-133a-3p. Theranostics. 2018;8(21):5855–69.
112. Divakaran V, Mann DL. The emerging role of microRNAs in cardiac remodeling and heart failure. Circ Res. 2008;103(10):1072–83.
113. Brown L, Ongusaha PP, Kim HG, Nuti S, Mandinova A, Lee JW, Khosravi-Far R, Aaronson SA, Lee SW. CDIP, a novel pro-apoptotic gene, regulates TNFalpha-mediated apoptosis in a p53-dependent manner. EMBO J. 2007;26(14):3410–22.
114. Deng Y, Zhang W, She J, Zhang L, Chen T, Zhou J, Yuan Z. GW27-e1167 circular RNA related to PPARγ function as ceRNA of microRNA in human acute myocardial infarction. J Am Coll Cardiol. 2016;68(16):51–2.
115. Bazan HA, Hatfield SA, Brug A, Brooks AJ, Lightell DJ Jr, Woods TC. Carotid plaque rupture is accompanied by an increase in the ratio of serum circR-284 to miR-221 levels. Circ Cardiovasc Genet. 2017;10(4):pii: e001720.
116. Salgado-Somoza A, Zhang L, Vausort M, Devaux Y. The circular RNA MICRA for risk stratification after myocardial infarction. Int J Cardiol Heart Vasc. 2017;17:33–6.
117. Li Y, Zheng Q, Bao C, Li S, Guo W, Zhao J, Chen D, Gu J, He X, Huang S. Circular RNA is enriched and stable in exosomes: a promising biomarker for cancer diagnosis. Cell Res. 2015;25(8):981–4.

118. Fanale D, Taverna S, Russo A, Bazan V. Circular RNA in Exosomes. Adv Exp Med Biol. 2018;1087:109–17.
119. Zhao Z, Li X, Gao C, Jian D, Hao P, Rao L, Li M. Peripheral blood circular RNA hsa_circ_0124644 can be used as a diagnostic biomarker of coronary artery disease. Sci Rep. 2017;7:39918.
120. Zhang Z, Yang T, Xiao J. Circular RNAs: promising biomarkers for human diseases. EBioMedicine. 2018;34:267–74.
121. Peng LC, Guanglin, Zhu Z, Shen Z, Du C, Zang R, Su Y, Xie H, Li H, Xu X, Xia Y, Tang W. Circular RNA ZNF609 functions as a competitive endogenous RNA to regulate AKT3 expression by sponging miR-150-5p in Hirschsprung's disease. Oncotarget. 2017;8(1):808–18.
122. Devaux Y, Vausort M, McCann GP, Zangrando J, Kelly D, Razvi N, Zhang L, Ng LL, Wagner DR, Squire IB. MicroRNA-150: a novel marker of left ventricular remodeling after acute myocardial infarction. Circ Cardiovasc Genet. 2013;6(3):290–8.
123. Aneja A, Tang WH, Bansilal S, Garcia MJ, Farkouh ME. Diabetic cardiomyopathy: insights into pathogenesis, diagnostic challenges, and therapeutic options. Am J Med. 2008;121(9):748–57.
124. Battiprolu PK, Gillette TG, Wang ZV, Lavandero S, Hill JA. Diabetic cardiomyopathy: mechanisms and therapeutic targets. Drug Discov Today Dis Mech. 2010;7(2):135–43.
125. Zhou B, Yu JW. A novel identified circular RNA, circRNA_010567, promotes myocardial fibrosis via suppressing miR-141 by targeting TGF-beta1. Biochem Biophys Res Commun. 2017;487(4):769–75.
126. Wang J, Liu L, Sun Y, Xue Y, Qu J, Pan S, Li H, Qu H, Wang J, Zhang J. miR-615-3p promotes proliferation and migration and inhibits apoptosis through its potential target CELF2 in gastric cancer. Biomed Pharmacother. 2018;101:406-13.
127. Boeckel JN, Jae N, Heumuller AW, Chen W, Boon RA, Stellos K, Zeiher AM, John D, Uchida S, Dimmeler S. Identification and characterization of hypoxia-regulated endothelial circular RNA. Circ Res. 2015;117(10):884–90.
128. Liu C, Yao MD, Li CP, Shan K, Yang H, Wang JJ, Liu B, Li XM, Yao J, Jiang Q, Yan B. Silencing of circular RNA-ZNF609 ameliorates vascular endothelial dysfunction. Theranostics. 2017;7(11):2863–77.
129. Legnini I, Di Timoteo G, Rossi F, Morlando M, Briganti F, Sthandier O, Fatica A, Santini T, Andronache A, Wade M, Laneve P, Rajewsky N, Bozzoni I. Circ-ZNF609 is a circular RNA that can be translated and functions in myogenesis. Mol Cell. 2017;66(1):22–37 e29.
130. Zheng C, Niu H, Li M, Zhang H, Yang Z, Tian L, Wu Z, Li D, Chen X. Cyclic RNA hsacirc000595 regulates apoptosis of aortic smooth muscle cells. Mol Med Rep. 2015;12(5):6656–62.
131. Dang RY, Liu FL, Li Y. Circular RNA hsa_circ_0010729 regulates vascular endothelial cell proliferation and apoptosis by targeting the miR-186/HIF-1alpha axis. Biochem Biophys Res Commun. 2017;490(2):104–10.
132. del Zoppo GJ, Hallenbeck JM. Advances in the vascular pathophysiology of ischemic stroke. Thromb Res. 2000;98(3):73–81.
133. Frizzell JP. Acute stroke: pathophysiology, diagnosis, and treatment. AACN Clin Issues. 2005;16(4):421–40.. quiz 597-428
134. Markus HS, Bevan S. Mechanisms and treatment of ischaemic stroke-insights from genetic associations. Nat Rev Neurol. 2014;10(12):723–30.
135. Bai Y, Zhang Y, Han B, Yang L, Chen X, Huang R, Wu F, Chao J, Liu P, Hu G, Zhang JH, Yao H. Circular RNA DLGAP4 ameliorates ischemic stroke outcomes by targeting miR-143 to regulate endothelial-mesenchymal transition associated with blood-brain barrier integrity. J Neurosci Off J Soc Neurosci. 2018;38(1):32–50.
136. Han B, Zhang Y, Zhang Y, Bai Y, Chen X, Huang R, Wu F, Leng S, Chao J, Zhang JH, Hu G, Yao H. Novel insight into circular RNA HECTD1 in astrocyte activation via autophagy by targeting MIR142-TIPARP: Implications for cerebral ischemic stroke. Autophagy. 2018;14:1164–84.
137. Sotoudeh Anvari M, Mortazavian Babaki M, Boroumand MA, Eslami B, Jalali A, Goodarzynejad H. Relationship between calculated total antioxidant status and atherosclerotic coronary artery disease. Anatol J Cardiol. 2016;16(9):689–95.
138. Liu X, Cheng Y, Zhang S, Lin Y, Yang J, Zhang C. A necessary role of miR-221 and miR-222 in vascular smooth muscle cell proliferation and neointimal hyperplasia. Circ Res. 2009;104(4):476–87.
139. Liu X, Cheng Y, Yang J, Xu L, Zhang C. Cell-specific effects of miR-221/222 in vessels: molecular mechanism and therapeutic application. J Mol Cell Cardiol. 2012;52(1):245–55.
140. Pan RY, Liu P, Zhou HT, Sun WX, Song J, Shu J, Cui GJ, Yang ZJ, Jia EZ. Circular RNAs promote TRPM3 expression by inhibiting hsa-miR-130a-3p in coronary artery disease patients. Oncotarget. 2017;8(36):60280–90.
141. Lin F, Zhao G, Chen Z, Wang X, Lv F, Zhang Y, Yang X, Liang W, Cai R, Li J, Li M, Zhang G. circRNAmiRNA association for coronary heart disease. Mol Med Rep. 2019;19(4):2527–36.
142. Naylor J, Li J, Milligan CJ, Zeng F, Sukumar P, Hou B, Sedo A, Yuldasheva N, Majeed Y, Beri D, Jiang S, Seymour VA, McKeown L, Kumar B, Harteneck C, O'Regan D, Wheatcroft SB, Kearney MT, Jones C, Porter KE, Beech DJ. Pregnenolone sulphate- and cholesterol-regulated TRPM3 channels coupled to vascular smooth muscle secretion and contraction. Circ Res. 2010;106(9):1507–15.
143. Li L, Wang Q, Yuan Z, Chen A, Liu Z, Wang Z, Li H. LncRNA-MALAT1 promotes CPC proliferation and migration in hypoxia by up-regulation of JMJD6 via sponging miR-125. Biochem Biophys Res Commun. 2018;499(3):711–8.

RNA Binding Proteins and Non-coding RNA's in Cardiovascular Diseases

5

Parveen Bansal and Malika Arora

Abstract

Cardiovascular disease (CVD) is the leading cause of mortality as well as morbidity worldwide. The disease has been reported to be chronic in nature and the symptoms of the disease worsen progressively over a long period of time. Inspite of noteworthy achievements have been made in the therapy of CVD yet the available drugs are associated with various undesirable factors including drug toxicity, complexity, resistance and many more. The versatility of RNAs makes them crucial therapeutics candidate for many human diseases. Deeper understanding of RNA biology, exploring new classes of RNA that possess therapeutic potential will help in its successful translation to the clinic. Understanding the mode of action of various RNAs such as miRNA, RNA binding proteins and siRNA in CVD will help in improved therapeutics among patients. Multiple strategies are being planned to determine the future potential of miRNAs to treat a disease. This review embodies the recent work done in the field of miRNA and its role in cardiovascular disease as diagnostic biomarker as well as therapeutic agents. In addition the review highlights the future of miRNAs as a potential therapeutic target and need of designing micronome that may reveal potential predictive targets of miRNA-mRNA interaction.

Keywords

Cardiovascular disease (CVD) · RNA Binding Proteins (RBPs) · Aptamer · microRNA

1 Introduction

Cardiovascular diseases (CVDs) have been found to be the leading cause of mortality around the globe. More than 80% of deaths are as a result of CVD, Ischemic heart disease and stroke. On an average, 235 per 100,000 deaths were reported to be due to the CVDs worldwide. In India the number is higher in comparison to other countries. The Global Burden of Disease has been estimated to be 272 per 100,000 population in India [1]. Among Indians, early disease onset, accelerated build-up and increased fatality have been observed. Numerous factors have been reported to be involved in the pathogenesis of the disease. These factors include both modifiable and non-modifiable factors such as genetic factors, lifestyle, obesity, excessive tobacco use, low fruit

P. Bansal (✉)
University Centre of Excellence in Research, Baba Farid University of Health Sciences, Faridkot, Punjab, India

M. Arora
Multidisciplinary Research Unit, Guru Gobind Singh Medical College, Faridkot, Punjab, India

J. Xiao (ed.), *Non-coding RNAs in Cardiovascular Diseases*, Advances in Experimental Medicine and Biology 1229, https://doi.org/10.1007/978-981-15-1671-9_5

and vegetable intake etc. Moreover, optimal therapy is not being received by the individuals from lower socioeconomic backgrounds frequently which have led to poorer outcomes. In the vicinity of poorer outcomes, such epidemic diseases can be counteracted by developing the strategies that includes formulation and effective implementation of evidence-based policy, reinforcement of health systems, as well as emphasis on prevention, early detection, along with treatment with the use of both conventional and innovative techniques. Most of such strategies are being tested in undergoing community-based studies. Among these studies, non-coding RNAs such as miRNA, aptamers and RNA binding proteins (RBPs) are also being explored for early detection of disease and good outcome among patients with cardiovascular disease [2].

The eukaryotic genome is comprised of both protein coding and non-protein coding DNA. Although there has been much agreement that a small fraction of these genomes has important biological functions, but it is still debatable that how the rest of the genome is contributing to the body. Hangauer et al. [3] demonstrated the fact that 85% of the human genome is actively transcribed into non-coding RNAs [3]. Due to the ambiguity, much of the speculation is centred that low level of DNA is transcribed into actual coding RNA yet the other non-coding RNA is arbitrarily assigned with various names such as micro RNA, silencing RNA, Long non coding RNA etc. RNA has become a spotlight of attention for developing novel therapeutic schemes and hence variety of therapeutic strategies is being coming into the picture that includes RNA interference, use of aptamers and role of microRNA (miRNA) that can alter the complex gene expression patterns [4]. The versatility of RNAs makes them crucial therapeutics candidate for many human diseases. Deeper understanding of RNA biology, exploring new classes of RNA that possess therapeutic potential will help in its successful translation to the clinic. Understanding the mode of action of various RNAs including long non-coding RNAs (lncRNAs), miRNA, siRNA, etc. in CVD will help in improved therapeutics among patients [5].

It is due to the fact that RNA offers various advantages in disease management as it can be edited and modified in its various forms such as secondary and tertiary structures. Although scientists are in process of manufacturing RNA-targeting therapies using variety of endogenous gene silencing regulators, Small interfering RNAs (Si RNAs), aptamers and microRNA for cardiovascular diseases yet the development of a novel, risk free therapeutic strategy is a major challenge and need of the hour in cardiovascular medicine [6]. Moreover, it has been observed that multiple cell types are being comprised by cardiovascular system which helps to amend the phenotypic response to any acute or chronic injury. The cellular phenotypic changes are controlled by various proteins such as RNA binding proteins (RBPs) and non coding RNAs such as miRNA etc. [7] which ultimately determine cardiovascular health and disease. While performing phenotypic conversions, RBPs are known to establish an impact on mRNA fates which is further responsible for mediating transcriptional/post-transcriptional modification. Similarly, it is well documented that an individual non coding RNA has capability to influence hundreds of transcripts and ultimately to affect complex programs of gene expression and thereby affecting the overall genotypic or phenotypic expressions of a cell [8, 9]. Moreover, it has been predicted that miRNA is a key player in regulating various cellular processes including cardiovascular development. It is pertinent to mention that in recent years RNA therapeutic strategies such as RNA binding proteins, miRNA, aptamers etc. are upcoming and witnessing huge progress in the field of cardiovascular diseases [10, 11]. The present manuscript has been compiled to summarize various approaches of RNA binding proteins and non-coding RNA in prognosis, diagnosis and therapeutics of cardiovascular diseases.

2 RNA and Its World of Therapeutics

Non coding DNA accounts for 98.5% of human genome. This non-coding DNA is transcribed to a wide range of functional RNA species widely called non coding RNAs [12]. These are classified into three different classes called small around19–25 nucleotides, intermediate-sized around 20–200 nucleotides and long around 200 nucleotides. It has been observed that the actual number of the non-coding RNA within the genome is unknown but the structure as well as function of them is being revealed using various bioinformatics software [13]. Many of the non-coding RNAs are not validated for their function and considered to be product of spurious transcription but as per current studies these are found to be highly potential biomarkers for CVD. In addition these so called spurious transcripts are emerging as next frontiers in the drug discovery.

According to the central dogma, different types of RNA passively convert the information encoded in the DNA to polypeptides via replication followed by transcription and translation respectively [14]. For such functions, RNA is not alone rather different types of RNA associate them with diversity of proteins· from the site of transcription i.e. nucleus to the outreaches i.e. cytoplasm. These proteins are classified under the category of RNA binding proteins that are helpful in performing various tasks such as transport, localization, translation and stability of mRNAs or other types of RNAs. In addition, these are the key factors to play important role in communication of crucial information to the translation machinery for critical surveillance of any kind of mutations. Hence RBPs possess the entire responsibility to shape the gene expression of a cell at multiple centres. In addition, it is well known fact that RBPs are keen factors in development, in various physical and chemical changes as well in context to development of heart. According to different studies, it has been demonstrated that RBPs have been placed in some specific stages of heart development and are involved in almost all stages of cardiogenesis such as formation, morphogenesis and maturation of heart [15]. The deeper insights into the function of RBPs may give rise to some specific targets that may provide attractive, novel targets for the prognosis, diagnosis and treatment of various heart diseases.

3 RNA Binding Proteins and Their Characteristics

RNA-binding proteins (RBPs) are very important interaction partners for all cellular RNAs. These proteins have been reported to regulate RNA processing at numerous levels including alternative splicing, mRNA stability, mRNA localisation and translation efficiency. The activities of RBPs in nucleus and cytoplasm are regulated through their cellular compartmentalisation. In the nuclear compartment, they function as splicing regulators often during development. In the cytoplasm, RBPs function in the regulation of mRNA localisation, mRNA stability and regulates the translational efficiency of mRNA. RNAs associate with RBPs to form dynamic ribonucleoprotein particles (RNPs) for execution of RNA function [16, 17]. Nascent pre-mRNA are covered with myriad of RBPs that collectively form RNPs. Previously, it has been reported that human genome encodes more than 700 RBPs. These proteins interact with the target mRNAs at 3′- and 5′- untranslated regions, intronic and exonic regions. Numerous sequencing-based RBP foot-printing studies have reported intricate and combinatorial interactions between RNA and RBPs [18]. Some of the general feature of RNA binding proteins are compiled and shown in Fig. 5.1.

4 RNA Binding Proteins in Cardiovascular Diseases

The function of RBPs can be disrupted in the disease. The competition for access of target mRNA by RBPs is determined by their expression level in a healthy and diseased individual. These can be either primary cause of the disease or a

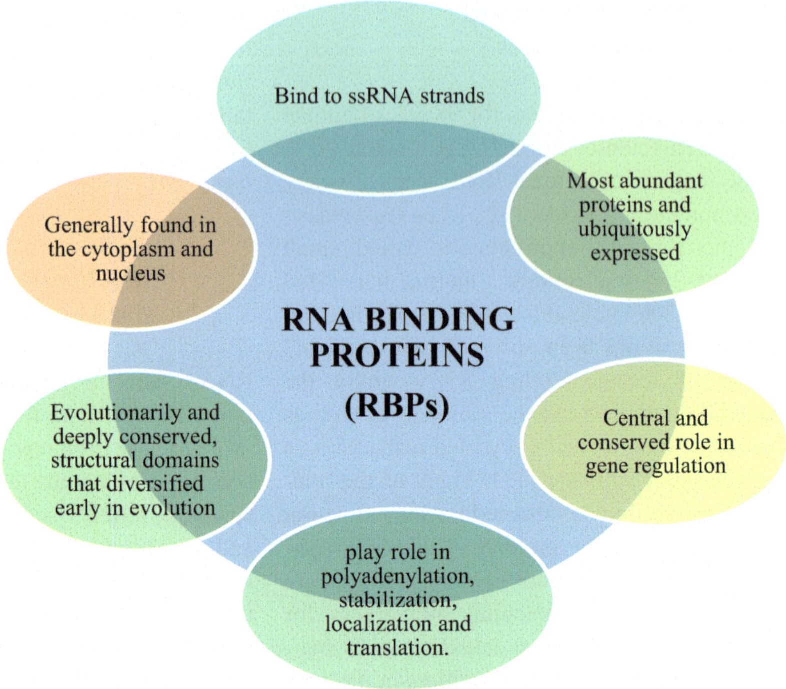

Fig. 5.1 Schematic representation of characteristics of RNA binding proteins

consequence. RBPs including quaking, HuR, muscle blind and SRSF1 have been found to be the major key players in cardiovascular disease. Homozygous alterations in these RBPs are reported to be associated with cardiac and vascular complications. These are crucial for maintaining mRNA transcript abundance and its translation into mature proteins.

Various studies have demonstrated the importance and co-ordinating role for RBPs in foetal, juvenile, and adult hearts. In addition, these studies have also demonstrated that how altered RBP levels can impact cardiac function in health and disease. During diseased conditions the expression of RBPs is varied that leads to defective splicing and causes translation of defective protein. Splicing defects can lead to heart dysfunction. Major RBPs that are associated with spliceosome and cardiovascular disease risk include Troponin T, SERCA2a/b and CETP [19, 20]. In addition, it as been observed that Celf1 and Muscleblind1 (MBNL) are associated with postnatal splicing for the effective organization of transverse tubules and calcium handling. However, Serine/Arginine rich splicing factor (SRSF1) has been found to guide the splicing pattern for maintaining electrical conductivity among cardiomyocytes during juvenile to adult transition. Another RBP of interest is RBM20 which is highly expressed in human heart. Even single nucleotide polymorphism (SNP) in exonic region of RBM20 results in increased risk of DCM due to altered expression of this RBP. It affects ion homeostasis, sarcomere organization and diastolic function including titin, tropomyosin I, PDZ and LIM domain 5. A variety of RNA binding proteins are engaged in different role and are helpful in the alleviation of CVD [21]. The availability of various RNA binding proteins and their role in CVD is compiled in Table 5.1.

RBPs have been reported to associate in repair of damaged vessels during vascular injury. For

Table 5.1 Various RNA binding proteins and their role in CVD

RBPs	Disease	Diagnostic criteria
Muscleblind1 (MBNL1)	Cardiomyocytes	Regulation of voltage gated channels responsible for cellular expression and splicing of the SCN5A, a voltage-gated sodium channel [22]
Poly (rc) binding protein (PCBP2)	Hypertrophy of cardiomyocytes	Inhibit hypertrophy of cardiomyocytes which is induced due to angiotensin II as it is responsible for degradation of GPR56 mRNA degradation [23, 24]
CIRP	Cardiac diseases	Enhances the translation of essential ion channel subunits Loss of CIRP results in defective voltage-gated potassium channel function and diminished bioelectric activity in mammalian hearts [25].
SRSF2	Cardiomyopathy	Extensive fibrosis, myofibril disarray, dilated cardiomyopathy evident after 5 weeks, decreased ventricle muscle contractility due to loss of this RBPs

the initiation of repair, RBPs co-ordinate important splicing events of mRNA of SM-myosin heavy chain, myosin light chain kinase, smoothelin, tropomyosin, metavinculin, calponin, and caldesmon. The actual procedure of repair used by these RBPs is largely unknown. Moreover, the impact of other RBPs has been found on expression of eNOS, enzyme involved in the synthesis of Nitric oxide (NO) by endothelial cells (EC) which triggers vasoconstriction. Experimental studies have been carried out to investigate the function of RBPs in human ECs. RBPs impact eNOS biology through hnRNP L, a protein that co-ordinates eNOS pre-mRNA alternative splicing that results in generation of a truncated, dominant negative eNOS isoform [26, 27]. Although evidences indicate that these alternative truncated eNOS isoforms affect NO production but the pathophysiological relevance in context with EC function in patients with CVD is unknown till date.

In addition, RNA-binding proteins have also been implicated in the posttranscriptional regulation of various other vital EC-derived factors, including VEGF, endoglin and HIF1a [28]. An isoform of RBP76/DRBP76/NF90 interacts with the 30 UTR of the VEGF mRNA and enhances VEGF production by human ECs whereas alterations in SRSF1 levels in senescent ECs alters splicing of VEGF and endoglin pre-mRNA [29, 30].

5 Micro RNAs and Its Biogenesis and General Properties

miRNA are considered to be potential post-transcriptional regulators and plays a vital role in gene expression. On an average, nearly 1000 miRNAs are encoded in the human genome and these are originated from various non-coding DNA/RNA regions. Depending upon the genomic location as well as gene structure, miRNA are classified as intergenic, intronic and exonic miRNA. According to this, more than 50% of the miRNA are located in the intergenic regions. The intergenic miRNA may exist either as single gene or may be as cluster of genes under the control of one promoter whereas intronic miRNA are located in introns of annotated genes that may be encoded from coding or non-coding genes. Exonic RNAs are originated from the overlapping region across an exon or intron of non-coding genes.

The biogenesis of miRNA involves various steps that convert a pre mature pre-miRNA to a mature miRNA. There is involvement of various

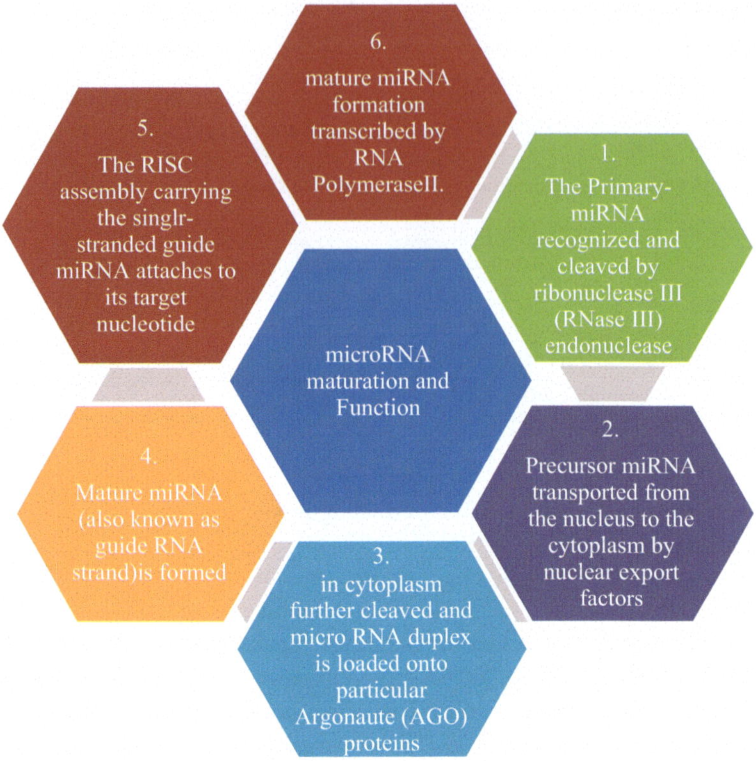

Fig. 5.2 Representation of biogenesis of miRNA

RNAs, RNA binding proteins and enzymes as well. The step by step process of miRNA biogenesis is shown in Fig. 5.2.

Structurally, miRNA are endogeneous, a class of highly abundant RNAs and are short nucleotides of length 19–22 nucleotides approximately. miRNA are endogenous but an exogenous miRNA can also be introduced into a cell by a viral vector that encodes pre-miRNA or by other synthetic vehicle carrying synthetic pre-miRNA or miRNA [31, 32]. The general properties of the miRNA are shown in Table 5.2.

6 miRNA in Cardiovascular Diseases

Recent advances in the field of miRNA have revealed its importance in numerous human diseases including coronary heart disease [33]. Deletion of specific region of dgcr8 gene, required of miRNA production in cardiomycotes results in ventricular malfunction and premature lethality [34]. Another miRNA, miRNA-21 (miR-21) has been found to be involved in patho-

Table 5.2 Representation of general properties of miRNA

Features	Property of miRNA
Prior to processing	Originated from a precursor miRNA (pre-miRNA) that contains 70–100 nucleotides with hairp in structure
Structure	19–25 nucleotide RNA duplex with 2 nucleotides 3′ overhang
Complementary	Partially complementary to mRNA, typically targets the untranslated mRNA regions at 3′ end
mRNA target	Multiple targets varying from 1–100 at a same time
Mechanism of gene regulation	Translational repression of mRNA, rarely endonucleolytic cleavage of mRNA, degradation of mRNA, mRNA de-adenylation and mRNA sequestration
Clinical applications	Potential biomarkers, diagnostic tools, therapeutic agent and drug target

genesis of cardiac fibrosis by upregulating the ERK-MAP kinase signalling pathway in cardiac fibroblasts [35]. Repression of miR21 significantly improves cardiac outcome. In addition, miRNA has also been reported to be involved in cardiac fibrosis [36]. Increased levels of miR21 have been found to mitigate fibrosis as they reduce collagen production. Similarly, decreased levels of miR-29 after MI induced production and deposition of collagen fibers. miRNAs are crucial for other regenerative processes in the heart [37]. Collectively, miRNA or anti-miR delivery has great therapeutic potential for a variety of diseases [38]. miRNAs based therapeutics in cardiovascular diseases can be used via different strategies. A reverse association of some miRNA and good outcome has been detected in patients with cardiovascular disease. It has been found that a decoy against miR-24 to reverse its inhibition on angiogenesis improves cardiac function in a mouse MI model [39]. Embryonic stem cells that overexpress miR-1 (ESCs) improved stem cell differentiation into cardiomyocytes and reduced levels of apoptosis following injection in the infarcted heart. miR-126 is expressed in mesenchymal stem cells and it improves angiogenesis and overall cardiac function in infracted myocardium. Further, treatment of infarcted heart cells with lentiviruses encoding miR-1/133/208/499 enables direct in vivo conversion of cardiac fibroblasts into cardiomyocyte-like cells in the infarcted heart [10]. A variety of miRNA are engaged in different role and are helpful in the alleviation of CVD either acting as diagnostic biomarker, therapeutic agents or as drug targets. The availability of various miRNA as biomarker reported in various studies is compiled in Table 5.3.

7 Commonly Expressed miRNA in Cardiovascular Diseases

miR-21 is first mammalian RNA identified and is one of the most commonly studied miRNA in a CVD. It is abundant in vessel wall and differentially expressed upon shear and mechanical stress to the vessel. Among humans, it is expressed in podocytes, dendritic cells and CD14+ monocytes [47] of normal cells rather highly expressed in various cancers and CVD [48] and human atherosclerotic plaque [49]. It is dynamically regulated in various pathological processes i.e. cell sur-

Table 5.3 Role of various miRNA as biomarker in cardiovascular diseases

miRNA	Disease	Diagnostic criteria
miR-122	Hyperlipidemia	Serves as a primary regulator of lipid biosynthesis. Aberrant levels is an indication of coronary artery disease (CAD) [40, 41]
miR-126, miR-9	Hypertension, CHF (cardiac heart failure), stroke	Regulation in vascular integrity and angiogenesis indicates disease [42, 43]
miR-143/145	Hypertension, CAD, stroke	Macrophage differentiation and polarized activation processes indicates disease [10]
miR-1254, miR-423, miR-30d	Chronic heart failure (CHF)	Increased level of miR-1254 represents the disease whereas miR-423 and miR-30d levels are decreased in CHF
miR-21, miR-210, miR-423, miR-1, miR-26b	Heart failure (HF)	Increased level of miR-21, 210, 423,1 and 26b represents the heart failure.
miR-1306, miR-30d, miR-126, miR-423, miR-18a	Acute heart failure (AHF)	Increased level of miR-1306 and mi-30d represents the disease whereas miR-126, miR-423 and miR-18a levels are decreased in acute heart failure
miR-30c, miR-146a	Heart failure with preserved ejection fraction	Decreased level of miR-1306 and mi-30d represents the heart failure with preserved ejection fraction disease
miR-26a	Cardiovascular repair; acute coronary syndromes	Up regulation in the patients' plasma [44]

(continued)

Table 5.3 (continued)

miRNA	Disease	Diagnostic criteria
miR-16, miR-27a, miR-101, and miR-150	Left ventricular contractility (LV)	Downregulation of miR-101 or miR-150 and upregulation of miR-16 or miR-27a correlate with higher risk of impaired LV contractility [45]
miR-1, miR-134, miR-186, miR-208, miR-223, and miR-499	Angina pectoris	Up regulation in serum samples [46]

vival, apoptosis and cell invasiveness [50]. Studies have reported that overexpression of miRNA21 in endothelial cells inhibits the expression of Peroxisome Proliferator-Activated Receptor-alpha (PPARα) that further results in increased expressions of VCAM-1 and MCP-1 [51]. Hydrogen peroxide and lipopolysaccharides alter the expression of various miRNAs, including miRNA21 in endothelial cells [52].

In addition, miR-155 is a "immuno-miR," with a pivotal role in both innate and adaptive immunity. It is second most commonly studied miRNA in atherosclerosis and hypertension. It is significantly expressed in hematopoietic stem cells and promotes B cell-related immunoglobulin production, T cell proliferation in response to antigen as well as cytokine production [53]. Various studies confirm that mineralocorticoid plays an important role in stimulation of hypertension. It has been observed that high serum levels of miR-155 in response to mineralocorticoid are available in the patient exhibiting greater reduction in systolic blood pressure. In contrast, levels of miR-155 were detected to be dramatically low in aorta of aged white mouse. In a cross sectional study of 932 Chinese patients, a negative co-relation was observed among plasma levels of miR-155 and severity of coronary atherosclerosis [54]. Moreover, miR-155 is found to be pro-inflammatory and predictive of worst outcome in patients with atherosclerosis.

miR-146 is another "immuno-miR" that primarily functions in innate immunity and negatively regulate the production of pro-inflammatory cytokines (Perry et al. 2008). As per a study of 50 patients, elevated expression of miR-146a, miR-146b and miR-21 was observed in plaque boarded arteries in comparison to normal vessels [50]. Moreover, it acts a potential mediator through which Apo E suppresses myeloid cell inflammation i.e. NF- κB activation [55]. Apo E is associated with normal physiologic removal of circulating triglyceride-rich particles e.g., VLDL. A strong anti-inflammatory and atheroprotective role of miR-146 family has been evidenced in various studies.

miR-143 and miR-145 form a classical cluster on chromosome 5 as these two are present in close proximity. Although miR-143 and miR-145 are available as cluster but expression level of miR-143 was found to be more than miR-145 due to an unknown mechanism. In a cohort (cohort that exhibited hyper-homocysteinemia (Hhcy) without carotid atherosclerosis, Hhcy with carotid atherosclerosis, and carotid atherosclerosis (without Hhcy) study, higher expression of miR143/145 was observed in patients with Hhcy in comparison with healthy controls [33]. Moreover, as per Santovito et al. 2013, miR-145 was up-regulated in carotid atheromas from hypertensive patients in comparison of carotid atherosclerosis without hypertension [56].

Another prototypical immune miR i.e. miR-223 is highly expressed in myeloid cells. Down-regulation of this miR is required for monocyte-to-macrophage differentiation [57] but miR-223 was found to be elevated in the visceral adipose of obese humans in the absence of hyperlipidemia and hypertension [57, 58]. A positive correlation was observed in increased miR-223 levels and the incidence of acute ischemic stroke [58]. Increased expression of miR-223 maybe because of hypomethylation of the miR-223 promoter and an increased hypomethylation of promoter region of miR223 was observed in atherosclerotic cerebral infarction patients. Apart above explained examples, a variety of miRNA are engaged in in the alleviation of CVD either as therapeutic agents or as drug targets. The availability of various miRNA as therapeutic agents and drug targets are compiled in Table 5.4.

Table 5.4 Role of various miRNA as therapeutic agent in cardiovascular diseases

miRNA	Therapeutic agent	Mechanism of action
miR-121	Hyperlipidemia	Reduces plasma cholesterol levels by 1. Repressing mRNA targets by binding to other regions including 5′ UTRs or protein-coding exons 2. Imperfect base pairing to the 3′ untranslated regions (3′ UTR) of messenger RNAs (mRNAs) thereby inducing repression of the target mRNA [59, 60]
miR-33	Atherosclerosis	Raised HDL and induced regression of atherosclerotic plaques by using 2′ F/MOE-modified anti-sense oligonucleotide; anti-miR-33 lentivirus [61, 62]
miR-34a	Myocardial infarction	Improve systolic pressure and increase angiogenesis and Akt activity with the use of LNA-anti-miR-34a [63]
miR-208	Obesity, diabetes, metabolic syndrome	Provides resistance to high-fat diet-induced obesity, improves systemic insulin sensitivity and glucose tolerance by imperfect base paring with the use of MGN-9103 (LNA modified anti-sense oligonucleotide) [64]
miR-29	Atrial fibrillation	Deregulation of miR-29 followed by targeting of mRNAs encoding fibrosis-promoting proteins by regulating genes involved in cardiac fibrosis and apoptosis [65]
miR-133 miR-30	Cardiac fibrosis	Direct interaction of both′ UTR of CTGF and down-regulate its expression followed by decreased production of collagen
miR-30	Myocardial infraction	Increased expression in MI and decreased expression in cardiac hypertrophy. In MI, it regulates several ion channel genes including gap junction protein alpha 1 (GJA1) that encode connexin 43, calcium channel beta-2 (CACNB2) etc.
miR-195	Cardiac hypertrophy	Up-regulated during cardiac hypertrophy. It regulates sodium channel (SCN)5A that encodes cardiac Na^+ channel etc.

8 Ongoing Clinical Trials in the Field of miRNA as Their Potential Role in CVD

Micro RNAs are considered as potential biomarkers, drug targets and novel therapeutic agents in cardiovascular disease. Their diagnostic value has been evaluated in various studies and hence these are emerging as novel drug targets, therapeutic targets with respect to coronary artery disease (CAD) and myocardial infarction (MI). As per current state of art, a number of clinical trials are being conducted on variety of miRNA of potential use. The first promising in vitro results are raising hope for future clinical application. A list of ongoing clinical trials in the field of cardiovascular diseases using various miRNA targets has been compiled in Table 5.5.

9 FDA Approved miRNA Drugs

Though the field of miRNA and its role in various diseases is not yet fully unfolded but the researchers are desperate and making critical steps for seeking approval for newly manufactured/to be manufactured new miRNA based medicines from

Table 5.5 Representation of list of ongoing clinical trials in the field of cardiovascular diseases using various miRNA targets [66]

Identification number	Recruiting status	Type of study	Conditions of diseases	Treatment	No of enrolments	Study completion date
NCT03792607	Recruiting	Observational	Type 2 diabetes mellitus Cardiovascular diseases	Mi RNA and Methylome	35	June 14, 2020
NCT03635255	Recruiting	Observational	Adverse cardiovascular	Mi RNA	450	September 21, 2020
NCT03395041	Recruiting	Observational	Coronary stenosis Periodontal diseases Acute coronary syndrome Non-ST elevation Myocardial infarction Unstable angina acute myocardial infarction Atherosclerosis Atheromatous plaques	Cardiac imaging tests	100	June 1, 2021
NCT03391908	Recruiting	Observational	Coronary stenosis Periodontal diseases Acute coronary syndrome Non-ST elevation Myocardial infarction Unstable angina acute myocardial infarction Atherosclerosis Atheromatous plaques	Cardiac imaging tests	100	January 2021
NCT03875495	Recruiting	Interventional (clinical trial)	Multiple myeloma	Temferon	9	March 2023
NCT03474614	Recruiting	Interventional (clinical trial)	Cerebral cavernous malformations	Propranolol	20	August 30, 2020
NCT03430583	Recruiting	Observational	Single ventricle heart disease	MZ101	100	December 31, 2020
NCT02267200	Completed	Observational	Hypertension,Pulmonary		100	September 2016
NCT02176395	Recruiting	Interventional (clinical trial)	Acute stroke	Danhong Placebo	46	June 2019

Table 5.6 List of miRNA based FDA approved drugs to be used for cardiovascular diseases

miRNA	Disease	Detection approach	References
miRNA -208a/b, miR-499	Acute myocardial infarction (AMI) and myocardial injury	Microarray and real time PCR	[66]
miRNA423-5p	Heart failure	Microarray and real time PCR	[67]
miR-328	Atrial fibrillation (adverse electrical remodelling)	Microarray and real time PCR	[68]
miR-1	AMI	Real time PCR	[69]
miR-26a	Cardiovascular repair, acute coronary syndromes	Real time PCR	[70]
miR-16, miR-27a, miR-101 and miR-150	Left ventricular contractility	Real time PCR	[5]
miR- 133	AMI and coronary artery stenosis	Real time PCR	[42]
miR-126, miR-17/ miR-92a, miR-155	Coronary artery disease	Microarray and real time PCR	[71]
miR-126	Congestive heart failure	Real time PCR	[46]
miR-203, miR-223, miR-499, miR-1, miR-134, miR-186	AMI and angina pectons	Deep sequencing	[48]
miR-21/590-5p family, miR-126, miR-451	Coronary artery disease	Microarray and real time PCR	[72]

US Food and Drug Administration (FDA). MiRNA has already made its way in the treatment of number of diseases and due to the positive outcomes various miRNA based drugs are entering to the market after seeking FDA approval. First anti-cancer miRNA-based drug, MRX-34 (a liposome-based miR-34 mimic) developed by Mirna Therapeutics came to the clinic in 2013 for the treatment of hepatocellular carcinoma (mirnarx.com; NCT01829971). The FDA approval for few of the miRNA has led the field to the new heights and it seems more promising that miRNA may contribute the disease alleviation by acting as a diagnostic as well as therapeutic modality. Few of such FDA approved drugs are enlisted in Table 5.6.

10 Future Prospects

miRNA and RNA binding proteins are two complex components of gene expression. Discovery of novel miRNAs and their utility in disease diagnosis and prognosis is highly appreciable that has been resulted as component of large and simultaneous research work of various branches such as molecular biology, biotechnology, bioinformatics, clinical-trial design, epidemiology, statistics as well as health-care economics. A number of miRNA biomarkers have been presented in various studies and these are emerging due to their attractive advantages over other molecular therapeutics such as small size along with conserved sequences and their stability in the body fluids. Such advantages and current achievements in the field of RNA are portraying a promising future for miRNA-based therapeutics in disease diagnosis and disease prevention as well. Although a huge amount of data has been gathered and evidencing the use of RNA in therapeutics but still the scientists has scratched the surface of the complex gene expression. Much more is yet to be done in the future with respect to miRNA and elucidating its potential. For implementation of this approach few new strategies needs to be designed for their effective delivery as well as several obstacles including their stability, renal clearance, off-target effects, inefficient endocytosis by target cells or the immunogenicity of delivery vehicles, need to be overcome. The RNA therapeutics have been depicted using various preclinical studies involving small animals rather involvement of large animals and patients will further explore their efficacy in future. In addition, development and improvement of RNA-based therapeutics requires robust design of the

RNA agents to avoid adverse effects and optimal delivery strategies to maximize their benefits.

Moreover, miRNA is targeting the mRNA which is structure specific as well as sequence specific. According to various bioinformatics based software, multiple databases are there which stores predicted microRNA to mRNA target relationships. These relationships are computed using diverse algorithms. Prediction databases generally compare the in vitro data to the data generated by bioinformatics tools which ultimately results in microRNA to mRNA transcript interactome generally referred as micronome. Now a days, micronome is developed to study the involvement of miRNA in well known signalling pathways and its role in diseases as well. The development of miRNA based micronome in Cardiovascular diseases will significantly improve the understanding of their involvement and the generation of novel therapeutic as well as drug targets in the field of RNA therapeutics in cardiovascular diseases.

References

1. de Bruin RG, Rabelink TJ, van Zonneveld AJ, Van der Veer EP. Emerging roles for RNA-binding proteins as effectors and regulators of cardiovascular disease. Eur Heart J. 2016;38(18):1380–8.
2. Adams BD, Parsons C, Walker L, Zhang WC, Slack FJ. Targeting noncoding RNAs in disease. J Clin Invest. 2017;127(3):761–71.
3. Hangauer MJ, Vaughn IW, McManus MT. Pervasive transcription of the human genome produces thousands of previously unidentified long intergenic noncoding RNAs. PLoS Genet. 2013;9(6):e1003569.
4. Miele E. Nanoparticle-based delivery of small interfering RNA: challenges for cancer therapy. Int J Nanomedicine. 2012;7:3637.
5. Devaux Y. Circular RNAs in heart failure. Eur J Heart Fail. 2017;19(6):701–9.
6. de Fougerolles A, Vornlocher HP, Maraganore J, Lieberman J. Interfering with disease: a progress report on siRNA-based therapeutics. Nat Rev Drug Discov. 2007;6(6):443.
7. Fu XD, Ares M Jr. Context-dependent control of alternative splicing by RNA-binding proteins. Nat Rev Genet. 2014;15(10):689.
8. Kong W. Upregulation of miRNA-155 promotes tumour angiogenesis by targeting VHL and is associated with poor prognosis and triple negative breast cancer. Oncogene. 2014;33(6):679–89.
9. Gasparini P. Protective role of miR-155 in breast cancer through RAD51 targeting impairs homologous recombination after irradiation. Proc Natl Acad Sci USA. 2014;111(12):4536–41.
10. Huang C, Li H, Wu W, Jiang T, Qiu Z. Regulation of miR155 affects pancreatic cancer cell invasiveness and migration by modulating the STAT3 signaling pathway through SOCS1. Oncol Rep. 2013;30:1223–30.
11. Krutzfeldt J. Silencing of microRNAs in vivo with 'antagomirs'. Nature. 2015;438:685–9.
12. ENCODE Project Consortium. An integrated encyclopedia of DNA elements in the human genome. Nature. 2012;489(7414):57.
13. Mattick JS, Makunin IV. Non-coding RNA. Hum Mol Genet. 2006;15(Suppl 1):R17–29.
14. Grosjean H. Modification and editing of RNA: historical overview and important facts to remember. In: Fine-tuning of RNA functions by modification and editing. Berlin/Heidelberg: Springer; 2005. p. 1–22.
15. Salehe BR. Predictive tools for the study of variations in ADP platelet responses: implications for personalised CVD risk and prevention strategies. Doctoral dissertation, University of Reading. 2017.
16. Castello A, Fischer B, Hentze MW, Preiss T. RNA-binding proteins in Mendelian disease. Trends Genet. 2013;29:318–27.
17. Chen CY, Shyu AB. Emerging mechanisms of mRNP remodeling regulation. Wiley Interdiscip Rev: RNA. 2014;5:713–22.
18. König J, Zarnack K, Luscombe NM, Ule J. Protein–RNA interactions: new genomic technologies and perspectives. Nat Rev Genet. 2012;13(2):77.
19. Keene JD. RNA regulons: coordination of post-transcriptional events. Nat Rev Genet. 2007;8(7):533.
20. Anderson PA, Greig A, Mark TM, Malouf NN, Oakeley AE, Ungerleider RM, Allen PD, Kay BK. Molecular basis of human cardiac troponin T isoforms expressed in the developing, adult, and failing heart. Circ Res. 1995;76(4):681–6.
21. Yang TP, Agellon LB, Walsh A, Breslow JL, Tall AR. Alternative splicing of the human cholesteryl Ester transfer protein Gene in transgenic mice exon exclusion modulates gene expression in response to dietary or developmental change. J Biol Chem. 1996;271(21):12603–9.
22. Freyermuth F. Splicing misregulation of SCN5A contributes to cardiac-conduction delay and heart arrhythmia in myotonic dystrophy. Nat Commun. 2016;7:11067.
23. Zhou A. mRNA stability hu proteins regulate human cardiac sodium channel expression. Circulation. 2014;130(Suppl 2):A15892.
24. Zhang Y, Si Y, Ma N, Mei J. The RNA-binding protein PCBP2 inhibits Ang II-induced hypertrophy of cardiomyocytes though promoting GPR56 mRNA degeneration. Biochem Biophys Res Commun. 2015;464(3):679–84.
25. Li J. Cold-inducible RNA-binding protein regulates cardiac repolarization by targeting transient outward potassium channels. Circ Res. 2015;116(10):1655–9.

26. Hui J, Stangl K, Lane WS, Bindereif A. HnRNP L stimulates splicing of the eNOS gene by binding to variable-length CA repeats. Nat Struct Mol Biol. 2003;10(1):33.
27. Lorenz M. Alternative splicing in intron 13 of the human eNOS gene: a potential mechanism for regulating eNOS activity. FASEB J. 2007;21(7):1556–64.
28. Osera C. Induction of VEGFA mRNA translation by CoCl2 mediated by HuR. RNA Biol. 2015;12(10):1121–30.
29. Galbán S. RNA-binding proteins HuR and PTB promote the translation of hypoxia-inducible factor 1α. Mol Cell Biol. 2008;28(1):93–107.
30. Vumbaca F, Phoenix KN, Rodriguez-Pinto D, Han DK, Claffey KP. Double-stranded RNA-binding protein regulates vascular endothelial growth factor mRNA stability, translation, and breast cancer angiogenesis. Mol Cell Biol. 2008;28(2):772–83.
31. Blanco FJ, Bernabeu C. Alternative splicing factor or splicing factor-2 plays a key role in intron retention of the endoglin gene during endothelial senescence. Aging Cell. 2011;10(5):896–907.
32. Liu K, Xuekelati S, Zhang Y, Yin Y, Li Y, Chai R, Li X, Peng Y, Wu J, Guo X. Expression levels of atherosclerosis-associated miR-143 and miR-145 in the plasma of patients with hyperhomocysteinaemia. BMC Cardiovasc Disord. 2017;17(1):163.
33. Henry JC, Azevedo-Pouly AC, Schmittgen TD. MicroRNA replacement therapy for cancer. Pharm Res. 2011;28(12):3030–42.
34. Quiat D, Olson EN. MicroRNAs in cardiovascular disease: from pathogenesis to prevention and treatment. J Clin Invest. 2013;123(1):11–8.
35. Rao SS. Engineering optimization: theory and practice. Hoboken: Wiley; 2009.
36. Thum T, et al. MicroRNA-21 contributes to myocardial disease by stimulating MAP kinase signalling in fibroblasts. Nature. 2008;456(7224):980.
37. Pan YZ, Zhou A, Hu Z, Yu AM. Small nucleolar RNA-derived microRNA hsa-miR-1291 modulates cellular drug disposition through direct targeting of ABC transporter ABCC1. Drug Metab Dispos. 2013;41(10):1744–51.
38. Seeger T, Boon RA. MicroRNAs in cardiovascular ageing. J Physiol. 2016;594(8):2085–94.
39. Condorelli G, Latronico MV, Cavarretta E. microRNAs in cardiovascular diseases: current knowledge and the road ahead. J Am Coll Cardiol. 2014;63(21):2177–87.
40. Meloni M. Local inhibition of microRNA-24 improves reparative angiogenesis and left ventricle remodeling and function in mice with myocardial infarction. Mol Ther. 2013;21(7):1390–402.
41. Wang P. Identification of resting and type I IFN-activated human NK cell miRNomes reveals microRNA-378 and microRNA-30e as negative regulators of NK cell cytotoxicity. J Immunol. 2012;189:211–21. https://doi.org/10.4049/jimmunol.1200609.
42. Valeri N. Modulation of mismatch repair and genomic stability by miR-155. Proc Natl Acad Sci USA. 2010;107:6982–7.
43. Icli B. MicroRNA-26a regulates pathological and physiological angiogenesis by targeting BMP/SMAD1 signaling. Circ Res. 2013;113(11):1231–41.
44. al DY. A panel of 4 microRNAs facilitates the prediction of left ventricular contractility after acute myocardial infarction. PLoS One. 2013;8(8):e70644.
45. Li HY, Zhang Y, Cai JH, Bian HL. MicroRNA-451 inhibits growth of human colorectal carcinoma cells via downregulation of Pi3k/Akt pathway. Asian Pac J Cancer Prev. 2013;14:3631–4.
46. Landgraf P, et al. A mammalian microRNA expression atlas based on small RNA library sequencing. Cell. 2007;129(7):1401–14.
47. Raitoharju E, et al. miR-21, miR-210, miR-34a, and miR-146a/b are up-regulated in human atherosclerotic plaques in the Tampere vascular study. Atherosclerosis. 2011;219(1):211–7.
48. Jazbutyte V, Thum T. MicroRNA-21: from cancer to cardiovascular disease. Curr Drug Targets. 2010;11(8):926–35.
49. Zhou J, et al. MicroRNA-21 targets peroxisome proliferators-activated receptor-α in an autoregulatory loop to modulate flow-induced endothelial inflammation. Proc Natl Acad Sci. 2011;108(25):10355–60.
50. Talepoor AG, Kalani M, Dahaghani AS, Doroudchi M. Hydrogen peroxide and lipopolysaccharide differentially affect the expression of microRNAs 10a, 33a, 21, 221 in endothelial cells before and after coculture with monocytes. Int J Toxicol. 2017;36(2):133–41.
51. Seddiki N, Brezar V, Ruffin N, Lévy Y, Swaminathan S. Role of mi R-155 in the regulation of lymphocyte immune function and disease. Immunology. 2014;142(1):32–8.
52. McCurley A. Direct regulation of blood pressure by smooth muscle cell mineralocorticoid receptors. Nat Med. 2012;18(9):1429.
53. Jia QW, Chen ZH, Ding XQ, Liu JY, Ge PC, An FH, Li LH, Wang LS, Ma WZ, Yang ZJ, Jia EZ. Predictive effects of circulating miR-221, miR-130a and miR-155 for coronary heart disease: a multi-ethnic study in China. Cell Physiol Biochem. 2017;42(2):808–23.
54. Li K, Ching D, Luk FS, Raffai RL. Apolipoprotein E enhances microRNA-146a in monocytes and macrophages to suppress nuclear factor-κB–driven inflammation and atherosclerosis. Circ Res. 2015;117(1):e1–e11.
55. Santovito D. Overexpression of microRNA-145 in atherosclerotic plaques from hypertensive patients. Expert Opin Ther Targets. 2013;17(3):217–23.
56. Fazi F, Rosa A, Fatica A, Gelmetti V, De Marchis ML, Nervi C, Bozzoni I. A minicircuitry comprised of microRNA-223 and transcription factors NFI-A and C/EBPα regulates human granulopoiesis. Cell. 2005;123(5):819–31.
57. Deiuliis JA. Visceral adipose microRNA 223 is upregulated in human and murine obesity and modulates

the inflammatory phenotype of macrophages. PLoS One. 2016;11(11):e0165962.
58. Chen Y. Increased circulating exosomal miRNA-223 is associated with acute ischemic stroke. Front Neurol. 2017;8:57.
59. Esau C. miR-122 regulation of lipid metabolism revealed by in vivo antisense targeting. Cell Metab. 2006;3:87–98.
60. Rayner KJ. Antagonism of miR-33 in mice promotes reverse cholesterol transport and regression of atherosclerosis. J Clin Investig. 2011;121:2921–31.
61. Banerjee J, Sen CK. MicroRNAs in skin and wound healing. Methods Mol Biol. 2013;936:343–56.
62. Montgomery RL. Therapeutic inhibition of miR-208a improves cardiac function and survival during heart failure. Circulation. 2011;124:1537–47.
63. Sassi Y. Cardiac myocyte miR-29 promotes pathological remodeling of the heart by activating Wnt signaling. Nat Commun. 2017;8(1):1614.
64. Laina A, Gatsiou A, Georgiopoulos G, Stamatelopoulos K, Stellos K. RNA therapeutics in cardiovascular precision medicine. Front Physiol. 2018;9:953.
65. Wang Y, Zhang X, Li H, Yu J, Ren X. The role of miRNA-29 family in cancer. Eur J Cell Biol. 2013;92(3):123–8.
66. Tijsen AJ. MiR423-5p as a circulating biomarker for heart failure. Circ Res. 2010;106(6):1035.
67. Wu. MiR-328 expression is decreased in high-grade gliomas and is associated with worse survival in primary glioblastoma. PLoS One. 2012;7(10):e47270.
68. Cheng C, Wang Q, You W, Chen M, Xia J. MiRNAs as biomarkers of myocardial infarction: a meta-analysis. PLoS One. 2014;9(2):e88566.
69. Yang Y, Li H, Hou S, Hu B, Liu J, Wang J. The noncoding RNA expression profile and the effect of lncRNA AK126698 on cisplatin resistance in non-small-cell lung cancer cell. PLoS One. 2013;8(5):e65309.
70. Fichtlscherer S, Zeiher AM, Dimmeler S. Circulating microRNAs: biomarkers or mediators of cardiovascular diseases? Arterioscler Thromb Vasc Biol. 2011;31(11):2383–90.
71. Fukushima Y, Nakanishi M, Nonogi H, Goto Y, Iwai N. Assessment of plasma miRNAs in congestive heart failure. Circ J. 2011;75(2):336–40.
72. Ren XL. MicroRNA-206 functions as a tumor suppressor in colorectal cancer by targeting FMNL2. J Cancer Res Clin Oncol. 2016;142(3):581–92.

Part III

Non-coding RNAs Regulation in Cardiovascular System

Involvement of Epigenetic Control and Non-coding RNAs in Cardiovascular System

6

Swati Sharma, Aastha Mishra, and Mohammad Zahid Ashraf

Abstract

Cardiovascular Diseases (CVDs) as a leading cause of death worldwide inflict major stress on morbidity and societal costs. Though the studies pertaining to pathophysiology and genetics of CVDs have helped in prevention, diagnosis and treatment of diseases, there are still lacunas in our knowledge. So, novel tools that can define genomic regulation under different conditions are needed to bridge this gap. 'Epigenetic' mechanism helps the cells to quickly respond to ever changing environment by molecular mechanisms like methylation, histone modifications, nc-RNAs. These mechanisms act as a new layer of regulation in CVDs. The role of epigenetics as a key regulatory player in prevention, diagnosis and treatment of CVDs is emerging. Thus, the focus of present chapter is to decipher the role of epigenetics in CVDs and its potential to be used in risk assessment or as biomarkers in devising and deploying better diagnosis and treatment for different CVDs.

Keywords

Epigenetics · Non-coding RNAs · DNA methylation · Cardiovascular diseases (CVDs) · Histone modifications

S. Sharma · A. Mishra · M. Z. Ashraf (✉)
Department of Biotechnology, Faculty of Natural Sciences, Jamia Millia Islamia, New Delhi, India
e-mail: zashraf@jmi.ac.in

1 Background

Cardiovascular system responsible for transportation of nutrients as well as cellular waste products comprises of the heart, blood and blood vessels. The term cardiovascular diseases (CVDs) refer to any disease of cardiovascular system. CVDs inflict major burden on mortality worldwide making it global epidemic even after the advances made in their prevention and management. CVDs are not only public health issue but also accounts for massive societal costs as healthcare expenditure. They as a group of multifactorial disorders are associated with various genetic and acquired risk factors. But the known genetic and environmental influences cannot fully explain the variability in CVD risk among different populations contributing to the major road blocks in its treatment and prevention. Though thorough studies pertaining to pathophysiology, epidemiology, gene polymorphism, genetic linkage maps and various environmental stresses have paved a way for better diagnosis and treatment of cardiovascular medicine, but still there is lacuna in our understanding of interaction between environment and genome, in development of CVD. As inherited genome contribute to only a part of individual's risk profile, '**epi**'genomics has emerged as a promising area of interest that can bridge gaps in our understanding pathophysiology to therapeutics of diseases. Epigenetic changes or modifications are the 'heritable changes in the genome that does not include changes in DNA sequences'

J. Xiao (ed.), *Non-coding RNAs in Cardiovascular Diseases*, Advances in Experimental Medicine and Biology 1229, https://doi.org/10.1007/978-981-15-1671-9_6

which includes various mechanisms like DNA methylation, demethylation, histone modifications, RNA mediated alterations (microRNAs, circulatory RNAs, long non-coding RNAs) etc. Epigenetic mechanisms collectively empower the cell to quickly respond to environmental changes. Various established risk factors for CVD such as stress, pollution, smoking, nutrition, circadian rhythm, hypoxia etc. are associated with modifications in epigenetic markers. Therefore, the examination of these markers as regulators in CVD may emerge as early preventive and novel therapeutic approach. This book chapter therefore focuses on acquainting the vascular biology community with the advent filed of epigenetics and its role in cardiovascular medicine. The chapter consists of a brief introduction of cardiovascular disease, epigenetic mechanisms and evidences linking various epigenetic mechanisms with CVD. The main emphasize of this chapter would be on epigenetic regulator of CVDs to understand their translational potential and clinical reality in cardiovascular medicine.

2 Cardiovascular Diseases (CVDs)

CVDs are wide spectrum of disorders that comprises of abnormalities related to heart and blood vasculature. They include: Coronary artery diseases (CAD) like angina and myocardial infarction (heart attack), stroke, heart failure, coronary heart disease, cerebrovascular disease, peripheral arterial disease, rheumatic heart disease cardiomyopathy, heart arrhythmia, congenital heart disease, congenital heart disease, thromboembolic disorders and thrombosis. The underlying molecular mechanism pertaining to different CVDs vary considerably as majority of CVDs are regulated by multiple factors. For example, CAD and stroke involve atherosclerosis and rheumatic heart disease involves damage to heart muscle and valves caused by streptococcal bacteria. Even with different molecular mechanisms, nevertheless, most CVDs share common risk factors that are, high blood pressure, high blood cholesterol, diabetes mellitus, smoking, obesity, lack of exercise, alcohol consumption, hypoxia, to name a few.

CVDs are the leading cause of death globally accounting for most of annual mortality as compared to any other disease [1]. Over the period of last 100 years the prevalence of CVDs has increased tremendously and for the coming two decades it is likely to remain a major health issue even with sophisticated techniques and improved medical care [2–4]. The deaths caused by CVDs have increased over the course of time from 12.3 million (25.8%) in 1990 to 17.9 million (32.1%) in 2015 [5, 6]. In 2016, 31% of the global deaths that reached up to 17.9 million people were due to Different CVDs. Heart attack and stroke contributed to 85% of these deaths [7]. Studies estimate that 90% of the CVDs may be preventable [8, 9] by improving the known risk factors like hypertension, diabetes, smoking, alcohol consumption by healthy eating, avoidance of smoke and alcohol, exercise and appropriate medical counselling [10]. Thus, people who are at high cardiovascular risk need early detection and management in order to prevent the occurrence of disease.

The CVDs appeared as a huge public health hazard during 1940s, that triggered the research associated with the factors that influence occurrence of the disease. The research programmes like Framingham Heart Study were initiated to find out common genetic, biochemical, environmental and life style related factors that lead to occurrence or predisposition to various CVDs [11]. This resulted in identification of several conditions like obesity, hypertension and diabetes to detect individuals at risk of CVD and their early treatment. It in turn lead to significant decline in CVD mortality in USA and Western Europe over the past 3 decades. Therefore, it is important to understand the risk factors associated with CVDs.

2.1 Types of Cardiovascular Diseases

CVDs are group of disorders involving heart, blood vessels or both. Thus, they are characterised either as vascular diseases that majorly affects blood vasculature or heart diseases that majorly affects heart.

2.1.1 Vascular Diseases

The common vascular diseases are coronary artery disease, peripheral arterial disease, cerebrovascular disease, renal artery stenosis, aortic aneurysm, stroke, thrombosis.

2.1.2 Heart Diseases

The common CVDs affecting heart are cardiomyopathy, hypertensive heart disease, heart failure, pulmonary heart disease, cardiac dysrhythmias, inflammatory heart disease, valvular heart disease, congenital heart disease, rheumatic heart disease.

2.2 The Risk Factors Associated with CVDs

The most contributing risk factors for stroke and heart disease are genetic predisposition, unhealthy diet, age, sex, excessive use of alcohol, obesity, hypertension, diabetes, hyperlipidemia, stress, air pollution etc. Though it is very difficult to access the individual contribution of each risk factor among different ethnic group or populations, but the overall impact of these risk factors is quite consistent [12].

2.2.1 Genetic Predisposition

Most CVDs are multifactorial in nature i.e. there are several genes or genetic factors that contribute to development and progression of the disease. There are many identified single nucleotide polymorphisms (SNPs) make individual susceptible to the disease [13, 14]. Even with the sophisticated techniques the contribution of all genetic factors and their influence of vascular diseases is poorly understood.

2.2.2 Age

Age is one of the most important contributing risk factors towards the development of heart diseases, with each passing decade it triples the risk of disease [15]. The case studies show that 82% coronary heart patients that die are either of 65 years or older [15]. Similarly, the risk of death by stroke doubles after every 10 passing years after the age of 55 [17]. There are multiple theories that explain the influence of age on CVDs, one relates to increased serum cholesterol level with age [18] other with the changes in vascular wall [15]. Age decreases the arterial elasticity and reduced arterial compliance that subsequently causes coronary artery disease.

2.2.3 Sex

Gender influences the prevalence of heart diseases. Men are more susceptible than premenopausal women [16]. Middle aged men are at 2–5 times higher risk of coronary heart diseases at compare to women [19]. A study by World Health Organisation (WHO) reveals that sex contributes to roughly 40% difference in the mortality rate caused by coronary heart diseases [20]. The influence of gender in CVDs may be due to hormonal differences between men and women [20].

2.2.4 Excessive Use of Alcohol

The effect of alcohol consumption on CVDs is complex and depends largely on the quantity of alcohol consumed. The high level of drinking is directly related to susceptibility to the disease [21].

2.2.5 Obesity

Another risk factor for developing CVDs is being overweight or obesity. An unhealthy diet and physical inactivity lead to high body mass index (BMI), that falls outside the normal range making a person obese. This may lead to diseases like coronary heart disease and congestive heart failure [22].

2.2.6 Hypertension

High blood pressure or hypertension cause stress on blood vasculature making them weak or cause them to clog. It is a potent risk factor that can lead to atherosclerosis as it causes narrowing of blood vessels which make them more prone to be blocked by blood clots or fatty deposits [23].

2.2.7 Diabetes

High blood glucose levels as experienced in diabetes make individual more vulnerable for developing CVDs. The high levels of glucose have damaging effect on arterial walls and more likely cause the build-up of fat deposits called atheroma. These fat depositions if occur in coronary arteries may lead to coronary heart disease and heart attacks [24].

2.2.8 Hyperlipidemia

Hyperlipidemia is presence of abnormal level of lipids (fats) in blood stream and is one of the major contributory risk factors for CVDs. The high levels of "bad cholesterol" i.e. low-density lipoprotein (LDL) cholesterol is associated with range of heart diseases as it results in fatty substance deposition on the vasculature leading to various complications [23].

2.2.9 Diet

Diet plays a crucial role in prevention and development of CVDs. A diet rich in saturated fatty acids increases the risk of stroke and heart diseases. It is estimated that 11% of stroke and 31% of coronary heart diseases worldwide are caused by high dietary saturated fatty acids [23].

2.2.10 Air Pollution

The effect of particulate matter present in the air for its short- and long-term exposure on CVDs has been accessed. It was found in recent studies that the long-term exposure of $PM_{2.5}$ results in increased 8–18% CVD mortality risk [24].

The majority of above-mentioned CVD risk factors are manageable and can be reduced by opting alternative lifestyle. For example, reduction of alcohol consumption, fatty food, salt, regular physical exercise, consumption of vegetables and fruits reduce the risk of CVDs drastically. In addition, the treatment of hypertension, diabetes and hyperlipidemia is essential for reducing the risk of heart diseases. Thus, there are choices by which people can adopt and sustain healthy way of living, but we need health policies and conducive environments that can make these choices affordable and available to masses. The other major forces driving occurrence of CVDs are stress, poverty, urbanization, socio-economic and cultural changes. With all the knowledge on contributing factors and advancement of genomic era, we still fail to answer the variability in CVD risk, role of individual risk factors, their cumulative effect. Also, the clinical utility of identified genetic markers has been limited in both prevention and prediction of diseases [25].With the translational disappointment of genomics field, the vascular community is now exploiting epigenomics as new avenue for assessing risk stratification, preventive measures and treatment. Epigenetics is the heritable changes in the genome that are not coded by the DNA sequence [26]. There are three broad mechanisms that define epigenetic changes: DNA methylation, post- translational histone modifications and RNA based mechanisms (microRNAs, circular RNAs and non-coding RNAs) [27]. DNA methylation is the most common epigenetic modification in the mammalian genome [28, 29]. The recent studies though suggest that all the three epigenetic modifications contribute to the pathogenesis of CVDs [30]. The international projects like Human Epigenome Project (HEP) and International Human Epigenome Consortium (IHEC) have been initiated to study and catalogue human epigenome along with correlation of its pathophysiology with several diseases including CVDs [31].The focus of this chapter is epigenetics in CVDs, and will be discussed under the following sections.

3 Leads from Genetics

Almost three decades ago the research on the genetic factors and genes that predispose an individual to CVDs has started. It was thought that the SNPs and mutations in the genome could be analogous to already known CVD risk factors. It was anticipated that they could be included in risk assessment model like Framingham score

[30] in order to calculate and determine the risk of an individual to develop CVD and adopt apt preventive therapeutic approaches. The traditional approach was to study the role of candidate gene as risk factor, but now the genome-wide association studies grouped with availability of large patient cohorts are used to uncover the novel genes and genetic factors that act like risk factors for various CVDs [31]. The genetic research has enabled the cardiovascular community to better understand the disease origin and its pathophysiology. It has progressively also helped in the risk stratification, direct and indirect diagnosis and therapeutic interventions. The novel GWAS has widened the understanding of pathophysiology of various CVDs. The genetic studies have also led to discovery of new drug targets that may considerably improve the current therapeutic approaches for CVDs. The genotyping studies have been used for diagnostic and prognostic assessment by clinicians. But still genetic studies are unable to find the "holy grail" for diagnosis of CVDs. So, there is a need of more profound knowledge that can answer dynamics of disease. 'Epi'genetics promises to deepen the present insights as it can well explain the influence of environment on the genome. It can unveil the interaction between the genetic variants and environment changes; thus, can elucidate the clinical drug responsiveness and patient outcome.

4 Epigenetic Revolutions – Genomics to Post-Genomic Era

Epigenetics has emerged as a post genomic era that can reveal the lacuna in our understanding of inheritance of common traits. It provides the link between environment and its effect on genome, thus deciphering the mechanism by which cells are able to respond quickly to environmental stimuli. The phenotypic variations seen in humans that cannot be solely defined by genotype, can be better explained in the light of epigenetic modifications [32]. Epigenetic mechanisms are stable cellular memory, which let the propagation of gene activities generation after generation without the changes in the DNA sequence. There are three broad mechanisms that define epigenetic changes: DNA methylation, post- translational histone modifications and RNA based mechanisms (microRNAs, circular RNAs and long non-coding RNAs). The simple and static evaluation of the genetic code has limited the understanding of genetic influence on CVDs. In this respect, epigenetics as a dynamic mechanism can explain and modify the genome's functionality under the influence of exogenous stimuli or environment condition. This would in turn help in identification of novel targets and mechanism of gene regulation with considerable acquisitions in CVD knowledge related to genetic risk and pathophysiology [33–35]. The environmental changes like pollution, diet, stress etc. leads to epigenetic modifications and impact the susceptibility to CVD (Fig. 6.1). There are reports that validate the role of epigenetic in various processes underlying CVDs like hypertension, inflammation and atherosclerosis [35].

The following sections of the chapters will deal with different epigenetic modifications and their role in progression, prevention, treatment and diagnosis of CVDs.

4.1 DNA Methylation

DNA methylation is the addition of the methyl group at the cytosine bases of the dinucleotide CpGs of eukaryotic DNA. As a result they are converted to 5-methylycytosine by de novo DNA methyltransferase (DNMT) enzymes such as DNMT1, DNMT3A and DNMT3B. In mammals, methylation is found sparsely but globally with the exception of CpG islands. Vertebrate CpG islands are short interspersed DNA sequences (>500 bp) generally found in the 5′ end of the gene that deviate significantly from the average genomic pattern by being GC-rich (G + C percentage greater than 55%), CpG rich (observed CpG/expected CpG of 0.65) and predominantly non-methylated [36].

Out of the several ways, the methylation of DNA is one of the most common ways of

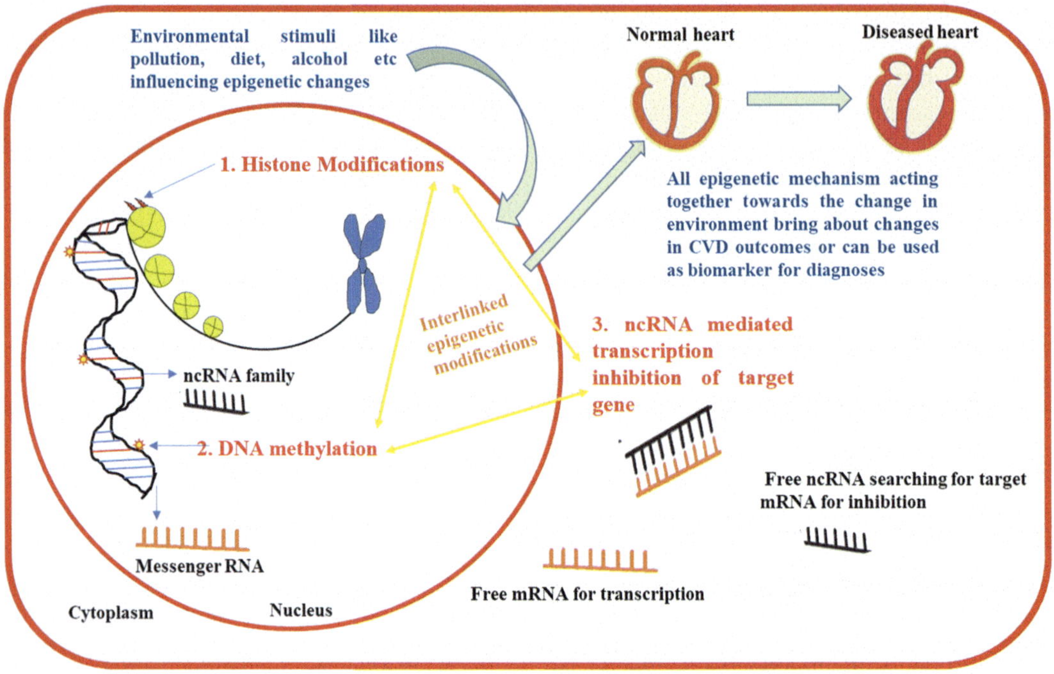

Fig. 6.1 Epigenetic modifications: The figure depicts the three most common epigenetic modifications that occur in mammalian genome namely, histone modification and chromatin remodelling, DNA methylation and modifications mediated by non-coding RNA (ncRNA) family like miRNA, circRNA and lncRNA. All these modifications are interlinked and enable cells to quickly respond to changing environment. The established risk factors of CVD like stress, pollution, age, diet, pollution etc. can act as environmental stimuli and triggers epigenetic modifications resulting in release of various regulatory molecules that can be used as biomarkers. The changes also influence the CVD outcomes

regulating gene expressions in eukaryotes [37]. It has emerged as an important process in numerous cellular processes like genomic imprinting, embryonic development, X-chromosome inactivation and many more. The first clue of the role of methylation in gene expression was provided by 5-azacytidine experiments in mouse studies [38]. The integration of 5-azacytidine in the growing strand of DNA severely inhibited the actions of DNMT enzymes to normally methylate DNA. Therefore, the comparisons of the cells before and after the treatment of 5-azacytidine allowed to see the impact of loss of methylation on gene expression [39]. The exact role of methylation in gene expression is unknown, perhaps it play a crucial role in repressing gene expression by blocking the promoters at which activating transcription factors bind. Approximately, 70% of annotated gene promoters are associated with CpG islands, making it the most common promoter type in the genome [36]. Not all CpG islands found are associated with the promoter. Recent works have found a large class of islands that are remote from the transcription start sites (TSSs) but still show evidence for the promoter function. The lack of CpG dinucleotides in the vertebrate genome except the CpG island is thought to be due to the loss of genomic CpGs due to deamination of methylated sequences [39].

Given the critical role of DNA methylation in gene expression and cell differentiation, it seems obvious that the errors in methylation could give rise to a number of devastating consequences, including various diseases. As a result, a growing number of human diseases have been found to be associated with aberrant DNA methylation [40]. The methylation of the promoter region bearing transcriptional start sites of many genes encoding tumor suppressors such as tumor protein p53, retinoblastoma-associated protein 1, tumor protein p16, breast cancer 1 and many more resulting in the reduced expression of these genes have been found in a large number of cancers like retinoblastoma, colon, lung and ovarian [40, 41]. 5-methylcytosine (5-mC) is spontaneously converted to thymine by deamination and is thought to be responsible for about one-third of all disease-causing mutations in the germline [39]. The mechanisms for establishing, maintaining and removing the methyl group are dependent on nucleosomal DNA and the histone modifications within the nucleosome [39]. Global methylation studies are the first ever epigenetics studies in the area of CVD research. The outcome of these studies though were conflicting as some studies highlighted decreased global DNA methylations with CVDs [40] while some associated increased global methylations with these disorders [41, 42]. Coronary heart disease have been associated with elevated homocystein and increased methylations [43]. DNA methylation studies include investigation of repetitive sequences across the genome such as Alu elements and long interspersed nucleotide element-1 (LINE)-1. Hypomethylation of LINE-1 was associated with cardiovascular risk factors such as higher serum vascular cell adhesion molecule [44] and higher low-density lipoprotein (LDL) and lower high-density lipoprotein (HDL) cholesterol [47]. LINE-1 hypomethylation has also been associated with higher prevalence of metabolic syndrome, and therefore elevated risk for CVD [48]. There are several genes responsible for DNA methylation and investigation of these candidate genes demonstrated some interesting results. *Fat mass and obesity-associated protein (FTO),* a prominent obesity-associated gene has been linked to levels of DNA methylation [49] and CVD risk independently of its effect on body mass index [50]. Similarly, other candidate genes such as *F2R Like Thrombin Or Trypsin Receptor 3, Insulin, GNAS Antisense RNA 1, Phospholipase A2 Group VII, Insulin Like Growth Factor 2,* to name a few has been associated with various CVDs [51–54]. With the advent of whole epigenome array several markers and novel distinct patterns of DNA methylations have been identified in the context of CVDs [55–58]. The outcome of all these studies could result in the novel therapeutic interventions in cardiovascular diseases.

4.2 Post-translation Histone Modifications and Chromatin Remodelling

Histone modification is a covalent post-translational modification, which includes methylation, phosphorylation, acetylation, sumoylation and ubiquitylation, to histone proteins. These modifications are known to play an important role in replication, transcription, heterochromatin formation, chromatin compaction, and DNA damage repair. Investigation of histone modifications in CVDs reveals the crucial role of histone deacetylases (HDACs). It is the most extensively studied family of histone-modifying enzymes in the cardiovascular system [59]. Studies have demonstrated the effect of its inhibition in attenuating hypertension [60] and in prevention of proliferation of vascular smooth muscle cells [61, 62]. Class III HDACs also known as sirtuins have been shown to participate in cardiac hypertrophy and myocardial ischemia [63]. The other class of enzyme, histone acetyl transferase has been associated in the settings of atherosclerosis through regulation of genes that inhibit endothelial cell inflammation [64]. Similarly, the loss-of-function studies of histone methyltransferase in the adult heart showed hypertrophy, dilation, and derepression of some cardiac disease genes [65]. The polycomb repressive complex, one of the best-studied gene silencing complexes, has been implicated in a wide variety of phenotypes in the cardiovascular system. They have been shown to be differentially involved in cardiac development and regeneration [66].

4.3 RNA Based Modifications (miRNAs, circRNAs, lncRNAs)

The RNA based modifications include microRNAs (miRNAs), circular RNAs (circRNAs) and recently discovered long non-coding RNAs (lncRNAs). They all are non-coding endogenous RNAs that regulate the genome without being translated into proteins. The recent studies show the implication of these non-coding RNAs in CVD pathophysiology. There is large number of growing evidences that show role of miRNAs and lncRNAs in both animal and cellular models of CVD. In the following sections, we will be studying the role of these non-coding RNAs in CVDs and how they can be used as either biomarker or for treatment in CVDs.

4.3.1 miRNAs in CVD Scenario

miRNAs are class of endogenous interfering RNAs that are coded by human genome. Mature miRNAs are 20–25 nucleotide long RNA sequence that are synthesised in canonical pathway from a large RNA precursor, pri-miRNA. In the nucleus pri-miRNA is transcribed and matured by RNA polymerase II. It is then subsequently cleaved by RNase III Drosha and associated protein, giving a 60–70 nucleotide long pre-miRNA, which is released into the cytoplasm. In cytoplasm it is cleaved by RNaseIII Dicer resulting in 21–25 nucleotide long double stranded miRNA/miRNA* duplex. This duplex is unwounded by RNA induced-silencing complex (RISC), which carries mature single stranded miRNA to target messenger RNA causing subsequent gene silencing. Thus, miRNAs decrease the expression of gene by binding to them and causing translational repression [67]. Non-coding RNAs like miRNAs have emerged as prime candidates for discovering novel biomarkers for CVDs. As there is correlation between the pathologies and blood miRNA levels, miRNAscan be great tool for being non-invasive biomarkers. The general hypothesis is that miRNAs would be differentially expressed in people having CVD and are at risk of CVD and in normal population. So, plasma miRNA levels can be promising avenue for evaluating early CVD risk and patient outcome, along with assessing individual patient response towards various surgical procedures or treatment. The pioneering work in this field is done by Dimmeler et al., they highlighted the change in serum miRNA levels of CAD patients Vs. control [42]. There are other studies that have shown miRNAs as potential biomarkers to predict CVD outcome. For instance, the work done by Seronde et al. has shown that low serum levels of miR-423-5p are associated with a poor long-term outcome in acute heart failure patients, emphasising the role of miR-423-5p as a prognostic biomarker for predicting acute heart failure [43]. The cardiovascular deaths caused by acute coronary syndrome were precisely predicted by the sericlevels of miR-132, miR-140-3p, and miR-210 in the study consisting of 1114 patients [44]. Several miRNAs are very sensitive to even small exogenous stimuli like changes in blood pressure that can be predictive of circulatory stress or hypertension (established risk factor for CVD) [45]. miR-22 is a potential biomarker candidate for predicting CVD in elderly patients asmiR-22 regulates cardiac autophagy specially in myocardium of elderly patients thus circulating levels this miRNA gives prognostic clue on eventual progression of disease ultimately leading to heart failure in elderly [46]. Regular exercise can reduce the outcomes of CVDs and several miRNAs have been proposed as biomarkers to monitor physiological effect of regular exercise in different populations. For example, decreased level of miR-146a and-miR-221, and increased level of miR-149 are seen after acute exercise [47]. Whereas the altered level of expression of miR-1, miR-133, and miR-206 is seen after the endurance exercise [48]. A recent study has highlighted the role of miR-145 in impeding the thrombus formation in vivo by targeting tissue factor in the case of venous thrombosis [49].

4.3.2 circRNAs in CVD Scenario

circular RNAs are single stranded RNAs that form a covalently closed continuous loop. They are expressed in mammalian tissues as transcriptional and translational regulators [50]. Just like miRNAs, circRNAs are stable and detectable in blood stream, making it possible to use them as non-invasive biomarker. It is seen that in aged human hearts the level of circAmotl1decreases dramatically [51]. The risk of atherosclerotic vascular diseases is correlated with the expression of the increased expression circANRILin CAD patients [52]. The diagnostic biomarkers for various CVDs identified in peripheral blood mononuclearcells (PBMCs) are Hsa_circ_0005836, hsa_circRNA_025016, andhsa_circ_0124644 [53, 54].

4.3.3 Long Non-coding (lnc)-RNAs in CVD Scenario

lncRNAs are the RNA sequences that exceed more than 200 nucleotides and don't code for any functional transcript. They differ from other non-coding RNAs like miRNAs as they are poorly conserved across the species also, they regulate gene expression at both transcription and post-transcriptional level. They allow microRNAs' target mRNA escape degradation as they act as decoy for microRNA [55]. The advancement in sequencing techniques like deep sequencing has made it possible to study the lncRNA profiles in different CVDs as well as normal healthy population. And it is found that lncRNAs regulate multiple biological pathways in aging and cardiac development [56]. The 9 lncRNAs namely CDKN2BAS1/ANRIL, RMRP, RNY5, SOX2-OT, SRA1 EGOT, H19, HOTAIR, and LOC285194/TUSC7 were significantly modulated in non-ischemic myocardial biopsies of patients suffering from heart failure and dilated ischemic cardiomyopathy. Also, in mouse model the expression level of RMRP, H19, and HOTAIRlncRNAs were upregulated when measured in hypertrophic heart sample [57]. MIAT (myocardial infarction-associated transcript) and SENCR (smooth muscle and endothelial cell enriched migration/differentiation-associated lncRNA), are other lncRNA markers that are associated with dysfunction and myocardial infarction [58, 59]. Nodal lncRNAs act as key regulators of cardiomyocte cell cycle as revealed by the data of single cardiomyocyte nuclear transcriptome analysis of normal and failing heart [60]. Interestingly, the severity of fibrosis in human diseased heart is directly correlated with a cardiac fibroblast enriched lncRNA- Wisper (Wisp2 super enhancer-associated RNA) [61]. Growing evidences show that majority of lncRNAs are localised in nucleus and are capable of triggering chromatin remodelling by recruitment of various epigenetic factors, thereby causing activation or repression of genes. The genes involved in cardiac hypertrophy are regulated by a cardiac-enriched lncRNA via its direct interaction with catalytic subunit of PRC2 causing inhibition of methylation of histone H3 lysine 27 [62].

At last we can conclude that non-coding RNAs play a role in controlling gene expression and shaping genome organisation. With increasingly more functions and roles of non-coding RNAs being discovered, we need to use better biochemical approaches along with deep sequencing analysis coupled with novel bioinformatics strategies so that a comprehensive understanding of their role in CVDs can be provided.

5 Perspective

The role of epigenetic alterations in the capacity of DNA methylation, chromatin remodelling and non coding-RNAs has been emerging in the development of CVDs. However, the results of epigenetic studies are inconsistent and contradictory. Epigenetic phenomenon, as we know, is not a stable or heritable event. It is dynamic in the sense that it gets altered by environmental factors and can vary with time. These all features have to be taken into considerations while designing the studies for any type of epigenetics research. Not just the nature of samples and the conditions they are exposed to are important but the numbers of times the samples are taken are equally critical. There are various upcoming combinatorial technologies through which researchers can explore epigenetic landscapes. Bisulfite-sequencing combined to ChIP, de novo methylation simultaneously examining nucleosome occupancy and CpG methylation can be utilized for studying multiple epigenetic marks simultaneously. Research in epigenetics is a relatively new approach but it has a remarkable potential to identify new biomarkers in the CVD field. These biomarkers would not be just helpful in CVD diagnosis, outcome, prognosis and treatment but could lead us to new avenues for novel targeted CVD therapies. However, more epigenomic studies are warranted that will help to decipher the complex link between genetics, epigenetics, and CVDs.

Competing Financial Interests The authors declare no competing financial interests.

References

1. Murray C, Lopez A. Alternative projections of mortality and disability by cause1990–2020: global burden of disease study. Lancet. 1997;349:1498–504.
2. Mathers CD, Loncar D. Projections of global mortality and burden of disease from 2002 to 2030. PLoS Med. 2006;3:e442.
3. MacKinnon AU. The origin of the modern epidemic of coronary artery disease in England. J R Coll Gen Pract. 1987;37:174–6.
4. Azambuja MI, Levins R. Coronary heart disease (CHD)—one or several diseases? Changes in the prevalence and features of CHD. Perspect Biol Med. 2007;50:228–42.
5. GBD. Mortality and causes of death collaborators (2014) Global, regional, and national age-sex specific all-cause and cause-specific mortality for 240 causes of death, 1990–2013: a systematic analysis for the Global Burden of Disease Study 2013. Lancet. 2013;385(9963):117–71.
6. GBD. Mortality and Causes of Death Collaborators (2017) Global, regional, and national life expectancy, all-cause mortality, and cause-specific mortality for 249 causes of death, 1980–2015: a systematic analysis for the Global Burden of Disease Study 2015. Lancet. 2015;388(10053):1459–544.
7. McGill HC, McMahan CA, Gidding SS. Preventing heart disease in the 21st century: implications of the Pathobiological Determinants of Atherosclerosis in Youth (PDAY) study. Circulation. 2008;117(9):1216–27.
8. O'Donnell MJ, Chin SL. Global and regional effects of potentially modifiable risk factors associated with acute stroke in 32 countries (INTERSTROKE): a case-control study. Lancet. 2016;388(10046):761–75.
9. Mendis S, Puska P, Norrving B, editors. Global atlas on cardiovascular disease prevention and control. Geneva: World Health Organization/World Heart Federation/World Stroke Organization; 2011.
10. GBD. Mortality and causes of death collaborators (2016) Global, regional, and national life expectancy, all-cause mortality, and cause-specific mortality for 249 causes of death, 1980–2015: a systematic analysis for the Global Burden of Disease Study 2015. Lancet. 2015;388(10053):1459–544.
11. Yusuf S, Hawken S, Ounpuu S, Dans T, Avezum A, Lanas F, Mc Queen M, Budaj A, Pais P, Varigos J, Lisheng L, INTERHEART Study Investigators. Effect of potentially modifiable risk factors associated with myocardial infarction in 52 countries (the INTERHEART study): case-control study. Lancet. 2004;364(9438):937–52.
12. Nikpay M, Goel A, Won H, Hall LM, Willenborg C, Kanoni S, Saleheen D, Kyriakou T, Nelson CP. A comprehensive 1000 Genomes–based genome-wide association meta-analysis of coronary artery disease. Nat Genet. 2015;47(10):1121–30.
13. MacRae CA, Vasan RS. The future of genetics and genomics: closing the phenotype gap in precision medicine. Circulation. 2016;133(25):2634–9.
14. Finegold JA, Asaria P, Francis DP. Mortality from ischaemic heart disease by country, region, and age: statistics from World Health Organisation and United Nations. Int J Cardiol. 2012;168(2):934–45.
15. World Health Organization. The atlas of heart disease and stroke/Judith Mackay and George Mensah with Shanthi Mendis and Kurt Greenland. World Health Organization. 2004.
16. Jousilahti P, Vartiainen E, Tuomilehto J, Puska P. Sex, age, cardiovascular risk factors, and coronary heart disease. Circulation. 1999;99(9):1165–72.
17. Jani B, Rajkumar C. Ageing and vascular ageing. Postgrad Med J. 2006;82(968):357–62.
18. Mukamal KJ, Chen CM, Rao SR, Breslow RA. Alcohol consumption and cardiovascular mortality among U.S. Adults, 1987 to 2002. J Am Coll Cardiol. 2010;55(13):1328–35.
19. Hubert HB, Feinleib M, McNamara PM, Castelli WP. Obesity as an independent risk factor for cardiovascular disease: a 26-year follow-up of participants in the Framingham Heart Study. Circulation. 1983;67(5):968–77.
20. Anderson KM, Odell PM, Wilson PW, Kannel WB. Cardiovascular disease risk profiles. Am Heart J. 1991;121:293–8.
21. Kannel WB, McGee DL. Diabetes and cardiovascular disease. the Framingham study. J Am Med Assoc. 1979;241(19):2035–8.
22. Finks SW, Airee A, Chow SL, Macaulay TE, Moranville MP, Rogers KC, Trujillo TC. Key articles of dietary interventions that influence cardiovascular mortality. Pharmacotherapy. 2012;32(4):e54–87.
23. Khallaf M. The impact of air pollution on health, economy, environment and agricultural sources. Rijeka: InTech; 2011. p. 69–92. ISBN 978-953-307-528-0
24. Di Angelantonio E, Butterworth AS. Clinical utility of genetic variants for cardiovascular risk prediction: a futile exercise or insufficient data? Circ Cardiovasc Genet. 2012;5:387–90.

25. Egger G, Liang G, Aparicio A, Jones PA. Epigenetics in human disease and prospects for epigenetic therapy. Nature. 2004;429:457–63.
26. Kaikkonen MU, Lam MT, Glass CK. Non-coding RNAs as regulators of gene expression and epigenetics. Cardiovasc Res. 2011;90:430–40.
27. Udali S, Guarini P, Moruzzi S, Choi SW, Friso S. Cardiovascular epigenetics: from DNA methylation to microRNAs. Mol Asp Med. 2013;34:883–901.
28. Abbott A. Project set to map marks ongenome. Nature. 2010;463:596–7.
29. Wilson PW, D'Agostino RB, Levy D, Belanger AM, Silbershatz H, Kannel WB. Prediction of coronary heart disease using risk factor categories. Circulation. 1998;97:1837–47.
30. Evans A, Salomaa V, Kulathinal S, Asplund K, Cambien F, Ferrario M, Perola M, Peltonen L, Shields D, Tunstall-Pedoe H, Kuulasmaa K. MORGAM (an international pooling of cardiovascular cohorts). Int J Epidemiol. 2005;34:21–7.
31. Turan N, Katari S, Coutifaris C, Sapienza C. Explaining inter-individual variability in phenotype:is epigenetics up to the challenge? Epigenetics. 2010;5:16–9.
32. Khalil CA. The emerging role of epigenetics in cardiovascular disease. Ther Adv Chronic Dis. 2014;5(4):178–87.
33. Webster AL, Yan MS, Marsden PA. Epigenetics andcardiovascular disease. Can J Cardiol. 2013;29(1):46–57.
34. Muka T, Koromani F, Portilla E, O'Connor A, Bramer WM, Troup J, Chowdhury R, Dehghan A, Franco OH. The role of epigeneticmodifications in cardiovascular disease: a systematic review. Int J Cardiol. 2016;212:174–83.
35. Bird A. CpG-rich islands and the function of DNA methylation. Nature. 1986;321:209–13.
36. Deaton AM, Bird A. CpG islands and the regulation of transcription. Genes Dev. 2011;25(10):1010–22.
37. McGhee JD, Ginder GD. Specific DNA methylation sites in the vicinity of the chicken beta-globin genes. Nature. 1979;280:419–20.
38. Han L, Su B, Li WH, Zhao Z. CpG island density and its correlations with genomic features in mammalian genomes. Genome Biol. 2008;9(5):R79.
39. Robertson KD. DNA methylation and human disease. Nat Rev Genet. 2005;6(8):597–610.
40. Gopalakrishnan S, Van Emburgh BO, Robertson KD. DNA methylation in development and human disease. Mutat Res. 2008;647(1–2):30–8.
41. Handy DE, Castro R, Loscalzo J. Epigenetic modifications: basic mechanisms and role in cardiovascular disease. Circulation. 2011;123:2145–56.
42. Huh I, Zeng J, Park T, Yi SV. DNA methylation and transcriptional noise. Epigenetics Chromatin. 2013;6(1):9.
43. Hsiung DT, Marsit CJ, Houseman EA, Eddy K, Furniss CS, McClean MD, Kelsey KT. Global DNA methylation level in whole blood as a biomarker in head and neck squamous cell carcinoma. Cancer Epidemiol Biomark Prev. 2007;16:108–14.
44. Sharma P, Kumar J, Garg G, Kumar A, Patowary A, Karthikeyan G, Ramakrishnan L, Brahmachari V, Sengupta S. Detection of altered global DNA methylation in coronary artery disease patients. DNA Cell Biol. 2008;27:357–65.
45. Baccarelli A, Tarantini L, Wright RO, Bollati V, Litonjua AA, Zanobetti A, Sparrow D, Vokonas PS, Schwartz J. Repetitive element DNA methylation and circulating endothelial and inflammation markers in the VA normative aging study. Epigenetics. 2010;5(3):222–8.
46. Cash HL, McGarvey ST, Houseman EA, Marsit CJ, Hawley NL, Lambert-Messerlian GM, Viali S, Tuitele J, Kelsey KT. Cardiovascular disease risk factors and DNA methylation at the LINE-1 repeat region in peripheral blood from Samoan Islanders. Epigenetics. 2011;6:1257–64.
47. Turcot V, Tchernof A, Deshaies Y, Pérusse L, Bélisle A, Marceau S, Biron S, Lescelleur O, Biertho L, Vohl MC. LINE-1 methylation in visceral adipose tissue of severely obese individuals is associated with metabolic syndrome status and related phenotypes. Clin Epigenetics. 2012;4:10.
48. Bell CG, Finer S, Lindgren CM, Wilson GA, Rakyan VK, Teschendorff AE, Akan P, Stupka E, Down TA, Prokopenko I, Morison IM, Mill J, Pidsley R, International Type 2 Diabetes 1q Consortium, Deloukas P, Frayling TM, Hattersley AT, MI MC, Beck S, Hitman GA. Integrated genetic and epigenetic analysis identifies haplotype-specific methylation in the FTO type 2 diabetes and obesity susceptibility locus. PLoS One. 2010;5:e14040.
49. Liu C, Mou S, Pan C. The FTO gene rs9939609 polymorphism predicts risk of cardiovascular disease: a systematic review and meta-analysis. PLoS One. 2013;8:e71901.
50. Breitling LP, Salzmann K, Rothenbacher D, Burwinkel B, Brenner H. Smoking, F2RL3 methylation, and prognosis in stable coronary heart disease. Eur Heart J. 2012;33:2841–8.
51. Talens RP, Jukema JW, Trompet S, Kremer D, Westendorp RG, Lumey LH, Sattar N, Putter H, Slagboom PE, Heijmans BT, PROSPER Group. Hypermethylation at loci sensitive to the prenatal environment is associated with increased incidence of myocardial infarction. Int J Epidemiol. 2012;41:106–15.
52. Jiang D, Zheng D, Wang L, Huang Y, Liu H, Xu L, Liao Q, Liu P, Shi X, Wang Z, Sun L, Zhou Q, Li N, Xu L, Le Y, Ye M, Shao G, Duan S. Elevated PLA2G7 gene promoter methylation as a gender-specific marker of aging increases the risk of coronary heart disease in females. PLoS One. 2013;8:e59752.
53. Perkins E, Murphy SK, Murtha AP, Schildkraut J, Jirtle RL, Demark-Wahnefried W, Forman MR, Kurtzberg J, Overcash F, Huang Z, Hoyo C. Insulin-like growth factor 2/H19 methylation at birth and risk of overweight and obesity in children. J Pediatr. 2012;161:31–9.

54. Irvin MR, Zhi D, Joehanes R, Mendelson M, Aslibekyan S, Claas SA, Thibeault KS, Patel N, Day K, Jones LW, Liang L, Chen BH, Yao C, Tiwari HK, Ordovas JM, Levy D, Absher D, Arnett DK. Epigenome-wide association study of fasting blood lipids in the genetics of lipid lowering drugs and diet network study. Circulation. 2014;130(7):565–72.
55. Guay SP, Voisin G, Brisson D, Munger J, Lamarche B, Gaudet D, Bouchard L. Epigenome-wide analysis in familial hypercholesterolemia identified new loci associated with high-density lipoprotein cholesterol concentration. Epigenomics. 2012;4:623–39.
56. Haas J, Frese KS, Park YJ, Keller A, Vogel B, Lindroth AM, Weichenhan D, Franke J, Fischer S, Bauer A, Marquart S, Sedaghat-Hamedani F, Kayvanpour E, Köhler D, Wolf NM, Hassel S, Nietsch R, Wieland T, Ehlermann P, Schultz JH, Dösch A, Mereles D, Hardt S, Backs J, Hoheisel JD, Plass C, Katus HA, Meder B. Alterations in cardiac DNA methylation in human dilated cardiomyopathy. EMBO Mol Med. 2013;5:413–29.
57. Movassagh M, Choy MK, Knowles DA, Cordeddu L, Haider S, Down T, Siggens L, Vujic A, Simeoni I, Penkett C, Goddard M, Lio P, Bennett MR, Foo RS. Distinct epigenomic features in end-stage failing human hearts. Circulation. 2011;124:2411–22.
58. Han P, Hang CT, Yang J, Chang CP, Bruneau B. Chromatin remodeling in cardiovascular development and physiology. Circ Res. 2011;108:378–96.
59. Cardinale JP, Sriramula S, Pariaut R, Guggilam A, Mariappan N, Elks CM, Francis J. HDAC inhibition attenuates inflammatory, hypertrophic, and hypertensive responses in spontaneously hypertensive rats. Hypertension. 2010;56:437–44.
60. Okamoto H, Fujioka Y, Takahashi A, Takahashi T, Taniguchi T, Ishikawa Y, Yokoyama M. Trichostatin A, an inhibitor of histone deacetylase, inhibits smooth muscle cell proliferation via induction of p21(WAF1). J Atheroscler Thromb. 2006;13:183–91.
61. Kong X, Fang M, Li P, Fang F, Xu Y. HDAC2 deacetylates class II transactivator and suppresses its activity in macrophages and smooth muscle cells. J Mol Cell Cardiol. 2009;46:292–9.
62. Matsushima S, Sadoshima J. The role of sirtuins in cardiac disease. Am J Physiol Heart Circ Physiol. 2015;309:H1375–89.
63. Zhang Y, Qiu J, Wang X, Zhang Y, Xia M. AMP-activated protein kinase suppresses endothelial cell inflammation through phosphorylation of transcriptional coactivator p300. Arterioscler Thromb Vasc Biol. 2011;31:2897–908.
64. Franklin S, Kimball T, Rasmussen TL, Rosa-Garrido M, Chen H, Tran T, Miller MR, Gray R, Jiang S, Ren S, Wang Y, Tucker HO, Vondriska TM. The chromatin-binding protein Smyd1 restricts adult mammalian heart growth. Am J Physiol Heart Circ Physiol. 2016;311:H1234–47.
65. Ai S, Yu X, Li Y, Peng Y, Li C, Yue Y, Tao G, Li C, Pu WT, He A. Divergent requirements for EZH1 in heart development versus regeneration. Circ Res. 2017;121:106–12.
66. Guo H, Ingolia NT, Weissman JS, Bartel DP. Mammalian microRNAs predominantly act to decrease target mRNA levels. Nature. 2010;466(7308):835–40.
67. Fichtlscherer S, Zeiher AM, Dimmeler S. Circulating microRNAs: biomarkers or mediators of cardiovascular diseases? Arterioscler Thromb Vasc Biol. 2011;31(11):2383–90.

7

Non-coding RNAs as Epigenetic Gene Regulators in Cardiovascular Diseases

Wanlin Jiang, Devendra K. Agrawal,
and Chandra Shekhar Boosani

Abstract

Epigenetic gene regulations can be considered as de-novo initiation of abnormal molecular signaling events whose regulation is otherwise required during normal or specific developmental stages of the organisms. Primarily, three different mechanisms have been identified to participate in epigenetic gene regulations which include, DNA methylation, non-coding RNA species (microRNAs [miRNA], and long non-coding RNAs [LNC-RNA]) and histone modifications. These de-novo epigenetic mechanisms have been associated with altered normal cellular functions which eventually facilitate normal cells to transition into an abnormal phenotype. Among the three modes of regulation, RNA species which are usually considered to be less stable, can be speculated to initiate instant alterations in gene expression compared to DNA methylation or histone modifications. However, LNC-RNAs appear to be more stable in the cells than the other RNA species. Moreover, there is increasing literature which clearly suggests that a single specific LNC-RNA can regulate multiple mechanisms and disease phenotypes. With specific focus on cardiovascular diseases, here we attempt to provide UpToDate information on the functional role of miRNAs and LNC-RNAs. Here we discuss the role of these epigenetic mediators in different components of cardiovascular disease which include physiopathological heart development, athersclerosis, retenosis, diabetic hearts, myocardial infarction, ischemia-reperfusion, heart valve disease, aortic aneurysm, osteogenesis, angiogenesis and hypoxia in the heart. While there is abundant literature support that shows the involvement of many LNC-RNAs and miRNAs in cardiovascular diseases, very few RNA species have been identified which regulate epigenetic mechanisms which is the current focus in this article. Understanding the role of these RNA species in regulating epigenetic mechanisms in different cell types causing cardiovascular disease, would advance the field and promote disease prevention approaches that are aimed to target epigenetic mechanisms.

Keywords

DNA methyltransferase · Histone modifications · Cardiovascular disease · Non-coding RNAs · Epigenetics

W. Jiang · D. K. Agrawal · C. S. Boosani (✉)
Department of Clinical & Translational Research,
Western University of Health Sciences,
Pomona, CA, USA
e-mail: cboosani@westernu.edu

J. Xiao (ed.), *Non-coding RNAs in Cardiovascular Diseases*, Advances in Experimental Medicine and Biology 1229, https://doi.org/10.1007/978-981-15-1671-9_7

1 Introduction

Several historical events in science have indicated the significance of epigenesis in gene regulation. Dr. Conrad Waddington's quest "How genotypes give rise to phenotypes during development", envisions the role of epigenetics in developmental stages. The study on mitotically and/or meiotically heritable changes in gene function by Dr. Arthur Riggs, could not explain the effects of non-heritable modifications on DNA. Maybe the most appropriate indications that can assign Epigenetics as an independent field of study came from Dr. Adrian Bird who defined epigenesis as "the structural adaptation of chromosomal regions so as to register, signal or perpetuate altered activity states" [1]. The current definitions of Epigenetics hold a much broader field of study which explores induced molecular expressions/modifications and their associations with normal and abnormal physiology in different cells.

Non-coding RNAs have contributed to a dramatic improvement in our understanding on disease progression and prevention. Based on the transcipt size, all non-coding RNAs can be divided as small non-coding RNAs which are less than 200 bp (includes miRNA, piRNA, tiRNAs, TSSa-RNAs, PROMPTs and snacRNA) and large non-coding RNAs which are more than 200 bp (LNC-RNAs, lincRNAs and T-UCRs) [2]. An exception to this would be the small nucleolar RNAs (snoRNAs) which are usually about 300 bp. Among these RNA species, miRNAs and LNC-RNAs have been identified to play an important role in epigenetic gene regulation through histone modifications and DNA methylation in addition to silencing or co-transcription of other miRNAs [3].

2 DNMTs and DNA Methylation

Specific methylation of the paired CG dinucleotide sequences (CpG) present on both strands of genomic DNA is strongly associated with gene silencing [4]. As a consequence, the cytosine residues get methylated (C5-methylcytosine, 5mC). This DNA methylation pattern is widely seen in eukaryotic genomes. The cystine methylation is mediated by specific group of enzymes called DNA methyltransferases (DNMTs), and in humans' different isoforms of these enzymes were identified which included DNMT1, DNMT2, DNMT3A, DNMT3B, and DNMT3L. Among these isoforms, DNMT1, which is often referred to as maintenance methylase, has the most significant role in regulating gene expression in normal conditions. Its unanticipated activity has been identified as the causative factor for the onset of disease phenotype in many proliferative diseases/disorders. The two isoforms DNMT3A and DNMT3B, are recognized as the next potent DNA methylases which have specific genomic targets and tissue or developmental specific functions [5]. The catalytic activity of other isoforms has been reported or speculated to be inter-regulatory or inter-dependent on other DNA methylases [6].

2.1 LNC-RNAs and miRNAs Regulate DNA Methylation

The LNC-RNA uc.4, regulates DNA methylation by targeting the Rap1 promoter and affects its down-stream signaling. In addition, it was also found to regulate gonadotropin-releasing hormone signaling pathway and Calcium signaling pathway during heart development [7]. Further, over expression of LNC-RNA uc.167 was found to decrease cellular levels of cardiac markers cTnT, MEF2C, and NKX2.5, and prevents the differentiation of P19 mouse teratocarcinoma epithelial cells. Notably, over expression of LNC-RNA uc.167 caused promoter hypermethylation at Opcm1, Mmp2, and Hspa13 genomic loci, and at the same time hypomethylation at the promoter regions of MEF2C, Strap, and Sufu was also noted[8, 9]. These studies indicate that the LNC-RNA uc.167 suppresses cellular differentiation into cardiomyocytes in which MEF2C plays a major role.

Intracellular levels of the microRNA miR-29, were found to increase during aging. In the turquoise killifish model, reduced levels of collagens and DNMTs were found associated with increased expression of the microRNA miR-29. In the transgenic zebrafish, knockdown of miR-

29 was identified to induce cardiac abnormalities which paralleled with impaired oxygen dependent pathways resulting in upregulation of several hypoxic markers such as lactate dehydrogenase, hypoxia inducible factor 1 alpha, hexokinase 2, erythropoietin A, heme oxygenase 1a and p27 [10]. Moreover, studies on the role of miR-29 in regulating DNA methylation in older mice aorta suggests another molecular regulatory mechanism of miR-29 that is associated with suppression of DNA demethylase activity which is mediated through down regulating Ten-Eleven Translocation (TET) family of proteins and Thymine DNA glycosylase [11].

2.2 miRNAs Regulating DNA Methylation During Progression of Atherosclerosis

In human aortic smooth muscle cells (HASMC) that were cultured in presence of oxidized low-density lipoprotein (oxLDL), elevated levels of the microRNA miR-29b that targets the 3′UTR of DNMT3b transcript was reported. As a result, the DNMT3b protein levels were lowered which subsequently induced MMP-2/MMP-9 HASMC cell migration [12]. In another report, the microRNA miR-152 was identified to play a protective role against atherosclerosis by inhibiting the expression of DNMT1. The reduced expression of DNMT1 restored athero-protective functions of ERα gene in HASMCs. Interesting was the SHXXT drug which is a traditional Chinese medicine, reported to restore the expression levels of miR-152 in HASMCs that were treated with LPS and also in the high fat diet-fed SD rats [13]. Further, migration of HASMCs was found to be affected in presence of the microRNA miR-210. The SPRED2 gene (sprouty-related EVH1 domain 2) was identified as a direct target for miR-210 in patients having carotid artery atherosclerosis and stroke. The oxLDL was reported as the inducer of miR-210 expression, and this induced expression of miR-210 occurs due to binding of the HiF-1α to the R2 region in the promoter of miR-210 which remained in an unmethylated state [14].

Connexin 43 (Cx43) is an important cell junction protein that controls proliferation and migrations of vascular SMCs. The microRNA miR-1298 was identified to prevent proliferation and migration of SMCs by targeting the 3′UTR of Cx43 [15]. We have recently reported that in presence of the microRNA miR-1264, proliferation of SMCs was facilitated. The important epigenetic mediator DNMT1 was identified as a direct target for miR-1264. Further, in presence of TNF-α and IGF-1, the expression of this microRNA was found to be drastically reduced [16].

Homocysteine (Hcy) was found to lower the expression of miR-125b. In ApoE null mice, the expression of DNMT3b was affected in presence of Hcy in vascular SMCs. In absence of the microRNA miR-125, DNMT3b was found to promote hypermethylation in the promoter region of p53 [17]. This resulted in the proliferation of vascular SMCs due to inhibition of p53. Another mechanism of Hcy mediated cell proliferation was reported to be mediated through the microRNA miR-143 where Hcy was found to induce the expression of DNMT3a. Subsequently, due to the activity of DNMT3a on the promoter region of the microRNA mir-143, its expression was found to be greatly reduced [18].

In Table 7.1, we summarized the list of miRNAs that have been reported to regulate expression of different genes which either promote or inhibit vascular SMCs proliferation and/or migration.

2.3 miRNAs Regulating Pulmonary Hypertension

Pulmonary hypertension results primarily due to vasoconstriction caused by pulmonary artery smooth muscle cells (PASMCs). PASMC proliferation was directly influenced by the microRNA miR-328, which prevents cell proliferation and migration by targeting the Ser/Thr-protein kinase-1 (PIM-1). In PDGFBB treated PASMCs, the levels of miR-328 were reported to be decreased. Further, an inverse correlation between the levels of miR-328 and DNMT1 was

Table 7.1 MicroRNAs that are associated with methylation dependent gene regulation in vascular SMCs

Methylation status	Associated miRNA	Genes regulated	Effect
Hypermethylation	miR-1298	cx43	Mitigates VSMCs proliferation and migration
Hypomethylation	miR-210	SPRED2	Prevents VSMCs migration
Hypermethylation	miR-143	DNMT3a	Prevents VSMCs proliferation
Hypermethylation	miR-328	PIM-1	Prevents VSMCs proliferation and migration
Hypermethylation	miR-126	Phosphorylation of RAF/MAPK	Improves microvessel density and RV function
Hypermethylation	miR-204	DNMT3a	Inhibits osteoblastic differentiation of VSMCs
Hypomethylation	miR-29b	MMP2/MMP9	Inducing VSMCs migration
Hypomethylation	miR-152	ERα	Protective role in atherosclerosis
Hypomethylation	miR-125b	p53	Inhibits VSMCs proliferation

deciphered which suggests the possibility of DNA methylation in the promoter region of miR-328 [19]. In the SD rat model for PAH disease, reduced levels of the microRNA miR-126 was reported. This was correlated with increased DNA methylation at the miR-126 locus in patients with uncompensated right ventricle failure. The reduced levels of miR-126 was attributed as a causative factor for the uncompensated RV failure resulting due to blocking of RAF phosphorylation regulated through MAPK and VEGF pathway [20].

2.4 DNA Methylation and Osteogenic Differentiation in Cardiac Cells

The LNC-RNA H19, was reported to induce osteogenic phenotype by inhibiting NOTCH1 pathway and by suppressing binding of p53 to its effector promoters. Consequently, upregulation of the osteogenesis promoting genes RUNX2 and BMP2 was observed in the heart valve interstitial cells. DNA hypomethylation at the promoter region of LNC-RNA H19 was identified as the causative factor that contributes to the elevated expression of LNC-RNA H19 in the mineralized aortic valves [20].

DNMT3a mediated DNA methylation appears to lower the cellular levels of the microRNA miR-204. This miR-204/DNMT3a regulatory circuit is required for osteoblastic differentiation of vascular SMCs [21]. This was further proved in uremia patients and in mice with calcified arteries, where the miR-204/DNMT3a mediated regulatory pathway was associated with osteogenic differentiation potential in vascular SMCs.

2.5 Regulating DNA Methylation in Endothelial Cells by Non-coding RNAs

In HUVEC cells, differential methylation at the LNC-RNA MEG3 locus was attributed to enriched presence of LNC-RNA MEG3. This was interpreted from the observation that in presence of DNMT inhibitors, no significant improvement in the expression levels of LNC-RNA MEG3 was noted. However, HIF-1α was found to upregulate the expression of LNC-RNA MEG3 and its downstream effector VEGFR2, which caused endothelial cell migration and angiogenesis [22]. Differential methylation at MEG3 locus may also have impacted the expression of the LNC-RNA MEG9, which was specifically induced by ionizing radiation. The ionizing radiation was shown to affect DNMTs by decreasing their protein expression levels at the treated site. Due to this, demethylation in the DLK1-DIO non-coding RNA cluster was noted in endothelial cells. This hypomethylation further led to induced expression of the LNC-RNA MEG9 originating from the DLK1-DIO3 cluster. As a result, the anti-apoptotic effects in endothelial cells was seen, indicating a direct correlation between the expression of LNC-RNA MEG9 and protection to the endothelial cells resulting due to inhibition of DNMTs [23].

Two specific miRNAs, miR-152 and miR-30a were found to promote differentiation of stem cells into endothelial cells, and these two miRNAs target two different isoforms of DNMTs. The miRNA miR-152 targets and affects DNMT1 expression while miR-30a targets and prevents the expression of DNMT3a. In human mesenchymal stem cells that were subjected to differentiation into endothelial cells, elevated levels of miR-152 and miR-30a were reported. Due to the inhibition of DNMT1 and DNMT3a by these two miRNAs, the transcription factor E2F1 was able to induce the expression of endothelial-specific genes (KDR, eNOS, and VE-cadherin) in addition to the arterial markers (Hey2, EphrinB2, and Dll4) [24].

2.6 Non-coding RNAs Regulate DNA Methylation in Cardiomyocytes and Myofibroblasts

The normal QT rhythm in the heart if affected can lead to atrial fibrillation. Several deleterious mutations in the ion channels have been detected. To fix these mutations, gene therapy approach has shown a promising path to address the associated postoperative sudden cardiac events [25, 26]. Differential methylation in the promoter region of the LNC-RNA KCNQ1OT1 and promoter polymorphism detected with an SNP rs11023840 which represents the AA genotype was observed in patients having symptomatic long QT rhythm [27] The study establishes a strong correlation between the DNA methylation events at the LNC-RNA KCNQ1OT1 locus and its resulting effects on the observed prolonged QT rhythm.

Phenanthrene treatment was shown to cause cardiac hypertrophy by inducing DNMTs which cause genomic DNA methylation at the miR-133a locus in rat heart tissues[28]. Due to the treatment with Phenanthrene, expression of CdC42 and RhoA were increased in H9C2 rat cardiomyoblast cells which suggests that CdC42 and RhoA are a direct targets of miR-133a. Of note, in diabetic hearts of Ins2 +/− Akita mouse model, decreased levels of DNMT1 and DNMT3b were observed, and at the same time, upregulated expression of DNMT3a and miR-133a were also noted. These studies suggest that in high glucose treated cardiomyocytes, DNMT1 prevents the expression of miR-133a to cause cardiac hypertrophy [29]. Two other microRNAs, miR-29 and miR-30 were found reduced due to the increased activity of DNMT3a in HL-1 cells and also in-vivo in a rat model of myocardial infarction and ischemia-reperfusion [30] In another study, the expression of the microRNA miR-29a was reported to be decreased in cardiac myofibroblasts of SD rats suggesting a direct role of miR-29a in cardiac fibrosis occurring possibly due to increased expression of DNMT3a [31].

2.7 Non-coding RNAs Regulating DNA Methylation in PBMCs

In PBMCs isolated from patients with carotid artery atherosclerosis, the endogenous levels of LNC-RNA NKILA was reported to be decreased. The LNC-RNA NKILA appears to confer a reduced inflammation by lowering the activity of NF-κB, which is a well know enhancer of cellular inflammation that functions by repressing the expression of KLF4. This mechanism apparently was found to be mediated through induced expression of DNMT3a and its DNA methylating effects on the KLF4 promoter sequence [32].

DNA hypomethylation at the promoter region of miR-223 locus was found to hold a strong association in patients who were diagnosed with atherosclerotic cerebral infarction (ACI) or were having atherosclerosis in carotid arteries. The genomic DNA isolated from the PBMCs of over 23 patients and 32 healthy subjects when subjected to bisulphite sequencing and real time PCR analysis enabled identification of 9 CpG dimers in the miR-223 promoter region. DNA hypomethylation observed in these patients was found to positively correlate with the total circulating cholesterol levels [33]. It would be interesting to see if SNPs or genetic polymorphisms exist at this locus in the disease patients and in healthy individuals from different ethnic groups. In addition, more detailed studies are required to analyze variations in the expression of the downstream targets.

3 Histone Modifications

Histone proteins coil DNA sequences and most modifications on the amino acid sequences on histones have been reported to either induce or inhibit transcription of the corresponding genes. Modifications on histone proteins are covalent in nature, and many different modifications have been described in the literature. Most post-translational modifications observed on histone proteins include methylation, phosphorylation, acetylation, ubiquitylation, and sumoylation on lysine, arginine, serine, threonine, and tyrosine. Among these, histone acetylation/deacetylation and histone methylation/demethylation are well characterized and their associations in different disease conditions have been widely studied. A class of enzymes called histone acetyltransferases (HATs) which include GNAT1, MYST, TAFII250, P300/CBP, and ACTR, add an acetyl group to the lysine residues on the histone proteins. Also, the group of enzymes called histone deacetylases (HDACs) which are classified into Class I, Class II and Class III, act by removing the acetyl groups from lysine residues on the histones. Similarly, the enzymes histone methyltransferases (HMTs), which add methyl groups to the lysine or arginine residues on histones have been described. These group of enzymes include G9a, SUV39-h1, SUV39-h2, SETDB1. In most of the methylation events, the methyl group was derived from S-adenosyl-L-methionine which is widely known as methyl group donor [34]. Proteins containing Jumonji C domains were found to participate in histone demethylation processes by directly removing methyl groups from the histones [35].

3.1 Non-coding RNAs Regulating Histone Modifications in Cardiac Stem Cells

Cellular reprograming to dedifferentiate fibroblasts into cardiomyocytes has received great attention, and gene therapy with stemness associated genes appears to be a promising approach [36–38]. The LNC-RNA HAND2 plays an important role in reprograming fibroblasts into cardiomyocytes during right ventricle development. Also, the LNC-RNA "upperhand" was speculated in sustaining the expression of HAND2 by inducing GATA4 expression [39]. Further, the expression of HAND2 was found to be dependent on upstream enhancer elements and are strongly influenced by H3K27 acetylation at this locus, as observed in the HAND2 deleted mice embryos [40]. The LNC-RNA "Fendrr" was reported to act as a dsDNA/RNA triplex to enable cardiac mesoderm differentiation via binding to PRC2 and TrxG/MLL Histone-Modifying Complexes. Loss of Fendrr was shown to reduce K27 trimethylation on Histone H3 which is bound to the promoter region of Foxf resulting in the expression of Foxf1. Also, K4 trimethylation on Histone 3 protein was reported to induce the exression of Gata6 and Nkx2-5 genes [41].

PDGF-BB and TGF-β mediated expression of microRNA miR-22, was found to target Methyl CpG– binding protein 2 (MECP2) and prevent its expression. Inhibition of MECP2 was found to promote differentiation of embryonic stem cells in the adventitia into SMCs, and this coincides with increased lysine methylation on Histone 3 (H3K9) which is at the promoter binding region of MECP2 [42]. Also, the microRNA miR-1, has been shown to induce cardiomyocyte progenitor cell differentiation into cardiomyocytes by inhibiting the expression of histone deacetylase 4 [43]. Further, both miR-1 and miR-133 were reported to be elevated in spontaneous myocardial differentiation in the mouse embryonic stem cells by preventing cyclin-dependent kinase-9 (Cdk9). This was further confirmed by the treatment with Trichostatin A, a histone deacetylase inhibitor, which favored myocardial differentiation [44]. In normal developmental and physiological conditions, miR-34a expression was found increased at one-week post-natal stage. On the contrary, after 7 days of myocardial infarction, miR-34a, which mediates cell cycle and cell death through inhibition of Sirt1, was reported to be increased in adult hearts [45].

3.2 Non-coding RNAs Regulate Histone Modification in Vascular SMCs During Atherosclerosis

In ApoE null mice, the LNC-RNA LincRNA-p21, notably decreased in the atherosclerotic plaques of patients with coronary artery disease. Knockdown of LincRNA-p21 was shown to induce proliferation of vascular SMCs. In the same mice, the interaction between mouse double minute 2 (MDM2), an E3 ubiquitin-protein ligase and p53 was reported. Blocking p300/p53 interaction led to reduced levels of the target genes p53 Puma, Bax, and Noxa. Also, LincRNA-p21 is a known transcriptional target of p53. Thus, blocking the interaction between p300 and p53 may have caused decreased expression of LincRNA-p21 [46]. In internal mammary arteries, the LNC-RNA LincRNA-p21 showed about seven-fold decrease in the coronary artery plaques. Further, the LNC-RNA FENDRR presented approximately two-fold decrease in expression in the coronary artery plaques. FENDRR also was found to stimulate Histone H3 Lysine 27 trimethylation in complex with PRC2. Therefore, it was presumed that the decrease in the expression of FENDRR may have led to the reduced levels of H3K27Me3, eventually contributing to VSMC cell proliferation and atherosclerotic plaque development [47].

The histone lysine methyltransferase enzyme, Suv39h1 causes H3K9 trimethylation on the inflammatory genes such as MCP-1, IL-6 and maintains normal state of the cells. A specific microRNA miR-125b was identified to inhibit the expression of Suv39h1 by targeting its 3′UTR, and this was found to induce proinflammatory signaling in diabetic vascular SMCs [48]. Also, oxLDL was identified to enhance the expression levels of microRNA-29b and at the same time, it also led to a significant decrease in HDAC1 expression by activating c-Fos and lysine acetylation at Lys9/Lys18 residues on H3 histone, in addition to methylation at Lys4, and subsequently inhibiting methylation at Lys9/Lys27 on histone H3 [49].

In Table 7.2, we summarized some of the non-coding RNAs that were reported to be associated with histone modifications in regulating gene expression during atherosclerosis.

Table 7.2 Non-coding RNAs that regulate specific gene expression through histone modifications in vascular SMCs

Non-coding RNA	Histone modifications and target gene	Genes regulated	Effect
miR-125b	H3K9me3; Suv39H1	MCP-1, IL-6	Inhibits monocyte binding and inflammatory
LincRNA-21	p300 (HAT)/p53 interaction; MDM2/p53 interaction	p53, Puma, Bax, Noxa	Inhibits VSMCs proliferation
FENDRR	H3K27Me3	-	Inhibits VSMCs proliferation and atherosclerotic plaque development
Giver	H3K27me3; Ccl2, Tnf, and Nox1	Ccl2, Tnf, and Nox1	Induces expression of inflammatory markers and oxidative markers
miR-2861	HDAC5	RunX2	Induces VSMCs osteogenic transdifferentiation
TUG1	EZH2	F-actin	Induces VSMCs phenotypic switch
miR-22	HDAC4; MECP2 and EVI1	PCNA, SMαA and SM-myh11	Inhibits VSMCs proliferation and phenotype switching

3.3 Non-coding RNAs Regulating Restenosis in Smooth Muscle Cells

The LNC-RNA TUG1, by forming TUG1/EZH2/α-actin complex, induces EZH2-mediated methylation of α-actin which is critical for F-actin polymerization. By modulating actin polymerization, the LNC-RNA promotes phenotype switch in vascular SMCs which exhibit phenotypic shift from contractile to synthetic type [50]. The above discussed LNC-RNA MEG3 and IRF-1 were shown to be decreased in the PDGFBB treated vascular SMCs, however at the same time, the expression of miR-125a-5p and HDAC4 was found increased which depicts an inverse correlation between these important targets of restenosis. The miR-125-5p inhibitor was shown to upregulate IRF-1 expression. Also, knockdown of HDAC4 was shown to promote MEG3 levels. In both these cases, the net effect was on vascular SMCs whose proliferation and migration got affected. These results establish an active MEG3/miR-125a-5p/HDAC4/IRF1 axis that plays a critical role in the development of neointimal hyperplasia and restenosis [51].

3.4 Non-coding RNA Regulating Aortic Aneurysm

Both PRC2 and EZH2 coordination is required for inducing H3-lysine 27 trimethylation to regulate smoothelin-1 (SMTN1), calponin (CNN1), vinculin (VCL1), and transgelin (SM22α) in vascular SMCs. Inhibition of these contractile proteins in human aortic vascular SMCs that were transfected with TGFR2G357W and ACTA2R179H lentiviral expression vectors, presented two aggressive genotypes of hereditary Thoracic aortic aneurysm. Knockdown of either MALAT1 or HDAC9 was shown to improve the expression of these contractile proteins in Fbn1C1039G/+ (Marfan) mice in which the phosphorylation of Smad2 and ERK was affected [52]. These results establish direct regulation of HDAC9–MALAT1–BRG1 complex in aortic aneurysm.

3.5 Non-coding RNAs Regulating Histone Modification in Endothelial Cells

Interaction of the LNC-RNA MANTIS with BRG1, which is chromatin-remodeling complex, assists in restoring the ATPase activity of BRG1 which is essential for transcription of critical genes such as SOX18, SMAD6, and COUPTFII in endothelial cells. In monkeys that were fed with high fat diet, simultaneous decrease in the expression of H3K4 lysine-specific demethylase 5B (JARID1B) and elevated expression of MANTIS was observed during atherosclerosis regression in carotid arteries [53]. These results show one of the many benefits of the LNC-RNA MANTIS in regressing the net atherosclerotic events. The Anti-Sense LNC-RNA of GATA6 (GATA6-AS), promotes the TGF-β2 induced endothelial to mesenchymal transition under hypoxic conditions, and this was negatively correlated with lysyl oxidase-like 2 protein. Further, the GATA6-AS affected trimethylation of lysine 4 of histone H3 (H3K4me3) by mobilizing LOXL2 onto the proinflammatory loci of cyclooxygenase-2 gene and favors inhibition of the pro-angiogenic genes [54, 55]. Treatment with the trypsin inhibitor, Ulinastatin was found to confer an anti-apoptotic effect and also decrease endothelial cell permeability in cardiac microvascular endothelial cells. In presence of induced sepsis conditions by treatment with lipopolysaccharide (LPS), Ulinastatin was reported to affect the expression of several apoptotic genes such as EZH2, ROS, caspase-3 and Bax. At the same time, it also promoted increased expression levels of MALAT1 and Bcl-2. Knockdown of MALAT1 was also found to inhibit the interaction of EZH2 and H3K27me3 with DAB2IP and Brachyury, which suggests that both DAB2IP and Brachyury are targets of EZH2 [55].

In HUVECs derived from the gestational diabetes patients, the precursor miRNA pre-miR-101 reduced the expression of EZH2 and also histone trimethylation at H3K27me3. Interesting was when the anti-miR anti-miR-101 was transfected into these cells, only the expression of EZH2 was found to be restored without affecting H3K27me3 [56]. The target microRNA of GATA6, miR-10a normally prevents the expression of VCAM-1 in endothelial cells. Under oscillatory shear stress (OS) conditions, HDAC-3/5/7–RARα hetero-repressor complex, was shown to prevent the binding of RARα with RARE to induce the expression of miR-10a [57]. In studying the role of gut microbiome in high fat diet supplemented mouse model of atherosclerosis, the expression of the microRNA miR-204 was found to hold an inverse correlation with Sirt1. When mice were treated with broad spectrum antibiotics to kill the gut microbiome, an increase in the expression of Sirt1 and Nitric oxide was observed which promoted vasorelaxation. The damage to the endothelium was restored when the anti-miR for miR-204 was used. These reports suggest a prominent role of gut microbiome in endothelial dysfunction under high fat diet supplementation [58]. In Table 7.3, we summarized specific miRNAs and LNC-RNAs that regulate cellular functions in endothelial cells during atherosclerosis.

3.6 Non-coding RNAs Regulating Histone Modifications in Cardiomyocytes and Cardio-Myofibroblasts

In the mouse model of transaortic constriction (TAC) that occurs in the heart due to pressure-overload, the LNC-RNA MyHEART (Myosin Heavy Chain Associated RNA Transcripts) not only was found to be decreased but along with it the other isoforms of myosin chains Myh6/7 were reduced, which is characteristic of cardiomyopathy. During TAC complex formation between Brg1, Hdac2/9 and Parp1 and its recruitment at the MyHEART locus was found to get affected. Moreover, MyHEART was found to interact with Brg1 and the helicase domain, to prevent Brg1 from binding to the chromatin bound DNA through competitive inhibition. This is considered as a supportive mechanism to protect the heart from hypertrophy and failure [59]. In the mouse model of transverse aortic constriction (TAC) with cardiac hypertrophy, the LNC-RNA TINCR was reportedly decreased. In addition, along with TINCR, Angiotensin II (Ang-II) was also reduced substantially in the cultured neonatal cardiomyocytes. In Ang-II induced cellular hypertrophy, Ca2+/calmodulin-

Table 7.3 Non-coding RNAs regulating histone dependent gene expression in vascular endothelial cells

Non-coding RNA	Role of Histone proteins	Genes affected	Effect
Pre-miR-101	Reduces EZH2 and downstream H3K27me3	miR-101	Impairs fetal endothelial cell functions
miR-34a	Directly inhibits the expression of Sirt1	miR-34a	Causes senescence in endothelial cells
miR-217	Directly reduces the expression of Sirt1	Upregulates FoxO1 acetylation	Promotes endothelial senescence
miR-204	Directly reduces the expression of sirt1	Downregulates eNOS signaling	Impairs endothelium-dependent vasorelaxation
GATA6-AS	Inhibits H3K4me3	PTGS2, POSTN	Inhibits proangiogenic factors
miR-10a	Promotes HDAC-3/5/7-RARα complex to prevent RARα binding to RARE	HDAC-3/5/7	Inhibits VCAM-1 in endothelial cells
MANTIS	H3K4me3	H3K4 lysine-specific demethylase 5B, JARID1B	Promotes angiogenesis
MALAT1	H3K27me3	EZH2	Inducing apoptosis and increasing the permeability of cardiac microvascular ECs.

dependent protein kinase II (CaMKII) expression was reported to be elevated. The LNC-RNA TINCR appears to mitigate myocardial hypertrophy. The underlying molecular mechanism appears to be mediated through recruitment of EZH2 stimulated trimethylated histones H3K27me3 onto the genomic regions of CaMKII, resulting in its inhibition during cellular hypertrophy [60]. Another LNC-RNA CHAER was reported in the cardiac hypertrophy model. By interacting with PRC2 complex, CHAER restricts H3K27me3 by EZH2. As a consequence, the expression of hypertrophy associated genes Myh7, Acta1 and Anf was enhanced. Further, this interaction was also reported to be triggered by mTORC1. In addition, treating the rat ventricular myocytes with Phenylephrine was shown to be a representative in-vitro model for TAC [61]. Lack of expression of the histone acetyl transferase p300 was paralleled with the reduced expression of LNC-RNA ANRIL. Further, when ANRIL-knockout mice were treated with streptozotocin to induce diabetes, both functional and structural improvements in diabetic nephropathy (DN) and diabetic cardiomyopathy (DCM) was observed. Suppression of p300 and EZH2 have contributed to inhibition of the growth promoting factor VEGF. Interestingly, p300 reduction was found to affect the transcription of ANRIL [62].

In the heart tissues of diabetic rats and neonatal rat cardiomyocytes, high glucose stimulated the expression of PKCβ2, and at the same time also caused a significant decrease in the expression of miR-150. In these cells, it was reported that the expression of miR-150 attenuates glucose-induced cardiomyocyte hypertrophy, and this was mediated through induction of histone acetyl transferase p300 which also acts as a transcriptional co-activator [63]. Also, in the cardiomyocytes of mice with miR-128 deleted, increased proliferation of neonatal cardiomyocytes was reported. On the contrary, overexpression of miR-128 affected the ability of the cardiomyocytes to proliferate. The induced cell proliferation observed in the miR-128 deleted cells can be attributed to the enhanced expression of SUZ12. The mechanism associated with this enhanced cell proliferation is by apparent inhibition of p27 by SUZ12, as a result, the cell cycle regulators Cyclin E and CDK2 were found activated [64].

Variations in the expression of different microRNAs was studied in the Transverse aortic constriction (TAC) mouse model. In these mice, cardiac hypertrophy and heart failure resulted due to pressure overload. The microRNA miR-208, was found to elevate *β-MHC* as well as reduce *α-MHC* gene expression which enhanced ventricular hypertrophy in mice [65]. In transgenic mice that overexpress microRNA miR-208a, arrhythmia and cardiac hypertrophy was observed. The indirect mechanism observed in these mice was HDAC2 mediated inhibition of the serum response factor [66]. By activating calcineurin, the microRNA miR-155 promoted cellular hypertrophy in cardiomyocytes and heart remodeling through inhibition of histone demethylase Jarid2/jumonji [67].

Three different microRNAs miR-133a, miR-21-3p and miR-22 were found to prevent the occurrence of cardiac hypertrophy. In CD1, after performing TAC and treatment with HDAC inhibitors, it was identified that the microRNA miR-133a expression was downregulated. Further, chromatin immunoprecipitation studies revealed that both the HDAC1 and HDAC2 were bound to the enhancer regions of miR-133a which clearly indicates the interdependence of HDACs and miR-133a in regulating cardiac hypertrophy [68]. Also, the microRNA miR-21-3p was found to prevent cardiac hypertrophy in mice after TAC and infusion of angiotensin (Ang II) in an HDAC8 dependent manner regulating the Akt/Gsk3β pathway [69]. Loss of miR-22 led to reduction in cardiac hypertrophy. The direct targets of microRNA miR-22 were Sirt1 and HDAC4 and this gene regulation is required to prevent cardiac hypertrophy [70].

In Table 7.4, we show microRNAs and LNC-RNAs that regulate histone modifications in cardiomyocytes during cardiac hypertrophy.

Table 7.4 Non-coding RNAs regulating target gene expression in cardiomyocytes

Non-coding RNA	Target genes of modified histones	Associated gene regulations	Effect
Pri-miR-208b	EZH2	Elevated levels of β-MHC and reduced levels of α-MHC	Promotes the expression of hypertrophic and fibrotic genes
miR-155	Jarid2/jumonji	Jarid2/jumonji inhibition of cyclin D1	Induces cardiac cell proliferation
miR-21-3p	HDAC8	Prevents activation of Akt/Gsk3β pathway	Prevents cardiac hypertrophy
miR-208a	HDAC2	Maintains the expression of hop; inhibits transcription of serum response factor	Induces cardiac hypertrophy
miR-214	EZH2	EZH2 repressed Six1 levels	Promotes cardiac hypertrophy
miR-22	Sirt1 and HDAC4	Inhibits MEF2C	Induces cardiac hypertrophy and remodeling
TINCR	EZH2	Inhibits CaMKII expression	Prevents cardiac hypertrophy
Chaer	EZH2 and PRC2 catalytic subunit	Induces Myh7, Acta1, Anf, and stimulates mTORC1 dependent pathway	Induces cardiac hypertrophy
miR-150	p300	Inhibits p300	Attenuates glucose-induced cardiomyocyte hypertrophy
ANRIL	Stimulates p300	Initiates VEGF signaling	Induces diabetic cardiomyopathy
miR-128	SUZ12and EZH2	Prevents the expression of p27	Impairs cardiomyocyte proliferation and cardiac function

4 LNC-RNAs Sequester miRNAs as Natural Sponges

Recent reports have identified additional roles of LNC-RNAs and suggests that they can also function as decoy microRNAs and compete for microRNA binding sites on the target transcripts [71]. The below described reports suggest a novel approach of using miRNA sponges for the prevention and treatment of atherosclerosis [72].

LNC-RNAs have also been reported to co-transcribe with miRNAs during disease development [73]. In knock-down experiments using lncRNA-AK131850 (miRNA sponge) in the osteoclasts from both newborn and mature subjects, induced expression of VEGFa was noted which stimulated proliferation, differentiation, migration and tube formation in endothelial progenitor cells. These reports identify that sequestering miR-93-5p using synthetic miRNA sponges promotes angiogenesis [74]. As discussed earlier, the SIRT1 antisense LNC-RNA (AS lncRNA) acts as a natural sponge for the microRNA miR-22, and increased Sirt1 expression stimulates proliferation and migration of the endothelial progenitor cells.

In endothelial cells, the LNC-RNA p21 was noted to act as a natural sponge for miR-130b and conferred reduced expression of miR-130b, which was evidenced through inhibition of cell proliferation and induction of apoptosis [75]. Also, the LNC-RNA HULC, prevented apoptosis by inducing TNF-α expression in endothelial cells. The underlying mechanism was primarily through down regulation of miR-9 mediated by DNA methylation activity of DNMTs [76]. Another similar report also suggests that the LNC-RNA, TCONS00024652 increases TNF-α and stimulates proliferation and angiogenesis in endothelial cells by sponging miR-21 [77]. In hypoxic conditions, increased expression of the LNC-RNA LINC00305 participates as an endogenous sponge for miR-136 and promotes apoptosis in endothelial cells [78, 79].

4.1 Interactions Between LNC-RNAs and miRNAs in Cardiovascular Diseases

Under chronic hypoxia, the LNC-RNA TUG1 was reported to interact with miR-29c to induce fibroblast to myofibroblast transformation. These observations were supported by simultaneous expression of myofibroblast markers collagen I and α-SMA [79]. In a mice ischemia and reperfusion model, decreased expression of the LNC-RNA CARL was found to restore the levels of miR-539 which CARL sequestered naturally. One of the main targets for miR-539 is Prohibitin 2 (PHB2) whose expression prevents mitochondrial fission and apoptosis in cardiomyocytes during myocardial infarction [80]. In the mouse model for myocardial infarction and cardiac fibrosis, the LNC-RNA PFL (NONMMUT022555) was reported to enhance fibrosis. Increased expression of PFL was found to lower the levels of microRNA miR-let-7d, which led to inhibition of platelet-activating factor receptor. The LNC-RNA PFL is a competitive target of let-7d. This endogenous target competition between PFL and let-7d promotes increased cell proliferation, fibroblast to myofibroblast transition and fibrosis [81]. In the rat model of diabetic cardiomyopathy (DCM) the LNC-RNA H19, which was down-regulated, affected cardiac structure and function, and alleviated inflammation and oxidative stress. The LNC-RNA H19 acts as a precursor for miR-675 and directly targets the pro-apoptotic gene "voltage-dependent anion channel 1" (VDAC1) to inhibit apoptosis in high glucose treated cardiomyocytes [82]. These studies describe additional novel biological functions of LNC-RNAs and their role in regulating different aspects of cardiovascular disease.

5 Conclusions

Epigenetically induced mechanisms have been described in many human diseases. Although the associated molecular mechanisms may have been normal at some developmental stage or specific to certain cell type or growth phase, their induced expression in disease conditions identifies them as potential targets for disease prevention. Primarily, these de-novo induced epigenetic mechanisms can be due to modifications to the genomic DNA, development of new RNA species and modifications to the expressed proteins. The end result normally caused by these epigenetic events is exacerbated disease progression. To identify such events, several high through-put and array-based platforms have been developed to unravel the varied expression of proteins which alter normal functions in the cells. The ever-increasing literature support that identifies new and additional intracellular regulations, supported by the development of improved and advanced analytical methods appears to be very favoring in understanding the disease progression. It is anticipated that with the technology advancements, a more comprehensive and deeper understanding of the molecular regulations can be perceived, and the future in identifying the disease and finding the appropriate target for disease prevention appears very promising.

References

1. Bird A. Perceptions of epigenetics. Nature. 2007;447(7143):396–8.
2. St Laurent G, Wahlestedt C, Kapranov P. The landscape of long noncoding RNA classification. Trends Genet. 2015;31(5):239–51.
3. Ghayor C, Weber FE. Epigenetic regulation of bone remodeling and its impacts in osteoporosis. Int J Mol Sci. 2016;17(9):1446.
4. Brenet F, Moh M, Funk P, Feierstein E, Viale AJ, Socci ND, Scandura JM. DNA methylation of the first exon is tightly linked to transcriptional silencing. PLoS One. 2011;6(1):e14524.
5. Boosani CS, Gunasekar P, Block M, Jiang W, Zhang Z, Radwan MM, Agrawal DK. Inhibition of DNA methyltransferase-1 instigates the expression of DNA methyltransferase-3a in angioplasty-induced restenosis. Can J Physiol Pharmacol. 2018;96(10):1030–9.
6. Lyko F. The DNA methyltransferase family: a versatile toolkit for epigenetic regulation. Nat Rev Genet. 2018;19(2):81–92.
7. Zhang Q, Feng M, Zhang H, Xu J, Zhang L, Wang X, Cheng Z, Qian L. Long noncoding RNA uc.4 inhibits cell differentiation in heart development by altering DNA methylation. J Cell Biochem. 2018;120(5):8061–8.
8. Yin A, Feng M, Cheng Z, Zhang Q, Li H, Xu J, Zhang H, Li Y, Qian L. Altered DNA methylation of long noncoding RNA uc.167 inhibits cell differentiation in heart development. Biomed Res Int. 2018;2018:4658024.
9. Song G, Shen Y, Ruan Z, Li X, Chen Y, Yuan W, Ding X, Zhu L, Qian L. LncRNA-uc.167 influences cell proliferation, apoptosis and differentiation of P19 cells by regulating Mef2c. Gene. 2016;590(1):97–108.
10. Heid J, Cencioni C, Ripa R, Baumgart M, Atlante S, Milano G, Scopece A, Kuenne C, Guenther S, Azzimato V, Farsetti A, Rossi G, Braun T, Pompilio G, Martelli F, Zeiher AM, Cellerino A, Gaetano C,

Spallotta F. Age-dependent increase of oxidative stress regulates microRNA-29 family preserving cardiac health. Sci Rep. 2017;7(1):16839.
11. Zhang P, Huang B, Xu X, Sessa WC. Ten-eleven translocation (Tet) and thymine DNA glycosylase (TDG), components of the demethylation pathway, are direct targets of miRNA-29a. Biochem Biophys Res Commun. 2013;437(3):368–73.
12. Chen KC, Wang YS, Hu CY, Chang WC, Liao YC, Dai CY, Juo SH. OxLDL up-regulates microRNA-29b, leading to epigenetic modifications of MMP-2/MMP-9 genes: a novel mechanism for cardiovascular diseases. FASEB J. 2011;25(5):1718–28.
13. Asghar MY, Viitanen T, Kemppainen K, Tornquist K. Sphingosine 1-phosphate and human ether-a'-go-go-related gene potassium channels modulate migration in human anaplastic thyroid cancer cells. Endocr Relat Cancer. 2012;19(5):667–80.
14. Chen KC, Liao YC, Wang JY, Lin YC, Chen CH, Juo SH. Oxidized low-density lipoprotein is a common risk factor for cardiovascular diseases and gastroenterological cancers via epigenomical regulation of microRNA-210. Oncotarget. 2015;6(27):24105–18.
15. Hu W, Wang M, Yin H, Yao C, He Q, Yin L, Zhang C, Li W, Chang G, Wang S. MicroRNA-1298 is regulated by DNA methylation and affects vascular smooth muscle cell function by targeting connexin 43. Cardiovasc Res. 2015;107(4):534–45.
16. Boosani CS, Dhar K, Agrawal DK. Down-regulation of hsa-miR-1264 contributes to DNMT1-mediated silencing of SOCS3.Molecular. Biol Rep. 2015;42(9):1365–76.
17. Cao C, Zhang H, Zhao L, Zhou L, Zhang M, Xu H, Han X, Li G, Yang X, Jiang Y. miR-125b targets DNMT3b and mediates p53 DNA methylation involving in the vascular smooth muscle cells proliferation induced by homocysteine. Exp Cell Res. 2016;347(1):95–104.
18. Zhang HP, Wang YH, Cao CJ, Yang XM, Ma SC, Han XB, Yang XL, Yang AN, Tian J, Xu H, Zhang MH, Jiang YD. A regulatory circuit involving miR-143 and DNMT3a mediates vascular smooth muscle cell proliferation induced by homocysteine. Mol Biol Rep. 2016;13(1):483–90.
19. Qian Z, Zhang L, Chen J, Li Y, Kang K, Qu J, Wang Z, Zhai Y, Li L, Gou D. MiR-328 targeting PIM-1 inhibits proliferation and migration of pulmonary arterial smooth muscle cells in PDGFBB signaling pathway. Oncotarget. 2016;7(34):54998–5011.
20. Potus F, Ruffenach G, Dahou A, Thebault C, Breuils-Bonnet S, Tremblay E, Nadeau V, Paradis R, Graydon C, Wong R, Johnson I, Paulin R, Lajoie AC, Perron J, Charbonneau E, Joubert P, Pibarot P, Michelakis ED, Provencher S, Bonnet S. Downregulation of MicroRNA-126 contributes to the failing right ventricle in pulmonary arterial hypertension. Circulation. 2015;132(10):932–43.
21. Lin X, Xu F, Cui RR, Xiong D, Zhong JY, Zhu T, Li F, Wu F, Xie XB, Mao MZ, Liao XB, Yuan LQ. Arterial calcification is regulated via an miR-204/DNMT3a regulatory circuit both in vitro and in female mice. Endocrinology. 2018;159(8):2905–16.
22. Ruan W, Zhao F, Zhao S, Zhang L, Shi L, Pang T. Knockdown of long noncoding RNA MEG3 impairs VEGF-stimulated endothelial sprouting angiogenesis via modulating VEGFR2 expression in human umbilical vein endothelial cells. Gene. 2018;649:32–9.
23. Espinosa-Diez C, Wilson R, Chatterjee N, Hudson C, Ruhl R, Hipfinger C, Helms E, Khan OF, Anderson DG, Anand S. MicroRNA regulation of the MRN complex impacts DNA damage, cellular senescence, and angiogenic signaling. Cell Death Dis. 2018;9(6):632.
24. Zhang R, Wang N, Zhang LN, Huang N, Song TF, Li ZZ, Li M, Luo XG, Zhou H, He HP, Zhang XY, Ma W, Zhang TC. Knockdown of DNMT1 and DNMT3a promotes the angiogenesis of human Mesenchymal stem cells leading to arterial specific differentiation. Stem Cells. 2016;34(5):1273–83.
25. Agrawal DK, Boosani CS. Gene therapy to keep the QT rhythms "on the QT". J Thorac Cardiovasc Surg. 2017;154(5):1641–3.
26. Liu Z, Hutt JA, Rajeshkumar B, Azuma Y, Duan KL, Donahue JK. Preclinical efficacy and safety of KCNH2-G628S gene therapy for postoperative atrial fibrillation. J Thorac Cardiovasc Surg. 2017;154(5):1644–51.. e1648
27. Coto E, Calvo D, Reguero JR, Moris C, Rubin JM, Diaz-Corte C, Gil-Pena H, Alosno B, Iglesias S, Gomez J. Differential methylation of lncRNA KCNQ1OT1 promoter polymorphism was associated with symptomatic cardiac long QT. Epigenomics. 2017;9(8):1049–57.
28. Huang L, Xi Z, Wang C, Zhang Y, Yang Z, Zhang S, Chen Y, Zuo Z. Phenanthrene exposure induces cardiac hypertrophy via reducing miR-133a expression by DNA methylation. Sci Rep. 2016;6:20105.
29. Chavali V, Tyagi SC, Mishra PK. MicroRNA-133a regulates DNA methylation in diabetic cardiomyocytes. Biochem Biophys Res Commun. 2012;425(3):668–72.
30. Wang JR, Zhou H, Yi XQ, Jiang ZH, Liu L. Total ginsenosides of Radix Ginseng modulates tricarboxylic acid cycle protein expression to enhance cardiac energy metabolism in ischemic rat heart tissues. Molecules. 2012;17(11):12746–57.
31. Qin RH, Tao H, Ni SH, Shi P, Dai C, Shi KH. microRNA-29a inhibits cardiac fibrosis in Sprague-Dawley rats by downregulating the expression of DNMT3A. Anatol J Cardiol. 2018;20(4):198–205.
32. Zhu X, Du J, Yu J, Guo R, Feng Y, Qiao L, Xu Z, Yang F, Zhong G, Liu F, Cheng F, Chu M, Lin J. LncRNA NKILA regulates endothelium inflammation by controlling a NF-kappaB/KLF4 positive feedback loop. J Mol Cell Cardiol. 2019;126:60–9.
33. Li Z, Yu F, Zhou X, Zeng S, Zhan Q, Yuan M, Yang Q, Liu Y, Xia J. Promoter hypomethylation of microRNA223 gene is associated with atherosclerotic cerebral infarction. Atherosclerosis. 2017;263:237–43.

34. Bannister AJ, Kouzarides T. Regulation of chromatin by histone modifications. Cell Res. 2011;21(3):381–95.
35. Klose RJ, Kallin EM, Zhang Y. JmjC-domain-containing proteins and histone demethylation. Nat Rev Genet. 2006;7(9):715–27.
36. Mathison M, Singh VP, Chiuchiolo MJ, Sanagasetti D, Mao Y, Patel VB, Yang J, Kaminsky SM, Crystal RG, Rosengart TK. In situ reprogramming to transdifferentiate fibroblasts into cardiomyocytes using adenoviral vectors: implications for clinical myocardial regeneration. J Thorac Cardiovasc Surg. 2017;153(2):329–39.. e323
37. Agrawal DK, Boosani CS. Cellular reprogramming in cardiac diseases: a feather in the hat of regenerative medicine. J Thorac Cardiovasc Surg. 2017;153(2):327–8.
38. Ieda M, Fu JD, Delgado-Olguin P, Vedantham V, Hayashi Y, Bruneau BG, Srivastava D. Direct reprogramming of fibroblasts into functional cardiomyocytes by defined factors. Cell. 2010;142(3):375–86.
39. Zhou H, Morales MG, Hashimoto H, Dickson ME, Song K, Ye W, Kim MS, Niederstrasser H, Wang Z, Chen B, Posner BA, Bassel-Duby R, Olson EN. ZNF281 enhances cardiac reprogramming by modulating cardiac and inflammatory gene expression. Genes Dev. 2017;31(17):1770–83.
40. Anderson KM, Anderson DM, McAnally JR, Shelton JM, Bassel-Duby R, Olson EN. Transcription of the non-coding RNA upperhand controls Hand2 expression and heart development. Nature. 2016;539(7629):433–6.
41. Grote P, Wittler L, Hendrix D, Koch F, Wahrisch S, Beisaw A, Macura K, Blass G, Kellis M, Werber M, Herrmann BG. The tissue-specific lncRNA Fendrr is an essential regulator of heart and body wall development in the mouse. Dev Cell. 2013;24(2):206–14.
42. Zhao H, Wen G, Huang Y, Yu X, Chen Q, Afzal TA, Luong Le A, Zhu J, Ye S, Zhang L, Xiao Q. MicroRNA-22 regulates smooth muscle cell differentiation from stem cells by targeting methyl CpG-binding protein 2. Arterioscler Thromb Vasc Biol. 2015;35(4):918–29.
43. Sluijter JP, van Mil A, van Vliet P, Metz CH, Liu J, Doevendans PA, Goumans MJ. MicroRNA-1 and -499 regulate differentiation and proliferation in human-derived cardiomyocyte progenitor cells. Arterioscler Thromb Vasc Biol. 2010;30(4):859–68.
44. Takaya T, Ono K, Kawamura T, Takanabe R, Kaichi S, Morimoto T, Wada H, Kita T, Shimatsu A, Hasegawa K. MicroRNA-1 and MicroRNA-133 in spontaneous myocardial differentiation of mouse embryonic stem cells. Circ J. 2009;73(8):1492–7.
45. Yang Y, Cheng HW, Qiu Y, Dupee D, Noonan M, Lin YD, Fisch S, Unno K, Sereti KI, Liao R. MicroRNA-34a plays a key role in cardiac repair and regeneration following myocardial infarction. Circ Res. 2015;117(5):450–9.
46. Wu G, Cai J, Han Y, Chen J, Huang ZP, Chen C, Cai Y, Huang H, Yang Y, Liu Y, Xu Z, He D, Zhang X, Hu X, Pinello L, Zhong D, He F, Yuan GC, Wang DZ, Zeng C. LincRNA-p21 regulates neointima formation, vascular smooth muscle cell proliferation, apoptosis, and atherosclerosis by enhancing p53 activity. Circulation. 2014;130(17):1452–65.
47. Cekin N, Ozcan A, Goksel S, Arslan S, Pinarbasi E, Berkan O. Decreased FENDRR and LincRNA-p21 expression in atherosclerotic plaque. Anatol J Cardiol. 2018;19(2):131–6.
48. Villeneuve LM, Kato M, Reddy MA, Wang M, Lanting L, Natarajan R. Enhanced levels of microRNA-125b in vascular smooth muscle cells of diabetic db/db mice lead to increased inflammatory gene expression by targeting the histone methyltransferase Suv39h1. Diabetes. 2010;59(11):2904–15.
49. Chen KC, Liao YC, Hsieh IC, Wang YS, Hu CY, Juo SH. OxLDL causes both epigenetic modification and signaling regulation on the microRNA-29b gene: novel mechanisms for cardiovascular diseases. J Mol Cell Cardiol. 2012;52(3):587–95.
50. Chen R, Kong P, Zhang F, Shu YN, Nie X, Dong LH, Lin YL, Xie XL, Zhao LL, Zhang XJ, Han M. EZH2-mediated alpha-actin methylation needs lncRNA TUG1, and promotes the cortex cytoskeleton formation in VSMCs. Gene. 2017;616:52–7.
51. Zheng X, Wu Z, Xu K, Qiu Y, Su X, Zhang Z, Zhou M. Interfering histone deacetylase 4 inhibits the proliferation of vascular smooth muscle cells via regulating MEG3/miR-125a-5p/IRF1. Cell Adhes Migr. 2019;13(1):41–9.
52. Lino Cardenas CL, Kessinger CW, Cheng Y, MacDonald C, MacGillivray T, Ghoshhajra B, Huleihel L, Nuri S, Yeri AS, Jaffer FA, Kaminski N, Ellinor P, Weintraub NL, Malhotra R, Isselbacher EM, Lindsay ME. An HDAC9-MALAT1-BRG1 complex mediates smooth muscle dysfunction in thoracic aortic aneurysm. Nat Commun. 2018;9(1):1009.
53. Leisegang MS, Fork C, Josipovic I, Richter FM, Preussner J, Hu J, Miller MJ, Epah J, Hofmann P, Gunther S, Moll F, Valasarajan C, Heidler J, Ponomareva Y, Freiman TM, Maegdefessel L, Plate KH, Mittelbronn M, Uchida S, Kunne C, Stellos K, Schermuly RT, Weissmann N, Devraj K, Wittig I, Boon RA, Dimmeler S, Pullamsetti SS, Looso M, Miller FJ Jr, Brandes RP. Long noncoding RNA MANTIS facilitates endothelial angiogenic function. Circulation. 2017;136(1):65–79.
54. Neumann P, Jae N, Knau A, Glaser SF, Fouani Y, Rossbach O, Kruger M, John D, Bindereif A, Grote P, Boon RA, Dimmeler S. The lncRNA GATA6-AS epigenetically regulates endothelial gene expression via interaction with LOXL2. Nat Commun. 2018;9(1):237.
55. Yu Z, Rayile A, Zhang X, Li Y, Zhao Q. Ulinastatin protects against lipopolysaccharide-induced cardiac microvascular endothelial cell dysfunction via down-

regulation of lncRNA MALAT1 and EZH2 in sepsis. Int J Mol Med. 2017;39(5):1269–76.
56. Floris I, Descamps B, Vardeu A, Mitic T, Posadino AM, Shantikumar S, Sala-Newby G, Capobianco G, Mangialardi G, Howard L, Dessole S, Urrutia R, Pintus G, Emanueli C. Gestational diabetes mellitus impairs fetal endothelial cell functions through a mechanism involving microRNA-101 and histone methyltransferase enhancer of zester homolog-2. Arterioscler Thromb Vasc Biol. 2015;35(3):664–74.
57. Lee DY, Lin TE, Lee CI, Zhou J, Huang YH, Lee PL, Shih YT, Chien S, Chiu JJ. MicroRNA-10a is crucial for endothelial response to different flow patterns via interaction of retinoid acid receptors and histone deacetylases. Proc Natl Acad Sci U S A. 2017;114(8):2072–7.
58. Vikram A, Kim YR, Kumar S, Li Q, Kassan M, Jacobs JS, Irani K. Vascular microRNA-204 is remotely governed by the microbiome and impairs endothelium-dependent vasorelaxation by downregulating Sirtuin1. Nat Commun. 2016;7:12565.
59. Han P, Li W, Lin CH, Yang J, Shang C, Nuernberg ST, Jin KK, Xu W, Lin CY, Lin CJ, Xiong Y, Chien H, Zhou B, Ashley E, Bernstein D, Chen PS, Chen HV, Quertermous T, Chang CP. A long noncoding RNA protects the heart from pathological hypertrophy. Nature. 2014;514(7520):102–6.
60. Shao M, Chen G, Lv F, Liu Y, Tian H, Tao R, Jiang R, Zhang W, Zhuo C. LncRNA TINCR attenuates cardiac hypertrophy by epigenetically silencing CaMKII. Oncotarget. 2017;8(29):47565–73.
61. Wang Z, Zhang XJ, Ji YX, Zhang P, Deng KQ, Gong J, Ren S, Wang X, Chen I, Wang H, Gao C, Yokota T, Ang YS, Li S, Cass A, Vondriska TM, Li G, Deb A, Srivastava D, Yang HT, Xiao X, Li H, Wang Y. The long noncoding RNA Chaer defines an epigenetic checkpoint in cardiac hypertrophy. Nat Med. 2016;22(10):1131–9.
62. Thomas AA, Feng B, Chakrabarti S. ANRIL regulates production of extracellular matrix proteins and vasoactive factors in diabetic complications. Am J Physiol Endocrinol Metab. 2018;314(3):E191–200.
63. Duan Y, Zhou B, Su H, Liu Y, Du C. miR-150 regulates high glucose-induced cardiomyocyte hypertrophy by targeting the transcriptional co-activator p300. Exp Cell Res. 2013;319(3):173–84.
64. Huang W, Feng Y, Liang J, Yu H, Wang C, Wang B, Wang M, Jiang L, Meng W, Cai W, Medvedovic M, Chen J, Paul C, Davidson WS, Sadayappan S, Stambrook PJ, Yu XY, Wang Y. Loss of microRNA-128 promotes cardiomyocyte proliferation and heart regeneration. Nat Commun. 2018;9(1):700.
65. Mathiyalagan P, Okabe J, Chang L, Su Y, Du XJ, El-Osta A. The primary microRNA-208b interacts with Polycomb-group protein, Ezh2, to regulate gene expression in the heart. Nucleic Acids Res. 2014;42(2):790–803.
66. Callis TE, Pandya K, Seok HY, Tang RH, Tatsuguchi M, Huang ZP, Chen JF, Deng Z, Gunn B, Shumate J, Willis MS, Selzman CH, Wang DZ. MicroRNA-208a is a regulator of cardiac hypertrophy and conduction in mice. J Clin Invest. 2009;119(9):2772–86.
67. Seok HY, Chen J, Kataoka M, Huang ZP, Ding J, Yan J, Hu X, Wang DZ. Loss of MicroRNA-155 protects the heart from pathological cardiac hypertrophy. Circ Res. 2014;114(10):1585–95.
68. Renaud L, Harris LG, Mani SK, Kasiganesan H, Chou JC, Baicu CF, Van Laer A, Akerman AW, Stroud RE, Jones JA, Zile MR, Menick DR. HDACs regulate miR-133a expression in pressure overload-induced cardiac fibrosis. Circ Heart Fail. 2015;8(6):1094–104.
69. Yan M, Chen C, Gong W, Yin Z, Zhou L, Chaugai S, Wang DW. miR-21-3p regulates cardiac hypertrophic response by targeting histone deacetylase-8. Cardiovasc Res. 2015;105(3):340–52.
70. Huang ZP, Chen J, Seok HY, Zhang Z, Kataoka M, Hu X, Wang DZ. MicroRNA-22 regulates cardiac hypertrophy and remodeling in response to stress. Circ Res. 2013;112(9):1234–43.
71. Ebert MS, Sharp PA. Emerging roles for natural microRNA sponges. Curr Biol. 2010;20(19):R858–61.
72. Ming GF, Wu K, Hu K, Chen Y, Xiao J. NAMPT regulates senescence, proliferation, and migration of endothelial progenitor cells through the SIRT1 AS lncRNA/miR-22/SIRT1 pathway. Biochem Biophys Res Commun. 2016;478(3):1382–8.
73. Kato M, Wang M, Chen Z, Bhatt K, Oh HJ, Lanting L, Deshpande S, Jia Y, Lai JY, O'Connor CL, Wu Y, Hodgin JB, Nelson RG, Bitzer M, Natarajan R. An endoplasmic reticulum stress-regulated lncRNA hosting a microRNA megacluster induces early features of diabetic nephropathy. Nat Commun. 2016;7:12864.
74. Quan H, Liang M, Li N, Dou C, Liu C, Bai Y, Luo W, Li J, Kang F, Cao Z, Yang X, Jiang H, Dong S. LncRNA-AK131850 sponges MiR-93-5p in newborn and mature osteoclasts to enhance the secretion of vascular endothelial growth factor a promoting Vasculogenesis of endothelial progenitor cells. Cell Physiol Biochem. 2018;46(1):401–17.
75. He C, Ding JW, Li S, Wu H, Jiang YR, Yang W, Teng L, Yang J, Yang J. The role of Long Intergenic noncoding RNA p21 in vascular endothelial cells. DNA Cell Biol. 2015;34(11):677–83.
76. Ma Y, Huang D, Yang F, Tian M, Wang Y, Shen D, Wang Q, Chen Q, Zhang L. Long noncoding RNA highly upregulated in liver Cancer regulates the tumor necrosis factor-alpha-induced apoptosis in human vascular endothelial cells. DNA Cell Biol. 2016;35(6):296–300.
77. Halimulati M, Duman B, Nijiati J, Aizezi A. Long noncoding RNA TCONS_00024652 regulates vascular endothelial cell proliferation and angiogenesis via microRNA-21. Exp Ther Med. 2018;16(4):3309–16.
78. Zhang BY, Jin Z, Zhao Z. Long intergenic noncoding RNA 00305 sponges miR-136 to regulate the

hypoxia induced apoptosis of vascular endothelial cells. Biomed Pharmacother. 2017;94:238–43.
79. Zhu Y, Feng Z, Jian Z, Xiao Y. Long noncoding RNA TUG1 promotes cardiac fibroblast transformation to myofibroblasts via miR29c in chronic hypoxia. Mol Med Rep. 2018;18(3):3451–60.
80. Wang K, Long B, Zhou LY, Liu F, Zhou QY, Liu CY, Fan YY, Li PF. CARL lncRNA inhibits anoxia-induced mitochondrial fission and apoptosis in cardiomyocytes by impairing miR-539-dependent PHB2 downregulation. Nat Commun. 2014;5:3596.
81. Liang H, Pan Z, Zhao X, Liu L, Sun J, Su X, Xu C, Zhou Y, Zhao D, Xu B, Li X, Yang B, Lu Y, Shan H. LncRNA PFL contributes to cardiac fibrosis by acting as a competing endogenous RNA of let-7d. Theranostics. 2018;8(4):1180–94.
82. Li X, Wang H, Yao B, Xu W, Chen J, Zhou X. lncRNA H19/miR-675 axis regulates cardiomyocyte apoptosis by targeting VDAC1 in diabetic cardiomyopathy. Sci Rep. 2016;6:36340.

Non-coding RNAs in Physiological Cardiac Hypertrophy

8

Lijun Wang, Jiaqi Wang, Guoping Li, and Junjie Xiao

Abstract

Non-coding RNA (ncRNA) is a class of RNAs that are not act as translational protein templates. They are involved in the regulation of gene transcription, RNA maturation and protein translation, participating in a variety of physiological and physiological processes. NcRNAs have important functions, and are recently one of the hotspots in biomedical research. Cardiac hypertrophy is classified into physiological cardiac hypertrophy and pathological cardiac hypertrophy. Different from pathological cardiac hypertrophy, physiological cardiac hypertrophy usually developed during exercise, pregnancy, normal postnatal growth, accompanied with preservation or improvement of systolic function, while no cardiac fibrosis. In this chapter, we will briefly introduce the definition, characteristics, and functions of ncRNAs, including miRNAs, lncRNAs, and circRNAs, as well as a summary of the existing bioinformatics online databases which commonly used in the study of ncRNAs. Specially, this chapter will be focused on the characteristics and the underlying mechanisms about physiological cardiac hypertrophy. Furthermore, the regulatory mechanism of ncRNAs in physiological hypertrophy and the latest research progress will be summarized. Taken together, exploring physiologic cardiac hypertrophy-specific ncRNAs might be a unique research perspective that provides new point of view for interventions in heart failure and other cardiovascular diseases.

Keywords

Physiological cardiac hypertrophy · NcRNAs · MiRNAs · LncRNAs · CircRNAs

L. Wang · J. Wang · J. Xiao (✉)
Cardiac Regeneration and Ageing Lab, Institute of Cardiovascular Sciences, School of Life Science, Shanghai University, Shanghai, China
e-mail: junjiexiao@shu.edu.cn

G. Li
Cardiovascular Division of the Massachusetts General Hospital and Harvard Medical School, Boston, MA, USA

1 Introduction

Non-coding RNAs (ncRNAs) are a class of RNAs that are not act as a template for translation proteins. They are involved in the regulation of mRNA translation, RNA splicing, DNA replication repair, gene transcription, development, and cell differentiation [1, 2]. Besides, it is closely related to the occurrence, development, progression, treatment, and diagnosis of various diseases [3–5]. NcRNAs can be divided into two broad categories depending on their biological functions: house keeping non-coding RNAs and regulatory

J. Xiao (ed.), *Non-coding RNAs in Cardiovascular Diseases*, Advances in Experimental Medicine and Biology 1229, https://doi.org/10.1007/978-981-15-1671-9_8

non-coding RNAs. Among them, house keeping non-coding RNAs include ribosomal RNAs (rRNAs), transfer RNAs (tRNAs), small nuclear RNAs (snRNAs), and small nucleolar RNAs (snoRNAs). Non-coding RNAs with regulatory effects can be divided into two subclasses (short non-coding RNAs and long non-coding RNAs) according to the length of the transcription product. Short non-coding RNAs include piRNAs, microRNAs (miRNAs, miRs), siRNAs, and among them, miRNAs are the most widely studied. Long non-coding RNA (lncRNA) refers to a class of non-coding RNAs that lack an >100 amino acids open reading frame and larger than 200 nucleotides, and their structure and function are diverse and complex [3]. In addition, linear products (miRNAs, lncRNAs) and circular RNA (circRNAs) can be classified according to the linearity or circularity of the transcription product. A large number of non-coding RNAs are detected in tissues and body fluids. In the cardiovascular system, ncRNAs are also key regulators involved in regulation of cardiac-related gene expression, and significantly affecting cardiac homeostasis maintenance and heart function [6–10].

Cardiac hypertrophy is classified as physiological cardiac hypertrophy and pathological cardiac hypertrophy [11]. Pathological cardiac hypertrophy is an injury response that occurs when the heart is overloaded, mainly due to increased myocardial cell volume, interstitial and perivascular fibrosis, loss of cardiomyocytes, increased collagen, and myofibroblasts activation. Eventually lead to myocardial structure disorder, reduced contractility, myocardial contraction and diastolic dysfunction. Pathological cardiac hypertrophy is considered to be an independent risk factor for increased morbidity and mortality of cardiovascular disease [12]. Different from pathological cardiac hypertrophy, physiological cardiac hypertrophy does not cause pathological changes such as loss of cardiomyocytes, decline of cardiac function, and aggravation of cardiac fibrosis [13, 14]. On the contrary, physiological cardiac hypertrophy is a protective response, which refers to the heart under the action of various physiological factors, such as regular exercise training and pregnancy [15]. During the progression of physiological hypertrophy, the area of cadiomyocytes, the volume of the heart, and the weight of the heart are increasing. In the meantime, the contractility function of heart also improved, however, there was no process of fibrosis. Previous studies have shown that physiological cardiac hypertrophy factors are resistant to persistent pathological stimuli, can inhibit ventricular remodeling and ameliorate heart failure [16–18]. Therefore, exploring the key regulatory factors of physiological cardiac hypertrophy is of great significance for the prevention and treatment of heart failure [15, 19].

2 Non-coding RNAs

2.1 MicroRNAs

MicroRNAs (miRNAs, miRs) are a class of ncRNAs of about 22 nucleotides in length that bind to messenger RNA via complementary or partial complementary base pairing. Degradation of mRNA, inhibition of mRNA translation is involved in the regulation of gene expression. MiRNAs need to undergo post-transcriptional modification [20]. The primary miRNAs (pri-miRNAs) transcribed by RNA polymerase II are processed to produce precursor miRNAs (pre-miRNAs), which are finally cleaved into mature miRNAs by RNase III enzyme DICER in the cytoplasm [21, 22]. MiRNAs can form RNA-induced silencing complexes (RISCs) with some proteins such as Argonaute protein family AGO2. Generally, the function of miRNAs is mainly determined by the function of their target genes. Different miRNAs can have different functions in the same tissue, and the same miRNA can also perform different functions in different tissues [4, 23, 24].

In cardiovascular system, miRNAs are involved in the cardiovascular development and the occurrence and development of cardiovascular diseases [7, 25, 26]. MiRNAs have been reported being involved in the regulation of almost all cardiovascular-related cells, such as endothelial cells, cardiomyocytes, smooth muscle cells, fibroblasts, etc., which play important regulatory roles in various cardiovascular diseases [27–29]. For example, miR-1, miR-133, miR-145, and miR-34 have been reported to negatively regulate the pathological hypertrophy of cardiomyocytes [30–36]. In contrast, miR-208a, miR-155, miR-199a have a pro-effect on the development pathological hypertrophy [37–41]. Besides, miRNAs can target specific transcription factors to indirectly regulate the expression of channel genes, thereby modulating cardiomyocytes excitability. MiR-122 can regulate the metabolism of NO by regulating its target gene L-arginine transporter 1 (SLC7A1), which leads to endothelial cells dysfunction [42]. MiR-122, as well as miR-33 may participate in the modulation of lipid homeostasis *in vivo*, and thus involved in the regulation of atherosclerosis [43, 44]. In addition, circulating miRNAs have been intensively studied as biomarkers in the cardiovascular system [6, 45]. Collectively, as potential biomarkers and therapeutic targets, miRNAs have prospective applications for cardiovascular diseases diagnosis and prognosis.

2.2 Long Non-coding RNAs

Long non-coding RNAs (LncRNAs) refer to a class of non-coding RNAs that are transcribed over 200 nucleotides in length. Similar to miRNAs, lncRNAs usually do not encoding proteins. LncRNAs are mostly transcribed by RNA polymerase II, can be spliced, and have 5′-terminal capped structure and 3′-terminal poly-A tail. Some lncRNAs also have splicing processes similar to mRNA biogenesis. The expression of lncRNAs are different among different tissues. Moreover, the same tissue or organ at different developmental stages, the expression of lncRNAs can also be different. Therefore, lncRNAs exhibit obvious tissue specificity and space-time specificity. Recent years, various functions of lncRNA have been discovered, which play an important role in gene transcription, protein translation, protein localization, stem cell pluripotency and modulation the progression of human diseases. It is valuable for diagnosis, treatment and prognosis evaluation of diseases [46]. Interestingly, recent studies have found that some lncRNAs can encode small peptides and exhibit their mode of action through translated products [47, 48].

In the cardiovascular system, lncRNAs have been reported to be involved in the occurrence and development of various diseases [10, 49–51]. For example, lncRNA Chaer was found to be enriched in the heart, and directly interacting with the catalytic subunit of PRC2, disrupting the PRC2-targeted genome site, thereby inhibiting histone H3K27 methylation in the promoter region of cardiac hypertrophy-related genes. Inhibition of Chaer in the heart can alleviate the pathogenesis of cardiac hypertrophy and improve cardiac function [52]. Besides, lncRNA Chrf, lncRNA mhrt have been reported to be involved in the regulation of pathological cardiac hypertrophy [53, 54]. Additionally, lncRNA Mexis, and lncRNA p21 regulate atherosclerosis [55, 56]. Furthermore, meg3, which is highly expressed in cardiac fibroblasts, is down-egulated in cardiac remodeling. And knockdown of meg3 would inhibit p53 binding to the promoter region of MMP-2, consequently blocking TGF-β1-induced MMP-2 expression and preventing cardiac fibrosis [57]. Moreover, lncRNA MIAT was found to promote cardiac fibrosis by up-regulating TGF-β1 by sponge miR-24 [58]. It is worth noting that, similar to miRNAs, the expression level of lncRNAs in serum have also been found to be closely associated with cardiovascular diseases. Therefore, lncRNAs can also be used as biomarkers for disease diagnosis. For instance, the expression level of lncRNA Lipcar was significantly different in patients with and without ventricular remodeling after myocardial infarction, suggesting that Lipcar might be a valuable biomarker of the progression of cardiac remodeling [59].

2.3 Circular RNAs

Circular RNAs (circRNAs) were first discovered in plant viruses in 1976, but did not receive much attention for decades. Due to the limitations of detection techniques and algorithms, it has long been believed that circular RNA is a small amount of splicing by-products present in mammals and does not have biological functions. Until recent years, with the breakthrough in high-throughput sequencing technology and bioinformatics analysis algorithms, a large number of circular RNAs were discovered in mammals [60–62]. In 2013, Hansen et al. discovered circRNA CDR1as has an important role. Since then, more and more circRNA studies have shown that circRNA is involved in the regulation of many important biological processes [63, 64]. Several mode of actions of circRNAs have been identified by multiple functional and mechanism studies [65–68]. Among them, the most well investigated action was that circRNA can be used as an endogenous miRNA sponge [63, 64, 69]. Besides, circRNA can interact with functional proteins and regulate gene transcription [70, 71]. What's more, some circRNAs have coding potential, which can be translated into small peptides or proteins [72–74]. The expression of circRNA in different species, tissues and cells is different, and it is closely related to the occurrence of various diseases such as tumors, nervous system diseases and metabolic diseases [75–77]. It is worth noting that because of its cell/tissue specificity and evolutionary conservation, circRNAs are of great potential as clinical therapeutic targets.

In cardiovascular, similar to miRNAs and lncRNAs, circRNAs are also involved in the regulation of many cardiovascular diseases [77, 78]. In the myocardial ischemia model, circRNA CDR1as (also known as ciRS-7) can be used as an endogenous sponge of miR-7a, aggravating myocardial apoptosis and myocardial infarct size [79]. CircRNA mm9_circ_016597 (MFACR) can also be used as miR-652-3p sponge to mediate mitochondrial division and cardiomyocytes apoptosis induced by myocardial ischemia-reperfusion injury [80]. CircRNA circ-Ttc3 plays a protective role in myocardial infarction, and reduces ATP depletion and apoptosis in cardiomyocytes [81]. The main mechanism is that circ-Ttc3 regulates the expression of downstream target genes Arl2, and protects cardiomyocytes from apoptosis via sponging miR-15b. CircRNA mm9_circ_012559 (also known as HRCR) is down-regulated in heart failure mice [82]. HRCR act as miR-223 sponge to inhibit miR-223 activity, which in turn aggravates the development of pathological cardiac hypertrophy and heart failure. In addition to cardiomyocytes, circRNAs also found to involved in the regulation of non-cardiomyocytes. Circ_000203, and circ_010567 have been reported to act as miRNA sponges that regulate cardiac fibroblasts or endothelial cells [83, 84]. However, act as miRNA sponge is only one of the mechanisms by which circRNAs take part in biological roles. CircRNAs function as protein sponges have also been investigated in cardiovascular system. In doxorubicin-induced cardiomyopathy, the circRNA Amotl1 can promote the phosphorylation of AKT and its nuclear transfer by binding AKT1 and PDK1, thereby alleviating cardiomyocytes apoptosis and myocardial injury [85]. In cardiac senescence, circRNA circ-Foxo3 binds and inhibits the migration of anti-aging and anti-stress proteins (ID-1, E2F1, FAK, HIF1α) from cytoplasm into nucleus and mitochondria, and thus mediating cardiac senescence [86]. In atherosclerosis, the circRNA circANRIL can bind to PES1 protein and promote p53 activation, play a role in aggravating apoptosis and suppression proliferation of vascular smooth muscle cells and macrophages, which ultimately play an important role in protecting atherosclerosis [70]. What is noteworthy is that except act as the key regulators of cardiac development and heart disease, circRNAs are also associated with cardiac regeneration. Super-enhancer (SEs)-related circRNA circNfix have been reported that knockdown of circNfix promotes cardiac regeneration by inhibiting Ybx1 ubiquitin-dependent degradation, increasing miR-214 activity [87].

3 Current Bioinformatics Tools in ncRNA Studies

A large number of ncRNAs have been identified, and the function of most ncRNAs has not been well documented. In ncRNA studies, RNA-sequencing and microarray are the most commonly used detection methods. A large number of statistically significant differential ncRNAs have been identified. Typically, sequencing data is validated by quantitative real-time PCR designed with specific primers. In the meantime, the application of bioinformatics is crucial for study of the function of ncRNA, especially in the prediction of function, exploration of interaction networks, and the relationship between ncRNAs and the occurrence and development of specific diseases. Therefore, a large number of Bioinformatic platforms have been developed and widely used. A summary about online databases is given in the Table 8.1.

4 NcRNAs Are Key Regulators of Physiological Cardiac Hypertrophy

4.1 Characteristics of Physiological Cardiac Hypertrophy

Endurance exercise have been reported to benefit whole body metabolism, however, the underlying mechanisms still largely remained unknown [15, 88–91]. Physiological cardiac hypertrophy usually occurs during exercise, pregnancy, and normal postnatal growth. Physiological hypertrophy includes exercise-induced physiological cardiac hypertrophy and pregnancy hypertrophy. Physiological cardiac hypertrophy is characterized by preservation or improvement of cardiac systolic function, without cardiac fibrosis. Especially, physiological hypertrophy is a reversible benign adaptive change that does not lead to pathological ventricular remodeling and heart failure [92]. When physiological cardiac hypertrophy occurs, the marker genes, such as ANP, BNP, β-MHC, of pathological remodeling do not increase. In addition, different from pathological cardiac hypertrophy, genes encoding Ca^{2+}-handling proteins did not change when physiological cardiac hypertrophy occurred.

The IGF1-PI3K-AKT signaling pathway is regarded as a key signaling pathway in regulating the development of physiological cardiac hypertrophy [93, 94]. Studies have shown that serum IGF1 levels are elevated in athletes with physiological cardiac hypertrophy, and also insulin-like growth factor-binding protein 2 (IGFBP2) plays an important role in the development of pregnancy hypertrophy [95, 96]. Insulin binds to and activates the insulin receptor, which recruits and phosphorylates the insulin receptor substrate 1 (IRS1) and insulin receptor substrate 2 (IRS2). These proteins activate the PI3K-AKT1 signaling pathway to promote cardiac physiological growth. Mouse-specific knockout of IRS1 or IRS2 can prevent exercise-induced physiological cardiac hypertrophy [97]. In addition, IGF1 activates the downstream signaling pathway by binding to and activating the IGF1 receptor IGF1R [98]. IGF1R is also essential for exercise-induced physiological cardiac hypertrophy. The catalytic subunit of PI3K, p110α, is a key molecule of physiological cardiac hypertrophy. When p110α knockout, IGF1R will not lead to the development of physiological hypertrophy. While activate p110α, the heart can demonstrate physiological growth spontaneously, and resist heart failure [99, 100]. Serine/threonine-protein kinases 1 (AKT1) is one of 3 closely related AKTs (AKT1, AKT2 and AKT3). The phosphorylation level of AKT1 is dynamically changed in exercised rats, AKT1 down-regulated in the first week, and then specifically increased phosphorylation level of AKT1 Ser-473 in the third week [101]. The expression of AKT decreased during pregnancy and then returned to normal levels after post portum delivery [102]. These all suggest that AKT plays an important role in physiological cardiac hypertrophy [103]. Besides, transcription factors C/EBPβ and CITED4 have been reported to be involved in the regulation of physiological cardiac hypertrophy. When physiological cardiac hypertrophy occurs, C/EBPβ is down-regulated, while CITED4 is up-regulated, which promotes cardiomyocytes proliferation and hypertrophy [18]. And moreover, thyroid hormone is also involved in the regulation of physiological cardiac hypertrophy [104, 105]. Thyroid hormone is closely associated with the development of physiological cardiac hypertrophy in cardiomyocytes via activating the PI3K/AKT/mTOR signaling pathway [106, 107].

Table 8.1 Summary of online databases associated with ncRNAs

NcRNAs	Database name	Description	Website	References
miRNAs	miRBase	MiRBase database is a comprehensive database that provides published miRNA sequence data, annotations, predicted target genes	http://www.mirbase.org	[116–118]
	RNAhybrid	RNAhybrid is a miRNA target gene prediction software developed based on the secondary structure of miRNA and target genes	https://bibiserv.cebitec.uni-bielefeld.de/rnahybrid/	[119]
	starBase	The database analyzed the interaction among miRNAs lncRNAs, circRNAs, protein and mRNAs, and analyzed the ceRNA mechanism. The database mainly contains information of three species: human, mouse and nematode	http://starbase.sysu.edu.cn/	[120, 121]
	ChIPBase	By integrating clip-seq and chip-seq data, the transcription and post-transcriptional regulation of microRNA were provided, and the regulatory network of transcription factor, microRNA and target genes was provided	http://rna.sysu.edu.cn/chipbase/	[122, 123]
	Targetscan	Targetscan database was developed for target prediction of miRNAs	http://www.targetscan.org/	[124]
lncRNAs	LNCipedia	LNCipedia includes a total of 146,742 human annotated lncRNA transcripts, all of which contain annotated information such as sequence, genomic location, and sources	https://lncipedia.org/	[125–127]
	Linc2GO	The database is intended to provide comprehensive functional annotations of human lncRNAs. MicroRNA-mRNA and microRNA-lncRNA interaction data were integrated to generate functional annotations of lncRNA based on the "ceRNA hypothesis"	https://omictools.com/linc2go-tool	[128]
	Noncode	NONCODE is intended to provide ncRNA annotation, which includes coding capability assessment, location information, expression information and potential functionality, and co-expression	http://www.noncode.org	[129–134]
circRNAs	circBase	This database collects thousands of circRNAs expressed in animals. This database allows users to search, browse, and download corresponding circRNAs	http://www.circbase.org/	[135]
	CIRCpedia v2	The database allows users to search, browse, and download circRNAs with expression characteristics of various cell types/tissues, including disease samples	http://www.picb.ac.cn/rnomics/circpedia/	[136]
	CircInteractome	The database allows users to prediction and map binding sites for RBPs and miRNAs on reported circRNAs	https://circinteractome.nia.nih.gov	[137, 138]
	circBank	The circBank database applied a novel nomenclature of human circRNAs and provides information about circRNAs sequences, miRNA-circRNA interactions, circRNA coding potential and conservation between human and mouse	http://www.circbank.cn/	[139]

4.2 NcRNAs and Physiological Cardiac Hypertrophy

To well investigate the underlying mechanism of physiological cardiac hypertrophy, it is usually use exercise training (running or swimming) to induce physiological cardiac hypertrophy. Currently, in the exercise-induced physiological cardiac hypertrophy model, miR-126, miR-144, miR-145, miR-21, miR-29a, miR-29c, miR-27a and miR-27b were found to be up-regulated, while miR-1, miR-124, miR-133a, miR-133b and miR-143 were found to be down-regulated [108–111]. However, none of these studies performed further mechanism researches to investigate why and whether these miRNAs are specific regulated during physiological hypertrophy. Moreover, none of those miRNAs have been checked their effects on cardiomyoytes growth and proliferation, which are considered to be the specific function in exercise-induced physiological hypertrophy [18]. The function of miR-222 and miR-17-3p on physiological cardiac hypertrophy is a relatively in-depth study of miRNAs [17, 112]. MiR-222 was significantly up-regulated in physiological cardiac hypertrophy both induced by swimming and running. Increased miR-222 can promote cardiomyocytes hypertrophy and proliferation through regulating its target genes p27, Hmbox1, HIPK1 and HIPK2. And it is necessary to increase the level of miR-222 in exercise-induced physiological cardiac hypertrophy. It is worth noting that cardiac-specific overexpression of miR-222 has a protective effect on ventricular remodeling induced by cardiac ischemia-reperfusion injury in mice, which can significantly improve cardiac function and ameliorate myocardial fibrosis [17]. In addition, miR-17-3p was also found to be significantly elevated in physiologically induced cardiac hypertrophy either induced by swimming or running. MiR-17-3p can also promote cardiomyocytes proliferation by directly acting on its target gene TIMP3, as well as indirectly inhibit PTEN and activate AKT signaling pathway to promote cardiomyocytes hypertrophy. Similar to miR-222, up-regulation of miR-17-3p can alleviate ventricular remodeling and heart failure caused by myocardial ischemia-reperfusion injury [112]. Besides, cardiac-specific overexpression of miR-223 exhibited significant physiological cardiac hypertrophy, and up-regulation of miR-223 in rat cardiomyocytes induced physiological growth through activation of AKT signaling pathway [113]. Moreover, miR-199-sponge transgenic mice can lead to physiological cardiac hypertrophy [114]. However, the roles of lncRNAs and circRNAs in physiological cardiac hypertrophy have not been reported. Therefore, further investigations to elucidate the underlying mechanisms of lncRNAs and circRNAs in physiological cardiac hypertrophy is of great significance.

5 Conclusion and Future Perspectives

With the deepening of research, more and more ncRNAs have been identified to be associated with cardiovascular physiology and pathology. The regulation of ncRNA expression levels is expected to become a new strategy for the treatment of heart diseases clinically in future. Although current experiments targeting ncRNAs for treatment of cardiac diseases that have been successfully used in animal models, the clinical treatment of pathological cardiac hypertrophy and heart failure progresses very slowly. Detailed studies about miR-222 and miR-17-3p specifically associated with physiological cardiac hypertrophy indicate that key factors of physiological cardiac hypertrophy might be resistant to sustained pathological hypertrophy stimuli, and changes in physiological hypertrophy-specific miRNAs can improve ventricular remodeling and further ameliorate heart failure. This suggests that exploring physiologic cardiac hypertrophy-specific ncRNAs might be a unique research perspective that provides new strategies for interventions in heart failure and other cardiovascular diseases. However, the research on key lncRNAs and circRNAs related to physiological cardiac hypertrophy has not been reported, and these still need to be further explored and studied in the future. Interestingly, it is worth mentioning that miR-222 and miR-17-3p are also sharing the same target gene TIMP3 in pulmonary arterial smooth muscle cells [115]. Although the specific relationship between miR-222 and miR-17-3p in cardiomyocytes is not clear, it is certain that there is definitely intrinsic connection between them. Therefore, future studies on the regulatory networks of ncRNAs among physiological specific miRNAs, lncRNAs and circRNAs will not only illuminate the molecular mechanisms but also provide us new therapeutic targets for cardiac diseases from the perspective of protecting the heart.

Acknowledgements This work was supported by the grants from National Natural Science Foundation of China (81722008, 91639101 and 81570362 to JJ Xiao, 81800358 to LJ Wang), Innovation Program of Shanghai Municipal Education Commission (2017-01-07-00-09-E00042 to JJ Xiao), the grant from Science and Technology Commission of Shanghai Municipality (17010500100, 18410722200 to JJ Xiao), Natural Science Foundation of Shanghai (19ZR1474100 to LJ Wang), National Key Research and Development Project (2018YFE0113500 to JJ Xiao), and the "Dawn" Program of Shanghai Education Commission (19SG34 to JJ Xiao).

Competing Financial Interests The authors declare no competing financial interests.

References

1. Chi KR. The dark side of the human genome. Nature. 2016;538(7624):275–7.
2. Li Y, Liang Y, Zhu Y, Zhang Y, Bei Y. Noncoding RNAs in cardiac hypertrophy. J Cardiovasc Transl Res. 2018;11(6):439–49.
3. Kopp F, Mendell JT. Functional classification and experimental dissection of long noncoding RNAs. Cell. 2018;172(3):393–407.
4. Treiber T, Treiber N, Meister G. Regulation of microRNA biogenesis and its crosstalk with other cellular pathways. Nat Rev Mol Cell Biol. 2019;20(1):5–20.
5. Sullenger BA, Nair S. From the RNA world to the clinic. Science. 2016;352(6292):1417–20.
6. Viereck J, Thum T. Circulating noncoding RNAs as biomarkers of cardiovascular disease and injury. Circ Res. 2017;120(2):381–99.
7. Barwari T, Joshi A, Mayr M. MicroRNAs in cardiovascular disease. J Am Coll Cardiol. 2016;68(23):2577–84.
8. Lucas T, Dimmeler S. RNA therapeutics for treatment of cardiovascular diseases: promises and challenges. Circ Res. 2016;119(7):794–7.
9. Creemers EE, van Rooij E. Function and therapeutic potential of noncoding RNAs in cardiac fibrosis. Circ Res. 2016;118(1):108–18.
10. Sallam T, Sandhu J, Tontonoz P. Long noncoding RNA discovery in cardiovascular disease: decoding form to function. Circ Res. 2018;122(1):155–66.
11. Nakamura M, Sadoshima J. Mechanisms of physiological and pathological cardiac hypertrophy. Nat Rev Cardiol. 2018;15(7):387–407.
12. Schiattarella GG, Hill JA. Inhibition of hypertrophy is a good therapeutic strategy in ventricular pressure overload. Circulation. 2015;131(16):1435–47.
13. Maillet M, van Berlo JH, Molkentin JD. Molecular basis of physiological heart growth: fundamental concepts and new players. Nat Rev Mol Cell Biol. 2013;14(1):38–48.
14. Bernardo BC, Weeks KL, Pretorius L, McMullen JR. Molecular distinction between physiological and pathological cardiac hypertrophy: experimental findings and therapeutic strategies. Pharmacol Ther. 2010;128(1):191–227.
15. Bernardo BC, Ooi JYY, Weeks KL, Patterson NL, McMullen JR. Understanding key mechanisms of exercise-induced cardiac protection to mitigate disease: current knowledge and emerging concepts. Phys Rev. 2018;98(1):419–75.
16. Bezzerides VJ, Platt C, Lerchenmuller C, Paruchuri K, Oh NL, Xiao C, Cao Y, Mann N, Spiegelman BM, Rosenzweig A. CITED4 induces physiologic hypertrophy and promotes functional recovery after ischemic injury. J Clin Investig. 2016;1(9)
17. Liu X, Xiao J, Zhu H, Wei X, Platt C, Damilano F, Xiao C, Bezzerides V, Bostrom P, Che L, Zhang C, Spiegelman BM, Rosenzweig A. miR-222 is necessary for exercise-induced cardiac growth and protects against pathological cardiac remodeling. Cell Metab. 2015;21(4):584–95.
18. Bostrom P, Mann N, Wu J, Quintero PA, Plovie ER, Panakova D, Gupta RK, Xiao C, MacRae CA, Rosenzweig A, Spiegelman BM. C/EBPbeta controls exercise-induced cardiac growth and protects against pathological cardiac remodeling. Cell. 2010;143(7):1072–83.
19. Vega RB, Konhilas JP, Kelly DP, Leinwand LA. Molecular mechanisms underlying cardiac adaptation to exercise. Cell Metab. 2017;25(5):1012–26.
20. Bartel DP. MicroRNAs: target recognition and regulatory functions. Cell. 2009;136(2):215–33.
21. Denli AM, Tops BB, Plasterk RH, Ketting RF, Hannon GJ. Processing of primary microRNAs by the Microprocessor complex. Nature. 2004;432(7014):231–5.
22. Lee Y, Ahn C, Han J, Choi H, Kim J, Yim J, Lee J, Provost P, Radmark O, Kim S, Kim VN. The nuclear RNase III Drosha initiates microRNA processing. Nature. 2003;425(6956):415–9.

23. Gebert LFR, MacRae IJ. Regulation of microRNA function in animals. Nat Rev Mol Cell Biol. 2019;20(1):21–37.
24. Pasquinelli AE. MicroRNAs and their targets: recognition, regulation and an emerging reciprocal relationship. Nat Rev Genet. 2012;13(4):271–82.
25. Tatsuguchi M, Seok HY, Callis TE, Thomson JM, Chen JF, Newman M, Rojas M, Hammond SM, Wang DZ. Expression of microRNAs is dynamically regulated during cardiomyocyte hypertrophy. J Mol Cell Cardiol. 2007;42(6):1137–41.
26. Cheng Y, Zhang C. MicroRNA-21 in cardiovascular disease. J Cardiovasc Transl Res. 2010;3(3):251–5.
27. Goretti E, Wagner DR, Devaux Y. miRNAs as biomarkers of myocardial infarction: a step forward towards personalized medicine? Trends Mol Med. 2014;20(12):716–25.
28. Schober A, Weber C. Mechanisms of MicroRNAs in Atherosclerosis. Annu Rev Phytopathol. 2016;11:583–616.
29. Zhou S, Lei D, Bu F, Han H, Zhao S, Wang Y. MicroRNA-29b-3p Targets SPARC gene to protect cardiocytes against autophagy and apoptosis in hypoxic-induced H9c2 cells. J Cardiovasc Trans Res. 2019;12(4):358–65.
30. Yin H, Zhao L, Zhang S, Zhang Y, Lei S. MicroRNA1 suppresses cardiac hypertrophy by targeting nuclear factor of activated T cells cytoplasmic 3. Mol Med Rep. 2015;12(6):8282–8.
31. Hua Y, Zhang Y, Ren J. IGF-1 deficiency resists cardiac hypertrophy and myocardial contractile dysfunction: role of microRNA-1 and microRNA-133a. J Cell Mol Med. 2012;16(1):83–95.
32. Care A, Catalucci D, Felicetti F, Bonci D, Addario A, Gallo P, Bang ML, Segnalini P, Gu Y, Dalton ND, Elia L, Latronico MV, Hoydal M, Autore C, Russo MA, Dorn GW 2nd, Ellingsen O, Ruiz-Lozano P, Peterson KL, Croce CM, Peschle C, Condorelli G. MicroRNA-133 controls cardiac hypertrophy. Nat Med. 2007;13(5):613–8.
33. Li R, Yan G, Zhang Q, Jiang Y, Sun H, Hu Y, Sun J, Xu B. miR-145 inhibits isoproterenol-induced cardiomyocyte hypertrophy by targeting the expression and localization of GATA6. FEBS Lett. 2013;587(12):1754–61.
34. Cha MJ, Jang JK, Ham O, Song BW, Lee SY, Lee CY, Park JH, Lee J, Seo HH, Choi E, Jeon WM, Hwang HJ, Shin HT, Choi E, Hwang KC. MicroRNA-145 suppresses ROS-induced Ca2+ overload of cardiomyocytes by targeting CaMKIIdelta. Biochem Biophys Res Commun. 2013;435(4):720–6.
35. Zaglia T, Ceriotti P, Campo A, Borile G, Armani A, Carullo P, Prando V, Coppini R, Vida V, Stolen, TO, Ulrik W, Cerbai E, Stellin G, Faggian G, De Stefani D, Sandri M, Rizzuto R, Di Lisa F, Pozzan T, Catalucci D, Mongillo M. Content of mitochondrial calcium uniporter (MCU) in cardiomyocytes is regulated by microRNA-1 in physiologic and pathologic hypertrophy. Proc Natl Acad Sci USA. 2017;114(43):E9006–15.
36. Ooi JYY, Bernardo BC, Singla S, Patterson NL, Lin RCY, McMullen JR. Identification of miR-34 regulatory networks in settings of disease and antimiR-therapy: Implications for treating cardiac pathology and other diseases. RNA Biol. 2017;14(5):500–13.
37. Tony H, Meng K, Wu B, Yu A, Zeng Q, Yu K, Zhong Y. MicroRNA-208a dysregulates apoptosis genes expression and promotes cardiomyocyte apoptosis during ischemia and its silencing improves cardiac function after myocardial infarction. Mediat Inflamm. 2015;2015:479123.
38. Diniz GP, Takano AP, Barreto-Chaves ML. MiRNA-208a and miRNA-208b are triggered in thyroid hormone-induced cardiac hypertrophy – role of type 1 Angiotensin II receptor (AT1R) on miRNA-208a/alpha-MHC modulation. J Mol Endocrinol. 2013;374(1–2):117–24.
39. Seok HY, Chen J, Kataoka M, Huang ZP, Ding J, Yan J, Hu X, Wang DZ. Loss of MicroRNA-155 protects the heart from pathological cardiac hypertrophy. Circ Res. 2014;114(10):1585–95.
40. Kong C, Sun L, Zhang M, Ding L, Zhang Q, Cheng X, Diao Z, Yan Q, Zhang H, Fang T, Zhen X, Hu Y, Sun H, Yan G. miR-133b reverses the hydrosalpinx-induced impairment of embryo attachment through down-regulation of SGK1. J Clin Endocrinol Metab. 2016;101(4):1478–89.
41. Li Z, Song Y, Liu L, Hou N, An X, Zhan D, Li Y, Zhou L, Li P, Yu L, Xia J, Zhang Y, Wang J, Yang X. miR-199a impairs autophagy and induces cardiac hypertrophy through mTOR activation. Cell Death Differ. 2017;24(7):1205–13.
42. Yang Z, Kaye DM. Mechanistic insights into the link between a polymorphism of the 3′UTR of the SLC7A1 gene and hypertension. Hum Mutat. 2009;30(3):328–33.
43. Aryal B, Singh AK, Rotllan N, Price N, Fernandez-Hernando C. MicroRNAs and lipid metabolism. Curr Opin Lipidol. 2017;28(3):273–80.
44. Novak J, Olejnickova V, Tkacova N, Santulli G. Mechanistic role of microRNAs in coupling lipid metabolism and atherosclerosis. Adv Exp Med Biol. 2015;887:79–100.
45. Creemers EE, Tijsen AJ, Pinto YM. Circulating microRNAs: novel biomarkers and extracellular communicators in cardiovascular disease? Circ Res. 2012;110(3):483–95.
46. Beermann J, Piccoli MT, Viereck J, Thum T. Non-coding RNAs in development and disease: background, mechanisms, and therapeutic approaches. Physiol Rev. 2016;96(4):1297–325.
47. Huang JZ, Chen M, Chen GXC, Zhu S, Huang H, Hu M, Zhu H, Yan GR. A peptide encoded by a putative lncRNA HOXB-AS3 suppresses colon cancer growth. Mol Cell. 2017;68(1):171–84.. e176
48. Nelson BR, Makarewich CA, Anderson DM, Winders BR, Troupes CD, Wu F, Reese AL, McAnally JR, Chen X, Kavalali ET, Cannon SC, Houser SR, Bassel-Duby R, Olson EN. A peptide encoded by a transcript annotated as long noncoding

RNA enhances SERCA activity in muscle. Science. 2016;351(6270):271–5.
49. Devaux Y, Zangrando J, Schroen B, Creemers EE, Pedrazzini T, Chang CP, Dorn GW 2nd, Thum T, Heymans S, Cardiolinc n. Long noncoding RNAs in cardiac development and ageing. Nat Rev Cardiol. 2015;12(7):415–25.
50. Viereck J, Thum T. Long Noncoding RNAs in Pathological Cardiac Remodeling. Circ Res. 2017;120(2):262–4.
51. Zhang D, Wang B, Ma M, Yu K, Zhang Q, Zhang X. lncRNA HOTAIR protects myocardial infarction rat by sponging miR-519d-3p. J Cardiovasc Transl Res. 2019;12(3):171–83.
52. Wang Z, Zhang XJ, Ji YX, Zhang P, Deng KQ, Gong J, Ren S, Wang X, Chen I, Wang H, Gao C, Yokota T, Ang YS, Li S, Cass A, Vondriska TM, Li G, Deb A, Srivastava D, Yang HT, Xiao X, Li H, Wang Y. The long noncoding RNA Chaer defines an epigenetic checkpoint in cardiac hypertrophy. Nat Med. 2016;22(10):1131–9.
53. Wang K, Liu F, Zhou LY, Long B, Yuan SM, Wang Y, Liu CY, Sun T, Zhang XJ, Li PF. The long noncoding RNA CHRF regulates cardiac hypertrophy by targeting miR-489. Circ Res. 2014;114(9):1377–88.
54. Han P, Li W, Lin CH, Yang J, Shang C, Nuernberg ST, Jin KK, Xu W, Lin CY, Lin CJ, Xiong Y, Chien H, Zhou B, Ashley E, Bernstein D, Chen PS, Chen HV, Quertermous T, Chang CP. A long noncoding RNA protects the heart from pathological hypertrophy. Nature. 2014;514(7520):102–6.
55. Sallam T, Jones M, Thomas BJ, Wu X, Gilliland T, Qian K, Eskin A, Casero D, Zhang Z, Sandhu J, Salisbury D, Rajbhandari P, Civelek M, Hong C, Ito A, Liu X, Daniel B, Lusis AJ, Whitelegge J, Nagy L, Castrillo A, Smale S, Tontonoz P. Transcriptional regulation of macrophage cholesterol efflux and atherogenesis by a long noncoding RNA. Nat Med. 2018;24(3):304–12.
56. Wu G, Cai J, Han Y, Chen J, Huang ZP, Chen C, Cai Y, Huang H, Yang Y, Liu Y, Xu Z, He D, Zhang X, Hu X, Pinello L, Zhong D, He F, Yuan GC, Wang DZ, Zeng C. LincRNA-p21 regulates neointima formation, vascular smooth muscle cell proliferation, apoptosis, and atherosclerosis by enhancing p53 activity. Circulation. 2014;130(17):1452–65.
57. Piccoli MT, Gupta SK, Viereck J, Foinquinos A, Samolovac S, Kramer FL, Garg A, Remke J, Zimmer K, Batkai S, Thum T. Inhibition of the cardiac fibroblast-enriched lncRNA Meg3 prevents cardiac fibrosis and diastolic dysfunction. Circ Res. 2017;121(5):575–83.
58. Qu X, Du Y, Shu Y, Gao M, Sun F, Luo S, Yang T, Zhan L, Yuan Y, Chu W, Pan Z, Wang Z, Yang B, Lu Y. MIAT Is a pro-fibrotic long non-coding RNA governing cardiac fibrosis in post-infarct myocardium. Sci Rep. 2017;7:42657.
59. de Gonzalo-Calvo D, Kenneweg F, Bang C, Toro R, van der Meer RW, Rijzewijk LJ, Smit JW, Lamb HJ, Llorente-Cortes V, Thum T. Circulating long-non coding RNAs as biomarkers of left ventricular diastolic function and remodelling in patients with well-controlled type 2 diabetes. Sci Rep. 2016;6:37354.
60. Burd CE, Jeck WR, Liu Y, Sanoff HK, Wang Z, Sharpless NE. Expression of linear and novel circular forms of an INK4/ARF-associated non-coding RNA correlates with atherosclerosis risk. PLoS Genet. 2010;6(12):e1001233.
61. Guo JU, Agarwal V, Guo H, Bartel DP. Expanded identification and characterization of mammalian circular RNAs. Genome Biol. 2014;15(7):409.
62. Jeck WR, Sharpless NE. Detecting and characterizing circular RNAs. Nat Biotechnol. 2014;32(5):453–61.
63. Hansen TB, Jensen TI, Clausen BH, Bramsen JB, Finsen B, Damgaard CK, Kjems J. Natural RNA circles function as efficient microRNA sponges. Nature. 2013;495(7441):384–8.
64. Memczak S, Jens M, Elefsinioti A, Torti F, Krueger J, Rybak A, Maier L, Mackowiak SD, Gregersen LH, Munschauer M, Loewer A, Ziebold U, Landthaler M, Kocks C, le Noble F, Rajewsky N. Circular RNAs are a large class of animal RNAs with regulatory potency. Nature. 2013;495(7441):333–8.
65. Zhang Y, Zhang XO, Chen T, Xiang JF, Yin QF, Xing YH, Zhu S, Yang L, Chen LL. Circular intronic long noncoding RNAs. Mol Cell. 2013;51(6):792–806.
66. Li Z, Huang C, Bao C, Chen L, Lin M, Wang X, Zhong G, Yu B, Hu W, Dai L, Zhu P, Chang Z, Wu Q, Zhao Y, Jia Y, Xu P, Liu H, Shan G. Exon-intron circular RNAs regulate transcription in the nucleus. Nat Struct Mol Biol. 2015;22(3):256–64.
67. Ebbesen KK, Hansen TB, Kjems J. Insights into circular RNA biology. RNA Biol. 2017;14(8):1035–45.
68. Li X, Yang L, Chen LL. The biogenesis, functions, and challenges of circular RNAs. Mol Cell. 2018;71(3):428–42.
69. Zheng Q, Bao C, Guo W, Li S, Chen J, Chen B, Luo Y, Lyu D, Li Y, Shi G, Liang L, Gu J, He X, Huang S. Circular RNA profiling reveals an abundant circHIPK3 that regulates cell growth by sponging multiple miRNAs. Nat Commun. 2016;7:11215.
70. Holdt LM, Stahringer A, Sass K, Pichler G, Kulak NA, Wilfert W, Kohlmaier A, Herbst A, Northoff BH, Nicolaou A, Gabel G, Beutner F, Scholz M, Thiery J, Musunuru K, Krohn K, Mann M, Teupser D. Circular non-coding RNA ANRIL modulates ribosomal RNA maturation and atherosclerosis in humans. Nat Commun. 2016;7:12429.
71. Zhu P, Zhu X, Wu J, He L, Lu T, Wang Y, Liu B, Ye B, Sun L, Fan D, Wang J, Yang L, Qin X, Du Y, Li C, He L, Ren W, Wu X, Tian Y, Fan Z. IL-13 secreted by ILC2s promotes the self-renewal of intestinal stem cells through circular RNA circPan3. Nat Immunol. 2019;20(2):183–94.
72. Yang Y, Gao X, Zhang M, Yan S, Sun C, Xiao F, Huang N, Yang X, Zhao K, Zhou H, Huang S, Xie B, Zhang N. Novel role of FBXW7 circular RNA in repressing glioma tumorigenesis. J Natl Cancer Inst. 2018;110(3):304–15.

73. Legnini I, Di Timoteo G, Rossi F, Morlando M, Briganti F, Sthandier O, Fatica A, Santini T, Andronache A, Wade M, Laneve P, Rajewsky N, Bozzoni I. Circ-ZNF609 Is a circular RNA that can be translated and functions in myogenesis. Mol Cell. 2017;66(1):22–37.. e29
74. Pamudurti NR, Bartok O, Jens M, Ashwal-Fluss R, Stottmeister C, Ruhe L, Hanan M, Wyler E, Perez-Hernandez D, Ramberger E, Shenzis S, Samson M, Dittmar G, Landthaler M, Chekulaeva M, Rajewsky N, Kadener S. Translation of CircRNAs. Mol Cell. 2017;66(1):9–21.. e27
75. Kristensen LS, Hansen TB, Veno MT, Kjems J. Circular RNAs in cancer: opportunities and challenges in the field. Oncogene. 2018;37(5):555–65.
76. Lu D, Xu AD. Mini review: circular RNAs as potential clinical biomarkers for disorders in the central nervous system. Front Genet. 2016;7:53.
77. Devaux Y, Creemers EE, Boon RA, Werfel S, Thum T, Engelhardt S, Dimmeler S, Squire I, Cardiolinc n. Circular RNAs in heart failure. Eur J Heart Fail. 2017;19(6):701–9.
78. Li M, Ding W, Sun T, Tariq MA, Xu T, Li P, Wang J. Biogenesis of circular RNAs and their roles in cardiovascular development and pathology. FEBS J. 2018;285(2):220–32.
79. Geng HH, Li R, Su YM, Xiao J, Pan M, Cai XX, Ji XP. The circular RNA Cdr1as promotes myocardial infarction by mediating the regulation of miR-7a on its target genes expression. PLoS One. 2016;11(3):e0151753.
80. Wang K, Gan TY, Li N, Liu CY, Zhou LY, Gao JN, Chen C, Yan KW, Ponnusamy M, Zhang YH, Li PF. Circular RNA mediates cardiomyocyte death via miRNA-dependent upregulation of MTP18 expression. Cell Death Differ. 2017;24(6):1111–20.
81. Cai L, Qi B, Wu X, Peng S, Zhou G, Wei Y, Xu J, Chen S, Liu S. Circular RNA Ttc3 regulates cardiac function after myocardial infarction by sponging miR-15b. J Mol Cell Cardiol. 2019;130:10–22.
82. Wang K, Long B, Liu F, Wang JX, Liu CY, Zhao B, Zhou LY, Sun T, Wang M, Yu T, Gong Y, Liu J, Dong YH, Li N, Li PF. A circular RNA protects the heart from pathological hypertrophy and heart failure by targeting miR-223. Eur Heart J. 2016;37(33):2602–11.
83. Tang CM, Zhang M, Huang L, Hu ZQ, Zhu JN, Xiao Z, Zhang Z, Lin QX, Zheng XL, Yang M, Wu SL, Cheng JD, Shan ZX. CircRNA_000203 enhances the expression of fibrosis-associated genes by derepressing targets of miR-26b-5p, Col1a2 and CTGF, in cardiac fibroblasts. Sci Rep. 2017;7:40342.
84. Zhou B, Yu JW. A novel identified circular RNA, circRNA_010567, promotes myocardial fibrosis via suppressing miR-141 by targeting TGF-beta1. Biochem Biophys Res Commun. 2017;487(4):769–75.
85. Zeng Y, Du WW, Wu Y, Yang Z, Awan FM, Li X, Yang W, Zhang C, Yang Q, Yee A, Chen Y, Yang F, Sun H, Huang R, Yee AJ, Li RK, Wu Z, Backx PH, Yang BB. A circular RNA binds to and activates AKT phosphorylation and nuclear localization reducing apoptosis and enhancing cardiac repair. Theranostics. 2017;7(16):3842–55.
86. Du WW, Yang W, Chen Y, Wu ZK, Foster FS, Yang Z, Li X, Yang BB. Foxo3 circular RNA promotes cardiac senescence by modulating multiple factors associated with stress and senescence responses. Eur Heart J. 2017;38(18):1402–12.
87. Huang S, Li X, Zheng H, Si X, Li B, Wei G, Li C, Chen Y, Chen Y, Liao W, Liao Y, Bin J. Loss of super-enhancer-regulated CircRNA Nfix induces cardiac regeneration after myocardial infarction in adult mice. Circulation. 2019;139(25):2857–76.
88. Wang L, Lv Y, Li G, Xiao J. MicroRNAs in heart and circulation during physical exercise. J Sport Health Sci. 2018;7(4):433–41.
89. Mach N, Fuster-Botella D. Endurance exercise and gut microbiota: A review. J Sport Health Sci. 2017;6(2):179–97.
90. Fiuza-Luces C, Santos-Lozano A, Joyner M, Carrera-Bastos P, Picazo O, Zugaza JL, Izquierdo M, Ruilope LM, Lucia A. Exercise benefits in cardiovascular disease: beyond attenuation of traditional risk factors. Nat Rev Cardiol. 2018;15(12):731–43.
91. Nieman DC, Wentz LM. The compelling link between physical activity and the body's defense system. J Sport Health Sci. 2019;8(3):201–17.
92. Weeks KL, McMullen JR. The athlete's heart vs. the failing heart: can signaling explain the two distinct outcomes? Physiology (Bethesda). 2011;26(2):97–105.
93. McMullen JR, Shioi T, Zhang L, Tarnavski O, Sherwood MC, Kang PM, Izumo S. Phosphoinositide 3-kinase(p110alpha) plays a critical role for the induction of physiological, but not pathological, cardiac hypertrophy. Proc Natl Acad Sci U S A. 2003;100(21):12355–60.
94. DeBosch B, Treskov I, Lupu TS, Weinheimer C, Kovacs A, Courtois M, Muslin AJ. Akt1 is required for physiological cardiac growth. Circulation. 2006;113(17):2097–104.
95. Neri Serneri GG, Boddi M, Modesti PA, Cecioni I, Coppo M, Padeletti L, Michelucci A, Colella A, Galanti G. Increased cardiac sympathetic activity and insulin-like growth factor-I formation are associated with physiological hypertrophy in athletes. Circ Res. 2001;89(11):977–82.
96. Olszanecka A, Dragan A, Kawecka-Jaszcz K, Fedak D, Czarnecka D. Relationships of insulin-like growth factor-1, its binding proteins, and cardiometabolic risk in hypertensive perimenopausal women. Metabolism. 2017;69:96–106.
97. Riehle C, Wende AR, Zhu Y, Oliveira KJ, Pereira RO, Jaishy BP, Bevins J, Valdez S, Noh J, Kim BJ, Moreira AB, Weatherford ET, Manivel R, Rawlings TA, Rech M, White MF, Abel ED. Insulin receptor substrates are essential for the bioenergetic and hypertrophic response of the heart to exercise training. Mol Cell Biol. 2014;34(18):3450–60.

98. Kim J, Wende AR, Sena S, Theobald HA, Soto J, Sloan C, Wayment BE, Litwin SE, Holzenberger M, LeRoith D, Abel ED. Insulin-like growth factor I receptor signaling is required for exercise-induced cardiac hypertrophy. J Mol Endocrinol. 2008;22(11):2531–43.
99. Weeks KL, Gao X, Du XJ, Boey EJ, Matsumoto A, Bernardo BC, Kiriazis H, Cemerlang N, Tan JW, Tham YK, Franke TF, Qian H, Bogoyevitch MA, Woodcock EA, Febbraio MA, Gregorevic P, McMullen JR. Phosphoinositide 3-kinase p110alpha is a master regulator of exercise-induced cardioprotection and PI3K gene therapy rescues cardiac dysfunction. Circ Heart Fail. 2012;5(4):523–34.
100. McMullen JR, Amirahmadi F, Woodcock EA, Schinke-Braun M, Bouwman RD, Hewitt KA, Mollica JP, Zhang L, Zhang Y, Shioi T, Buerger A, Izumo S, Jay PY, Jennings GL. Protective effects of exercise and phosphoinositide 3-kinase(p110alpha) signaling in dilated and hypertrophic cardiomyopathy. Proc Natl Acad Sci U S A. 2007;104(2):612–7.
101. Gosselin H, Beliveau L, Burelle Y, Clement R, Lajoie C, El-Helou V, Calderone A. Disparate regulation of signaling proteins after exercise and myocardial infarction. Med Sci Sports Exerc. 2006;38(3):455–62.
102. Gonzalez AM, Osorio JC, Manlhiot C, Gruber D, Homma S, Mital S. Hypertrophy signaling during peripartum cardiac remodeling. Am J Phys Heart Circ Phys. 2007;293(5):H3008–13.
103. O'Neill BT, Kim J, Wende AR, Theobald HA, Tuinei J, Buchanan J, Guo A, Zaha VG, Davis DK, Schell JC, Boudina S, Wayment B, Litwin SE, Shioi T, Izumo S, Birnbaum MJ, Abel ED. A conserved role for phosphatidylinositol 3-kinase but not Akt signaling in mitochondrial adaptations that accompany physiological cardiac hypertrophy. Cell Metab. 2007;6(4):294–306.
104. Fisher DA, Klein AH. Thyroid development and disorders of thyroid function in the newborn. N Engl J Med. 1981;304(12):702–12.
105. Chang KC, Figueredo VM, Schreur JH, Kariya K, Weiner MW, Simpson PC, Camacho SA. Thyroid hormone improves function and Ca2+ handling in pressure overload hypertrophy. Association with increased sarcoplasmic reticulum Ca2+-ATPase and alpha-myosin heavy chain in rat hearts. J Clin Investig. 1997;100(7):1742–9.
106. Trivieri MG, Oudit GY, Sah R, Kerfant BG, Sun H, Gramolini AO, Pan Y, Wickenden AD, Croteau W, Morreale de Escobar G, Pekhletski R, St Germain D, Maclennan DH, Backx PH. Cardiac-specific elevations in thyroid hormone enhance contractility and prevent pressure overload-induced cardiac dysfunction. Proc Natl Acad Sci U S A. 2006;103(15):6043–8.
107. Belke DD, Gloss B, Swanson EA, Dillmann WH. Adeno-associated virus-mediated expression of thyroid hormone receptor isoforms-alpha1 and -beta1 improves contractile function in pressure overload-induced cardiac hypertrophy. Endocrinology. 2007;148(6):2870–7.
108. Fernandes T, Hashimoto NY, Magalhaes FC, Fernandes FB, Casarini DE, Carmona AK, Krieger JE, Phillips MI, Oliveira EM. Aerobic exercise training-induced left ventricular hypertrophy involves regulatory MicroRNAs, decreased angiotensin-converting enzyme-angiotensin ii, and synergistic regulation of angiotensin-converting enzyme 2-angiotensin (1-7). Hypertension. 2011;58(2):182–9.
109. Ramasamy S, Velmurugan G, Shanmugha Rajan K, Ramprasath T, Kalpana K. MiRNAs with apoptosis regulating potential are differentially expressed in chronic exercise-induced physiologically hypertrophied hearts. PLoS One. 2015;10(3):e0121401.
110. Ma Z, Qi J, Meng S, Wen B, Zhang J. Swimming exercise training-induced left ventricular hypertrophy involves microRNAs and synergistic regulation of the PI3K/AKT/mTOR signaling pathway. Eur J Appl Physiol. 2013;113(10):2473–86.
111. Martinelli NC, Cohen CR, Santos KG, Castro MA, Biolo A, Frick L, Silvello D, Lopes A, Schneider S, Andrades ME, Clausell N, Matte U, Rohde LE. An analysis of the global expression of microRNAs in an experimental model of physiological left ventricular hypertrophy. PLoS One. 2014;9(4):e93271.
112. Shi J, Bei Y, Kong X, Liu X, Lei Z, Xu T, Wang H, Xuan Q, Chen P, Xu J, Che L, Liu H, Zhong J, Sluijter JP, Li X, Rosenzweig A, Xiao J. miR-17-3p contributes to exercise-induced cardiac growth and protects against myocardial ischemia-reperfusion injury. Theranostics. 2017;7(3):664–76.
113. Yang L, Li Y, Wang X, Mu X, Qin D, Huang W, Alshahrani S, Nieman M, Peng J, Essandoh K, Peng T, Wang Y, Lorenz J, Soleimani M, Zhao ZQ, Fan GC. Overexpression of miR-223 tips the balance of pro- and anti-hypertrophic signaling cascades toward physiologic cardiac hypertrophy. J Biol Chem. 2016;291(30):15700–13.
114. Li Z, Liu L, Hou N, Song Y, An X, Zhang Y, Yang X, Wang J. miR-199-sponge transgenic mice develop physiological cardiac hypertrophy. Cardiovasc Res. 2016;110(2):258–67.
115. Xu Y, Bei Y, Shen S, Zhang J, Lu Y, Xiao J, Li X. MicroRNA-222 promotes the proliferation of pulmonary arterial smooth muscle cells by targeting P27 and TIMP3. Cell Physiol Biochem. 2017;43(1):282–92.
116. Griffiths-Jones S, Grocock RJ, van Dongen S, Bateman A, Enright AJ. miRBase: microRNA sequences, targets and gene nomenclature. Nucleic Acids Res. 2006;34(Database issue):D140–4.
117. Kozomara A, Birgaoanu M, Griffiths-Jones S. miRBase: from microRNA sequences to function. Nucleic Acids Res. 2019;47(D1):D155–62.
118. Kozomara A, Griffiths-Jones S. miRBase: integrating microRNA annotation and deep-sequencing data. Nucleic Acids Res. 2011;39(Database issue):D152–7.

119. Kruger J, Rehmsmeier M. RNAhybrid: microRNA target prediction easy, fast and flexible. Nucleic Acids Res. 2006;34(Web Server issue):W451–4.
120. Li JH, Liu S, Zhou H, Qu LH, Yang JH. starBase v2.0: decoding miRNA-ceRNA, miRNA-ncRNA and protein-RNA interaction networks from large-scale CLIP-Seq data. Nucleic Acids Res. 2014;42(Database issue):D92–7.
121. Yang JH, Li JH, Shao P, Zhou H, Chen YQ, Qu LH. starBase: a database for exploring microRNA-mRNA interaction maps from Argonaute CLIP-Seq and Degradome-Seq data. Nucleic Acids Res. 2011;39(Database issue):D202–9.
122. Yang JH, Li JH, Jiang S, Zhou H, Qu LH. ChIPBase: a database for decoding the transcriptional regulation of long non-coding RNA and microRNA genes from ChIP-Seq data. Nucleic Acids Res. 2013;41(Database issue):D177–87.
123. Zhou KR, Liu S, Sun WJ, Zheng LL, Zhou H, Yang JH, Qu LH. ChIPBase v2.0: decoding transcriptional regulatory networks of non-coding RNAs and protein-coding genes from ChIP-seq data. Nucleic Acids Res. 2017;45(D1):D43–50.
124. Lewis BP, Burge CB, Bartel DP. Conserved seed pairing, often flanked by adenosines, indicates that thousands of human genes are microRNA targets. Cell. 2005;120(1):15–20.
125. Volders PJ, Anckaert J, Verheggen K, Nuytens J, Martens L, Mestdagh P, Vandesompele J. LNCipedia 5: towards a reference set of human long non-coding RNAs. Nucleic Acids Res. 2019;47(D1):D135–9.
126. Volders PJ, Helsens K, Wang X, Menten B, Martens L, Gevaert K, Vandesompele J, Mestdagh P. LNCipedia: a database for annotated human lncRNA transcript sequences and structures. Nucleic Acids Res. 2013;41(Database issue):D246–51.
127. Volders PJ, Verheggen K, Menschaert G, Vandepoele K, Martens L, Vandesompele J, Mestdagh P. An update on LNCipedia: a database for annotated human lncRNA sequences. Nucleic Acids Res. 2015;43(8):4363–4.
128. Liu K, Yan Z, Li Y, Sun Z. Linc2GO: a human LincRNA function annotation resource based on ceRNA hypothesis. Bioinformatics. 2013;29(17):2221–2.
129. Zhao Y, Li H, Fang S, Kang Y, Wu W, Hao Y, Li Z, Bu D, Sun N, Zhang MQ, Chen R. NONCODE 2016: an informative and valuable data source of long non-coding RNAs. Nucleic Acids Res. 2016;44(D1):D203–8.
130. Liu C, Bai B, Skogerbo G, Cai L, Deng W, Zhang Y, Bu D, Zhao Y, Chen R. NONCODE: an integrated knowledge database of non-coding RNAs. Nucleic Acids Res. 2005;33(Database issue):D112–5.
131. Xiyuan L, Dechao B, Liang S, Yang W, Shuangsang F, Hui L, Haitao L, Chunlong L, Wenzheng F, Runsheng C, Yi Z. Using the NONCODE database resource. Curr Protoc Bioinformatics. 2017;58:12 16 11–9.
132. Fang S, Zhang L, Guo J, Niu Y, Wu Y, Li H, Zhao L, Li X, Teng X, Sun X, Sun L, Zhang MQ, Chen R, Zhao Y. NONCODEV5: a comprehensive annotation database for long non-coding RNAs. Nucleic Acids Res. 2018;46(D1):D308–14.
133. Bu D, Yu K, Sun S, Xie C, Skogerbo G, Miao R, Xiao H, Liao Q, Luo H, Zhao G, Zhao H, Liu Z, Liu C, Chen R, Zhao Y. NONCODE v3.0: integrative annotation of long noncoding RNAs. Nucleic Acids Res. 2012;40(Database issue):D210–5.
134. He S, Liu C, Skogerbo G, Zhao H, Wang J, Liu T, Bai B, Zhao Y, Chen R. NONCODE v2.0: decoding the non-coding. Nucleic Acids Res. 2008;36(Database issue):D170–2.
135. Glazar P, Papavasileiou P, Rajewsky N. circBase: a database for circular RNAs. RNA. 2014;20(11):1666–70.
136. Dong R, Ma XK, Li GW, Yang L. CIRCpedia v2: an updated database for comprehensive circular RNA annotation and expression comparison. Genomics Proteomics Bioinformatics. 2018;16(4):226–33.
137. Panda AC, Dudekula DB, Abdelmohsen K, Gorospe M. Analysis of circular RNAs using the web tool circInteractome. Methods Mol Biol. 2018;1724:43–56.
138. Dudekula DB, Panda AC, Grammatikakis I, De S, Abdelmohsen K, Gorospe M. CircInteractome: A web tool for exploring circular RNAs and their interacting proteins and microRNAs. RNA Biol. 2016;13(1):34–42.
139. Liu M, Wang Q, Shen J, Yang BB, Ding X. Circbank: a comprehensive database for circRNA with standard nomenclature. RNA Biol. 2019;16(7):899–905.

9 Non-coding RNAs in Cardiac Regeneration

C. F. T. van der Ven, B. C. R. Hogewoning, A. van Mil, and Joost P. G. Sluijter

1 Introduction

Cardiovascular disease is a leading cause of death worldwide, and with the dramatically increasing numbers of heart failure patients in the next 10 years, mortality will only increase [1]. For patients with end-stage heart failure, heart transplantation is the sole option. Regrettably, the number of available donor hearts is drastically lower than the number of patients waiting for heart transplantation. Despite evidence of cardiomyocyte renewal in adult human hearts, regeneration of functional myocardium after injury can be neglected. The limited regenerative capacity due to inadequate proliferation of existing cardiomyocytes is insufficient to repopulate areas of lost myocardium [2]. As a solution, the hypothesis that adult stem cells could be employed to generate functional cardiomyocytes was proposed. One of the early studies that supported this hypothesis involved direct injection of hematopoietic c-kit-positive cells derived from bone marrow into the infarcted heart [3]. However, in sharp contrast, more recent evidence emerged demonstrating that these hematopoietic stem cells only differentiate into cells down the hematopoietic lineage rather than into cardiomyocytes [4, 5], and the focus shifted towards stem cells residing in the heart, called cardiac progenitor cells. These CPCs were extracted and injected into the myocardium to regenerate the heart [6]. In recent years, over 80 pre-clinical studies employing cardiac stem cells in vivo in large and small animals to evaluate the effect on functional parameters were systematically reviewed, identifying differences between large and small animals [7]. Despite the positive outcome of these stem cell therapies on functional parameters, c-kit-positive cardiac progenitor cells were shown to contribute minimally to the generation of functional cardiomyocytes [8, 9]. This heavily debated topic is summarized concisely by van Berlo and Molkentin [10]. Recently, single-cell sequencing and genetic lineage tracing of proliferative cells in the murine heart in both homeostatic and regenerating conditions did not yield a quiescent cardiac stem cell population or other cell types that support transdifferentiation into cardiomyocytes, nor did it support proliferation of cardiac myocytes [11, 12]. Now, the focus is shifting towards exploiting the limited regenera-

C. F. T. van der Ven · B. C. R. Hogewoning · A. van Mil
Laboratory of Experimental Cardiology, UMC Utrecht Regenerative Medicine Center, University Utrecht, University Medical Center Utrecht, Utrecht, The Netherlands

J. P. G. Sluijter (✉)
Laboratory of Experimental Cardiology, UMC Utrecht Regenerative Medicine Center, University Utrecht, University Medical Center Utrecht, Utrecht, The Netherlands

Department of Cardiology, Regenerative Medicine Centre, UMC Utrecht, Utrecht, The Netherlands
e-mail: j.sluijter@umcutrecht.nl

J. Xiao (ed.), *Non-coding RNAs in Cardiovascular Diseases*, Advances in Experimental Medicine and Biology 1229, https://doi.org/10.1007/978-981-15-1671-9_9

tive capacity of the cardiomyocytes themselves, by re-activating proliferation of existing cardiomyocytes through dedifferentiation, reentry into the cell cycle, and cytokinesis. This process is the new focus of research to promote cardiac regeneration, and can be controlled on multiple levels, including cell-cycle manipulation, reprogramming, small molecules, extra-cellular matrix (ECM), proteins, and RNA regulation [13].

Cardiac neovascularization, the new blood vessels formation in the heart, is an essential part of cardiac regeneration. Neovascularization is distinct from vasculogenesis, which is considered de novo primitive vascular network formation, and occurs when angioblast precursors differentiate into endothelial cells in the developmental stages [14]. Angiogenesis is the formation of a new blood vessel from the existing blood vessels. In the past the focus has been on mechanisms influencing the inhibition of angiogenesis, relating to its role in the spread of tumors [15]. However, there has been a growing interest in tackling ischemic disorders by promoting neovascularization in an attempt to regenerate tissues [16].

This chapter will focus on findings regarding the role of non-coding RNAs in cardiac regeneration. Cardiac regeneration is defined as the repair of cardiac tissue, which in turn enhances or restores the functional capabilities of the heart. Studying the role of these non-coding RNAs in species with inherent cardiac regenerative capacity uncovers and helps to understand the mechanisms that drive cardiac regeneration, such as cardiomyocyte proliferation and neovascularization. First, we elaborate on the regenerative capacity in lower vertebrates and rodents and their role as scientific models, then we elucidate the role of non-coding RNAs in cardiomyocyte proliferation and neovascularization.

2 Cardiac Regeneration in Various Scientific Model Species

Regenerative capacity varies between species. Lower vertebrate species have a high regenerative capacity throughout life, whereas in higher vertebrate species this regenerative capacity decreases after birth. Teleost fish like zebrafish and urodeles like newts or axolotls display robust cardiac regeneration, making them excellent model systems to study the underlying processes for cardiac regeneration. In zebrafish, after apical resection, bleeding is halted by blood clotting in the wound. Then fibrin is deposited, and where mammalian hearts become fibrotic through collagen deposition and scarring, the zebrafish heart replaces lost myocardium by proliferation of cardiomyocytes [17, 18]. Cardiomyocyte proliferation is highest 2 weeks after injury, and 2 months after injury the majority of the lost myocardium has been renewed and cardiac output restored [18, 19]. By employing Cre-based genetic fate mapping it was shown that resident cardiomyocytes dedifferentiate, proliferate, and mature similar to the developmental program to replace the lost myocardium, indicating that stem cells are not the source of regenerated myocardium [20, 21]. Similarly, in urodeles complete regeneration without scarring was observed two to 3 months after the injury [22], and it was demonstrated that sarcomeric gene expression is downregulated during regeneration which supports the notion that adult cardiomyocytes can generate more cardiomyocytes via dedifferentiation, proliferation, and redifferentiation. This concept is known as the dedifferentiation hypothesis [23, 24]. A concise recapitulation of the evolution of the scientific view on cardiomyocyte proliferation was published by Yutzey [25].

Rodent models like mice and rats display full growth and regeneration before and shortly after birth, yet have a reduced cardiac regenerative capacity as adult mammals [19]. Thus, neonatal rodents are excellent models for studying the mechanisms, and adult rodents are a suitable model to test stimulation of regeneration. To study the regenerative capacity of the fetal mice heart, an X-linked mutation, deadly to cardiomyocytes was introduced in female embryos. Due to random X inactivation half of the cardiomyocytes were lost, though at birth the hearts were fully functional. The fetal hearts compensated for the effective loss of 50% of cardiomyocytes by increased healthy cardiac cells proliferation [26]. High regenerative capacity in neonatal mice hearts has been demonstrated in multiple cardiac damage models: myocardial infarction [27], ventricular resection [28], cryoinfarction [29, 30], and clamping [31]. The human heart can also fully recover from injury as demonstrated in a case study of myocardial infarction in neonatal humans as a result of coronary artery occlusion. The infants fully recovered from the ischemic injury [32].

3 Non-coding RNA in Cardiomyocyte Proliferation

In contrast to the aforementioned lower vertebrate species, cardiomyocyte proliferation in adult mammals is, though present [2], insufficient to replenish lost cardiomyocytes due to injury. The proliferative state of cardiomyocytes as observed in embryonic stages of development quickly diminishes as the cells differentiate into the mature phenotype characterized by binucleation and hypertrophy. This development and maturation is regulated by many different factors. The capability of mature cardiomyocytes to again become proliferative is small [33–35]. Consequently, after the significant loss of cardiomyocytes as seen in ischemic injury, the heart cannot replace the lost cardiomyocytes and regenerate the myocardium. To increase the regenerative capacity of the heart, revealing the mechanisms underlying the development and proliferation of cardiomyocytes is essential. Recently, non-coding RNAs have been found playing important roles in regulating cardiomyocyte proliferation. These non-coding RNAs and their effect on cardiomyocyte proliferation are listed in Table 9.1. Here, we aim to highlight the discoveries of these non-coding RNAs and their role, organized per non-coding RNA class. At the time of writing the knowledge on the role of non-coding RNA in cardiac regeneration is limited to microRNAs (miRNAs) and long non-coding RNAs (lncRNAs). Other non-coding RNAs such as circular RNA, PIWI-interacting RNAs, or small inhibitory RNAs are not covered, as their functions in cardiac regeneration are still to be further studied.

3.1 MicroRNA

With their function as post-transcriptional regulators and their broad spectrum of targets due to partially complementary binding, miRNAs are potential candidates to regulate cardiomyocyte proliferation. Both the aforementioned models, fish and rodent, are widely used to study the involvement of miRNAs in cardiac regeneration, and cardiomyocyte proliferation specifically. A common approach to characterize miRNAs that could potentially regulate cardiomyocyte regeneration is to compare miRNA expression levels in different stages of development in prenatal and postnatal rodent hearts. Candidate miRNAs are then validated in one or multiple in vivo models of cardiac injury in either or both neonatal and adult rodents. Oftentimes, a model of cardiac injury is employed to replicate the disease as observed in humans. These models are based on either surgical induction, via ischemia or ischemia/reperfusion, or on genetic induction of heart failure (HF). Here, the role of the different miRNAs in cardiomyocyte proliferation is illustrated per disease model.

3.1.1 Surgical Cardiac Injury Models

Through ligation of the left anterior descending coronary artery (LAD), ischemia is induced in the left ventricle, inducing a myocardial infarction (MI), thereby resulting in a loss of cardiomyocytes [36]. The following miRNAs were found to play a role in increasing the regenerative capacity of the heart using this approach.

Table 9.1 Overview of identified non-coding RNAs validated in vivo for their role in cardiomyocyte proliferation

ncRNA	Target	Effect on Cardiac Function	Species	References
Let-7a/c	FNTß, SMARCA5	Negative	Zebrafish	Aguirre et al. [37]
miR-1-2	lrx5	Positive	Mice	Zhao et al. [46]
miR-15	Chek1	Negative	Mice	Porrello et al. [44, 45]
miR-17-92, miR-19a/b	PTEN	Positive	Mice	Chen et al. [48]
miR-31a	RhoBTB1	Positive	Rats	Xiao et al. [49]
miR-34a	Sirt1, Cyclin D1, Bcl2	Negative	Mice	Yang et al. [39]
miR-99/100	FNTß, SMARCA5	Negative	Zebrafish	Aguirre et al. [37]
miR-128	SUZ12, CDK2, Cyclin E, GATA4	Negative	Mice	Huang et al. [38]
miR-133a-1/2	SRF, Cyclin D2	Positive	Mice	Liu et al. [47]
miR-195	Chek1	Negative	Mice	Porrello et al. [44]
miR-199a	Homer1, Hopx	Positive	Mice, rats	Eulalio et al. [42]
miR-296	Trip53inp1, Itm2a	Positive	Mice	Cai et al. [55]
miR-302	Hippo, spec.: Lats2, Mob1, Mst1	Positive	Mice	Tian et al. [40] and Wang et al. [41]
miR-590	Homer1, Hopx	Positive	Mice, rats	Eulalio et al. [42]
CAREL	Trip53inp1, Itm2a	Negative	Mice	Cai et al. [55]
CRRL	miR-199a - Hopx	Negative	Rat	Chen et al. [59]
ECRAR	ERK1/2, Cyclin D1, Cyclin E1	Positive	Rat	Chen et al. [50]
LINCM3 (*Gas5)*	*Nppa, Dstan, Cyclin G1, Cyclin D2*		Mice	Yin et al. [54] and See [51]
LINCM9 (*Sghrt)*	*Cyclin G1, Cyclin D2*		Mice	See et al. [51]
MALAT-1	Nkx2.5, GATA4	Negative	Zebrafish	Wu et al. [56]
NR_045363	miR-216a	Positive	Mice	Wang et al. [58]
Sirt1 antisense lncRNA	Sirt1 mRNA	Positive	Mice	Li et al. [57]

Initially miR-99/100 and Let-7a/c were identified as key players in cardiomyocyte dedifferentiation in a cardiac apical resection model in zebrafish that naturally regenerate. They were both validated in mice subjected to LAD ligation causing MI. Blocking these miRNAs increased expression of their target proteins farnesyl transferase-beta (FNTß) and SWI/SNF-related matrix associated actin-dependent regulator of chromatin-subfamily A, number 5 (SMARCA5). Upon blocking, increased left ventricular ejection fraction and fractional shortening indicated functional improvements. The resulting cardiac regeneration, induced via dedifferentiation and proliferation of cardiomyocytes, and improved functional effects in both species proved that this mechanism is conserved between species [37].

Over-expression of miR-128 in cardiomyocytes in a neonatal apical resection model, suppressed cardiomyocyte proliferation and hampering cardiac function, thereby inhibiting cardiac regeneration, which can be observed after apical resection in untreated neonatal mice. Additionally, the role of miR-128 in cardiac regeneration was validated by deletion in cardiomyocytes in adult mice demonstrating improved cardiomyocyte proliferation after myocardial infarction induced by permanent LAD ligation. By deleting miR-128 the expression of SUZ12, a chromatin modifier, was enhanced. This in turn suppressed cyclin-dependent kinase inhibitor p27 and activated cell cycle regulators Cyclin E and cyclin dependent kinase 2 (CDK2), promoting cell cycle re-entry in adult cardiomyocytes.

Additionally, increased levels of GATA4 were observed, indicative of dedifferentiated cardiomyocytes [38].

In neonatal mice, miR-34a levels were found to be low and in adult mice, miR-34a levels were high, even after cardiac injury. Increasing miR-34a expression levels in neonatal mice resulted in a decreased regenerative capacity and hampered recovery. Inhibiting miR-34a in adult mice hearts after inducing MI increased the regenerative capacity and improved cardiac function, reduced adverse remodeling, decreased fibrosis, and increased cell cycle activity. Further investigation demonstrated that this miR-43a inhibition resulted in higher protein levels of Sirt1, Cyclin D1, and Bcl2. These proteins have been implicated in cell cycle activity, cellular aging, and cell survival. The former was merely protective against cell death, whereas the latter two maintained proliferative and cell cycle capacities [39].

Similarly, the miRNA cluster miR-302-367 was found to be elevated in pre-natal stages compared to post-natal stages. Reactivating the cluster in adult hearts led to cardiomyocyte proliferation, though persistent, prolonged expression resulted in cardiomegaly and ultimately in heart failure. The positive effect of reactivation of the cluster on cardiomyocyte proliferation was confirmed in mice with MI induced by LAD ligation. Transient transfection with the miRNA cluster however prevented the adverse effects of persistent over-expression without compromising the positive effect of increased cardiomyocyte proliferation on the regenerative capacity of the heart. This cluster was found to target components of the Hippo pathway. Specifically, proliferation-associated gene Ccnd1, and consequently Cyclin G1, was elevated, and kinases Mst1 and Mob1b were decreased [40]. In a more recent study, miR-302 was injected intramyocardially using a hydrogel delivery system for local and sustained delivery in adult Confetti mice with a MI. Due to the lineage labeling it was possible to distinguish newly generated cardiomyocytes as a result of clonal expansion. In addition, infarcted mice treated with the miR-302 showed comparable cardiac function to non-infarcted mice, as measured by ejection fraction and fractional shortening. Mice treated with miR-302 mimic demonstrated knock-down of Lats2, Mob1, and Mst1, all components of the Hippo signaling pathway, which controls cell proliferation mediated by YAP [41].

Additionally, miR-199a and miR-590 were identified by using a high-throughput functional screening with a human whole-genome miRNA library, and validated in vivo. Neonatal rats received injections of one of the two miRNAs together with a lipid transfection agent directly in the heart. Four days after treatment the ventricular wall thickness had increased, proliferating cardiomyocytes were found, and no fibrosis was observed. Next, adult mice were treated with AAV9 vectors expressing the two miRNAs after induction of a MI through permanent LAD ligation. Infarct size was significantly decreased in mice treated with miRNAs and cardiac function measured by left ventricular ejection fraction, fractional shortening, and end-systolic anterior wall thickness was preserved [42]. Expanding on these results, miR-199a was overexpressed using AAVs in pigs subjected to MI and reperfusion. Functional parameters improved, such as overall and local contractility. Muscle mass increased while scar tissue decreased, demonstrating that it is possible to regenerate the myocardium in larger mammals by stimulating endogenous repair via cardiomyocyte proliferation [43]. In all, expression of miR-199a and miR-590 after MI reduced infarct size and improved cardiac function by actively stimulating cardiomyocyte proliferation. Both miRs suppressed Homer1 and Hopx, genes involved in calcium signaling and in regulating proliferation, respectively [42, 43]. After inducing MI on day 1 after birth through LAD ligation, the mouse heart recovered fully within 3 weeks, through proliferation of existing cardiomyocytes. This regenerative response was impaired by over-expression of miR-195, one of the members of the miR-15 family, leading to adverse remodeling as observed in adult mice. Next, in an ischemia-reperfusion model of MI the miR-15 family was inhibited during postnatal development into adulthood. This led to an increase in cardiomyocyte proliferation and improved systolic function. Thus, inhibition of the miR-15 family increases the regenerative capacity [44]. In an earlier study by the same group, miR-195 was shown to directly affect cell cycle genes Chek1, Cdc2a, Birc5, Nusap1, and *Spag5*, supposedly increasing mitotic and cell cycle entry, and cell cycle progression. However, of these, Chek1 is the only gene with a miR-15 binding site that is conserved between mice and humans [45].

3.1.2 Genetic Cardiac Injury Models

When *Dicer,* which is required for pre-miR processing to mature miRNAs, was deleted in the hearts of embryonic mice using Cre recombinase and under the control of the *Nkx2.5* promotor this led to death as a result of heart failure. Thus proper miRNA functioning is required in cardiac development. In the *Dicer* mutant hearts, miR-1 was dysregulated. Using homologous recombination, miR-1-2 was deleted in mouse embryonic stem cells. Heterozygous animals were intercrossed to create offspring lacking miR-1-2. These mice died early, mostly due to ventricular septum defects, and those that survived suffered from cardiac arrhythmias and hyperplasia due to abnormalities in the cardiomyocyte cell cycle. Loss of miR-1-2 resulted in a loss of lrx5, leading to abnormal repolarization of cardiomyocytes and consequently cardiac arrhythmias. Furthermore, miR-1-2 mutants were hyperplastic as a result of increased mitotic activity in cardiomyocytes. This indicates a potential role for miR-1-2 in stimulating the regenerative capacity, though the observation in this study may be a result of increased proliferation in the early stages of development rather than in adult animals, for cytokinesis was not observed in adult animals [46].

Another example of complete knockout of a miRNA resulting in abnormal cardiomyocyte proliferation is the double knockout of miRNA-133a-1 and miRNA-133a-2 in mice, targeting Cyclin D2 and serum response factor (SRF). Mice lacking genes for one of the variants were normal, but deletion of both genes led to ventricular septal defects and consequently death in embryonic and neonatal animals, as a result of dysregulated cardiomyocyte proliferation, apoptosis, and abnormal expression of smooth muscle genes in the heart. Mice surviving into adulthood perished from heart failure and sudden death. Thus, miR-133a-1 and − 2 are essential for normal cardiac growth and function [47].

Similarly, complete knockout of the miR-17-92 cluster in embryonic, postnatal, and adult mice resulted in smaller hearts and lower proliferation rates in postnatal animals, a reduced number of cardiomyocytes in adult hearts, and decreased cardiac function, demonstrating that this cluster is essential for cardiomyocyte proliferation in embryonic and postnatal hearts. Overexpression of the cluster in a transgenic mouse model demonstrated enlargement of the hearts and thickening of the ventricle walls due to proliferation rather than hypertrophy. Overexpression of miR-17-92 using tamoxifen-inducible Cre recombinase in mice, subjected to MI, attenuated the effects of MI-induced damage and adverse remodeling. miR-17-92 was found to affect phosphatase and tensin homolog (PTEN), and overexpression of PTEN diminished miR-19 (a member of the miR-17-92 cluster) promoted cardiomyocyte proliferation. These results confirmed that the miR-17-92 cluster, and miR-19 specifically, can induce proliferation by suppressing PTEN in cardiomyocytes [48].

Some miRNAs have been validated in vivo without cardiac validation. For example, miRNA array on post-natal day 0 and day 10 rat cardiomyocytes revealed upregulated miR-31a levels on day 10. Inhibition of miR-31a on days 0, 1, and 2 resulted in reduced cardiomyocyte proliferation through RhoBTB1, a subfamily of the Rho small GTPases, suggesting that upregulating miR-31 might increase the generative capacity of the heart through stimulating cardiomyocyte proliferation [49].

Overall, evidence that miRNAs can influence cardiomyocyte proliferation is accumulating. Multiple miRNAs have been identified and validated in vivo. However, it is not yet fully understood how these miRNAs in turn are regulated, nor is it evident that miRNA are the sole regulatory RNAs in cardiac regeneration. Long non-coding RNAs are emerging as regulators of RNAs (mRNA, miRNA, circRNA) as well as

DNA and proteins. Their broad complex roles in gene regulation is a popular current topic, and there is evidence for involvement of several lncRNAs in cardiomyocyte proliferation.

3.2 Long Non-coding RNA

Long non-coding RNAs are a class of RNA molecules consisting of over 200 nucleotides that can regulate gene expression, both at transcriptional and post-transcriptional level, in a range of cellular processes, including (de)differentiation and proliferation. The research field of lncRNAs is relatively young and only a limited number of lncRNAs have been explored in the context of cardiovascular regeneration. How the lncRNAs listed in Table 9.1 was identified and how they affect cardiomyocyte proliferation is elaborated on in the following paragraphs.

Three lncRNAs have been identified that influence cardiomyocyte proliferation through affecting cell cycle genes. Endogenous cardiac regeneration-associated regulator (ECRAR) [50], LINCM3 (Gas5), and LINCM9 (Sghrt) [51] exert their function indirectly on one or more Cyclin proteins.ECRAR binds to extracellular signal-regulated kinases 1 and 2 (ERK1/2) activating cyclin D1 and cyclin E1, which both activate E2F transcription factor 1 (E2F1). E2F1 can upregulate ECRAR, creating a positive feedback loop that stimulates cell cycle progression, promoting proliferation in cardiomyocytes. Over-expression of ECRAR stimulated cardiomyocyte proliferation in vivo in the adult rat heart. To assess the effect of ECRAR over-expression in a disease environment, rats with MI from LAD ligation were injected with Adenovirus-mediated ECRAR. Over-expression of ECRAR led to increased proliferation resulting in cardiomyogenesis. Furthermore, infarct size was significantly smaller in rats that were treated with ECRAR, scar formation measured by fibrotic area was less, and functional parameters were improved, suggesting ECRAR enhances the regenerative capacity of the myocardium. This was confirmed by knockdown of ECRAR in naturally regenerative neonatal rat hearts, preventing recovery after MI. ECRAR showed a 12-fold increased expression from the analysis of four datasets of RNA-sequencing in fetal compared to adult human cardiac tissues. This finding was confirmed in rat fetal hearts, where ECRAR expression is high on embryonic day 12 and decreased after birth [50].

Similarly, nuclear RNA-sequencing of single cardiomyocytes from failing and healthy human heart tissue identified heterogeneity in the transcriptomic stress-response [51]. Key nodal lncRNA surfaced that regulate dedifferentiation and cell cycle genes in certain subsets of cardiomyocytes that can potentially regulate cardiac repair. In the diseased cells of a trans-aortic constriction (TAC) mice model, LINCM3 (*Gas5*) and LINCM9 (*Sghrt*) were upregulated, and LINCM5 was down-regulated compared to sham operated mice. Both *Gas5* and *Sghrt* are part of signaling pathways related to translation, precursor metabolites generation, oxidative stress response, oxidative phosphorylation, cell proliferation, and cardiac muscle tissue development. This indicated that both lncRNAs could be the main effectors regulating other genes within the same gene regulatory network. This hypothesis was tested by knocking down either of these lncRNAs in adult cardiomyocytes from TAC operated mice. Knockdown of *Gas5* down-regulated the expression of *Nppa* (fetal reprogramming), *Dstn* (dedifferentiation marker), *Ccng1* (cell cycle gene, coding for Cyclin G1), and *Ccnd2* (cell cycle gene, coding for Cyclin D2). *Gas5* has previously been shown to accumulate in the heart [52] and regulate apoptosis [53] and proliferation [54] in other cell types. *Sghrt,* at the time of writing, has no previously described function. Suppression of *Sghrt* did not have any significant effects on either *Nppa* or *Dstn,* increased *Ccng1,* and decreased *Ccnd2.* Thus, these experiments demonstrated that both lncRNAs can regulate genes in the same regulatory network at a transcriptional level [51].

Three other lncRNAs have been identified to be involved in cardiomyocyte regeneration, though not through affecting cell cycle genes. CAREL [55], MALAT1 [56], and Sirt1 antisense lncRNA [57] influence cardiomyocyte proliferation through anti-proliferative and pro-apoptotic pathways, through inhibiting transcription factors in developmental pathways, and through stabilization of mRNA, respectively.

Microarray analysis revealed that lncRNA CAREL was upregulated in postnatal mouse hearts. Over-expression of CAREL in cardiomyocytes of mice diminished their division and proliferation, and the regenerative capacity of neonatal hearts was lost. In contrast, silencing CAREL stimulated cardiac regeneration and promoted cardiac function after injury in both neonatal and adult mice. CAREL binds competitively to the targets of miR-296, Trip53inp1 and Itm2a. In line with previous results, over-expression of miR-296 induced cardiomyocyte proliferation and increased the regenerative capacity. In CAREL transgenic mice, the regenerative capacity was decreased, and could be restored by over-expressing miR-296 [55].

LncRNA MALAT-1 is expressed in adult zebrafish hearts [56]. MALAT-1 knock-out zebrafish showed an enlarged pericardium and other cardiac developmental abnormalities. Cardiac progenitor cell genes *nkx2.5* and *gata4* were upregulated, hinting at a regulatory role for MALAT-1 [56].

Expression patterns of Silent information regulator factor 2 related enzyme 1 (Sirt1) antisense lncRNA are higher in embryonic and neonatal compared to adult mouse hearts [57]. Sirt1 antisense lncRNA can bind Sirt1 messengerRNA, stabilizing it, and enhancing its translation into Sirt1 protein. Isolated neonatal cardiomyocytes were transfected with Sirt1 antisense lncRNA to examine its role in proliferation. Over-expression resulted in higher cell cycle activity, increased mitosis, and a higher cell number, indicating a positive influence on proliferation. In contrast, knocking down Sirt1 antisense lncRNA decreased the number of cardiomyocytes, cell cycle activity, and mitosis, and increased apoptosis. Next, intra-myocardial injections of LNA targeting Sirt1 antisense lncRNA resulted in decreased levels of proliferation in neonatal mice. Following these experiments, Sirt1 antisense lncRNA was over-expressed in both healthy and LAD-MI adult mice, leading to increased cardiomyocyte proliferation compared to their respective controls and a higher survival rate in the treated LAD-MI mice compared to untreated mice. In the latter group, cardiac output parameters, left ventricular ejection fraction and fractional shortening, improved, and the infarct size was smaller compared to untreated LAD-MI animals. These outcomes indicate that Sirt1 antisense lncRNA positively affects the regenerative capacity in ischemic adult hearts [57].

In addition to affecting gene expression through the aforementioned mechanisms, lncRNAs can act as sponges to miRNAs. Two lncRNAs have been identified that function thusly in affecting cardiomyocyte proliferation.

Recently, lncRNA NR_045363 was discovered to be mainly expressed in cardiomyocytes compared to non-cardiomyocytes, and more in embryonic mouse hearts than in adult mouse hearts [58]. Over-expression of this lncRNA in neonatal mice cardiomyocytes significantly increased proliferation in vitro and in vivo. Knockdown in primary embryonic cardiomyocytes led to decreased proliferation. Furthermore, over-expression in mice subjected to MI resulted in significantly ameliorated left ventricular ejection fraction and fractional shortening. Additionally, using EdU staining cardiomyocyte proliferation was shown to have increased in the animals over-expressing NR_045363. In silico target prediction showed miR-216a as a potential targets of NR_045363. Mir-216a is also a target of LOC101927497, the human ortholog of NR_045363. These predictions were validated in vitro and it showed that knockdown of NR_045363 led to increased miR-216a expression, and over-expression of NR_045363 resulted in decreased miR-216a expression levels. The researchers concluded that NR_045363 may function as a miRNA sponge for miR-216a, thereby preventing down-regulation of the targets of miR-216a, and consequently promoting proliferation [58].

Interestingly, one lncRNA has been identified that affects one of the cardiomyocyte proliferation-associated miRNAs. Cardiomyocyte regeneration related lncRNA (CRRL) has been identified from RNA-sequencing data of human fetal and adult heart tissues. CRRL promotes the expression of Hopx, the gene coding for Homeodomain-only protein, by directly binding miR-199a-3p, thereby removing the inhibition of miR-199a-3p on Hopx mRNA expression [59]. Loss of CRRL in adult rats preserved cardiac function and diminished adverse remodeling post infarct. Knockdown of CRRL in neonatal rat cardiomyocytes promoted proliferation in vitro and in vivo [59]. Thus, downregulation of the Hopx gene by removing the miR-199a-3p sponge CRRL via knockdown has a comparable effect to adding miR-199a as described previously [42].

4 Non-coding RNAs in Neovascularization

The growth of new blood vessels requires proangiogenic stimuli, including growth factors such as vascular endothelial growth factor (VEGF-A) [60]. Certain non-coding RNAs, for example, have the ability to influence these proangiogenic factors. Therefore, non-coding RNAs have the potential to become a therapeutic tool for treating ischemic cardiac tissue [61].

The following part provides an overview of advances in non-coding RNA research on cardiac regeneration through neovascularization. The non-coding RNAs listed in Table 9.2 are also shown in Fig. 9.1, to illustrate the pathways they affect, and their effect on cell cycle progression or apoptosis, respectively.

4.1 MiRNA

The first example of involvement of miRNA in the regulation of neovascularization was shown by Yang [39]. Their discovery demonstrated that knocking out the miRNA processing enzyme Dicer in mice would result in early death during embryonic development, due to impaired angiogenesis [39, 62]. Following up on that discovery,

Table 9.2 Overview of identified non-coding ribonucleic acids validated in vivo for their role in neovascularization

ncRNA	Target	Effect on neovascularisation	Species	References
miR-24	PAK4, GATA2	Positive	Zebrafish	Fiedler et al. [68] and Meloni et al. [69]
miR-26a	SMAD1	Negative	Mice	Icli et al. [72]
miR-92a	nMKK4, KLF4	Negative	Mice, Pigs	Bonauer et al. [66] and Hinkel et al. [67]
miR-126	SPRED1, PI3K/Akt	Negative	Mice	Qian et al. [70]
miR-132/212	SPRED1, RASA1	Positive	Mice	Lei et al. [76]
miR-150	VEGF	Negative	Rat	He et al. [78]
miR-210	Ptp1b, Efna3	Negative	Mice	Hu et al. [63], Arif et al. [64] and Fan et al. [65]
miR-214	QKI	Positive	Mice	van Mil et al. [77]
miR-377	STK35	Positive	Rat	Wen et al. [73] and Fan et al. [65]
ALIEN	503 unspecified genes	Negative		Kurian et al. [84] and Gomes et al. [85]
MALAT1	VEGFR2	Positive	Mice	Michalik et al. [80] and Zhang et al. [81]
MANTIS	BRG1, SOX18, SMAD, COUP-TFII	Positive	Mice	Leisegang et al. [82]
MIAT	miR-150	Negative	Rat cell (in vitro)	Yan et al. [79]
PUNISHER	Unknown	Positive	Zebrafish	Kurian et al. [84]

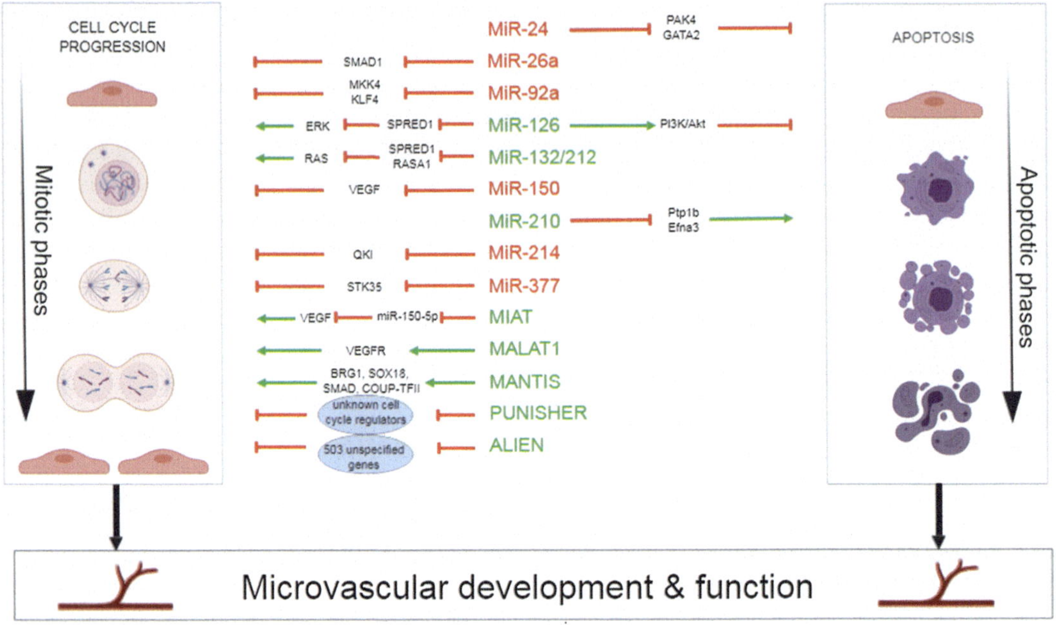

Fig. 9.1 Schematic representation of non-coding ribonucleic acids (RNA) and their respective targets that affect microvascular development and function through either stimulation (green) or repression (red) of cell cycle progression or apoptosis

numerous studies have shown the critical roles of miRNAs in neovascularization.

Over-expression of miR-210 on MI-injured cardiac tissue, showed an increase in neovascularization and angiogenic processes [63]. MiR-210 is known as a hypoxamiR, a label given to miRNAs that have an important role in hypoxic conditions [64]. Improved contractility in mammalian acute cardiac ischemia (ACI) models was observed when exposed to over-expression of miR-210, through the stimulation of hepatocyte growth factor (HGF) expression as well as the effect of miR-210 on left ventricular (LV) remodeling. This study concluded that through administration of miR-210 agonists, increased micro-vessel density was observed, indicating a potential therapeutic tool for patients with ACI [65].

In mice, miR-92a has been observed to control recovery of ischemic tissue and has been noticed to play a role in angiogenesis. Both in vitro and in vivo, over-expression of miR-92a in endothelial cells blocked neovascularization. In MI models, miR-92a antagonists demonstrated enhanced angiogenesis and resulted into recovery of the injured tissue. MiR-92a affects numerous proteins that promote angiogenesis, including integrin subunit α5. An abundance of miR-92a in endothelial cell caused a decline in endothelial cell migration, decreased vascular network formation, blocking of sprouting in a 3D neovascularization model, as well as reduced adhesion of the endothelial cell to fibronectin. MiR-92a influences MAP kinase kinase 4 (MKK4) and Kruppel-like factors-4 (KLF4) by targeting integrin subunit alpha-5, thereby inhibiting cell cycle progression in endothelial cells, and consequently the formation of new blood vessels. MiR-92a can therefore be categorized as an anti-angiogenic factor [62, 66]. Most of these studies were solely conducted in small animal models, and Hinkel et al. [67] took the next step and tested the efficacy of using the therapeutic potential of miR-92a inhibition in a pre-clinical porcine model of ischemia and reperfusion (I/R). The study showed that by using LNA-modified antisense miR-92a (miR-92a inhibitor), when applied regionally with the use of a catheter, the infarct size could be reduced significantly. This consequence resulted in enhanced cardiac function, as measured by LV ejection fraction and LV end-diastolic pressure. Histochemistry in the models confirmed an increased density of capillaries in the post-ischemic MI porcine hearts [67]. This study indicates that *anti-angiogenic* non-coding RNAs have the potential to be used as therapeutic targets in regenerative blood vessel formation.

MiR-24 is an additional anti-angiogenic miRNA, validated in a MI model in mice. MiR-24 has multiple effects on cardiac vascularization was shown to be upregulated as a consequence of cardiac ischemia. By acting on transcription factor GATA2, usually enriched in EC, as well as affecting PAK4, a p21-activated kinase, miR-24 promotes apoptosis of EC, limits cell sprouting (branching of vessels), and inhibits capillary network formation. Silencing of miR-24-targets as well as over-expression of miR-24, significantly restricted and halted angiogenesis in zebrafish embryos. Complete block of miR-24 decreased the damaged myocardial infarct size in mice, through increased vascularization and reduced apoptosis of the endothelial tissue. This resulted in improved cardiac function and thus miR-24 could be a potential therapeutic candidate for the regeneration of damaged tissue [62, 68]. In a mouse LAD-MI model, miR-24 expression showed increased expression levels in ECs. By blocking miR-24 specifically through local delivery of an adenovirus-mediated decoy, angiogenesis and blood perfusion of the myocardial tissue surrounding the infarcted area increased. In addition, there was a reduction in the infarct size, miR-24 induced fibroblast apoptosis, and overall cardiac function improved. Despite these potentially regenerative measures and effects, miR-24 decoy also increased cardiomyocyte apoptosis. In vitro, miR-24 inhibition supported endothelial cell survival, proliferation, and blood-vessel forming capabilities. Additionally, it led to fibroblast apoptosis, which could result in a reduction in scar formation in vivo, and CM apoptosis. These results were confirmed in vivo 14 days post-MI [69]. Both inhibition [68] and over-expression [70] of miR-24 have yielded positive results in mice with acute MI. Meloni et al. [69] set out to test the results of inhibiting miR-24 on cardiac function in a MI model and observed, 14 days after MI, that cardiac function had improved. These results indicated that the initial positive effect on endothelial cells is stronger than the apoptotic effect in CMs, resulting in a pro-angiogenic response and improved cardiac function 2 weeks after MI. It must be noted that that extended inhibition of miR-24 could lead to increased apoptosis in CMs and have a destructive effect on cardiac function and infarct size.

Wang et al. [71] discovered the importance of miR-126 in ensuring vascular integrity and function. The observation of mutant mice lacking the gene encoding for miR-126 resulted in dead embryos, or embryos suffering from ruptured blood vessels, hemorrhages and systemic edema. These abnormalities can be linked to reduced pro-angiogenic growth factor signaling, through e.g. VEGF and fibroblast growth factor (FGF). A lack of these angiogenic factors can lead to decreased endothelial cell growth, sprouting, and adhesion. MiR-126 as a pro-angiogenic stimulator is linked to the inhibition of Spred-1, which is an inhibiting regulator of MAP kinase signaling. If Spred-1 is over-expressed, it decreases pro-angiogenic signals by VEGF and FGF. In the absence of miR-126, there is no regulation of Spred-1. The group of mutant animals that survived showed malfunctioning cardiac neovascularization following MI induced by permanent LAD ligation, indicating the essential function of miR-126 [71].

In mice that suffer from ACI and in humans with acute coronary syndromes, increased levels of miR-26a has been observed [72]. Expression of miR-26a resulted in endothelial cell cycle arrest, inhibition of endothelial cell migration, sprouting angiogenesis, and blood vessel network formation in Matrigel. Blocking of miR-26a has the opposite effects. Over-expression of miR-26a in vivo in mice inhibited endothelial cell SMAD1 expression. It also resulted into a decrease in exercise-induced angiogenesis. Additionally, miR-26a inhibitor given intravenously resulted in increased levels of SMAD1 expression and readily induced significant levels of angiogenesis within 2 days. The pathway of miR-26a consists of the inhibition of the bone morphogenic protein/SMAD1 signaling pathway in ECs through directly targeting SMAD1. Through this blockage, Id1 expression is decreased, resulting in increased levels of p21 and p27 (regulators of the cell-cycle). leading to reduced infarct size and damage [72].

MiR-377 was found to play a role in paracrine-mediated angiogenesis [73]. In vivo evidence proved that, by knockdown of miR-377, mesenchymal stem cell (MSC) mediated angiogenesis increased, as well as the recovery of cardiac function after MI. Through the transplantation of these MSCs in MI rat hearts, the genetic over-expression of miR-377, its knockdown and a control were compared. Anti-MiR-377 treated hearts showed most myocardial angiogenesis post-MI. Through computational miRNA prediction analysis, VEGF was determined to be a potential target affected by miR-377. Verification of this assumption was performed through Western Blotting as well as through dual luciferase reporter assay. Wen et al. [73] determined that miR-377 can bind to the VEGF untranslated-region (UTR), resulting in its negative regulation on expression [73]. STK35, also known as CLP36-interacting kinase 1, was found to be one of the top targets for miR-377. Indeed knockdown of STK35 resulted into a decreased angiogenic potential of ECs [74]. Goyal et al. concluded that VEGF stimulation in ECs increased STK35 expression, so targeting STK35 would have an antagonistic effect to VEGF. Subsequent studies have demonstrated that myocardial tissue, derived via human cardiac biopsies from patients that suffered from heart failure (HF), showed a significant increase in miR-377 expression compared to non-failing control hearts [74]. The transplantation of miR-377 knockdown hCD34+ cells into ischemic myocardium enhanced the proangiogenic capabilities of the tissue, stimulating LV remodeling and reducing cardiac fibrosis [75].

Not all miRNAs relevant to angiogenesis have been validated in cardiac disease models. Other models have been employed to demonstrate the role of miRNAs in angiogenesis in other tissues such as the eye, muscle tissue, or cerebral tissue. These miRs could potentially be used to play a therapeutic role in cardiac tissue with regards to cardiac regeneration.

For example, miR-132/212 was knocked out in mice subjected to hind-limb ischemia. These animals displayed slower recovery compared to wild-type animals. These results were validated in vitro in a human umbilical vein endothelial cell (HUVEC)/pericyte co-culture by transfection of miR-132 and miR-212i. Addition of these miRs resulted in improved tubule formation, additional junctions, and longer tubule length, whereas inhibiting these miRs resulted in the opposite. By directly inhibiting SPRED1 and RASA1, miR 132/212 modulates the Ras-MAP-kinase pathway and promotes arteriogenesis [76]. MiR-214 has been proven to have an influence on developmental angiogenesis in vivo and in vitro, as well as in adult angiogenesis of mice. Specifically, van Mil et al. [77] demonstrated that miR-214 directly targets Quaking (QKI), a protein instrumental for vascular development. QKI transcript levels were increased in various tissues of mice transfected with antagomiR-214, and QKI knockdown by siRNA as well as miR-214 over-expression demonstrated abnormal vascular sprouting, confirming its importance on vascular formation. Additionally, the role of miR-214 on developmental angiogenesis was shown as antagomir-mediated miR-214 knockdown enhanced mouse retinal developmental angiogenesis. Mechanistic studies indicated that by silencing miR-214, more potent pro-angiogenic growth factors, such as VEGF-A, were secreted and the pro-angiogenic activity of EC-derived conditioned medium was increased, introducing a new pathway to possibly improve therapeutic vascular growth [77].

Established in the study above as well, miRNA influence on VEGF is a determining factor towards the neovascularization of respective tissues. A study by He et al. [78] demonstrated the regulatory function miR-150 has on post-stroke cerebral ischemia in rats via its interaction with VEGF. Through the upregulation of miR-150, the study resulted into decreased levels of vascular density of near-infarcted zones of the brain after middle cerebral artery occlusion. Additionally, miR-150 was seen to counter-effect tube formation, proliferation and migration of brain microvascular endothelial cells. All these results could be linked to the interaction of miR-150 and VEGF, leading to reduced expression. Using a dual-luciferase assay, VEGF was determined to be a direct target of miR-150 [78].

The aforementioned miRNAs play crucial roles in neovascularization and are consequently potential opportunities for therapy. Naturally, expression of miRNAs can be controlled by lncRNAs as illustrated in the subchapter on cardiomyocyte proliferation. Several lncRNAs have been identified to play a role in regulating neovascularization. These are highlighted in the next section.

4.2 LncRNA

LncRNAs have been established as regulators of various mechanisms involving neovascularization. This group of lncRNAs is also known as "Angio-lncRs" [14]. Due to the relative novelty of lncRNAs, lncRNAs that have not been directly validated in cardiac disease models are included in this part if the mechanism plays a role in neovascularization and has the potential to be relevant for cardiac regeneration.

The interplay between previously introduced miR-150 and the lncRNA MIAT was demonstrated with regards to their role in cardiac neovascularization [79]. In cardiac as well as in retinal cells, MIAT functions as a reliever to miR-150-5p repression of the pro-angiogenic growth factor VEGF. By functioning as a sponge to miR-150, it has proven to enhance cardiac hypertrophy in rat derived heart H9c2 cells. MIAT can therefore be labelled as a competitive endogenous RNA. Knockdown of MIAT results in depleted levels of vascular forming networks that result from reduced TNF-α and VEGF. Taken together, this study showed that MIAT functions as an inducer of in pathological angiogenesis [14, 79].

In vivo genetic deletion of MALAT1 as well as pharmacological inhibition of MALAT1 reduced vascular growth, indicating its significance in neovascularization. Using a genetic ablation mouse model, Michalik et al. [80] determined that the lack of MALAT1 resulted in lower neonatal retina vascularization and delayed vessel extension, as opposed to wild-type mice from the same litter. Furthermore, pharmacologically inhibiting MALAT1 with GapmeRs in a hind limb ischemia mouse model hampered blood flow recovery and reduced capillary density. MALAT1 controls the transition between proliferative and migratory phenotypes of ECs, and its silencing through small interfering RNA (siRNA) resulted in the reduction of the number of proliferating ECs. Zhang et al. [81] additionally conducted RNA-immunoprecipitation experiments. These tests demonstrated how MALAT1 has an immediate effect on vascular endothelial growth factor receptor 2 (VEGFR2) to facilitate angiogenesis, indicating that MALAT1 controls intrinsic angiogenesis through direct regulating VEGFR2. The silencing of MALAT1 reduced tube formation, proliferation as well as cell migration in skeletal muscle microvascular endothelial cell [80, 81]. Even though the aforementioned experiments employed the hind limb ischemia model, the results are relevant for cardiac endothelial cells that are in similar pathological remodeling conditions [62].

The lncRNA named MANTIS also affects angiogenesis [82, 83]. In particular HUVECs were used in a Matrigel angiogenesis assay in mice. CRISPR/Cas9-facilitated knockout of MANTIS, or silencing through siRNAs or GapmeRs, decreased angiogenic sprouting and tube formation. MANTIS was discovered to target the endothelial genes *SMAD6*, *SOX18*, and *COUP-TFII*, all important pro-angiogenic genes. Silencing of MANTIS using GapmeRs and siRNAs resulted in decreased protein expression of SMAD6, SOX18, and COUP-TFII in human aortic smooth muscle cells, human coronary artery smooth muscle cells, and in human aortic ECs. Furthermore, depression of any of these three proteins in a spheroid outgrowth assay resulted in poor endothelial sprouting. MANTIS was found to interact with BRG1, part of an ATP-dependent transcription activator family of proteins [82, 83]. MANTIS increases ATP-ase activity of BRG1 by acting as a promoter for BAF155, a subunit of the complex. The BRG1 protein family regulates the alteration and remodeling of the chromatin structure of the genes it acts on, namely *SOX18*, *SMAD6*, and *COUP-TFII* in this particular example. MANTIS can therefore be seen as a promoter of angiogenesis by stimulating transcription of these genes. Leisegang et al. concluded from their data that a decrease in MANTIS levels impaired the endothelial angiogenic function ex vivo as well as in vivo, opening more doors for the relatively unknown domain of lncRNA influence on angiogenic functions [82].

An antisense lncRNA named PUNISHER was found to have a large effect on neovascularization, as its inhibition led to severe vascular defects with problematic branching and decreased vessel formation [83]. These observations were made with the help of human pluripotent stem cell differentiation models. In zebrafish, PUNISHER supports and maintains EC function, yet its particular mechanism is still unknown.

In addition, knockdown of the lncRNA ALIEN resulted into observed down-regulation of 503 genes that contributed to angiogenesis and blood vessel development [83, 84].

5 Discussion

This chapter outlines various non-coding RNAs, their targets, and their effects on cardiac regeneration. By focusing on cardiomyocyte proliferation and cardiac neovascularization as hallmarks of regeneration, research involving the inhibition or enhanced expression of certain non-coding RNAs that resulted in significant alterations in the regenerative abilities of the heart was used to highlight the role non-coding RNAs can play in cardiac regeneration. These results open doors for new research into potential therapeutics based on the influence of non-coding RNAs on cellular pathways.

For non-coding RNAs to be used clinically several challenges have to be overcome and several requirements have to be met. The non-coding RNAs need to be stable, specific, and with high binding affinity, and they need to be delivered efficiently to the target tissue. Modification of non-coding RNAs to improve stability, specificity, and uptake, as well as delivery strategies are reviewed elsewhere [86–89]. Briefly, non-coding RNAs are modified with chemical modifications, such as 2′ sugar modifications, locked nucleic acids, or phosphodiester and phosphorothioate linkages, to improve stability, specificity, and uptake. Delivery strategies include (biodegradable) biomaterials, lipid-based vehicles, viruses, exosomes, nanoparticles, microbubbles, and (cationic) polymeric drug delivery devices [90, 91]. Their advantages include small size, stability, reduced degradation, improved uptake, and specificity. Local delivery may be facilitated by targeting ligands or localized injections. These strategies need to be investigated in models that allow for inclusion of delivery and surgical practices akin to surgery in humans, and that adequately resemble human pathophysiology. Additional to delivery, bio-distribution and pharmacokinetics/pharmacodynamics of these delivery vehicles need to be characterized. Furthermore, modulation of expression by non-coding RNAs can have profound effects in both the short and the long term. Their targets not only have to be identified and validated in short-term studies, the effect of non-coding RNA modulation also has to be assessed in long-term in vivo studies. As illustrated by Tian et al. and Gabisonia et al. [40, 43], persistent and uncontrolled expression can result in death. Besides these short and long-term effects, off-target effects have to be identified and investigated, for non-coding RNAs can have multiple targets. Only after these rigorous tests have been performed to a satisfactory level, the safety and efficacy of ncRNA therapeutics can be assessed in humans [92, 43]. Therefore, to bring non-coding RNA therapeutics one step closer to clinical applications, research needs to move forward into more representative models of human disease that encompass all aspects of treatment.

Acknowledgments This work was funded by the Netherlands CardioVascular Research Initiative (CVON: The Dutch Heart Foundation, Dutch Federation of University Medical Centers, the Netherlands Organization for Health Research and Development, and the Royal Netherlands Academy of Science) and Vrienden UMC Utrecht (C.V., J.S.); an unrestricted grant from CELLINK to Vrienden UMC Utrecht (C.V., J.S.).

References

1. Benjamin, E.J. Muntner, P. Alonso, A. Bittencourt, M.S. Callaway, C.W. Carson, A.P. Chamberlain, A.M. Chang, A.R. Cheng, S. Das, S.R. Delling, F.N. Djousse, L. Elkind, M.S.V. Ferguson, J.F. Fornage, M. Jordan, L.C. Khan, S.S. Kissela, B.M. Knutson, K.L. Kwan, T.W. Lackland, D.T. Lewis, T.T. Lichtman, J.H. Longenecker, C.T. Loop, M.S. Lutsey, P.L. Martin, S.S. Matsushita, K. Moran, A.E. Mussolino, M.E. O'Flaherty, M. Pandey, A. Perak, A.M. Rosamond, W.D. Roth, G.A. Sampson, U.K.A. Satou, G.M. Schroeder, E.B. Shah, S.H. Spartano, N.L. Stokes, A. Tirschwell, D.L. Tsao, C.W. Turakhia, M.P. VanWagner, L.B. Wilkins, J.T. Wong, S.S. Virani, S. S (2019) American Heart Association Council on Epidemiology and Prevention Statistics Committee and Stroke Statistics Subcommittee. Heart disease and stroke statistics-2019 update: a report from the American Heart Association. Circulation 139 (10): e56-e528.
2. Bergmann O, Bhardwaj RD, Bernard S, Zdunek S, Barnabé-Heider F, Walsh S, Zupicich J, Alkass K, Buchholz BA, Druid H, Jovinge S, Frisén J. Evidence for cardiomyocyte renewal in humans. Science. 2009;324(5923):98–102.
3. Orlic D, Kajstura J, Chimenti S, Jakoniuk I, Anderson SM, Li B, Pickel J, McKay R, Nadal-Ginard B, Bodine DM, Leri A, Anversa P. Bone marrow cells regenerate infarcted myocardium. Nature. 2001;410(6829):701–5.
4. Balsam LB, Wagers AJ, Christensen JL, Kofidis T, Weissman IL, Robbins RC. Haematopoietic stem cells adopt mature haematopoietic fates in ischaemic myocardium. Nature. 2004;428(6983):668–73.
5. Murry CE, Soonpaa MH, Reinecke H, Nakajima H, Nakajima HO, Rubart M, Pasumarthi KB, Virag JI, Bartelmez SH, Poppa V, Bradford G, Dowell JD, Williams DA, Field LJ. Haematopoietic stem cells do not transdifferentiate into cardiac myocytes in myocardial infarcts. Nature. 2004;428:664–8.
6. Beltrami AP, Barlucchi L, Torella D, Baker M, Limana F, Chimenti S, Kasahara H, Rota M, Musso E, Urbanek K, Leri A, Kajstura J, Nadal-Ginard B, Anversa P. Adult cardiac stem cells are multipotent and support myocardial regeneration. Cell. 2003;114(6):763–76.
7. Zwetsloot PP, Végh AM, Jansen of Lorkeers SJ, van Hout GP, Currie GL, Sena ES, Gremmels H, Buikema JW, Goumans MJ, Macleod MR, Doevendans PA, Chamuleau SA, Sluijter JP. Cardiac stem cell treatment in myocardial infarction: a systematic review and meta-analysis of preclinical studies. Circ Res. 2016;118(8):1223–32.
8. van Berlo JH, Kanisicak O, Maillet M, Vagnozzi RJ, Karch J, Lin SC, Middleton RC, Marbán E, Molkentin JD. c-kit+ cells minimally contribute cardiomyocytes to the heart. Nature. 2014;509(7500):337–41.
9. Sultana N, Zhang L, Yan J, Chen J, Cai W, Razzaque S, Jeong D, Sheng W, Bu L, Xu M, Huang GY, Hajjar RJ, Zhou B, Moon A, Cai CL. Resident c-kit(+) cells in the heart are not cardiac stem cells. Nat Commun. 2015;6:8701.
10. van Berlo JH, Molkentin JD. Most of the dust has settled: cKit+ progenitor cells are an irrelevant source of cardiac myocytes in vivo. Circ Res. 2016;118(1):17–9.
11. Kretzschmar K, Post Y, Bannier-Hélaouët M, Mattiotti A, Drost J, Basak O, Li VSW, van den Born M, Gunst QD, Versteeg D, Kooijman L, van der Elst S, van Es JH, van Rooij E, van den Hoff MJB, Clevers H. Profiling proliferative cells and their progeny in damaged murine hearts. Proc Natl Acad Sci. 2018;115(52):E12245–54.
12. Li Y, He L, Huang X, Bhaloo SI, Zhao H, Zhang S, Pu W, Tian X, Li Y, Liu Q, Yu W, Zhang L, Liu X, Liu K, Tang J, Zhang H, Cai D, Ralf AH, Xu Q, Lui KO, Zhou B. Genetic lineage tracing of nonmyocyte population by dual recombinases. Circulation. 2018;1389(8):793–805.
13. Bergmann O. Clearing up the mist: cardiomyocyte renewal in human hearts. Eur Heart J. 2019;40(13):1037–8.
14. Yu B, Wang S. Angio-LncRs: LncRNAs that regulate angiogenesis and vascular disease. Theranostics. 2018;8(13):3654–75.
15. Folkman J. Tumor angiogenesis. Adv Cancer Res. 1985;43:175–203.
16. Tabibiazar R, Rockson SG. Angiogenesis and the ischaemic heart. Eur Heart J. 2001;22(11):903–18.
17. Lepilina A, Coon AN, Kikuchi K, Holdway JE, Roberts RW, Burns CG, Poss KDA. Dynamic epicardial injury response supports progenitor cell activity during zebrafish heart regeneration. Cell. 2006;127(3):607–19.
18. Poss KD, Wilson LG, Keating MT. Heart regeneration in zebrafish. Science. 2002;298(5601):2188–90.
19. Kikuchi K, Poss KD. Cardiac regenerative capacity and mechanisms. Annu Rev Cell Dev Biol. 2012;28(1):719–41.
20. Jopling C, Sleep E, Raya M, Martí M, Raya A, Izpisúa Belmonte JC. Zebrafish heart regeneration occurs by cardiomyocyte dedifferentiation and proliferation. Nature. 2010;464(7288):606–9.
21. Kikuchi K, Holdway JE, Werdich AA, Anderson RM, Fang Y, Egnaczyk GF, Evans T, MacRae CA, Stainier DYR, Poss KD. Primary contribution to zebrafish heart regeneration by gata4+ cardiomyocytes. Nature. 2010;464(7288):601–5.
22. Witman N, Murtuza B, Davis B, Arner A, Morrison JI. Recapitulation of developmental cardiogenesis governs the morphological and functional regenera-

tion of adult newt hearts following injury. Dev Biol. 2011;354(1):67–76.

23. Laube F, Heister M, Scholz C, Borchardt T, Braun T. Re-programming of newt cardiomyocytes is induced by tissue regeneration. J Cell Sci. 2006;119(22):4719–29.
24. Wang WE, Li L, Xia X, Fu W, Liao Q, Lan C, Yang D, Chen H, Yue R, Zeng C, Zhou L, Zhou B, Duan DD, Chen X, Houser SR, Zeng C. Dedifferentiation, proliferation, and redifferentiation of adult mammalian cardiomyocytes after ischemic injury. Circulation. 2017;136(9):834–48.
25. Yutzey K. Cardiomyocyte proliferation: teaching an old dogma new tricks. Circ Res. 2017;120:627–9.
26. Drenckhahn J-D, Schwarz QP, Gray S, Laskowski A, Kiriazis H, Ming Z, Harvey RP, Du X-J, Thorburn DR, Cox TC. Compensatory growth of healthy cardiac cells in the presence of diseased cells restores tissue homeostasis during heart development. Dev Cell. 2008;15(4):521–33.
27. Haubner BJ, Adamowicz-Brice M, Khadayate S, Tiefenthaler V, Metzler B, Aitman T, Penninger JM. Complete cardiac regeneration in a mouse model of myocardial infarction. Aging. 2012;4(12):966–77.
28. Porrello ER, Mahmoud AI, Simpson E, Hill JA, Richardson JA, Olson EN, Sadek HA. Transient regenerative potential of the neonatal mouse heart. Science. 2011;331(6020):1078–80.
29. Jesty SA, Steffey MA, Lee FK, Breitbach M, Hesse M, Reining S, Lee JC, Doran RM, Nikitin AY, Fleischmann BL, Kotlikoff MI. c-kit+ precursors support postinfarction myogenesis in the neonatal, but not adult, heart. Proc Natl Acad Sci. 2012;109(33):13380–5.
30. Strungs, E.G. Ongstad, E.L. O'Quinn, M.P. Palatinus, J.A. Jourdan, L.J. Gourdie, R.G (2013) Cryoinjury models of the adult and neonatal mouse heart for studies of scarring and regeneration. Methods Mol Biol 1037:343–353.
31. Bryant, D.M. O'Meara, C.C. Ho, N.N. Gannon, J. Cai, L. Lee, R.T (2015) A systematic analysis of neonatal mouse heart regeneration after apical resection. J Mol Cell Cardiol 79:315–318.
32. Haubner BJ, Schneider J, Schweigmann U, Schuetz T, Dichtl W, Velik-Salchner C, Stein JI, Penninger JM. Functional recovery of a human neonatal heart after severe myocardial infarction. Circ Res. 2016;118(2):16–221.
33. Ahuja P, Sdek P, MacLellan WR. Cardiac myocyte cell cycle control in development, disease, and regeneration. Physiol Rev. 2007;87(2):521–44.
34. van Amerongen MJ, Engel FB. Features of CM proliferation and its potential for cardiac regeneration. J Cell Mol Med. 2008;12:2233–44.
35. Bicknell KA, Coxon CH, Brooks G. Can the CM cell cycle be reprogrammed? J Mol Cell Cardiol. 2007;42(4):706–21.
36. Muthuramu I, Lox M, Jacobs F, De Geest B. Permanent ligation of the left anterior descending coronary artery in mice: a model of post-myocardial infarction remodeling and heart failure. J Vis Exp. 2014;94
37. Aguirre A, Montserrat N, Zacchigna S, Nivet E, Hishida T, Krause MN, Kurian L, Ocampo A, Vazquez-Ferrer E, Rodriquez-Esteban C, Kumar S, Moresco JJ, Yates JR III, Campistol JM, Sancho-Martinez I, Giacca M, Izpisua Belmonte JC. In vivo activation of a conserved microRNA program induces mammalian heart regeneration. Cell Stem Cell. 2014;15(5):589–604.
38. Huang W, Feng Y, Liang J, Yu H, Wang C, Wang B, Wang M, Jiang L, Meng W, Cai W, Medvedovic M, Chen J, Paul C, Davidson WS, Sadayappan S, Stambrook P, Yu X, Wang Y. Loss of microRNA-128 promotes cardiomyocyte proliferation and heart regeneration. Nat Commun. 2018;9(1):700.
39. Yang Y, Cheng HW, Qiu Y, Dupee D, Noonan M, Lin YD, Fisch S, Unno K, Sereti KI, Liao R. MicroRNA-34a plays a key role in cardiac repair and regeneration following myocardial infarction. Circ Res. 2015;117(5):450–9.
40. Tian Y, Liu Y, Wang T, Zhou N, Kong J, Chen L, Snitow M, Morley M, Li D, Petrenko N, Zhou S, Lu M, Gao E, Koch WJ, Stewart KM, Morrisey EE. A microRNA-Hippo pathway that promotes cardiomyocyte proliferation and cardiac regeneration in mice. Sci Transl Med. 2015;7(279):279–89.
41. Wang LL, Liu Y, Chung JJ, Wang T, Gaffey AC, Lu M, Cavanough CA, Zhou S, Kanade R, Atluri P, Morrisey EE, Burdick J. Sustained miRNA delivery from an injectable hydrogel promotes cardiomyocyte proliferation and functional regeneration after ischaemic injury. Nat Biomed Eng. 2017;1(12):983–92.
42. Eulalio A, Mano M, Dal Ferro M, Zentilin L, Sinagra G, Zacchigna S, Giacca M. Functional screening identifies miRNAs inducing cardiac regeneration. Nature. 2012;492(7429):376–81.
43. Gabisonia K, Prosdocimo G, Aquaro GD, Carlucci L, Zentilin L, Secco I, Ali H, Braga L, Gorgodze N, Bernini F, Burchielli S, Collesi C, Zandonà L, Sinagra G, Piacenti M, Zacchigna S, Bussani R, Recchia FA, Giacca M. MicroRNA therapy stimulates uncontrolled cardiac repair after myocardial infarction in pigs. Nature. 2019;569(7756):418.
44. Porrello ER, Mahmoud AI, Simpson E, Johnson BA, Grinsfelder D, Canseco D, Mammen PP, Rothermel BA, Olson EN, Sadek HA. Regulation of neonatal and adult mammalian heart regeneration by the miR-15 family. Proc Natl Acad Sci. 2013;110(1):187–92.
45. Porrello ER, Johnson BA, Aurora AB, Simpson E, Nam YJ, Matkovich SJ, Dorn GW 2nd, van Rooij E, Olson EN. MiR-15 family regulates postnatal mitotic arrest of cardiomyocytes. Circ Res. 2011;109(6):670–9.
46. Zhao Y, Ransom J, Li A, von Vedantham C, Drehle M, Muth AN, Tsuchihashi T, McManus MT, Schwartz RJ, Srivastava D. Dysregulation of cardiogenesis, cardiac conduction, and cell cycle in mice lacking miRNA-1-2. Cell. 2007;129(2):303–17.

47. Liu N, Bezprozvannaya S, Williams AH, Qi X, Richardson JA, Bassel-Duby R, Olson EN. MicroRNA-133a regulates cardiomyocyte proliferation and suppresses smooth muscle gene expression in the heart. Genes Dev. 2008;22(23):3242–54.
48. Chen J, Huang ZP, Seok HY, Ding J, Kataoka M, Zhang Z, Hu X, Wang G, Lin Z, Wang S, Pu WT, Liao R, Wang DZ. mir-17-92 cluster is required for and sufficient to induce cardiomyocyte proliferation in postnatal and adult hearts. Circ Res. 2013;112(12):1557–66.
49. Xiao J, Liu H, Cretoiu D, Toader DO, Suciu N, Shi J, Shen S, Bei Y, Sluijter JP, Das S, Kong X, Li X. miR-31a-5p promotes postnatal cardiomyocyte proliferation by targeting RhoBTB1. Exp Mol Med. 2017;49(10):e386.
50. Chen Y, Li X, Li B, Wang H, Li M, Huang S, Sun Y, Chen G, Si X, Huang C, Liao W, Liao Y, Bin J. Long non-coding RNA ECRAR triggers post-natal myocardial regeneration by activating ERK1/2 signaling. Mol Ther. 2019;27(1):29–45.
51. See K, Tan WLW, Lim EH, Tiang Z, Lee LT, Li PYQ, Luu TDA, Ackers-Johnson M, Foo RS. Single cardiomyocyte nuclear transcriptomes reveal a lincRNA-regulated de-differentiation and cell cycle stress-response in vivo. Nat Commun. 2017;8(1):225.
52. Coccia EM, et al. Regulation and expression of a growth arrest-specific gene (gas5) during growth, differentiation, and development. Mol Cell Biol. 1992;12(8):3514–21.
53. Mourtada-Maarabouni M, Pickard MR, Hedge VL, Farzaneh F, Williams GT. GAS5, a non-protein-coding RNA, controls apoptosis and is downregulated in breast cancer. Oncogene. 2009;28(2):195–208.
54. Yin D. Long noncoding RNA GAS5 affects cell proliferation and predicts a poor prognosis in patients with colorectal cancer. Med Oncol. 2014;31(11):253.
55. Cai B, Ma W, Ding F, Zhang L, Huang Q, Wang X, Hua B, Xu J, Li J, Bi C, Guo S, Yang F, Han Z, Li Y, Yan G, Yu Y, Bao Z, Yu M, Li F, Tian Y, Pan Z, Yang B. The long noncoding RNA CAREL controls cardiac regeneration. J Am Coll Cardiol. 2018;72(5):534–50.
56. Wu M, Zhang S, Chen X, Xu H, Li X. Expression and function of lncRNA MALAT-1 in the embryonic development of zebrafish. Gene. 2019;680:65–71.
57. Li B, Hu Y, Li X, Jin G, Chen X, Chen G, Chen Y, Huang S, Liao W, Liao Y, Teng Z, Bin J. Sirt1 antisense long noncoding RNA promotes cardiomyocyte proliferation by enhancing the stability of Sirt1. J Am Heart Assoc. 2018;7(21)
58. Wang J, Chen X, Shen D, Ge D, Chen J, Pei J, Li Y, Yue Z, Feng J, Chu M, Nie Y. A long non-coding RNA NR_045363 controls cardiomyocyte proliferation and cardiac repair. J Mol Cell Cardiol. 2019;127:105–14.
59. Chen G, Li H, Li X, Li B, Zhong L, Huang S, Zheng H, Li M, Jin G, Liao W, Liao Y, Chen Y, Bin J. Loss of long non-coding RNA CRRL promotes cardiomyocyte regeneration and improves cardiac repair by functioning as a competing endogenous RNA. J Mol Cell Cardiol. 2018;122:152–64.
60. Adair TH, Montani JP. Angiogenesis. San Rafael (CA): Morgan & Claypool Life Sciences Chapter 1, overview of angiogenesis; 2010.
61. Choong OK, Lee DS, Chen CY, Hsieh P. The roles of non-coding RNAs in cardiac regenerative medicine. Non-coding RNA Research. 2017;2(2):100–10.
62. Juni R, Abreu R, da Costa Martins P. Regulation of microvascularization in heart failure – an endothelial cell, non-coding RNAs and exosome liaison. Non-coding RNA Research. 2017;2(1):45–55.
63. Hu S, Huang M, Li Z, Jia F, Ghosh Z, Lijkwan MA, Fasanaro P, Sun N, Wang X, Martelli F, Robbins RC, Wu JC. MicroRNA-210 as a novel therapy for treatment of ischemic heart disease. Circulation. 2010;122(11 Suppl):S124–31.
64. Arif M, Pandey R, Alam P, Jiang S, Sadayappan S, Paul A, Ahmed R. MicroRNA-210-mediated proliferation, survival, and angiogenesis promote cardiac repair post myocardial infarction in rodents. J Mol Med (Berl). 2017;95(12):1369–85.
65. Fan ZG, Qu XL, Chu P, Gao YL, Gao XF, Chen SL, Tian NL. MicroRNA-210 promotes angiogenesis in acute myocardial infarction. Mol Med Rep. 2018;17(4):5658–65.
66. Bonauer A, Carmona G, Iwasaki M, Mione M, Koyanagi M, Fischer A, Burchfield J, Fox H, Doebele C, Ohtani K, et al. MicroRNA-92a controls angiogenesis and functional recovery of ischemic tissues in mice. Science. 2009;324(5935):1710–3.
67. Hinkel R, Penzkofer D, Zahlke S, Fischer A, Husada W, Xu QF, Baloch E, Van Rooij E, Zeiher AM, Kupatt C, et al. Inhibition of microRNA-92a protects against ischemia/reperfusion injury in a large-animal model. Circulation. 2013;128(10):1066–75.
68. Fiedler J, Jazbutyte V, Kirchmaier BC, Gupta SK, Lorenzen J, Hartmann D, Galuppo P, Kneitz S, Pena JTG, Sohn-Lee C. MicroRNA-24 regulates vascularity after myocardial infarction. Circulation. 2011;124(6):720–30.
69. Meloni M, Marchetti M, Garner K, Littlejohns B, Sala-Newby G, Xenophontos N, Floris I, Suleiman MS, Madeddu P, Caporali A, Emanueli C. Local inhibition of microRNA-24 improves reparative angiogenesis and left ventricle remodeling and function in mice with myocardial infarction. Mol Ther. 2013;21(7):1390–402.
70. Qian L, Van Laake LW, Huang Y, Liu S, Wendland MF, Srivastava D. miR-24 inhibits apoptosis and represses Bim in mouse cardiomyocytes. J Exp Med. 2011;208(3):549–60.
71. Wang S, Aurora AB, Johnson BA, Qi X, Mcanally J, Hill JA, Richardson JA, Bassel-duby R, Olson EN, Hill A, et al. The endothelial-specific MicroRNA miR-126 governs vascular integrity and angiogenesis. Dev Cell. 2008;15(2):261–71.
72. Icli B, Wara AKM, Moslehi J, Sun X, Plovie E, Cahill M, Marchin JF, Schissler A, Padera RF, Shi J, et al. MicroRNA-26a regulates pathological and physiological angiogenesis by targeting BMP/SMAD1 signaling. Circ Res. 2013;113(11):1231–41.

73. Wen Z, Huang W, Feng Y, et al. MicroRNA-377 regulates mesenchymal stem cell-induced angiogenesis in ischemic hearts by targeting VEGF. PLoS One. 2014;9(9):e104666.
74. Goyal A, Behring A, Kumar A, Siess W. STK35L1 associates with nuclear actin and regulates cell cycle and migration of endothelial cells. PLoS One. 2011;6(1):E16249.
75. Joladarashi D, Garikipati VNS, Thandavarayan RA, et al. Enhanced cardiac regenerative ability of stem cells after ischemia-reperfusion injury: role of human CD34+ cells deficient in microRNA-377. J Am Coll Cardiol. 2015;66(20):2214–26.
76. Lei Z, van Mil A, Brandt MM, Grundmann S, Hoefer I, Smits M, El Azzouzi H, Fukao T, Cheng C, Doevendans PA, Sluijter JP. MicroRNA-132/212 family enhances arteriogenesis after hindlimb ischemia through modulation of the Ras-MAPK pathway. J Cell Mol Med. 2015;19(8):1994–2005.
77. van Mil A, Grundmann S, Goumans M, Lei Z, Oerlemans M, Jaksani S, Doevendans P, Sluijter J. MicroRNA-214 inhibits angiogenesis by targeting quaking and reducing angiogenic growth factor release. Cardiovasc Res. 2012;93(4):655–65.
78. He Q, Li Q, Jin H, Zhi F, Suraj B, Zhu Y, Xia Y, Mao L, Chen X, Hu B. MiR-150 regulates poststroke cerebral angiogenesis via vascular endothelial growth factor in rats. CNS Neurosci Ther. 2016;22(6):507–17.
79. Yan B, Yao J, Liu JY. lncRNA-MIAT regulates microvascular dysfunction by functioning as a competing endogenous RNA. Circ Res. 2015;116(7):1143–56.
80. Michalik KM, You X, Manavski Y. Long noncoding RNA MALAT1 regulates endothelial cell function and vessel growth. Circ Res. 2014;114(9):1389–97.
81. Zhang X, Tang X, Hamblin MH, Yin KJ. Lcong non-coding RNA Malatl regulates angiogenesis in hindlimb ischemia. Int J Mol Sci. 2018;19(6):1723.
82. Leisegang MS, Fork C, Josipovic I, Richter FM, Preussner J, Hu J, Miller MJ, Epah J, Hofmann P, Günther S, Moll F, Valasarajan C, Heidler J, Ponomareva Y, Freiman TM, Maegdefessel L, Plate KH, Mittelbronn M, Uchida S, Künne C, Stellos K, Schermuly RT, Weissmann N, Devraj K, Wittig I, Boon RA, Dimmeler S, Pullamsetti SS, Looso M, Miller FJ, Brandes RP. Long noncoding RNA MANTIS facilitates endothelial angiogenic function. Circulation. 2017;136(1):65–79.
83. Trotter KW, Archer TK. The BRG1 transcriptional coregulator. Nucl Recept Signal. 2008;6(1):e004.
84. Kurian L, Aguirre A, Sancho-Martinez I, Benner C, Hishida T, Nguyen TB, Reddy P, Nivet E, Krause MN, Nelles DA, Esteban CR, Campistol JM, Yeo GW, Belmonte J. Identification of novel long noncoding RNAs underlying vertebrate cardiovascular development. Circulation. 2015;131(14):1278–90.
85. Gomes C, Spencer H, Ford K, Michel L, Baker A, Emanueli C, Balligand J, Devaux Y. The function and therapeutic potential of long non-coding RNAs in cardiovascular development and disease. Mol Ther Nucleic Acids. 2017;8:494–507.
86. Lei Z, Sluijter JP, van Mil A. MicroRNA therapeutics for cardiac regeneration. Mini Rev Med Chem. 2015;15(6):441–51.
87. Tibbitt MW, Dahlman JE, Langer R. Emerging frontiers in drug delivery. J Am Chem Soc. 2016;138(3):704–17.
88. Van der Ven CFT, Wu PJ, Tibbit MW, van Mil A, Sluijter JPG, Langer R, Aikawa E. *In vitro* 3D model and miRNA drug delivery to target calcific aortic valve disease. Clin Sci. 2017;131(3):181–95.
89. Fenton OS, Olafson KN, Pillai PS, Mitchell MJ, Langer R. Advances in biomaterials for drug delivery. Adv Mater. 2018;30
90. Kwekkeboom RF, Lei Z, Bogaards SJ, Aiazian E, Kamp O, Paulus WJ, Sluijter JP, Musters RJ. Ultrasound and microbubble-induced local delivery of MicroRNA-based therapeutics. Ultrasound Med Biol. 2015;41(1):163–76.
91. Kwekkeboom RF, Sluijter JP, van Middelaar BJ, Metz CH, Brans MA, Kamp O, Paulus WJ, Musters R. Increased local delivery of antagomir therapeutics to the rodent myocardium using ultrasound and microbubbles. J Control Release. 2016;222:18–31.
92. Kwekkeboom RF, Lei Z, Doevendans PA, Musters RJ, Sluijter JP. Targeted delivery of miRNA therapeutics for cardiovascular diseases: opportunities and challenges. Clin Sci (Lond). 2014;127(6):351–65.

Role of Non-coding RNA in Diabetic Cardiomyopathy

10

Lu Xia and Meiyi Song

Abstract

Diabetic cardiomyopathy (DCM) is the leading cause of morbidity and mortality in diabetic population worldwide, characteristic by cardiomyocyte hypertrophy, apoptosis and myocardial interstitial fibrosis and eventually developing into heart failure. Non-coding RNAs, such as microRNAs (miRNAs), circular RNAs (circRNAs), long non-coding RNAs (lncRNAs) and other RNAs without the protein encoding function were emerging as a popular regulator in various types of processes during human diseases. The evidences have shown that miRNAs are regulators in diabetic cardiomyopathy, such as insulin resistance, cardiomyocytes apoptosis, and inflammatory, especially their protective effect on heart function. Besides that, the functions of lncRNAs and circRNAs have been gradually confirmed in recent years, and their functions in DCM have become increasingly prominent. We highlighted the nonnegligible roles of non-coding RNAs in the pathological process of DCM and showed the future possibilities of these non-coding RNAs in DCM treatment. In this chapter, we summarized the present advance of the researches in this filed and raised the concern and the prospect in the future.

Keywords

Non-coding RNA · Diabetic cardiomyopathy · Heart failure · Diabetes mellitus

Diabetic cardiomyopathy (DCM) was the specific abnormality of myocardial structure and function in diabetic patients, and does not coexist with cardiovascular diseases such as coronary artery disease and hypertension [1]. DCM was characterized by myocardial dilation, hypertrophy, decreased left ventricular diastolic, systolic function, and eventually develops into heart failure. About 75% of the human genomic DNA sequence can be transcribed, and nearly 74% of the transcripts are non-coding RNAs, which play an important role in maintaining the normal physiological function and the occurrence and progress of diseases in organisms. Various non-coding RNAs have been shown to be involved in regulating the occurrence of DCM, including miRNA and other types of non-coding RNA. In this review, we summarized current studies of non-coding RNA and DCM.

L. Xia · M. Song (✉)
Division of Gastroenterology and Hepatology, Digestive Disease Institute, Shanghai Tongji Hospital, Tongji University School of Medicine, Shanghai, China

J. Xiao (ed.), *Non-coding RNAs in Cardiovascular Diseases*, Advances in Experimental Medicine and Biology 1229, https://doi.org/10.1007/978-981-15-1671-9_10

1 Introduction of Diabetic Cardiomyopathy

There were two types of diabetes which named type 1 and type 2 diabetes. Type 1 diabetes was caused by insufficient insulin secretion and type 2 diabetes was caused by insulin resistance and gestational-related diabetes mellitus. The complications of diabetes, including diabetic microangiopathy and diabetic macroangiopathy, were the main causes of disability and death of diabetes mellitus. The incidence of diabetes was increased year by year due to the increased obesity population and rapid ageing population. According to the data from International Diabetes Alliance research project, near 451 million people worldwide suffer from diabetes in 2017. And it was estimated that 693 million people around the world will be diagnosed as diabetes by 2045. As the complication of diabetes mellitus, diabetic cardiomyopathy (DCM) received more attention by clinicians [2]. In 1972, Rubler observed 4 diabetic patients with congestive heart failure, and found that these patients had no other potential causes of heart failure, such as coronary artery disease, dilated cardiomyopathy or hypertension, except diabetes mellitus [3]. Both type 1 and type 2 diabetes could be complicated with DCM, associated with the main pathological changes, including cardiomyocyte hypertrophy, extracellular matrix deposition, myocardial microvascular basement membrane thickening, and interstitial fibrosis [4, 5]. Until now, there is no corresponding clinical guidelines or consensus for diagnosis and management of patients with DCM [6]. The diagnosis of DCM still belongs to exclusive diagnosis, mainly diagnosed by clinical history of diabetes mellitus, manifestations and symptoms of cardiac dysfunction, combined with laboratory examinations such as echocardiography [7]. With the excluded of coronary heart disease, hypertensive heart disease, dilated cardiomyopathy and other heart diseases. According to the changes of cardiac structure and cardiac function, DCM can be divided into three stages. Stage 1, there are changes in cardiac structure and no changes in diastolic function. Left ventricular ejection fraction (EF) is normal and subclinical. Changes of cardiac structure are aggravated in stage 2, with ventricular hypertrophy, myocardial fibrosis, decreased ventricular diastolic function in cardiac function, and gradually abnormal systolic function, EF value < 50%. Cardiac structural changes further aggravated in stage 3, cardiac microvascular changes, ventricular hypertrophy and myocardial fibrosis further aggravated, with global diastolic and systolic disorders occurred [8, 9].

Comprehensive treatment, including lifestyle interventions, were currently used in the treatment of DCM [10]. Quitting smoking, limiting alcohol, controlling salt intake, optimizing diet and moderate exercise were first proposed [11–15]. The injection of metformin, thiazolidinediones and glucagon-like polypeptide (GLP-1) analogues not only made effects on diabetes mellitus, especially improved insulin resistance and promoted glucose uptake and utilization, but also resisted myocardial cell damage and prevented cardiac remodeling [16]. Other medications that were used in cardiovascular system were also considered to have therapeutic effects on DCM, including renin-angiotensin-aldosterone system (RASS) inhibitors, beta-blockers, calcium channel antagonists, statins, and trimetazidine. According to the latest ADA/AHA guidelines, RASS inhibitors should be used as first-line drugs in patients with diabetes mellitus and hypertension [17]. Although drug therapy could improve the progression of DCM, the negative effects of drug could not be avoided. A comprehensive treatment was still in an urgent need.

2 Current Research on the Pathogenesis of DCM

The pathogenesis of DCM has not been fully elucidated till now. Abnormal insulin signal transduction, metabolic disorders, microangiopathy, myocardial interstitial fibrosis, imbalance of calcium regulation, and cardiac autonomic neuropathy might be involved in the occurrence and development of DCM. Thus, enhanced understanding of DCM will provide clues to prevent the occurrence and diagnosis of DCM.

2.1 Insulin Resistance and Abnormal Insulin Metabolic Signaling

Insulin resistance in myocardial was a metabolic and functional disorder accompanied by the development of DCM. In normal heart, insulin affected the mammalian target of rapamycin (mTOR)–S6 kinase 1(S6K1) pathway to regulate myocardial metabolism through the targeting of phosphatidylinositol 3 kinase/protein kinase B signaling pathway [18, 19]. Insulin could also regulate glucose transport, glycolysis, glycogen synthesis, protein synthesis, lipid metabolism in cardiac myocytes, and affect myocardial contractile function [20]. Different from the regulation of cardiomyocyte in physiological states, insulin resistance leaded to the imbalance between myocardial metabolism and growth activity, which was mainly regulated by mitogen-activated protein kinase signaling pathway [21]. It has been found that impaired insulin-mediated glucose uptake occurs before impaired insulin-activated protein kinase B signaling pathway in insulin-resistant animal models, and this defect was caused by the decrease of glucose transporter 4 and abnormal translocation of glucose transporter 4 membrane (GLUT4) [22, 23]. Insulin resistance in cardiomyocytes could lead to functional disorders and metabolic changes. The inhibition of insulin signal transduction in cardiomyocytes was one of the markers of DCM. Insulin resistance during the development of DCM was associated with the increased risk of left ventricular hypertrophy and heart failure.

2.2 Direct Myocardium Injury by Metabolic Disorder

Metabolic disorder, mainly referred to hyperglycemia and glucotoxicity, was an important factor to trigger DCM [24]. Metabolic disorder, could first cause the biological changes on cardiac myocytes, which lead to subclinical myocardial dysfunction. Then the dysfunction developed into myocardial small vessel disease, microcirculation disorder and cardiac autonomic neuropathy, and eventually heart failure occurred. Glycolipid metabolism disorder that owing to interactions between lipid metabolic disorder and hyperglycemia in diabetic patients could directly affect the function of mitochondria, and the dysfunction of mitochondria future affected the metabolism of cardiac myocytes and caused the dysfunction of cardiomyocytes, which was an important reason for the occurrence and development of DCM [25–27].

Hyperglycemia can induce myocardial injury through direct and indirect pathways, which was the key factor in the progression of DCM. Mitochondrial damage, which was induced by hyperglycemia, was mainly related to abnormal polyol pathway activation. This damage future increased the expression of advanced glycation end products (AGEs), the activation of hexamine pathway and protein kinase C pathway. AGEs accumulation leaded to development of cardiac fibrosis and stiffness, increased connective tissue cross-linking, and impaired diastolic relaxation. AGE receptors (AGERs) on the cell surface were activated by AGEs, and then the expression of various inflammatory mediators was increased. Ultimately, these lead to the deposition of matrix components through the mitogen-activated protein kinase (MAPK) and Janus kinase (JAK) signaling pathways [28, 29].

In addition, dysfunction of cardiac myocytes and accumulation of abnormal substances caused by energy utilization disorders could also lead to DCM. In physiological state, fatty acid oxidation (FAO) provided nearly 70% of the energy required for cardiomyocytes, and glycolysis was another 30–40% source of energy, while almost all of the energy of diabetic patients came from the oxidation of non-esterified fatty acids due to the impairment of glucose utilization [30, 31]. These leaded to accumulation of lipid metabolites, such as diacylglycerols, ceramides, uncoupling protein 3, and the production of reactive oxygen species in mitochondria and peroxidase bodies in cardiac myocytes affecting myocardial energy supply, inducing inflammation, and leading to myocardial fibrosis, myocardial cell necrosis and myocardial dysfunction. In addition, ceramide was the intracellular apoptotic messenger, which induced cardiomyocyte apoptosis by activating NF-κB translocation to the nucleus, up-regulating inducible nitric oxide synthase and activating cysteine protease [32, 33]. Besides, ceramide directly activated atypical PKCs to phosphorylate and inhibit the insulin metabolic through Akt signaling, attenuating GLUT4 translocation and insulin-induced glucose uptake [34].

2.3 Calcium Ion Regulation Imbalance

The mechanism of calcium regulation was related to early concealed ventricular systolic dysfunction in DCM. Calcium ion levels in cardiac myocytes mainly depend on the calcium channels in cell membranes and sarcoplasmic reticulum. In diabetic individuals, oxidative stress caused by accumulation of toxic metabolites from disordered lipid metabolism might be the main cause of the imbalance of calcium regulation [35]. Lipid toxicity weakened calcium uptake in sarcoplasmic reticulum and other calcium exchange activities, and decreased calcium processing capacity in cardiomyocytes through inhibited ATPase activity on the cardiomyocyte membranes [36]. Some studies shown that the activities of sarcoplasmic reticulum calcium ATPase isomer 2, carnitine receptor and sodium-calcium exchanger in DCM patients are significantly reduced, which further reduced the release of sarcoplasmic reticulum stored calcium ions and the recovery of calcium ions from diastolic sarcoplasmic reticulum, resulting in the accumulation of calcium ions in the cytoplasm of end-diastolic myocardial cells, the decrease of myocardial compliance, and the impairment of myocardial diastolic and systolic functions [37]. In addition, the increase of AGEs induced by hyperglycemia could also lead to imbalance of calcium regulation in cardiac myocytes and affect myocardial contractile function ultimately [38, 39].

2.4 Mitochondrial Dysfunction and Oxidative Stress

The swelling and fragmentation of mitochondria in diabetic patients might impaired mitochondrial function, suggesting the involvement of impaired mitochondrial morphology and dysfunction in the pathogenesis of DCM. The function of mitochondrial has been altered due to metabolic disorder in DCM patients. As mentioned above, increased fatty acid uptake and beta-oxidation during diabetic cardiomyopathy might exceed mitochondrial respiratory capacity. Hence, mitochondria played an important role in abnormal energy metabolism and accumulation of toxic lipid products in cardiomyocytes [40].

Cardiomyocytes not only decomposed fatty acids, but also accumulated intermediate products and phospholipids of glycolysis pathway. The increased fatty acid concentration in cardiomyocyte of DCM patients could induce the activation of peroxisome proliferator-activated receptor alpha (PPAR-alpha) [41]. These promoted the expression of fatty acid oxidation and its uptake genes, which inhibited the pyruvate dehydrogenase kinase activation and impaired the oxidative capacity of glucose, in order to increase the uptake of fatty acids by mitochondria, increase myocardial oxygen consumption and reduce heart rate [42]. Therefore, mitochondria metabolized fatty acids accompanied with the increased cardiac oxygen consumption, resulting in changes in cardiac structure and function, leading to DCM.

ROS came from NADPH oxidases, xanthine oxidase, uncoupling of nitric oxide synthase, the process of arachidonic acid metabolism and microsomal P-450 enzymes [43]. Diabetes mellitus resulted in a large number of ROS aggregation, due to the rapid increase of ROS production and the relative inadequacy of antioxidant capacity [44]. ROS induced by diabetes could lead to structural damage of myocardial mitochondria, and further damage mitochondrial function by inducing the opening of mitochondrial membrane permeability channels [45]. ROS produced by mitochondria could also induced DCM mainly through PKC signaling pathways and hexosamine pathway [46, 47].

2.5 Other Pathophysiological Mechanisms of DCM

Microangiopathy and vascular injury DCM were independent of coronary artery disease, which were mainly manifested as microangiopathy. Microangiopathy was an important pathological change in the development of diabetes mellitus [48], which mainly included morphological changes of vascular endothelial cells, reduction of mitochondria and capillary basement membrane thickening, small artery thickening, capillary microaneurysm and decrease of capillary density [49]. The typical characteristics of microangiopathy were microcirculation disturbance. Cardiac microangiopathy might occur prior to clinical symptoms in DCM patients, leading to chronic myocardial ischemia, extensive focal myocardial necrosis, and even heart failure, cardiogenic shock and sudden death. The damage of vascular endothelial cells and vascular smooth muscle cells that were caused by oxidative stress were the main cause of pathological changes of blood vessels in diabetic patients, and might be the most important initiating events of cascade reaction of vascular pathological changes [50].

Autophagy was inhibited at high glucose concentration (e.g. diabetes), which might be related to the development of DCM [51]. Autophagy in response to cardiac energy stress was mediated by a network of AMPK and insulin signaling pathways, which were the main regulator of cellular and systemic energy balance [52]. As a response to exercise, hypoxia, oxidative stress and glucose deficiency, the AMPK and insulin signaling pathways were activated to accommodate the increase in intracellular insulin and AMP/ATP ratios. New evidence suggested that AMPK regulated not only cell energy, but also other cellular processes, including protein synthesis, cell growth and autophagy [53–55]. The activity of AMPK decreased at high glucose concentration, leading to autophagy disorder [56]. In streptozotocin-induced type 1 diabetic mice, overexpression of alpha-MHC-Beclin 1could activate autophagy of cardiomyocytes, thus further accelerate the diabetes mellitus induced cardiomyocytes damage [57]. However, there existed debate in the autophagic changes that were found in diabetes and its complications, different results were observed in different tissues. Therefore, further research was needed before potential drugs could be used clinically.

3 Non-coding RNAs and DCM

Non-coding RNAs were mainly defined as a class of RNA that did not encode proteins, including RNAs with definite functions, such as rRNAs, tRNAs, snRNAs, snoRNAs, and microRNAs (miRNAs), as well as RNAs with unknown functions. These RNAs shared some common features, such as they could perform biological functions at the RNA level without being translated into proteins after their transcribed from the genome. Long non-coding RNAs (lncRNAs) and circular RNAs (circRNAs) were the novel members of non-coding RNA family, whose functions and regulatory approaches have not been completely revealed. This suggested that non-coding RNA was still of great values in the diagnosis, evaluation and treatment of DCM. The current research progress in this field will be introduced here.

3.1 miRNA and Pathogenesis of DCM

Among all non-coding RNAs, miRNAs were one of most concerned regulatory RNAs. The classical way of miRNAs function was through binding to complementary sequences on the target gene mRNA to take effect as a post-transcriptional inhibitor of target gene expression [58]. Although the latest research reported the non-canonical molecular mechanisms of miRNA, the follow-up functional researches were still underway [59]. Their functions covered a wide range of aspects, including organism growth, development, maintenance of homeostasis and disease occurrence. In the past decade, there have been continuous studies on the role of miRNAs in the development and progression of DCM. The expression pattern of miRNAs during diabetic cardiomyopathy were revealed in 2011. 19 miRNAs and 16 miRNAs expression were detected by miRNA array and real-time RT-PCR in diabetic heart. GO pathway analyze and target gene analyze also showed the close relationship above miRNA and the Typical pathological process of DCM, such as cardiac hypertrophy and myocardial fibrosis [60]. In 2013, researchers identified 43 different expression miRNAs in mice heart from streptozotocin induced DCM, which 37 miRNAs were downregulated and 6 miRNAs were upregulated. Ultimately, the decrease of miR-1, miR-499, miR-133a, and miR-133b and increase of miR-21 were identified by RT-qPCR. Interestingly, miR-1, miR-499, miR-133a, and miR-133b were also involved in the antioxidant effect that were produced by N-acetylcysteine (NAC)-treatment in DCM [61].

3.1.1 miRNAs were Involved in Cardiomyocytes Injury or Cell Survival

Among the members of the miR-30 family, miR-30d and miR-30c have been reported to play different roles in DCM. It was reported that decreased expression of miR-30c could lead to the activation of p53/p21 pathway and cardiomyocyte apoptosis. Downregulation of miR-30c was a mediator of myocardial hypertrophy in response to high glucose condition by upregulation of Cdc42 and Pak1 genes [62]. Through its target gene PGC-1β miR-30c could also affect cardiomyocyte apoptosis, which was produced by affecting the utilization of glucose and the accumulation of lipids in cardiomyocytes [63]. Interestingly, miR-30d was identified as a regulator of cardiomyocyte pyroptosis, the pro-inflammatory programmed cardiomyocyte death in DCM rat model. Beside miR-30 family, miR-9 was another regulating miRNA of ventricular cardiomyocytes pyroptosis, whose rised a potential therapeutic target for DCM [64]. In addition, knockdown MiR-195 could extenuated the cardiac dysfunction and cardiomyocytes apoptosis in diabetic mice [65].

3.1.2 miRNA Related to DCM Induced Cardiac Injury

As the second found miRNA family in C. elegans, Let-7 functioned during tissue development, metabolic process, aging and immunology function [66]. lin28/let-7 was a typical regulator of insulin-PI3K-mTOR signaling in skeletal muscles, which was the largest metabolic organ in the human body [67]. Let-7 also restrained the amino acid-sensing pathway to inhibit mTOR-induced anabolism and autophagic catabolism [68]. The overexpression of let-7 revealed glucose intolerance and insulin insensitivity in mice [67, 69]. Inhibition of let-7 family was found as a therapeutic method against ischemia-reperfusion injury in diabetic rats via improving glucose uptake and insulin resistance.

miR-21 was a novel miRNA related to virous pathological changes in the heart, such as miR-21-3p regulated sepsis-associated or aging induced cardiac dysfunction. Overexpression of miR-21 that was induced by high glucose increased macrophage apoptosis, which participated in atherosclerosis. The inhibition of miR-21 leaded to weight loss in db/db mice by targeting TGFRB2, PTEN, and Sprouty1 and 2, which provided a safety and effective method to get a weight control in animal model. Long-term miR-21 knockout also abolished the effect on heart induced by obesity, reduced cardiac function and cardiac fibrosis [70]. In addition to disorders of lipid metabolism induced cardiomyopathy, cardiomyocyte apoptosis associated with glucose metabolism was also regulated by miR-21. Under the high glucose-stimulated, miR-21 targeted DSFP8 to activate the p38 pathway and c-Jun N-terminal kinase (JNK)/stress-activated kinase (SAPK) pathway, resulting in cardiac fibroblast proliferation and collagen synthesis [71].

Hyperglycemia could affect the action potential of cardiomyocytes and lead to abnormal systolic and diastolic function of myocardium through induce the expression of miR-1/133 in cardiomyocytes and inhibit the genes encoding slowly activating delayed rectifier potassium channel- KCNE1 and KCNQ1. miR-133a overexpression in heart reversed the diabetes collagen synthesis induced cardiac fibrosis and repaired the heart function. The expression of miR-133a in cardiomyocytes was negatively correlated with the expression of fibronectin 1, collagen type IV α1, connective tissue growth factor, fibroblast growth factor and TGF-β1. In diabetic hearts, the expression of miR-133a was down-regulated, resulting in an increased risk of myocardial fibrosis [72]. Cardiac-specific miR-133a overexpression mice alleviated diabetes mellitus induced cardiac fibrosis by inhibiting ERK1/2 and SMAD-2 phosphorylation [73]. Application of miR-133a treatment in vivo. could significantly extenuated cardiac hypertrophy, fibrosis and Type 1 diabetes mellitus induced systolic dysfunction [74].

miR-143/145 cluster was an effector of activin A, whose released from epicardial adipose tissue was closely related to T2DM. Precursor-miR-143 overexpression decreased insulin-stimulated glucose uptake in cardiomyocytes due to Akt phosphorylation. On the contrary, miR-145 had no effect on the glucose uptake and utilization in cardiomyocytes. An activin A-p38-miR-143/145-ORP8 axis was built in regulating glucose uptake by insulin, which was directly related to insulin resistance during the development of T2DM [75]. However, the function of this pathway in heart failure and remodeling during DCM was still needed to be discussed.

miR-451 expression level was upregulated in T2DM heart, and this upregulation of miR-451 expression was time and dose dependent. Knockdown miR-451 alleviated the lipotoxicity in cardiomyocytes by suppression of the LKB1/AMPK pathway. Cardiac function recovery accompanied by decreasingthe concentration of lipid metabolism intermediate and reactive oxygen species production [76]. miR-503 participated in the protective effect of phase II enzyme inducer in DCM rat, and related to the antioxidant effect on cardiomyocytes [77].

It was reported that miR-155 is involved in metabolic diseases and inflammation disease [78–81]. miR-155 was a direct blocker of IL-13-induced anti-inflammatory type 2 macrophage by inhibiting the expression of IL-13Rα1. As an important contributor of excessive inflammatory response, miR-155 overexpression was also detected in the virus infected heart [82]. A covalent complex of gold nanoparticle (AuNP) and thiol-modified antago-miR-155 was made in a resent study, which transported miR-155 directly to macrophages. As a high specificity messenger of macrophage, AuNP-based miR-155 antagonist was injected into the ovariectomized female mice diabetic mouse model, which promoted M2 macrophages polarization in vivo. Then, recovered DCM induced cardiac function, mitigated coordinating inflammation, apoptosis, and fibrosis [83].

Endothelial to mesenchymal transition (EMT) was a phenotypic change during endothelial injury, which was closely related to cardiac fibrosis and existed in the pathogenesis of DCM. Specific overexpression of miR-200b in endothelial cells were detected to be induced in diabetic mice heart. Meanwhile, endothelial miR-200b overexpression blocked the EMT, further protected cardiac systolic function in diabetic mice.

3.2 Other Non-coding RNAs and DCM

3.2.1 lncRNAs in the Diagnose and Pathological Process of DCM

Long non-coding RNAs (lncRNAs) was a class longer than 200 nucleotides RNA, which without protein-coding function. lncRNAs had many epigenetic forms of regulation, including DNA methylation, histone modification and regulation of miRNA [84, 85]. lncRNAs played important roles in chromosome modification, X-chromosome silencing, genomic imprinting, transcriptional interference, transcriptional activation and intranuclear transport [86]. According to the mechanism of action of lncRNA, lncRNAs had the following functions according to the mechanisms of action: (1) Transcription occured in the upstream promoter region of the protein-coding gene, which interfered with the expression of downstream genes (e.g. SER3 gene in yeast). (2) Regulated the expression of downstream gene expression by means of RNA polymerase II inhibition or mediating chromatin remodeling and histone modification (e.g. p15AS in mice) [87]. (3) By forming complementary double-stranded with the mRNA of coding genes, lncRNAs interfered with the cleavage of RNA, thus produced different forms of cleavage. (4) By forming complementary double-stranded with transcripts of protein-coding genes, the expression level of genes was regulated by attracting endogenous siRNA through DICER. (5) By binding to specific proteins, lncRNAs transcripts could regulate the activity of corresponding proteins. (6) As a structural component, lncRNAs forms nucleic acid-protein complexes with proteins [88]. (7) By binding to a specific protein, changed the localization of this protein. (8) As a precursor molecule of small RNA, such as miRNA and piwi-interacting RNA (piRNA) [89–91].

As a research hotspot in the field of non-coding RNAs, the role of lncRNAs in DCM has been gradually revealed [92]. Downregulated expression of lncRNA homeobox transcript antisense RNA (HOTAIR) was detected in the heart and serum of DCM patients. Further studies have found that HOTAIR enhances the viability of cardiomyocytes by activating PI3K/Akt pathway, which may provide a possible treatment of DCM. The latest research focused on the involvement of HOTAIR in animal DCM model and the molecular mechanism. In STZ-induced mouse DCM model, specific overexpression of HOTAIR in cardiac myocytes could improve cardiac function, reduce myocardial death, inflammation and oxidative stress [93].

As one of the first reported lncRNAs, lncRNA-H19 was well studied on its biological functions and the mechanism of its interaction with other molecules [94]. The encoding gene of lncRNA-H19 and the insulin-like growth factor 2 were from the same gene cluster, indicating the potential relationship of lncRNA-H19 with metabolism and blood glucose regulation [95]. Decreased IGF2 and lncRNA-H19 in pancreatic might play a key role in the repair of islet ultrastructure and function in offspring of gestational diabetes mellitus [96]. Interestingly, there was a double negative feedback between lncRNA-H19 and its target miRNA let-7 in participating the glucose metabolism in muscle cells. More concretely, as a sponge of let-7, lncRNA-H19 was decreased in the muscle of DM patients, while let-7 was increased. lncRNA H19-miR-675-VDAC1 was recognized as the mediate axis in regulating the function of lncRNA H19 in cardiomyocytes [97]. In DCM, overexpression of lncRNA-H19 reduced inflammation and oxidative stress, protected myocardial cells from apoptosis, inhibited autophagy. The inhibitory effect of lncRNA H19 on autophagy of cardiomyocytes was mediated by its direct binding with EZH2 and restraining DIRAS3 transcription [98].

Metastasis-associated lung adenocarcinoma transcript 1 (MALAT1) was related to tumor cell growth invasion and metastasis. It was also recognized as a significantly upregulated lncRNA in diabetic rats. Inhibition of MALAT1 in rat heart could protect heart from DCM induced dysfunction by significant reducing the cardiomyocytes apoptosis [99]. Besides that, MALAT1 knockdown also alleviated the DCM early characteristic inflammation response [100]. The up-regulation of MALAT1 in cardiomyocytes and hearts of hyperglycemic mice could be counteracted by nitric oxide [101].

Other lncRNAs have also been found to be involved in the development of DCM. Most of the studies are concerned about the effects of lncRNA on cardiomyocyte survival, including apoptosis, pyroptosis or autophagy. Overexpression of myocardial infarction associated transcript (MIAT) was detected in the DCM mice and showed protective effect on cardiac function. Similar to other LncRNA, MIAT functioned as a competing endogenous of miR-22-3p, resulting in the activation of target gene DAPK2 [102]. Inhibition of Kcnq1ot1 reduced cardiomyocytes pyroptosis hence affecting the function of cardiac function in mice DCM model, which was also identified as a sponge lncRNA of miR-214-3p, leading to the increase of caspase-1 and IL-1β [103].

Although lncRNAs have been found to be associated with ventricular remodeling, especially cardiac fibrosis, the relationship between lncRNAs and DCM-induced myocardial fibrosis has been less discussed [104, 105]. As an cardiac fibroblasts (CFs) enriched lncRNA in heart, lncRNA Crnde (CRNDE) was significantly negatively related to cardiac fibrosis in patients with cardiac fibrosis or in DCM mice. Overexpression CRNDE could reduce the marker gene of myofibroblast expression in TGF-β induced CFs and alleviate DCM-related cardiac fibrosis. At the same time, left ventricular function was partial recovery by CRNDE overexpression through formatting a Smad3-Crnde negative feedback [106].

lncRNAs were specific markers to predict the occurrence of DCM in well-controlled type 2 diabetes patients. Circulating long intergenic non-coding RNA predicting cardiac remodeling (LIPCAR) was negatively correlated with diastolic function(E/A peak flow), while serum smooth muscle and endothelial cell-enriched migration/differentiation-associated long non-coding RNA (SENCR) were significantly related to cardiac remodeling in patient with uncomplicated type 2 diabetes. All the above motioned results demonstrated that lncRNAs was valuable tools for recognizing the cardiomyopathy at a preclinical stage, especially for the screening for the first diagnosis patients or the well-controlled patients [107].

3.2.2 CircRNAs as Potential Tools for DCM

Circular RNAs (circRNAs) were the important members of non-coding RNAs. Although circRNAs werediscovered in organisms as early as 1979, the functional research of circRNAs has been zigzag [108]. Because most of the circRNAs were derived from gene exons, researchers used probes to capture known exon sequences and then conducted in-depth sequencing. Through this way, more than 3000 circRNAs were identified in 2000 clinical samples. However, because this method retained linear RNA, the researchers also found that the expression of circRNAs has no obvious relationship with the number of RNA produced by parent gene. Thus, the change of expression of cyclic RNA could not be simply attributed to the change of the expression of the mother gene. It might contain more complex generation and regulation mechanisms. In the past 10 years, the function of circRNAs has been gradually revealed. circRNAs were implicated in the development of metabolic disease and cardiovascular disease such as coronary heart disease, pathological cardiac hypertrophy and cardiac remodeling [109, 110]. Studies described the circRNAs expression pattern in human endothelial cells after high glucose stimulation. 95 circRNAs different expressed were observed in different group, which may be involved in the process of the endothelial dysfunction in diabetes mellitus. But unfortunately, there was no research to explain the role of a specific circRNA in the pathogenesis of DCM.

4 Conclusion

Different models will have certain influence during the process of studying the pathogenesis of DCM. TIDM and T2DM have the greatest impact on cardiomyopathy. Although both of them involve oxidative stress, inflammation, cardiomyocyte apoptosis and high glucose stimulation induced hypertrophy, the role of insulin resistance could not be ignored [111]. In addition, high fat and lipid metabolism disorders also played a role in the pathogenesis of DCM, which needed further clarification. Considering the current research situation of the relationship between non-codingRNAs and DCM, there were still many valuable problems need to be further discussed.

Based on the results of the current study, there was no doubt that miRNAs could regulate DCM. This regulation ran through the entire process of DCM from initial to advanced heart failure. DCM shared a common pathological process with many cardiac injury diseases. High glucose and oxidative stress damaged cardiomyocytes in early stage of disease, which leading to apoptosis or even necrosis of cardiomyocytes. At the late stage of DCM induced heart failure, the main pathological manifestations were cardiac hypertrophy and ventricular remodeling. In addition, metabolic changes in the heart were closely related to DCM, including abnormal glycometabolism and lipid metabolism, which was also related to the discovery of miRNAs function in the above pathological processes. For example, the miR-155 described above was a classical metabolic syndrome-related miRNA [112, 113]. MiR-133a was a muscle-specific miRNA, and its association with cardiac fibrosis has been reported already. These conclusions were confirmed in the cardiac fibrosis that was induced by DCM. We made it clear that these miRNAs were closely related to DCM. However, almost no miRNA was obtained that was specific related to DCM. Indicated that no breakthrough has been made either in solving the specific target of miRNAs treatment or in finding specific markers again. According to the classical definition, noncoding RNA was a kind of RNA without coding function in transcriptome. However, recent studies found that some non-coding RNAs or its precursors can also be translated [114, 115]. This brought more possibilities in exploring the function and mechanism of non-coding RNA in human diseases. The functions of circRNAs and its relationship with diseases were the hotspots of current research, especially after the redefinition of circRNA as a functional RNA. The potential of circRNAs was not only embodied in its subunits, but also in its coding and homeopathic regulation of nearby genes [116].

However, the research on non-coding RNAs as a biomarker of DCM was relatively rare, which may be due to the following reasons: (1) In clinical, compared with other diseases such as myocardial infarction, the diagnosis of diabetic cardiomyopathy often required comprehensive clinical history, cardiac ultrasonography and other results to diagnose. Also, fewer cases of definite diagnosis were obtained. (2) Diagnosed patients have often entered the stage of heart failure, that too many confounding factors existed. (3) DCM was mostly developed on the basis of type 2 diabetes mellitus in clinical patients. However, more attention has been paid to type 1 diabetes mellitus induced DCM in experimental research, which was different between clinical and basic research.

In addition, conservativeness of non-coding RNAs among species was also one of the bottlenecks to its application in clinical treatment in the future. This made it more difficult for the transformation from animal model to clinical practice. Therefore, a small amount of non-coding RNAs, which was found to be highly conservative among species, could be the target of future therapeutic strategies developing.

In conclusion, the pathogenesis of DCM is not completely clear at present. The research on the relationship between non-coding RNAs and DCM has revealed the strong role of non-coding RNAs in the pathogenesis of DCM. Research on this direction is a meaningful perspective to explore the pathogenesis of DCM in the future.

Competing Financial Interests The authors declare no competing financial interests.

References

1. Tao L, Shi J, Yang X, Yang L, Hua F. The exosome: a new player in diabetic cardiomyopathy. J Cardiovasc Transl Res. 2019;12(1):62–7.
2. Ernande L, Audureau E, Jellis CL, Bergerot C, Henegar C, Sawaki D, Czibik G, Volpi C, Canoui-Poitrine F, Thibault H, Ternacle J, Moulin P, Marwick TH, Derumeaux G. Clinical implications of echocardiographic phenotypes of patients with diabetes mellitus. J Am Coll Cardiol. 2017;70(14):1704–16.
3. Rubler S, Dlugash J, Yuceoglu YZ, Kumral T, Branwood AW, Grishman A. New type of cardiomyopathy associated with diabetic glomerulosclerosis. Am J Cardiol. 1972;30(6):595–602.
4. Rawshani A, Rawshani A, Sattar N, Franzen S, McGuire DK, Eliasson B, Svensson AM, Zethelius B, Miftaraj M, Rosengren A, Gudbjornsdottir S. Relative prognostic importance and optimal levels of risk factors for mortality and cardiovascular outcomes in type 1 diabetes mellitus. Circulation. 2019;139(16):1900–12.
5. Armstrong AC, Ambale-Venkatesh B, Turkbey E, Donekal S, Chamera E, Backlund JY, Cleary P, Lachin J, Bluemke DA, Lima JA, Group DER. Association of Cardiovascular Risk Factors and Myocardial Fibrosis with Early Cardiac Dysfunction in type 1 diabetes: the diabetes control and complications trial/epidemiology of diabetes interventions and complications study. Diabetes Care. 2017;40(3):405–11.

6. Arnett DK, Blumenthal RS, Albert MA, Buroker AB, Goldberger ZD, Hahn EJ, Himmelfarb CD, Khera A, Lloyd-Jones D, McEvoy JW, Michos ED, Miedema MD, Munoz D, Smith SC, Jr., Virani SS, Williams KA, Sr., Yeboah J, Ziaeian B (2019) 2019 ACC/AHA guideline on the primary prevention of cardiovascular disease. Circulation:CIR0000000000000678.
7. Wu S, Lu Q, Ding Y, Wu Y, Qiu Y, Wang P, Mao X, Huang K, Xie Z, Zou MH. Hyperglycemia-driven inhibition of AMP-activated protein kinase alpha2 induces diabetic cardiomyopathy by promoting mitochondria-associated endoplasmic reticulum membranes in vivo. Circulation. 2019;139(16):1913–36.
8. Dillmann WH. Diabetic cardiomyopathy. Circ Res. 2019;124(8):1160–2.
9. Kenny HC, Abel ED. Heart failure in type 2 diabetes mellitus. Circ Res. 2019;124(1):121–41.
10. Palomer X, Pizarro-Delgado J, Vazquez-Carrera M. Emerging actors in diabetic cardiomyopathy: heartbreaker biomarkers or therapeutic targets? Trends Pharmacol Sci. 2018;39(5):452–67.
11. Aaron CP, Tandri H, Barr RG, Johnson WC, Bagiella E, Chahal H, Jain A, Kizer JR, Bertoni AG, Lima JA, Bluemke DA, Kawut SM. Physical activity and right ventricular structure and function. The MESA-right ventricle study. Am J Respir Crit Care Med. 2011;183(3):396–404.
12. Redberg RF, Greenland P, Fuster V, Pyorala K, Blair SN, Folsom AR, Newman AB, O'Leary DH, Orchard TJ, Psaty B, Schwartz JS, Starke R, Wilson PW. Prevention conference VI: diabetes and cardiovascular disease: writing group III: risk assessment in persons with diabetes. Circulation. 2002;105(18):e144–52.
13. Song G, Chen C, Zhang J, Chang L, Zhu D, Wang X. Association of traditional Chinese exercises with glycemic responses in people with type 2 diabetes: a systematic review and meta-analysis of randomized controlled trials. J Sport Health Sci. 2018;7(4):442–52.
14. Le S, Mao L, Lu D, Yang Y, Tan X, Wiklund P, Cheng S. Effect of aerobic exercise on insulin resistance and central adiposity disappeared after the discontinuation of intervention in overweight women. J Sport Health Sci. 2016;5(2):166–70.
15. Li L, Zhang S, Dobson J. The contribution of small and large sensory afferents to postural control in patients with peripheral neuropathy. J Sport Health Sci. 2019;8(3):218–27.
16. Barakat GM, Nuwayri-Salti N, Kadi LN, Bitar KM, Al-Jaroudi WA, Bikhazi AB. Role of glucagon-like peptide-1 and its agonists on early prevention of cardiac remodeling in type 1 diabetic rat hearts. Gen Physiol Biophys. 2011;30(1):34–44.
17. Cryer MJ, Horani T, DiPette DJ. Diabetes and hypertension: a comparative review of current guidelines. J Clin Hypertens (Greenwich). 2016;18(2):95–100.
18. Suhara T, Baba Y, Shimada BK, Higa JK, Matsui T. The mTOR Signaling pathway in myocardial dysfunction in type 2 diabetes mellitus. Curr Diab Rep. 2017;17(6):38.
19. Bar L, Feger M, Fajol A, Klotz LO, Zeng S, Lang F, Hocher B, Foller M. Insulin suppresses the production of fibroblast growth factor 23 (FGF23). Proc Natl Acad Sci U S A. 2018;115(22):5804–9.
20. Wang Q, Ren J. mTOR-independent autophagy inducer trehalose rescues against insulin resistance-induced myocardial contractile anomalies: role of p38 MAPK and Foxo1. Pharmacol Res. 2016;111:357–73.
21. Kumphune S, Chattipakorn S, Chattipakorn N. Roles of p38-MAPK in insulin resistant heart: evidence from bench to future bedside application. Curr Pharm Biotechnol. 2013;19(32):5742–54.
22. Ginion A, Auquier J, Benton CR, Mouton C, Vanoverschelde JL, Hue L, Horman S, Beauloye C, Bertrand L. Inhibition of the mTOR/p70S6K pathway is not involved in the insulin-sensitizing effect of AMPK on cardiac glucose uptake. Am J Phys Heart Circ Phys. 2011;301(2):H469–77.
23. Schwenk RW, Angin Y, Steinbusch LK, Dirkx E, Hoebers N, Coumans WA, Bonen A, Broers JL, van Eys GJ, Glatz JF, Luiken JJ. Overexpression of vesicle-associated membrane protein (VAMP) 3, but not VAMP2, protects glucose transporter (GLUT) 4 protein translocation in an in vitro model of cardiac insulin resistance. J Biol Chem. 2012;287(44):37530–9.
24. Shao Y, Chernaya V, Johnson C, Yang WY, Cueto R, Sha X, Zhang Y, Qin X, Sun J, Choi ET, Wang H, Yang XF. Metabolic diseases downregulate the majority of histone modification enzymes, making a few Upregulated enzymes novel therapeutic targets—"sand out and gold stays". J Cardiovasc Transl Res. 2016;9(1):49–66.
25. Gu J, Yan X, Dai X, Wang Y, Lin Q, Xiao J, Zhou S, Zhang J, Wang K, Zeng J, Xin Y, Barati MT, Zhang C, Bai Y, Li Y, Epstein PN, Wintergerst KA, Li X, Tan Y, Cai L. Metallothionein preserves Akt2 activity and cardiac function via inhibiting TRB3 in diabetic hearts. Diabetes. 2018;67(3):507–17.
26. Jia G, Hill MA, Sowers JR. Diabetic cardiomyopathy: an update of mechanisms contributing to this clinical entity. Circ Res. 2018;122(4):624–38.
27. Yin Y, Zheng Z, Jiang Z. Effects of lycopene on metabolism of glycolipid in type 2 diabetic rats. Biomed Pharmacother. 2019;109:2070–7.
28. Pei Z, Deng Q, Babcock SA, He EY, Ren J, Zhang Y. Inhibition of advanced glycation endproduct (AGE) rescues against streptozotocin-induced diabetic cardiomyopathy: role of autophagy and ER stress. Toxicol Lett. 2018;284:10–20.
29. Saleh A, Smith DR, Tessler L, Mateo AR, Martens C, Schartner E, Van der Ploeg R, Toth C, Zochodne DW, Fernyhough P. Receptor for advanced glycation end-products (RAGE) activates divergent signaling pathways to augment neurite outgrowth of adult sensory neurons. Exp Neurol. 2013;249:149–59.

30. Fang YH, Piao L, Hong Z, Toth PT, Marsboom G, Bache-Wiig P, Rehman J, Archer SL. Therapeutic inhibition of fatty acid oxidation in right ventricular hypertrophy: exploiting Randle's cycle. J Mol Med. 2012;90(1):31–43.
31. Bergman HM, Lindfors L, Palm F, Kihlberg J, Lanekoff I. Metabolite aberrations in early diabetes detected in rat kidney using mass spectrometry imaging. Anal Bioanal Chem. 2019;411(13):2809–16.
32. He L, Kim T, Long Q, Liu J, Wang P, Zhou Y, Ding Y, Prasain J, Wood PA, Yang Q. Carnitine palmitoyltransferase-1b deficiency aggravates pressure overload-induced cardiac hypertrophy caused by lipotoxicity. Circulation. 2012;126(14):1705–16.
33. Feuerstein GZ. Apoptosis in cardiac diseases--new opportunities for novel therapeutics for heart diseases. Cardiovasc Drugs Ther. 1999;13(4):289–94.
34. Simon JN, Chowdhury SA, Warren CM, Sadayappan S, Wieczorek DF, Solaro RJ, Wolska BM. Ceramide-mediated depression in cardiomyocyte contractility through PKC activation and modulation of myofilament protein phosphorylation. Basic Res Cardiol. 2014;109(6):445.
35. Ilatovskaya DV, Blass G, Palygin O, Levchenko V, Pavlov TS, Grzybowski MN, Winsor K, Shuyskiy LS, Geurts AM, Cowley AW Jr, Birnbaumer L, Staruschenko A. A NOX4/TRPC6 pathway in Podocyte calcium regulation and renal damage in diabetic kidney disease. J Am Soc Nephrol. 2018;29(7):1917–27.
36. Liu Y, Steinbusch LKM, Nabben M, Kapsokalyvas D, van Zandvoort M, Schonleitner P, Antoons G, Simons PJ, Coumans WA, Geomini A, Chanda D, Glatz JFC, Neumann D, Luiken J. Palmitate-induced Vacuolar-type H(+)-ATPase inhibition feeds forward into insulin resistance and contractile dysfunction. Diabetes. 2017;66(6):1521–34.
37. Bugger H, Riehle C, Jaishy B, Wende AR, Tuinei J, Chen D, Soto J, Pires KM, Boudina S, Theobald HA, Luptak I, Wayment B, Wang X, Litwin SE, Weimer BC, Abel ED. Genetic loss of insulin receptors worsens cardiac efficiency in diabetes. J Mol Cell Cardiol. 2012;52(5):1019–26.
38. Hegab Z, Mohamed TMA, Stafford N, Mamas M, Cartwright EJ, Oceandy D. Advanced glycation end products reduce the calcium transient in cardiomyocytes by increasing production of reactive oxygen species and nitric oxide. FEBS Open Bio. 2017;7(11):1672–85.
39. Yan D, Luo X, Li Y, Liu W, Deng J, Zheng N, Gao K, Huang Q, Liu J. Effects of advanced glycation end products on calcium handling in cardiomyocytes. Cardiology. 2014;129(2):75–83.
40. Tong M, Saito T, Zhai P, Oka SI, Mizushima W, Nakamura M, Ikeda S, Shirakabe A, Sadoshima J. Mitophagy is essential for maintaining cardiac function during high fat diet-induced diabetic cardiomyopathy. Circ Res. 2019;124(9):1360–71.
41. Liu F, Song R, Feng Y, Guo J, Chen Y, Zhang Y, Chen T, Wang Y, Huang Y, Li CY, Cao C, Zhang Y, Hu X, Xiao RP. Upregulation of MG53 induces diabetic cardiomyopathy through transcriptional activation of peroxisome proliferation-activated receptor alpha. Circulation. 2015;131(9):795–804.
42. Pedersen MT, Vorup J, Bangsbo J. Effect of a 26-month floorball training on male elderly's cardiovascular fitness, glucose control, body composition, and functional capacity. J Sport Health Sci. 2018;7(2):149–58.
43. Rezende F, Prior KK, Lowe O, Wittig I, Strecker V, Moll F, Helfinger V, Schnutgen F, Kurrle N, Wempe F, Walter M, Zukunft S, Luck B, Fleming I, Weissmann N, Brandes RP, Schroder K. Cytochrome P450 enzymes but not NADPH oxidases are the source of the NADPH-dependent lucigenin chemiluminescence in membrane assays. Free Radic Biol Med. 2017;102:57–66.
44. Elbatreek MH, Pachado MP, Cuadrado A, Jandeleit-Dahm K, Schmidt H. Reactive oxygen comes of age: mechanism-based therapy of diabetic end-organ damage. Trends Endocrinol Metab. 2019;30(5):312–27.
45. Munzel T, Gori T, Bruno RM, Taddei S. Is oxidative stress a therapeutic target in cardiovascular disease? Eur Heart J. 2010;31(22):2741–8.
46. Yang YC, Tsai CY, Chen CL, Kuo CH, Hou CW, Cheng SY, Aneja R, Huang CY, Kuo WW. Pkcdelta activation is involved in ROS-mediated mitochondrial dysfunction and apoptosis in Cardiomyocytes exposed to advanced Glycation end products (Ages). Aging Dis. 2018;9(4):647–63.
47. Rajamani U, Essop MF. Hyperglycemia-mediated activation of the hexosamine biosynthetic pathway results in myocardial apoptosis. Am J Phys Cell Phys. 2010;299(1):C139–47.
48. Adameova A, Dhalla NS. Role of microangiopathy in diabetic cardiomyopathy. Heart Fail Rev. 2014;19(1):25–33.
49. McGrath GM, McNeill JH. Cardiac ultrastructural changes in streptozotocin-induced diabetic rats: effects of insulin treatment. Can J Cardiol. 1986;2(3):164–9.
50. Yuan J, Tan JTM, Rajamani K, Solly EL, King EJ, Lecce L, Simpson PJL, Lam YT, Jenkins AJ, Bursill CA, Keech AC, Ng MKC. Fenofibrate rescues diabetes-related impairment of ischemia-mediated angiogenesis by PPARalpha-independent modulation of Thioredoxin-interacting protein. Diabetes. 2019;68(5):1040–53.
51. Niu C, Chen Z, Kim KT, Sun J, Xue M, Chen G, Li S, Shen Y, Zhu Z, Wang X, Liang J, Jiang C, Cong W, Jin L, Li X. Metformin alleviates hyperglycemia-induced endothelial impairment by downregulating autophagy via the Hedgehog pathway. Autophagy. 2019;15(5):843–70.
52. Kjobsted R, Roll JLW, Jorgensen NO, Birk JB, Foretz M, Viollet B, Chadt A, Al-Hasani H, Wojtaszewski JFP. AMPK and TBC1D1 regulate muscle glucose uptake after – but not during – exercise and contraction. Diabetes. 2019;292(5):1308–17.

53. Yoon KJ, Zhang D, Kim SJ, Lee MC, Moon HY. Exercise-induced AMPK activation is involved in delay of skeletal muscle senescence. Biochem Biophys Res Commun. 2019;512(3):604–10.
54. Sanchez-Lopez E, Zhong Z, Stubelius A, Sweeney SR, Booshehri LM, Antonucci L, Liu-Bryan R, Lodi A, Terkeltaub R, Lacal JC, Murphy AN, Hoffman HM, Tiziani S, Guma M, Karin M. Choline uptake and metabolism modulate macrophage IL-1beta and IL-18 production. Cell Metab. 2019;29(6):1350–1362.e7.
55. Zhao H, Li T, Wang K, Zhao F, Chen J, Xu G, Zhao J, Li T, Chen L, Li L, Xia Q, Zhou T, Li HY, Li AL, Finkel T, Zhang XM, Pan X. AMPK-mediated activation of MCU stimulates mitochondrial Ca(2+) entry to promote mitotic progression. Nat Cell Biol. 2019;21(4):476–86.
56. Wang Y, Xiong H, Liu D, Hill C, Ertay A, Li J, Zou Y, Miller P, White E, Downward J, Goldin RD, Yuan X, Lu X. Autophagy inhibition specifically promotes epithelial-mesenchymal transition and invasion in RAS-mutated cancer cells. Autophagy. 2019;15(5):886–99.
57. Xie Z, Lau K, Eby B, Lozano P, He C, Pennington B, Li H, Rathi S, Dong Y, Tian R, Kem D, Zou MH. Improvement of cardiac functions by chronic metformin treatment is associated with enhanced cardiac autophagy in diabetic OVE26 mice. Diabetes. 2011;60(6):1770–8.
58. Wang L, Lv Y, Li G, Xiao J. MicroRNAs in heart and circulation during physical exercise. J Sport Health Sci. 2018;7(4):433–41.
59. Dragomir MP, Knutsen E, Calin GA. SnapShot: unconventional miRNA functions. Cell. 2018;174(4):1038–1038.e1031.
60. Diao X, Shen E, Wang X, Hu B. Differentially expressed microRNAs and their target genes in the hearts of streptozotocin-induced diabetic mice. Mol Med Rep. 2011;4(4):633–40.
61. Yildirim SS, Akman D, Catalucci D, Turan B. Relationship between downregulation of miRNAs and increase of oxidative stress in the development of diabetic cardiac dysfunction: junctin as a target protein of miR-1. Cell Biochem Biophys. 2013;67(3):1397–408.
62. Raut SK, Kumar A, Singh GB, Nahar U, Sharma V, Mittal A, Sharma R, Khullar M. miR-30c mediates upregulation of Cdc42 and Pak1 in diabetic cardiomyopathy. Cardiovasc Drugs Ther. 2015;33(3):89–97.
63. Yin Z, Zhao Y, He M, Li H, Fan J, Nie X, Yan M, Chen C, Wang DW. MiR-30c/PGC-1beta protects against diabetic cardiomyopathy via PPARalpha. Cardiovasc Diabetol. 2019;18(1):7.
64. Jeyabal P, Thandavarayan RA, Joladarashi D, Suresh Babu S, Krishnamurthy S, Bhimaraj A, Youker KA, Kishore R, Krishnamurthy P. MicroRNA-9 inhibits hyperglycemia-induced pyroptosis in human ventricular cardiomyocytes by targeting ELAVL1. Biochem Biophys Res Commun. 2016;471(4):423–9.
65. Zheng D, Ma J, Yu Y, Li M, Ni R, Wang G, Chen R, Li J, Fan GC, Lacefield JC, Peng T. Silencing of miR-195 reduces diabetic cardiomyopathy in C57BL/6 mice. Diabetologia. 2015;58(8):1949–58.
66. Bussing I, Slack FJ, Grosshans H. Let-7 microRNAs in development, stem cells and cancer. Trends Mol Med. 2008;14(9):400–9.
67. Zhu H, Shyh-Chang N, Segre AV, Shinoda G, Shah SP, Einhorn WS, Takeuchi A, Engreitz JM, Hagan JP, Kharas MG, Urbach A, Thornton JE, Triboulet R, Gregory RI, Consortium D, Investigators M, Altshuler D, Daley GQ. The Lin28/let-7 axis regulates glucose metabolism. Cell. 2011;147(1):81–94.
68. Dubinsky AN, Dastidar SG, Hsu CL, Zahra R, Djakovic SN, Duarte S, Esau CC, Spencer B, Ashe TD, Fischer KM, MacKenna DA, Sopher BL, Masliah E, Gaasterland T, Chau BN, Pereira de Almeida L, Morrison BE, La Spada AR. Let-7 coordinately suppresses components of the amino acid sensing pathway to repress mTORC1 and induce autophagy. Cell Metab. 2014;20(4):626–38.
69. Frost RJ, Olson EN. Control of glucose homeostasis and insulin sensitivity by the Let-7 family of microRNAs. Proc Natl Acad Sci U S A. 2011;108(52):21075–80.
70. Seeger T, Fischer A, Muhly-Reinholz M, Zeiher AM, Dimmeler S. Long-term inhibition of miR-21 leads to reduction of obesity in db/db mice. Obesity (Silver Spring). 2014;22(11):2352–60.
71. Liu S, Li W, Xu M, Huang H, Wang J, Chen X. Micro-RNA 21Targets dual specific phosphatase 8 to promote collagen synthesis in high glucose-treated primary cardiac fibroblasts. Am J Cardiol. 2014;30(12):1689–99.
72. Nandi SS, Duryee MJ, Shahshahan HR, Thiele GM, Anderson DR, Mishra PK. Induction of autophagy markers is associated with attenuation of miR-133a in diabetic heart failure patients undergoing mechanical unloading. Am J Transl Res. 2015;7(4):683–96.
73. Chen S, Puthanveetil P, Feng B, Matkovich SJ, Dorn GW 2nd, Chakrabarti S. Cardiac miR-133a overexpression prevents early cardiac fibrosis in diabetes. J Cell Mol Med. 2014;18(3):415–21.
74. Nandi SS, Shahshahan HR, Shang Q, Kutty S, Boska M, Mishra PK. MiR-133a mimic alleviates T1DM-induced systolic dysfunction in Akita: an MRI-based study. Front Physiol. 2018;9:1275.
75. Blumensatt M, Greulich S, Herzfeld de Wiza D, Mueller H, Maxhera B, Rabelink MJ, Hoeben RC, Akhyari P, Al-Hasani H, Ruige JB, Ouwens DM. Activin a impairs insulin action in cardiomyocytes via up-regulation of miR-143. Cardiovasc Res. 2013;100(2):201–10.
76. Kuwabara Y, Horie T, Baba O, Watanabe S, Nishiga M, Usami S, Izuhara M, Nakao T, Nishino T, Otsu K, Kita T, Kimura T, Ono K. MicroRNA-451 exacerbates lipotoxicity in cardiac myocytes and high-fat diet-induced cardiac hypertrophy in mice through suppression of the LKB1/AMPK pathway. Circ Res. 2015;116(2):279–88.

77. Miao Y, Wan Q, Liu X, Wang Y, Luo Y, Liu D, Lin N, Zhou H, Zhong J. miR-503 is involved in the protective effect of phase II enzyme inducer (CPDT) in diabetic cardiomyopathy via Nrf2/ARE Signaling pathway. Biomed Res Int. 2017;2017:9167450.
78. Virtue A, Johnson C, Lopez-Pastrana J, Shao Y, Fu H, Li X, Li YF, Yin Y, Mai J, Rizzo V, Tordoff M, Bagi Z, Shan H, Jiang X, Wang H, Yang XF. MicroRNA-155 deficiency leads to decreased atherosclerosis, increased White adipose tissue obesity, and non-alcoholic fatty liver disease: a NOVEL MOUSE MODEL OF OBESITY PARADOX. J Biol Chem. 2017;292(4):1267–87.
79. Johnson C, Ct D, Virtue A, Gao T, Wu S, Hernandez M, Singh L, Wang H, Yang XF. Increased expression of Resistin in MicroRNA-155-deficient White adipose tissues may be a possible driver of metabolically healthy obesity transition to classical obesity. Front Physiol. 2018;9:1297.
80. Wang L, Zhang N, Wang Z, Ai DM, Cao ZY, Pan HP. Decreased MiR-155 level in the peripheral blood of non-alcoholic fatty liver disease patients may serve as a biomarker and may influence LXR activity. Vitro Cell Dev Biol Plant. 2016;39(6):2239–48.
81. Miller AM, Gilchrist DS, Nijjar J, Araldi E, Ramirez CM, Lavery CA, Fernandez-Hernando C, McInnes IB, Kurowska-Stolarska M. MiR-155 has a protective role in the development of non-alcoholic hepatosteatosis in mice. PLoS One. 2013;8(8):e72324.
82. Corsten MF, Papageorgiou A, Verhesen W, Carai P, Lindow M, Obad S, Summer G, Coort SL, Hazebroek M, van Leeuwen R, Gijbels MJ, Wijnands E, Biessen EA, De Winther MP, Stassen FR, Carmeliet P, Kauppinen S, Schroen B, Heymans S. MicroRNA profiling identifies microRNA-155 as an adverse mediator of cardiac injury and dysfunction during acute viral myocarditis. Circ Res. 2012;111(4):415–25.
83. Jia C, Chen H, Wei M, Chen X, Zhang Y, Cao L, Yuan P, Wang F, Yang G, Ma J. Gold nanoparticle-based miR155 antagonist macrophage delivery restores the cardiac function in ovariectomized diabetic mouse model. Int J Nanomedicine. 2017;12:4963–79.
84. Li D, Kular L, Vij M, Herter EK, Li X, Wang A, Chu T, Toma MA, Zhang L, Liapi E, Mota A, Blomqvist L, Serezal IG, Rollman O, Wikstrom JD, Bienko M, Berglund D, Stahle M, Sommar P, Jagodic M, Landen NX. Human skin long noncoding RNA WAKMAR1 regulates wound healing by enhancing keratinocyte migration. Proc Natl Acad Sci U S A. 2019;116(19):9443–52.
85. Cheedipudi SM, Matkovich SJ, Coarfa C, Hu X, Robertson MJ, Sweet M, Taylor M, Mestroni L, Cleveland J, Willerson JT, Gurha P, Marian AJ. Genomic reorganization of Lamin-associated domains in cardiac Myocytes is associated with differential gene expression and DNA methylation in human dilated cardiomyopathy. Circ Res. 2019;124(8):1198–213.
86. Wang CY, Jegu T, Chu HP, Oh HJ, Lee JT. SMCHD1 merges chromosome compartments and assists formation of super-structures on the inactive X. Cell. 2018;174(2):406–21.. e425
87. Lin N, Chang KY, Li Z, Gates K, Rana ZA, Dang J, Zhang D, Han T, Yang CS, Cunningham TJ, Head SR, Duester G, Dong PD, Rana TM. An evolutionarily conserved long noncoding RNA TUNA controls pluripotency and neural lineage commitment. Mol Cell. 2014;53(6):1005–19.
88. Wang P, Xue Y, Han Y, Lin L, Wu C, Xu S, Jiang Z, Xu J, Liu Q, Cao X. The STAT3-binding long noncoding RNA lnc-DC controls human dendritic cell differentiation. Science. 2014;344(6181):310–3.
89. Xu M, Chen X, Lin K, Zeng K, Liu X, Pan B, Xu X, Xu T, Hu X, Sun L, He B, Pan Y, Sun H, Wang S. The long noncoding RNA SNHG1 regulates colorectal cancer cell growth through interactions with EZH2 and miR-154-5p. Mol Cancer. 2018;17(1):141.
90. Wilusz JE, Sunwoo H, Spector DL. Long noncoding RNAs: functional surprises from the RNA world. Genes Dev. 2009;23(13):1494–504.
91. Mohammad F, Pandey RR, Nagano T, Chakalova L, Mondal T, Fraser P, Kanduri C. Kcnq1ot1/Lit1 noncoding RNA mediates transcriptional silencing by targeting to the perinucleolar region. Mol Cell Biol. 2008;28(11):3713–28.
92. Ma C, Luo H, Liu B, Li F, Tschope C, Fa X. Long noncoding RNAs: a new player in the prevention and treatment of diabetic cardiomyopathy? Diabetes Metab Res Rev. 2018;34(8):e3056.
93. Gao L, Wang X, Guo S, Xiao L, Liang C, Wang Z, Li Y, Liu Y, Yao R, Liu Y, Zhang Y. LncRNA HOTAIR functions as a competing endogenous RNA to upregulate SIRT1 by sponging miR-34a in diabetic cardiomyopathy. J Cell Physiol. 2019;234(4):4944–58.
94. Liu R, Li X, Zhu W, Wang Y, Zhao D, Wang X, Gurley EC, Liang G, Chen W, Lai G, Pandak WM, Lippman HR, Bajaj JS, Hylemon PB, Zhou H. Cholangiocyte-derived exosomal LncRNA H19 promotes hepatic stellate cell activation and cholestatic liver fibrosis. Hepatology. 2019;70(4):1317–35.
95. Tarnowski M, Tkacz M, Czerewaty M, Poniewierska-Baran A, Grymula K, Ratajczak MZ. 5Azacytidine inhibits human rhabdomyosarcoma cell growth by downregulating insulinlike growth factor 2 expression and reactivating the H19 gene product miR675, which negatively affects insulinlike growth factors and insulin signaling. Int J Oncol. 2015;46(5):2241–50.
96. Ding GL, Wang FF, Shu J, Tian S, Jiang Y, Zhang D, Wang N, Luo Q, Zhang Y, Jin F, Leung PC, Sheng JZ, Huang HF. Transgenerational glucose intolerance with Igf2/H19 epigenetic alterations in mouse islet induced by intrauterine hyperglycemia. Diabetes. 2012;61(5):1133–42.
97. Li X, Wang H, Yao B, Xu W, Chen J, Zhou X. lncRNA H19/miR-675 axis regulates cardiomyocyte apoptosis by targeting VDAC1 in diabetic cardiomyopathy. Sci Rep. 2016;6:36340.

98. Zhuo C, Jiang R, Lin X, Shao M. LncRNA H19 inhibits autophagy by epigenetically silencing of DIRAS3 in diabetic cardiomyopathy. Oncotarget. 2017;8(1):1429–37.
99. Zhang M, Gu H, Xu W, Zhou X. Down-regulation of lncRNA MALAT1 reduces cardiomyocyte apoptosis and improves left ventricular function in diabetic rats. Int J Cardiol. 2016;203:214–6.
100. Zhang M, Gu H, Chen J, Zhou X. Involvement of long noncoding RNA MALAT1 in the pathogenesis of diabetic cardiomyopathy. Int J Cardiol. 2016;202:753–5.
101. Bacci L, Barbati SA, Colussi C, Aiello A, Isidori AM, Grassi C, Pontecorvi A, Farsetti A, Gaetano C, Nanni S. Sildenafil normalizes MALAT1 level in diabetic cardiomyopathy. Endocr Rev. 2018;62(1):259–62.
102. Zhou X, Zhang W, Jin M, Chen J, Xu W, Kong X. lncRNA MIAT functions as a competing endogenous RNA to upregulate DAPK2 by sponging miR-22-3p in diabetic cardiomyopathy. Cell Death Dis. 2017;8(7):e2929.
103. Yang F, Qin Y, Wang Y, Li A, Lv J, Sun X, Che H, Han T, Meng S, Bai Y, Wang L. LncRNA KCNQ1OT1 mediates Pyroptosis in diabetic cardiomyopathy. Cell Physiol Biochem. 2018;50(4):1230–44.
104. Qu X, Du Y, Shu Y, Gao M, Sun F, Luo S, Yang T, Zhan L, Yuan Y, Chu W, Pan Z, Wang Z, Yang B, Lu Y. MIAT is a pro-fibrotic Long non-coding RNA governing cardiac fibrosis in post-infarct myocardium. Sci Rep. 2017;7:42657.
105. Chen Z, Li C, Lin K, Cai H, Ruan W, Han J, Rao L. Non-coding RNAs in cardiac fibrosis: emerging biomarkers and therapeutic targets. Am J Cardiol. 2018;25(6):732–41.
106. Zheng D, Zhang Y, Hu Y, Guan J, Xu L, Xiao W, Zhong Q, Ren C, Lu J, Liang J, Hou J. Long noncoding RNA Crnde attenuates cardiac fibrosis via Smad3-Crnde negative feedback in diabetic cardiomyopathy. FEBS J. 2019;286(9):1645–55.
107. de Gonzalo-Calvo D, Kenneweg F, Bang C, Toro R, van der Meer RW, Rijzewijk LJ, Smit JW, Lamb HJ, Llorente-Cortes V, Thum T. Circulating long-non coding RNAs as biomarkers of left ventricular diastolic function and remodelling in patients with well-controlled type 2 diabetes. Sci Rep. 2016;6:37354.
108. Hsu MT, Coca-Prados M. Electron microscopic evidence for the circular form of RNA in the cytoplasm of eukaryotic cells. Nature. 1979;280(5720):339–40.
109. Wang K, Long B, Liu F, Wang JX, Liu CY, Zhao B, Zhou LY, Sun T, Wang M, Yu T, Gong Y, Liu J, Dong YH, Li N, Li PF. A circular RNA protects the heart from pathological hypertrophy and heart failure by targeting miR-223. Eur Heart J. 2016;37(33):2602–11.
110. Gomes CPC, Salgado-Somoza A, Creemers EE, Dieterich C, Lustrek M, Devaux Y, Cardiolinc network. Circular RNAs in the cardiovascular system. Noncoding RNA Res. 2018;3(1):1–11.
111. Leonska-Duniec A, Jastrzebski Z, Zarebska A, Maciejewska A, Ficek K, Cieszczyk P. Assessing effect of interaction between the FTO A/T polymorphism (rs9939609) and physical activity on obesity-related traits. J Sport Health Sci. 2018;7(4):459–64.
112. Mahdavi R, Ghorbani S, Alipoor B, Panahi G, Khodabandehloo H, Esfahani EN, Razi F, Meshkani R. Decreased serum level of miR-155 is associated with obesity and its related metabolic traits. Clin Lab Med. 2018;64(1):77–84.
113. Bacci M, Giannoni E, Fearns A, Ribas R, Gao Q, Taddei ML, Pintus G, Dowsett M, Isacke CM, Martin LA, Chiarugi P, Morandi A. miR-155 drives metabolic reprogramming of ER+ breast Cancer cells following Long-term Estrogen deprivation and predicts clinical response to aromatase inhibitors. Cancer Res. 2016;76(6):1615–26.
114. Lauressergues D, Couzigou JM, Clemente HS, Martinez Y, Dunand C, Becard G, Combier JP. Primary transcripts of microRNAs encode regulatory peptides. Nature. 2015;520(7545):90–3.
115. Yang Y, Fan X, Mao M, Song X, Wu P, Zhang Y, Jin Y, Yang Y, Chen LL, Wang Y, Wong CC, Xiao X, Wang Z. Extensive translation of circular RNAs driven by N(6)-methyladenosine. Cell Res. 2017;27(5):626–41.
116. Liu CX, Li X, Nan F, Jiang S, Gao X, Guo SK, Xue W, Cui Y, Dong K, Ding H, Qu B, Zhou Z, Shen N, Yang L, Chen LL. Structure and degradation of circular RNAs regulate PKR activation in innate immunity. Cell. 2019;177(4):865–80.

11 Comprehensive Overview of Non-coding RNAs in Cardiac Development

Enrico Pozzo, Yoke Chin Chai, and Maurilio Sampaolesi

Abstract

Cardiac development in the human embryo is characterized by the interactions of several transcription and growth factors leading the heart from a primordial linear tube into a synchronous contractile four-chamber organ. Studies on cardiogenesis showed that cell proliferation, differentiation, fate specification and morphogenesis are spatiotemporally coordinated by cell-cell interactions and intracellular signalling cross-talks. In recent years, research has focused on a class of inter- and intra-cellular modulators called non-coding RNAs (ncRNAs), transcribed from the non-coding portion of the DNA and involved in the proper formation of the heart. In this chapter, we will summarize the current state of the art on the roles of three major forms of ncRNAs [microRNAs (miRNAs), long ncRNAs (lncRNAs) and circular RNAs (circRNAs)] in orchestrating the four sequential phases of cardiac organogenesis.

Keywords

lncRNAs · miRNAs · circRNAs · Cardiac development · Embryology

Abbreviations

circRNAs	circular RNAs
CS	Carnegie Stage
dpc	days post coitum
ESCs	embryonal stem cells
FHF	first heart field
lncRNAs	long non-coding RNAs
miRNAs	microRNAs
ncRNAs	non-coding RNAs
RNA-seq	RNA sequencing
SHF	secondary heart field

1 Background

Successful development of the embryonic heart sees the cardiac progenitor cells proliferate and differentiate into beating cardiomyocytes (CMs). Cardiac organogenesis requires exquisite modulation of gene expression, and transcriptional

E. Pozzo · Y. C. Chai
Translational Cardiomyology Laboratory, Stem Cell Research Institute, Stem Cell Biology and Embryology Unit, Department of Development and Regeneration, KU Leuven, Leuven, Belgium

M. Sampaolesi (✉)
Translational Cardiomyology Laboratory, Stem Cell Research Institute, Stem Cell Biology and Embryology Unit, Department of Development and Regeneration, KU Leuven, Leuven, Belgium

Human Anatomy Unit, Department of Public Health, Experimental and Forensic Medicine, University of Pavia, Pavia, Italy
e-mail: maurilio.sampaolesi@kuleuven.be

J. Xiao (ed.), *Non-coding RNAs in Cardiovascular Diseases*, Advances in Experimental Medicine and Biology 1229, https://doi.org/10.1007/978-981-15-1671-9_11

dysregulation in this process underpins congenital heart diseases. Most of the literature to be discussed in this chapter will mainly focus on murine studies, as heart development has been mainly investigated using transgenic mouse models. From a clinical standpoint, a comparison between mouse and human cardiac development by means of episcopic fluorescence image capture revealed the relevance of this model, as the cellular events leading to the formation of the heart are comparable in both mammals.

The early stage embryo is a disc formed by the three sheets of ectoderm, mesoderm and endoderm known as the three germ layers. The tissues forming the heart mainly come from the mesoderm germ layer. However, some of the cells migrate from the ectoderm and form the cardiac neural crest cells. The latter will participate in the septation of the cardiac outflow tract into aorta and pulmonary artery, remodel the pharyngeal arch arteries, develop the valves, and take part in the formation of the cardiac conduction system.

The phases of cardiac development in human and mouse have different timings, as summarized in Fig. 11.1. Following gastrulation, the heart muscle cells start developing from a pool of mesodermal cardiac precursor cells found in the anterior lateral plate of the embryonic mesoderm. These progenitors will then migrate to the cranial and cranio-lateral regions of the developing embryo. The subsequent phases of cardiac development can be divided into the following key steps, which warrant the correct formation and maturation of the three-dimensional structures of the heart: cardiac crescent (CS8), linear heart tube (CS9), cardiac looping (CS10), chamber formation (CS11-19), and maturation (CS20-birth).

In order to regulate the fate of the several progenitor cells to eventually form the heart, noncoding RNAs (ncRNAs) have been recognized to play a fundamental role in cardiac development and pathologies [1, 2], thanks to recent technological advances in sequencing and computational algorithms. Additionally, the discovery of ncRNAs has also expanded the functional complexity of transcriptome, adding new molecular dimension to temporal regulation, cellular and

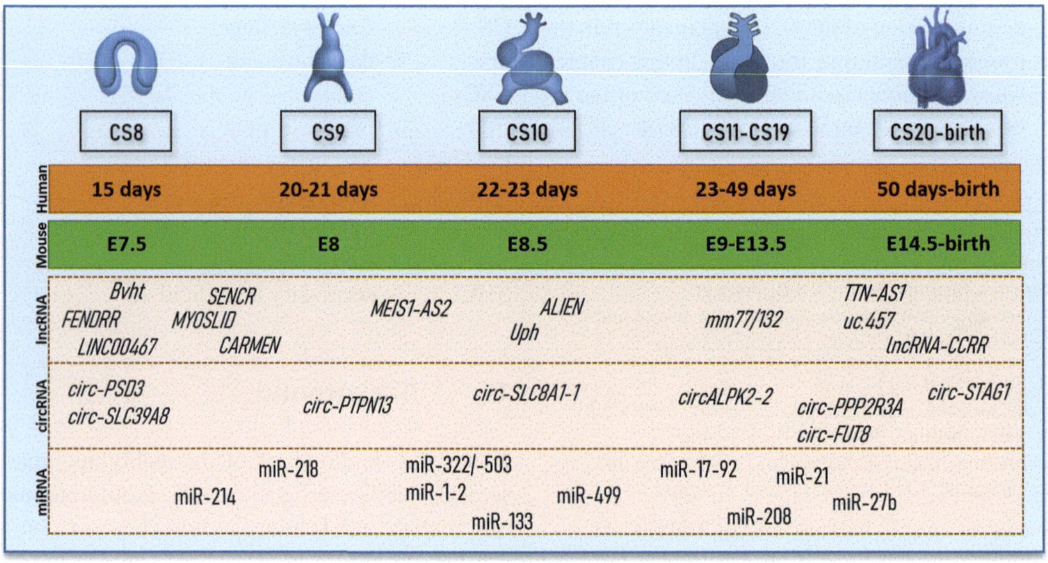

Fig. 11.1 The interactions among miRNAs, lncRNAs and circRNAs during cardiac development: Cardiac crescent (CS8), linear heart tube (CS9), cardiac looping (CS10), chamber formation (CS11–19), and maturation (CS20-birth)

tissue specificities and functional diversity in heart organogenesis [3, 4]. At genetic level, ncRNAs modulate gene expression patterns by interrogating transcription, chromatin modification and post-transcriptional alterations [2]. First referred to as the 'junk DNA', a large part of the non-coding portion of the human genome (up to 90%) has now been proven to be actively transcribed into several types of ncRNAs which hold several biological functions throughout prenatal development and post-natal life [5, 6]. Based on the molecular length and function, three main categories of ncRNAs have been identified: long ncRNAs (lncRNAs; longer than 200 nucleotides), microRNAs (miRNAs; maximum 22 nucleotides long), and circular RNAs (circRNAs; formed by 1-5 exons).

The widest subgroup of ncRNAs consists of lncRNAs [7], mostly transcribed by RNA polymerase II, which causes them to undergo capping at 5′ end and polyadenylation at 3′ end. lncRNAs have a limited to absent protein-coding potential due to the lack of open reading frames. LncRNAs appeared to be critical regulators of gene expression in both transcription and post-transcription gene regulation events, with the majority of them exhibiting developmental stage-specific regulation paralleling mRNA expression patterns [8]. They can act either in *cis*, in order to regulate the nearby genes, or in *trans*, which let them modulate the expression of the target genes by means of several mechanisms. These mechanisms include: DNA looping, recruiting chromatin modifiers and transcription factors, miRNA sponges, and influencing mRNA splicing, translation or degradation. Through genome-wide RNA sequencing, more than 100 annotated and newly described IncRNAs have been defined in the cardiac differentiation and maturation signatures [9]. Nevertheless, the exact transcriptomic profiling and roles of lncRNAs during heart development (i.e. CMs differentiation, heart wall development, cardiac chamber and outflow tract formation, and cardiac cell electricphysiology and conduction) have not yet been detailed.

The mechanism of gene expression regulation by miRNAs, on the other hand, is at the post-transcriptional level, with silencing of genes that occurs via targeting the protein-coding and non-coding genes. Following synthesis of pri-miRNAs by RNA polymerase II and III in the nucleus, the microprocessor complex Drosha-Dgcr8 cleaves the pri-miRNAs into pre-miRNAs. These are then transported into the cytosol, where the Dicer-TRBP complex cleaves pre-miRNAs to form the mature 22 nucleotide-long miRNA molecules. Here, miRNAs will go through the RNA-induced silencing complex, formed by the Argonaute proteins, which guides the miRNAs towards the target mRNA for its degradation [10, 11]. The fundamental role played by miRNAs in cardiac development was proved by Dicer knock-down in murine ESCs which, among other effects, led to cardiac development defects [12].

circRNAs are single-stranded circular RNAs predominantly found in the cytoplasm. Thanks to the absence of 5′ and 3′ ends, they have a more stable structure making them more resistant to the exonuclease-mediated degradation to which the other ncRNAs undergo. Based on the derivation sources, circRNAs can be categorized into: (1) circRNA derived from exons (ecircRNA; the most abundant form of circRNAs), (2) circRNA derived from lariat introns (ciRNA), and (3) circRNA derived from exons wih retained introns (ElciRNA) [13–15]. circRNA length ranges between 100–1000 bases and, although their abundance is relatively low, some are expressed at higher levels compared to their linear transcripts. Although circRNAs are ubiquitously expressed, they accumulate in fully differentiated somatic cells while being quite diluted in proliferating cells including tumour cells. Mechanistically, it has been shown that circRNAs can act as miRNA sponges to counteract the inhibition induced by the latter. Indeed, the phenotype induced by gain and loss of function esperiments in zebrafish indicated that a specific circRNA could have functions beyond sequestering specific miRNAs [16]. As a single-stranded

RNA, circRNAs can bind the trans 3' UTRs of target mRNAs to concur in gene expression regulation. In addition, circRNAs can be involved in the regulation of RNA-binding proteins [17]. Compared to lncRNAs and miRNAs, however, the functions of thousands of described circRNAs remain limited. Interestingly, based on deep RNA sequencing analysis, the top-expressed circRNAs in the human heart were associated with cardiac- or skeletal muscle genes including TTN, RYR2 and DMD [18].

Since ncRNAs regulators have only been recently related to cardiac development and disease, a detailed understanding on the expression dynamic of these ncRNAs during each stages of the embryonic heart development is quintessential. Thus, in this chapter we will summarize the roles that ncRNAs play in the development of the heart.

2 From Cardiac Crescent to Looping Heart Tube: The Role of ncRNAs

In the early stages of development, the cardiac precursor cell population is found in the two symmetrical sides of the lateral plate mesoderm of the flat tri-laminar disc. At CS8 (human 15–20 days, mouse E7.5), the lateral plate gets divided by the intraembryonic coelom in two layers, i.e. the somatic and the splanchnic mesoderm. Once the two sides start merging, the splanchnic mesoderm merges cranially and forms a horseshoe-shaped field named the cardiac crescent. The cells that form the cardiac crescent are termed the first heart field (FHF) and will contribute to the left ventricle and atrioventricular canal [19]. At the medial sides of the cardiac crescent processes, a separate population of cells forms the second heart field (SHF) which will contribute to the outflow tract myocardium, right ventricle and both atria. Cells derived from the FHF will first fuse at the midline to form the linear heart tube at CS9, after which SHF cells will add to the heart tube and increase it in size. Subsequently, the heart tube loops at CS10 [20].

Several genes are expressed in the committed mesodermal cells towards cardiac lineage. The earliest genes involved in commitment of embryonic stem cells (ESCs) towards cardiac mesoderm are the transcription factor *Brachyury* and *eomesodermin* (*Eomes*). Both *Brachyury* and *Eomes* are critical for the primitive streak patterning and the mesendoderm specification in the early embryo. In particular, *Eomes* is the key transcription factor required for the formation of either endoderm or cardiovascular mesoderm according to a high or low level of Activin, respectively. Following commitment to mesoderm, *Eomes* will then induce the expression of *Mesp1* [21], which will eventually start the cardiovascular differentiation [22].

Several ncRNAs collaborate with *Eomes* in the early commitment of ESCs towards cardiac mesoderm. For instance, the exon 2 of lncRNA *linc1405* was shown to co-localize with *Eomes* in the primitive streak and played a major role in the activation of *Mesp1*-mediated cardiac mesoderm specification of ESCs [23]. The lncRNA *Fendrr* (ENSMUSG00000097336) was shown to be expressed in *EOMES*-positive cells at E6.5-7, with its loss resulted in embryonic lethality in mice [24]. Finally, it has been reported that other lncRNAs and circRNAs are either transcriptionally regulated (*LINC00467*) or co-expressed (*RP3428L16.2*, *RP11829H16.3*; *circPSD3*, *circSLC39A8*, *circALMS1*) with *EOMES* in human cardiac progenitors [25].

Mesp1-expressing cells contribute to FHF and SHF derivatives, which will eventually give rise to the three main compartments of the heart, i.e. cardiac muscle (made by CMs), vessels (endothelial cells) and epicardium [26, 27]. Downstream of *Mesp1*, the FHF expresses the transcription factors *Nkx2.5, Hand1* and *Tbx5* [28, 29], while SHF expresses *Nkx2.5, Gata4/6, Hand2*, *Tbx1/2*, *Mef2c* and *Isl1* [30–36].

Upon fusion at the midline of the cell populations derived from the FHF, the heart tube forms

(CS9, mouse E8, human day 21), and CMs arrest the proliferation process. SHF precursor cells simultaneously migrate from the pericardium to the heart tube at the venous and arterial poles [36]. As they are mediated by WNT/β-catenin signaling [37], they proliferate at high rates and thus contribute to the heart tube's growth. During their addition to the heart tube, the SHF-derived CMs temporarily stop proliferating. Noncanonical WNT and Notch signaling also regulate differentiation during second heart field deployment [38, 39].

For the expression of *Mesp1*, the downregulation of miR-142-3p during ESC differentiation is required. Conversely, *Mesp1* activates the miR-322/-503 cluster during the heart looping [40]. In mice, the lncRNA *Braveheart* (*Bvht*, AK143260) is required to induce *Mesp1*, and the depletion of *Bvht* in mouse ESCs impairs the formation of CMs. Intriguingly, to date the transcript of *Bvht* has not yet been identified in human. Conversely, the lncRNA *Carmen* was seen to be conserved from mouse to human, and its expression is induced between the mesodermal and cardiac progenitor stage. Similar to *Bvht*, depletion of *Carmen* was associated with a significant reduction in the expression of differentiation makers and cardiac transcription factors, including NKX2.5, TBX5, GATA4, MYH6, MYH7, and TNNI [41]. Moreover, the expression of the master cardiac transcription factor – Nkx2.5 was modulated by novlnc6 which influenced the expression of BMP10 (a key signaling ligand for cardiogenesis during embryonic stem cell cardiac differentiation) [42].

Mesp2 has redundant functions compensating for *Mesp1* upon knock-out of the latter [43, 44]. However, *Mesp1* plays a major role in the motility of progenitors required for the correct cell migration and cardiac development [45]. A group of ncRNAs were reported to be co-expressed with *MESP2* in the early cardiac mesoderm (*circPSD3*; *RP11445F12.1*, *RP11445F12.2*, *RP3428L16.2*, *LINC00467*) [25].

The T-box family genes start being expressed in the FHF and SHF. In the FHF, *Tbx5* expression is modulated by miR-218 family, with the over-expression of *Tbx5* affecting heart development in both humans and mice, resulting in heart chamber abnormalities and heart-looping defects [46]. Intriguingly, the ectopic expression of *Gata4* and *Tbx5*, combined with chromatin remodeling component Baf60c/Smarcd3, was shown to induce beating myocardium in mesoderm [47]. Conversely, in the SHF TBX1 interferes with BMP signaling cascade components and has a negative regulatory effect on *Mef2c* transcript and SRF protein levels [48–50]. The subsequent differentiation of the myocardium at the arterial pole of the heart tube is reinforced by BMP which drives the miRNA 17-92-mediated repression of *Isl1* and *Tbx1* [25]. Repression of *Tbx1* during heart maturation is of utmost importance, as its overexpression leads to *Gata4* and *Mef2c* downregulation with subsequent blockage of the cardiac differentiation pathway [51]. This finding is corroborated by the required upregulation of MEF2C during induction of cardiac differentiation of the human embryonic stem cells which was found to be modulated via overexpression of miRNA-499 and miRNA-1 [52].

SHF and neural crest cells involved in cardiac development are characterized by the expression of *Isl1* [53, 54] although it has been shown to be transiently expressed in FHF cells as well, albeit with no related function [33, 55]. A group of ncRNAs were shown to be co-expressed (*MEIS1-AS2; circ-PTPN13, circ-ENC1, circ-PPP2R3A, circ-FUT8*) or transcriptionally regulated (*LINC01021, AC009518.4*) with *ISL1* in human cardiac progenitors [25, 55]. *ISL1* is targeted by miR-17-92 to promote differentiation of the myocardium at the arterial pole in the final stages of maturation [51]. Finally, the expression of HAND2 – critical for ventricular CMs expansion – is initially discovered in the cardiac crescent at E7.75 and will continue throughout the linear heart tube at E8.5. It has been recently shown that the lncRNA Uph (also named Hand2as or lncHand2), playing critical roles in the regulation of the precise expression of HAND2, together with miR-1-2 family in looping heart, to eventually lead to chamber formation [56, 57].

Myocardin (*Myocd*) is a master regulator of the smooth muscle cell phenotype. It is expressed in cardiac crescent and it coactivates several factors including *Gata4, Tbx5,* serum response factor (*Srf*) – which regulates BMP10 in cardiac maturation – and MEF2 [58, 59]. MYOCD is activated by lncRNAs MYOSLID [60] and SENCR, although the latter has an indirect influence on it. In mice, *mm67* and *mm85* have been shown to activate *Myocd*. In subsequent stages, *Myocd* is shown to be modulated by miR-1 [61], and miR-214 has been shown to indirectly regulate its expression [62, 63]. *Myocardin* is required for CMs survival and heart function maintenance after birth [64]. Finally, for the correct formation of heart and vessels the lncRNA ALIEN was identified in mesendodermal tissues between cardiac crescent and heart tube [3].

In the looping heart, miR-1-2 family targets NOTCH ligands, HDAC4, Hand2, MEF2 and SRF to eventually allow the progenitor cells to proliferate and differentiate. The miR-1/133a cluster is positively regulated by *Myocd*, which aids in the specification of immature embryonic CMs into fetal ones [61, 65]. miR-1 is polycistronically clustered on the same chromosome with miR-133, however they have different – and sometimes opposing – effects during cardiac differentiation. The deletion of miR-133a genes led to ventricular septal defects and abnormal cardiomyocytic proliferation which eventually leading to neonatal death [66]. However, its overexpression in mouse and human ESCs caused the repression of cardiac markers [67, 68].

Another miRNA involved in the looping of the heart is miR-499, encoded by Myh7b. In vitro, its overexpression was shown to speed up the beating embryoid bodies formation while its inhibition blocked cardiac differentiation [65].

During cardiac differentiation, several circRNAs were seen to be overexpressed. *Circ-SLC8A1-1* is expressed from the gene *NCX1* (Na^{+}/Ca^{++} exchanger, also known as *SLC8A1*) during CMs differentiation in hESC and mouse [69]. In a study comparing human, mice and rat hearts, circSLC8A1-1 was shown to be the most abundant circRNA in the hearts [70]. Intriguingly, upregulation of *circ-SLC8A1* was observed in the DCM [71]. Other reported circRNAs during cardiac differentiation include *circ-TTN-90, circ-TTN-275, circ-TPM1-1, circ-HIPK3-2, circ-EXOC6B-14, circ-MB-2, circ-ALPK2-2, circ-MYBPC3-3, circ-NEBL-19* and *circ-RYR2-113* in hESC differentiating towards CMs [18]. On the contrary, the *circr-Foxo3* was found to interact with multiple stress- and senescence-related factors (e.g. ID-1, E2F1 and FAK), which was highly associated with heart samples from both aged patients and mice [72].

3 Chamber Formation and the Final Phases of Heart Maturation

It is perceivable that heart being a mechanical pump requires three-dimensionality (in term of chambers, valves, septation and blood vessels) to fullfil its biological functions, and cardiac function dictates its form to a large extent. Hence, the formation and maturation of the heart structure are highly associated with the contractile force and hemodynamic demands towards the systemic circulation, in addition to influences by other factors such as oxygen gradient and nutrient enviroment. In the final stages of heart formation, the major contribution in cardiac growth comes from the intracardiac myocardial cells. In particular, the ventricular and atrial myocardium arises from the outer curvature of the heart, whereas the cardiac cushion develops from the endocardium beneath the atrioventricular canals and outflow tract myocardium [73].

Many transcriptional regulation in organogenesis involve members of the ancient family of T-box transcription factors, including the specification of cardiac chambers and the conduction system [74]. Herein, the T-box activators and repressors work together for the cardiac ballooning by inducing cardiac cushions (TBX2 and TBX3) limited to the atrioventricular canal (TBX20 and TBX5). Several circRNAs have been seen to co-express with TBX5, including *circ-HIPK3*, *circ-PLOD2_1*, *circ-RHOBTB3*, *circ-PSMB1*, *circ-SLC8A1_1* and *circ-MYH6/7_1*. Similarly, the expression of TBX2 was seen to co-express with several lncRNAs and circRNAs, including TTN-AS1, RP11-617F23.1, *circ-PHKB_1*, *circ-HIPK3*, *circ-SLC8A1_1*, *circ-MYH6/7_1* and *circ-PALM2* [25]. Cells that are originating from TBX2-expressing prognitors will contribute to right and left ventricular walls [19], and the repressive interaction of *Tbx20* upstream of *Tbx2* underlie the primary lineage specification to chamber and non-chamber myocardium, thereby determining heart integrity and contractile function [75]. Moreover, the chamber formation is also mediated by the expression of several key regulators, including *Gata4*, *Nkx2.5*, *Tbx5*, *dHand*, *eHand*, *Pitx2*, *MEF2C*, and *Irx4* [76]. Intriguingly, analysis of paired human atrial and ventricular samples revealed that 17–28% of the total lncRNA transcripts were differentially regulated in the four chambers, vastly attributed to their distinctive roles in cardiac functions [77]. The lncRNA uc.457 has also been associated with ventricular septal defect in human, and was recently revealed to regulate proliferation and differentiation of CMs by inhibiting the protein expression of histone cell cycle regulation defective homolog a, cardiac muscle troponin T, natriuretic peptide A and mef2C, respectively [78].

Chamber-specific expression of miRNA signatures in human heart has also been reported recently [79]. By performing miRNA deep sequencing, Kakimoto Y et al. revealed that the miRNA-1 was the most abundant in both atrial (21%) and ventricular (26%) chambers, and the miRNA-208 family showed prominent chamber specificity in the atrial (miRNA-208b-3p and miRNA-208a-3p) and ventricle (miRNA-208-3p and miRNA-208b-5p). In zebrafish, it has been shown that the miRNA-143-adducin3 is essential for chamber morphogenesis through direct inhibition of adducin3 which encodes an F-actin capping protein. Disruption of this miRNA led to ventricular collapse and decreased contractility [80]. The miRNA-138 is another molecule that is required to establish appropriate gene expression restricted to the atrio-ventricular valve region, and its dysregulation caused abnormal ventricular formation [81]. For cardiac valvulogenesis, Kopla HJ et al. reported that the miRNA-21 was necessary for proper development of the atrioventricular valve by repressing the tumor suppressor programmed cell death 4 (PDCD4b) expression, since miRNA-21 expression is known to be restricted to valvular endothelium and implicated in the response to several forms of cardiac stress [82].

During perinatal transition of heart, maturation of the cardiac tissue is required to warrant functional adaptation of the changes in nutrient environment and hemodynamic load after birth. The maturation and final septation of the heart requires, together with *Gata4*, *Nkx2-5* and *Tbx5*, the expression of *RxRa*, *FOG-2*, *Pitx2*, *Sox4*, *NF-Atc*, *TEF-1*, *Tbx1*, *Hey2*, *CITED*, and *ZIC3* [76]. At the cellular level, majority of CMs undergo dramatic changes in the morphology, proliferation, gene expression and metabolism. Therefore, any abberant transcriptional pertubation occur at this stage often lead to congenital heart defects. In fact, during CM maturation many lncRNAs are strictly regulated by maturation stage-specific transcription factors. For instances, it has been reported that approximately 70% of the lncRNAs that were highly expressed at CM maturation stage could bind to *NFAT* – an important CM maturation regulator when coupled with calcineurin [25]. Abnormal *NFAT* signaling causes pathological cardiac hypertrophy and heart failure. Of all lncRNAs, 90% of them are enriched for the *MEIS1* motif which has been implicated in heart development [83].

Furthermore, a recent study reported a high-resolution landscape on neonatal cardiac lncRNAs interactions with neighboring transcriptomic molecules during cardiac maturation and postnatal stress in murine [8]. Specifically, the study revealed the *Ppp1r1b-lncRNA* as a regulator of its partner gene *Tcap* which encodes the muscle protein titin and the expression ratio of *Ppp1r1b-lncRNA/Tcap* could be used as a molecular signature for ventricular septum defect in human infantile hearts. Impuls conduction through the heart is the fundamental phenomenon of a synchronized muscle fiber contraction, proper transcriptional regulation of muscle fiber assembly and maturation is of quintessential. In this context, the cardiac conduction regulatory RNA (lncRNA-CCRR) was found to control cardiac conduction by promoting binding of connexin43 to the interacting protein CIP85. Silencing or knockdown lncRNA-CCRR causes malformation of intercalated discs and gap junctions that slow longitudinal cardiac conduction [84]. Other examples of lncRNAs that regulates CMs proliferation, differentiation and maturation includes uc. 40, uc.167, uc.245 and TUC40 [85–88].

In term of miRNA modulation, miRNA-27b has been reported to play critical roles in skeletal muscle development [89], and it is robustly expressed within the myocardium in the adult heart [90]. Via microarray analysis, Chinchilla A et al. found that relatively few miRNAs display discrete peak of decreasing or increasing expression profiles during ventricular maturation. In particular, the miRNA-27b (an early stage marker of ventricular chamber formation) displays an overt myocardial expression during cardiogenesis, and it regulates the cardiac myogenesis transcription factor – *Mef2c* without disturbing the expression of other cardiac genes [91]. This specific role of miRNA-27b on *Mef2c* suggests potential therapeutic for cardiac hypertrophy. Interestingly, the miRNA-27a exhibited a strongly upregulatory role on the *β-MHC* gene by targeting the thyroid hormone receptor β1 (TRβ1) in ventricular CMs [92]. The miRNA-143 plays an essential role in mechanotransduction pathway, in particular on circulatory adaptation and regulation between the outflow tracts and ventricles by suppressing retinoic acid signaling [93]. Besides miRNA itself, the miRNA-processing enzyme Dicer also plays a critical role in promoting cardiac outflow tract aligment and chamber septation by upregulating the morphogen *Pitx2c* and *Sema3c*. Due to impairment of miRNA processing at later-stage, cardiac-specific Dicer deficiency mice exhibited misexpression of cardiac contractile proteins and rapidly developed dilated cardiomyopathy, heart failure and postnatal lethality [94]. Moreover, the miRNA-208a is reported as a novel modulator of cardiac hypertrophy and electrical conduction. Overexpression of miRNA-208a (which is encoded within an intron of α-cardiac muscle myosin heavy chain gene (Myh6)) in mice induced muscle hypertrophy and arrhythmias, whereas sufficient level of miRNA-208a expression was required for proper cardiac conduction and the expression of cardiac genes such as GATA4 and connexin 40 [95].

The miRNAs also play important roles in cardiac extracellular matrix remodeling. For instances, the miRNA-133 and miRNA-30 were reported to directly downregulate connective tissue growth factor (CTGF), which is a key molecule in maintaining proper extracellular matrix remodeling in myocardium [96]. Overexpression of these miRNAs resulted in low CTGF level accompanied by decreased production of collagen, whereas knocking down their expression causing cardiac fibrosis. Furthermore, in CMs derived from rats at 4 weeks, the miRNA-29a was found to be differentially upregulated which inversely regulated CMs proliferation by targeting to Cyclin D2 (CCND2) [97]. This finding suggest an inhibition role of miRNAs in CMs proliferation during postnatal development. The circRNAs play a critical role in cardiac cell specification from cardiac progenitor cells to CMs. It is reported that nearly 500 and 200 circRNAs were positively (e.g. *circ-SLC8A1-1*, *circ-TTN-275*, and *circ-ALPK2-1*) and negatively (e.g. *circ-DNMT3B-4*, *circ-OSBPL10* and *circ-FGD4-7*) correlated to the differentiation of human embryonic stem cells to CMs [13, 18]. Of interest, the *circ-TTN* was differentially expressed in neonatal and adult rat hearts [70] and revealed to be co-expressed with MYL4 – mutation of which leads to abberant sarcomere formation, atrial enlargement and fibrillation [98]. By circRNA profiling, *circ-TTN* expression was dynamically regulated in mice with dilated cardiomyopathy, and largely downregulated in mice lacking the RNA-binding motif protein 20 (RBM20), suggesting a novel mechanistic insights for diated cardiomyopathy [99]. Expression of other circRNAs, such as *circ-SLC8A1*, *circ-CHD7*, *circ-ATXN10* and *circ-DNAJC6* was also found to be prominent in patients with dilated cardiomyopathy [100].

4 Future Perspectives

ncRNAs have gained interest in the past decades due to their role in modulating cell fate at a post-transcriptional level. The modulation occurring in the prenatal life at the embryo level helps us shedding a light on the tuning required for the proper formation of the heart and the other organs. More importantly, it gives us the possibility to better understand how congenital heart diseases occur.

Potentially, ncRNAs could be used both for diagnostic and therapeutic purposes. In this view, the fact that circRNA concentration profiles change during cardiac development and disease independently from their host gene expression, they represent novel and more stable biological markers. Although they are still at their infancy, artificial circRNAs similarly to miRNA mimics and antagomirs could represent promising tools in regenerative medicine since they are highly stable and can regulate a wide range of cellular functions. Recent studies have highlighted the extensive network of interactions among microRNAs, lncRNAs and circRNAs, forming crucial regulatory axis participating in the modulation of cardiac differentiation [101].

In order to obtain mature CMs from induced pluripotent stem cells (iPSCs), Miyamoto has recently shown that the use of *Gata4-Mef2c-Tbx5*, or GMT, led to the correct formation of cardiac cells [102, 103]. Emerging literature is showing the cardiac differentiation potential of PSCs but also the limitations to generate fully mature CMs to model cardiac diseases or for drug screening porpuses. Specific ncRNAs control and promote the differentiation of PSCs and mesodermal progenitors into CMs and the use of microvesicles to transfer those peculiar ncRNAs is a fascinating possibility to better coordinate cardiogenic maturation of healthy and pathological progenitor cells. This will be critical to better understand the role of ncRNAs in the regulation of cardiovascular system development and eventually in the progression of cardiovascular disease.

World-leading laboratories are investing in gene editing, mainly in CRISPR/Cas9 technology, to edit efficiently any genomic locus with high DNA sequence specificity and possibly without undesired byproducts. However, CRISPR/Cas9 technology is still a very young gene-editing technology that can result in off-target effects with unexpected consequence and the long-term impact of genetic alteration on future generations is yet unknown. In addition, small indels generated by CRISPR/Cas9 system can alter or prevent functional modifications of ncRNAs or affect overlapping/adjacent genes in loci characterized by bidirectional promoters or sense/antisense genes (where lncRNAs are generated) [104]. Although a prudent path should be considered for CRISPR/Cas9-based *in vivo* applications, these novel gene editing approaches will allow us to perform more precise perturbation studies to uncover the basic principles of cardiac development and better collocate transcription factors, ncRNA networks and molecular pathways that contribute to CM maturation (Table 11.1).

Table 11.1 ncRNAs involved in cardiac development

	Cardiac Crescent	Linear heart tube	Looping heart tube	Chamber formation	Final maturation
Genes	EOMES, Mesp 1/2, Myocd	Hand1, Tbx5, Nkx2–5, Gata4/6,Hand2, Tbx1/2, Mef2c, Isl1	Nkx2–5, dHand, HAND2, Cspg2, FOG-2, BMP 2/4, TBX1, ISL, Mef2c, SRF	Nkx2–5, Tbx5, RXRα, FOG-2, SRF	GATA4, TEF-1, Hey2, Sox4, chek1, Myh7b, Thrap1, Myostatin, Myh6, Myh7
miRNAs	miR-142-3p (downregulate), miR-214	miR-218	miR-322/−503, miR-1-2, miR-133, miR-499	miR-17-92, miR-208	miR-21, miR-27b
lncRNAs	linc1405, Bvht, lncRNA-uc.167, RP11829H16.3, RP3428L16.2, LINC00467, FENDRR, mm67, mm85, MYOSLID, SENCR	CARMEN, LINC01021 AC009518.4, MEIS1-AS2	ALIEN, Uph	mm77/132	TTN-AS1, AC159540.1, AC007740.1, LINC00881, RP11-617F23.1, MIR133A1HG, CTD-2545 M3.8
circRNAs	circ-PSD3, circ-ALMS1, circ-SLC39A8	circ-PTPN13, circ-ENC1, circ-PPP2R3, circ-FUT8	circ-ALPK2–1, circ-SLC8A1–1, circ-TTN-275	circTPM1–1, circTTN-90, circTTN-275, circHIPK3–2, circEXOC6B-14, circALPK2–2, circMB-2, circNEBL-19, circMYBPC3–3 and circRYR2–113	circ-PPP2R3A, circ-FUT8, circ-ENC1, circ-PTPN13, circ-NEIL3, circ-DLG1, circ-STAG1, circ-ASH1L, circ-HIPK3, circ-PLOD2_1, circ-MAN1A2_1, circ-DDX26B_1, circ-RHOBTB3, circ-PSMB1, circ-SLC8A1_1, circ-SLC8A1_2, circ-MYH6/7_2, circ-TTN_1, circ-MYH6/7_1, circ-UNC45B, circ-GUCY1A3, circ-PALM2

Acknowledgements Funding: Fonds Wetenschappelijk Onderzoek (#G088715N and #G0D4517N to MS, #1S90718N to EP), CARIPLO Foundation #2015_0634 and C1-KUL 3DMUSYC (#C14/17/111) grants.

References

1. Mercer TR, Dinger ME, Mattick JS. Long non-coding RNAs: insights into functions. Nat Rev Genet. 2009;10(3):155–9.
2. Mercer TR, Mattick JS. Structure and function of long noncoding RNAs in epigenetic regulation. Nat Struct Mol Biol. 2013;20(3):300–7.
3. Kurian L, Aguirre A, Sancho-Martinez I, Benner C, Hishida T, Nguyen TB, Reddy P, Nivet E, Krause MN, Nelles DA, Esteban CR, Campistol JM, Yeo GW, Belmonte JCI. Identification of novel long non-coding RNAs underlying vertebrate cardiovascular development. Circulation. 2015;131(14):1278–90.
4. Matkovich SJ, Edwards JR, Grossenheider TC, de Guzman Strong C, Dorn GW 2nd. Epigenetic coordination of embryonic heart transcription by dynamically regulated long noncoding RNAs. Proc Natl Acad Sci U S A. 2014;111(33):12264–9.
5. Carninci P, Kasukawa T, Katayama S, Gough J, Frith MC, Maeda N, Oyama R, Ravasi T, Lenhard B, Wells C, Kodzius R, Shimokawa K, Bajic VB, Brenner SE, Batalov S, Forrest AR, Zavolan M, Davis MJ, Wilming LG, Aidinis V, Allen JE, Ambesi-Impiombato A, Apweiler R, Aturaliya RN, Bailey TL, Bansal M, Baxter L, Beisel KW, Bersano T, Bono H, Chalk AM, Chiu KP, Choudhary V, Christoffels A, Clutterbuck DR, Crowe ML, Dalla E, Dalrymple BP, de Bono B, Della Gatta G, di Bernardo D, Down T, Engstrom P, Fagiolini M, Faulkner G, Fletcher CF, Fukushima T, Furuno M, Futaki S, Gariboldi M, Georgii-Hemming P, Gingeras TR, Gojobori T, Green RE, Gustincich S, Harbers M, Hayashi Y, Hensch TK, Hirokawa N, Hill D, Huminiecki L, Iacono M, Ikeo K, Iwama A, Ishikawa T, Jakt M, Kanapin A, Katoh M, Kawasawa Y, Kelso J, Kitamura H, Kitano H, Kollias G, Krishnan SP, Kruger A, Kummerfeld SK, Kurochkin IV, Lareau LF, Lazarevic D, Lipovich L, Liu J, Liuni S, McWilliam S, Madan Babu M, Madera M, Marchionni L, Matsuda H, Matsuzawa S, Miki H, Mignone F, Miyake S, Morris K, Mottagui-Tabar S, Mulder N, Nakano N, Nakauchi H, Ng P, Nilsson R, Nishiguchi S, Nishikawa S, Nori F, Ohara O, Okazaki Y, Orlando V, Pang KC, Pavan WJ, Pavesi G, Pesole G, Petrovsky N, Piazza S, Reed J, Reid JF, Ring BZ, Ringwald M, Rost B, Ruan Y, Salzberg SL, Sandelin A, Schneider C, Schonbach C, Sekiguchi K, Semple CA, Seno S, Sessa L, Sheng Y, Shibata Y, Shimada H, Shimada K, Silva D, Sinclair B, Sperling S, Stupka E, Sugiura K, Sultana R, Takenaka Y, Taki K, Tammoja K, Tan SL, Tang S, Taylor MS, Tegner J, Teichmann SA, Ueda HR, van Nimwegen E, Verardo R, Wei CL, Yagi K, Yamanishi H, Zabarovsky E, Zhu S, Zimmer A, Hide W, Bult C, Grimmond SM, Teasdale RD, Liu ET, Brusic V, Quackenbush J, Wahlestedt C, Mattick JS, Hume DA, Kai C, Sasaki D, Tomaru Y, Fukuda S, Kanamori-Katayama M, Suzuki M, Aoki J, Arakawa T, Iida J, Imamura K, Itoh M, Kato T, Kawaji H, Kawagashira N, Kawashima T, Kojima M, Kondo S, Konno H, Nakano K, Ninomiya N, Nishio T, Okada M, Plessy C, Shibata K, Shiraki T, Suzuki S, Tagami M, Waki K, Watahiki A, Okamura-Oho Y, Suzuki H, Kawai J, Hayashizaki Y, Consortium F, Group RGER, Genome Science G. The transcriptional landscape of the mammalian genome. Science. 2005;309(5740):1559–63.
6. Kapranov P, Cheng J, Dike S, Nix DA, Duttagupta R, Willingham AT, Stadler PF, Hertel J, Hackermuller J, Hofacker IL, Bell I, Cheung E, Drenkow J, Dumais E, Patel S, Helt G, Ganesh M, Ghosh S, Piccolboni A, Sementchenko V, Tammana H, Gingeras TR. RNA maps reveal new RNA classes and a possible function for pervasive transcription. Science. 2007;316(5830):1484–8.
7. Scheuermann JC, Boyer LA. Getting to the heart of the matter: long non-coding RNAs in cardiac development and disease. EMBO J. 2013;32(13):1805–16.
8. Touma M, Kang X, Zhao Y, Cass AA, Gao F, Biniwale R, Coppola G, Xiao X, Reemtsen B, Wang Y. Decoding the long noncoding RNA during cardiac maturation: a roadmap for functional discovery. Circ Cardiovasc Genet. 2016;9(5):395–407.
9. Devaux Y, Zangrando J, Schroen B, Creemers EE, Pedrazzini T, Chang CP, Dorn GW 2nd, Thum T, Heymans S, Cardiolinc network. Long noncoding RNAs in cardiac development and ageing. Nat Rev Cardiol. 2015;12(7):415–25.
10. Rotini A, Martinez-Sarra E, Pozzo E, Sampaolesi M. Interactions between microRNAs and long non-coding RNAs in cardiac development and repair. Pharmacol Res. 2018;127:58–66.
11. Quattrocelli M, Sampaolesi M. The mesmiRizing complexity of microRNAs for striated muscle tissue engineering. Adv Drug Deliv Rev. 2015;88:37–52.
12. Zhao Y, Ransom JF, Li A, Vedantham V, von Drehle M, Muth AN, Tsuchihashi T, McManus MT, Schwartz RJ, Srivastava D. Dysregulation of cardiogenesis, cardiac conduction, and cell cycle in mice lacking miRNA-1-2. Cell. 2007;129(2):303–17.
13. Bei Y, Yang T, Wang L, Holvoet P, Das S, Sluijter JPG, Monteiro MC, Liu Y, Zhou Q, Xiao J. Circular RNAs as potential Theranostics in the cardiovascular system. Mol Ther Nucleic Acids. 2018;13:407–18.
14. Jeck WR, Sorrentino JA, Wang K, Slevin MK, Burd CE, Liu J, Marzluff WF, Sharpless NE. Circular RNAs are abundant, conserved, and associated with ALU repeats. RNA. 2013;19(2):141–57.
15. Li Z, Huang C, Bao C, Chen L, Lin M, Wang X, Zhong G, Yu B, Hu W, Dai L, Zhu P, Chang Z, Wu Q, Zhao Y, Jia Y, Xu P, Liu H, Shan G. Exon-intron

circular RNAs regulate transcription in the nucleus. Nat Struct Mol Biol. 2015;22(3):256–64.
16. Memczak S, Jens M, Elefsinioti A, Torti F, Krueger J, Rybak A, Maier L, Mackowiak SD, Gregersen LH, Munschauer M, Loewer A, Ziebold U, Landthaler M, Kocks C, le Noble F, Rajewsky N. Circular RNAs are a large class of animal RNAs with regulatory potency. Nature. 2013;495(7441):333–8.
17. Ashwal-Fluss R, Meyer M, Pamudurti NR, Ivanov A, Bartok O, Hanan M, Evantal N, Memczak S, Rajewsky N, Kadener S. circRNA biogenesis competes with pre-mRNA splicing. Mol Cell. 2014;56(1):55–66.
18. Tan WL, Lim BT, Anene-Nzelu CG, Ackers-Johnson M, Dashi A, See K, Tiang Z, Lee DP, Chua WW, Luu TD, Li PY, Richards AM, Foo RS. A landscape of circular RNA expression in the human heart. Cardiovasc Res. 2017;113(3):298–309.
19. Aanhaanen WT, Brons JF, Dominguez JN, Rana MS, Norden J, Airik R, Wakker V, de Gier-de Vries C, Brown NA, Kispert A, Moorman AF, Christoffels VM. The Tbx2+ primary myocardium of the atrioventricular canal forms the atrioventricular node and the base of the left ventricle. Circ Res. 2009;104(11):1267–74.
20. Gunthel M, Barnett P, Christoffels VM. Development, proliferation, and growth of the mammalian heart. MolTher. 2018;26(7):1599–609.
21. Costello I, Pimeisl IM, Drager S, Bikoff EK, Robertson EJ, Arnold SJ. The T-box transcription factor Eomesodermin acts upstream of Mesp1 to specify cardiac mesoderm during mouse gastrulation. Nat Cell Biol. 2011;13(9):1084–91.
22. van den Ameele J, Tiberi L, Bondue A, Paulissen C, Herpoel A, Iacovino M, Kyba M, Blanpain C, Vanderhaeghen P. Eomesodermin induces Mesp1 expression and cardiac differentiation from embryonic stem cells in the absence of Activin. EMBO Rep. 2012;13(4):355–62.
23. Guo X, Xu Y, Wang Z, Wu Y, Chen J, Wang G, Lu C, Jia W, Xi J, Zhu S, Jiapaer Z, Wan X, Liu Z, Gao S, Kang J. A Linc1405/Eomes complex promotes cardiac mesoderm specification and Cardiogenesis. Cell Stem Cell. 2018;22(6):893–908.. e896
24. Grote P, Wittler L, Hendrix D, Koch F, Wahrisch S, Beisaw A, Macura K, Blass G, Kellis M, Werber M, Herrmann BG. The tissue-specific lncRNA Fendrr is an essential regulator of heart and body wall development in the mouse. Dev Cell. 2013;24(2):206–14.
25. Li Y, Zhang J, Huo C, Ding N, Li J, Xiao J, Lin X, Cai B, Zhang Y, Xu J. Dynamic organization of lncRNA and circular RNA regulators collectively controlled cardiac differentiation in humans. EBioMedicine. 2017;24:137–46.
26. Bondue A, Tannler S, Chiapparo G, Chabab S, Ramialison M, Paulissen C, Beck B, Harvey R, Blanpain C. Defining the earliest step of cardiovascular progenitor specification during embryonic stem cell differentiation. J Cell Biol. 2011;192(5):751–65.
27. Lescroart F, Chabab S, Lin X, Rulands S, Paulissen C, Rodolosse A, Auer H, Achouri Y, Dubois C, Bondue A, Simons BD, Blanpain C. Early lineage restriction in temporally distinct populations of Mesp1 progenitors during mammalian heart development. Nat Cell Biol. 2014;16(9):829–40.
28. Devine WP, Wythe JD, George M, Koshiba-Takeuchi K, Bruneau BG. Early patterning and specification of cardiac progenitors in gastrulating mesoderm. elife. 2014;3:e03848.
29. Ivanovitch K, Temino S, Torres M. Live imaging of heart tube development in mouse reveals alternating phases of cardiac differentiation and morphogenesis. elife. 2017;6:e30668.
30. Tsuchihashi T, Maeda J, Shin CH, Ivey KN, Black BL, Olson EN, Yamagishi H, Srivastava D. Hand2 function in second heart field progenitors is essential for cardiogenesis. Dev Biol. 2011;351(1):62–9.
31. Greulich F, Rudat C, Kispert A. Mechanisms of T-box gene function in the developing heart. Cardiovasc Res. 2011;91(2):212–22.
32. Laugwitz KL, Moretti A, Caron L, Nakano A, Chien KR. Islet1 cardiovascular progenitors: a single source for heart lineages? Development. 2008;135(2):193–205.
33. Dodou E, Verzi MP, Anderson JP, Xu SM, Black BL. Mef2c is a direct transcriptional target of ISL1 and GATA factors in the anterior heart field during mouse embryonic development. Development. 2004;131(16):3931–42.
34. Molkentin JD, Lin Q, Duncan SA, Olson EN. Requirement of the transcription factor GATA4 for heart tube formation and ventral morphogenesis. Genes Dev. 1997;11(8):1061–72.
35. Harrelson Z, Kelly RG, Goldin SN, Gibson-Brown JJ, Bollag RJ, Silver LM, Papaioannou VE. Tbx2 is essential for patterning the atrioventricular canal and for morphogenesis of the outflow tract during heart development. Development. 2004;131(20):5041–52.
36. van den Berg G, Abu-Issa R, de Boer BA, Hutson MR, de Boer PA, Soufan AT, Ruijter JM, Kirby ML, van den Hoff MJ, Moorman AF. A caudal proliferating growth center contributes to both poles of the forming heart tube. Circ Res. 2009;104(2):179–88.
37. Kwon C, Arnold J, Hsiao EC, Taketo MM, Conklin BR, Srivastava D. Canonical Wnt signaling is a positive regulator of mammalian cardiac progenitors. Proc Natl Acad Sci U S A. 2007;104(26):10894–9.
38. High FA, Jain R, Stoller JZ, Antonucci NB, Lu MM, Loomes KM, Kaestner KH, Pear WS, Epstein JA. Murine Jagged1/Notch signaling in the second heart field orchestrates Fgf8 expression and tissue-tissue interactions during outflow tract development. J Clin Invest. 2009;119(7):1986–96.
39. Rochais F, Dandonneau M, Mesbah K, Jarry T, Mattei MG, Kelly RG. Hes1 is expressed in the second heart field and is required for outflow tract development. PLoS One. 2009;4(7):e6267.

40. Shen X, Soibam B, Benham A, Xu X, Chopra M, Peng X, Yu W, Bao W, Liang R, Azares A, Liu P, Gunaratne PH, Mercola M, Cooney AJ, Schwartz RJ, Liu Y. miR-322/−503 cluster is expressed in the earliest cardiac progenitor cells and drives cardiomyocyte specification. Proc Natl Acad Sci U S A. 2016;113(34):9551–6.
41. Ounzain S, Micheletti R, Arnan C, Plaisance I, Cecchi D, Schroen B, Reverter F, Alexanian M, Gonzales C, Ng SY, Bussotti G, Pezzuto I, Notredame C, Heymans S, Guigo R, Johnson R, Pedrazzini T. CARMEN, a human super enhancer-associated long noncoding RNA controlling cardiac specification, differentiation and homeostasis. J Mol Cell Cardiol. 2015;89(Pt A):98–112.
42. Ounzain S, Micheletti R, Beckmann T, Schroen B, Alexanian M, Pezzuto I, Crippa S, Nemir M, Sarre A, Johnson R, Dauvillier J, Burdet F, Ibberson M, Guigo R, Xenarios I, Heymans S, Pedrazzini T. Genome-wide profiling of the cardiac transcriptome after myocardial infarction identifies novel heart-specific long non-coding RNAs. Eur Heart J. 2015;36(6):353–368a.
43. Saga Y. Genetic rescue of segmentation defect in MesP2-deficient mice by MesP1 gene replacement. Mech Dev. 1998;75(1–2):53–66.
44. Saga Y, Miyagawa-Tomita S, Takagi A, Kitajima S, Miyazaki J, Inoue T. MesP1 is expressed in the heart precursor cells and required for the formation of a single heart tube. Development. 1999;126(15):3437–47.
45. Chiapparo G, Lin X, Lescroart F, Chabab S, Paulissen C, Pitisci L, Bondue A, Blanpain C. Mesp1 controls the speed, polarity, and directionality of cardiovascular progenitor migration. J Cell Biol. 2016;213(4):463–77.
46. Liberatore CM, Searcy-Schrick RD, Yutzey KE. Ventricular expression of tbx5 inhibits normal heart chamber development. Dev Biol. 2000;223(1):169–80.
47. Takeuchi JK, Bruneau BG. Directed transdifferentiation of mouse mesoderm to heart tissue by defined factors. Nature. 2009;459(7247):708–11.
48. Fulcoli FG, Huynh T, Scambler PJ, Baldini A. Tbx1 regulates the BMP-Smad1 pathway in a transcription independent manner. PLoS One. 2009;4(6):e6049.
49. Chen L, Fulcoli FG, Tang S, Baldini A. Tbx1 regulates proliferation and differentiation of multipotent heart progenitors. Circ Res. 2009;105(9):842–51.
50. Pane LS, Zhang Z, Ferrentino R, Huynh T, Cutillo L, Baldini A. Tbx1 is a negative modulator of Mef2c. Hum Mol Genet. 2012;21(11):2485–96.
51. Wang J, Greene SB, Bonilla-Claudio M, Tao Y, Zhang J, Bai Y, Huang Z, Black BL, Wang F, Martin JF. Bmp signaling regulates myocardial differentiation from cardiac progenitors through a MicroRNA-mediated mechanism. Dev Cell. 2010;19(6):903–12.
52. Wilson KD, Hu S, Venkatasubrahmanyam S, Fu JD, Sun N, Abilez OJ, Baugh JJ, Jia F, Ghosh Z, Li RA, Butte AJ, Wu JC. Dynamic microRNA expression programs during cardiac differentiation of human embryonic stem cells: role for miR-499. Circ Cardiovasc Genet. 2010;3(5):426–35.
53. Cai CL, Liang X, Shi Y, Chu PH, Pfaff SL, Chen J, Evans S. Isl1 identifies a cardiac progenitor population that proliferates prior to differentiation and contributes a majority of cells to the heart. Dev Cell. 2003;5(6):877–89.
54. Engleka KA, Manderfield LJ, Brust RD, Li L, Cohen A, Dymecki SM, Epstein JA. Islet1 derivatives in the heart are of both neural crest and second heart field origin. Circ Res. 2012;110(7):922–6.
55. Dorn T, Goedel A, Lam JT, Haas J, Tian Q, Herrmann F, Bundschu K, Dobreva G, Schiemann M, Dirschinger R, Guo Y, Kuhl SJ, Sinnecker D, Lipp P, Laugwitz KL, Kuhl M, Moretti A. Direct nkx2-5 transcriptional repression of isl1 controls cardiomyocyte subtype identity. Stem Cells. 2015;33(4):1113–29.
56. Anderson KM, Anderson DM, McAnally JR, Shelton JM, Bassel-Duby R, Olson EN. Transcription of the non-coding RNA upperhand controls Hand2 expression and heart development. Nature. 2016;539(7629):433–6.
57. Han X, Zhang J, Liu Y, Fan X, Ai S, Luo Y, Li X, Jin H, Luo S, Zheng H, Yue Y, Chang Z, Yang Z, Tang F, He A, Shen X. The lncRNA Hand2os1/Uph locus orchestrates heart development through regulation of precise expression of Hand2. Development. 2019;146(13):dev176198.
58. Huang J, Elicker J, Bowens N, Liu X, Cheng L, Cappola TP, Zhu X, Parmacek MS. Myocardin regulates BMP10 expression and is required for heart development. J Clin Invest. 2012;122(10):3678–91.
59. Belian E, Noseda M, Abreu Paiva MS, Leja T, Sampson R, Schneider MD. Forward programming of cardiac stem cells by homogeneous transduction with MYOCD plus TBX5. PLoS One. 2015;10(6):e0125384.
60. Wang K, Long B, Liu F, Wang JX, Liu CY, Zhao B, Zhou LY, Sun T, Wang M, Yu T, Gong Y, Liu J, Dong YH, Li N, Li PF. A circular RNA protects the heart from pathological hypertrophy and heart failure by targeting miR-223. Eur Heart J. 2016;37(33):2602–11.
61. Wystub K, Besser J, Bachmann A, Boettger T, Braun T. miR-1/133a clusters cooperatively specify the cardiomyogenic lineage by adjustment of myocardin levels during embryonic heart development. PLoS Genet. 2013;9(9):e1003793.
62. Sahoo S, Meijles DN, Al Ghouleh I, Tandon M, Cifuentes-Pagano E, Sembrat J, Rojas M, Goncharova E, Pagano PJ. MEF2C-MYOCD and Leiomodin1 suppression by miRNA-214 promotes smooth muscle cell phenotype switching in pulmonary arterial hypertension. PLoS One. 2016;11(5):e0153780.
63. Wu Y, Li Z, Yang M, Dai B, Hu F, Yang F, Zhu J, Chen T, Zhang L. MicroRNA-214 regulates smooth muscle cell differentiation from stem cells by tar-

geting RNA-binding protein QKI. Oncotarget. 2017;8(12):19866–78.
64. Huang J, Min Lu M, Cheng L, Yuan LJ, Zhu X, Stout AL, Chen M, Li J, Parmacek MS. Myocardin is required for cardiomyocyte survival and maintenance of heart function. Proc Natl Acad Sci U S A. 2009;106(44):18734–9.
65. Sluijter JP, van Mil A, van Vliet P, Metz CH, Liu J, Doevendans PA, Goumans MJ. MicroRNA-1 and -499 regulate differentiation and proliferation in human-derived cardiomyocyte progenitor cells. Arterioscler Thromb Vasc Biol. 2010;30(4):859–68.
66. Liu N, Bezprozvannaya S, Williams AH, Qi X, Richardson JA, Bassel-Duby R, Olson EN. microRNA-133a regulates cardiomyocyte proliferation and suppresses smooth muscle gene expression in the heart. Genes Dev. 2008;22(23):3242–54.
67. Ivey KN, Muth A, Arnold J, King FW, Yeh RF, Fish JE, Hsiao EC, Schwartz RJ, Conklin BR, Bernstein HS, Srivastava D. MicroRNA regulation of cell lineages in mouse and human embryonic stem cells. Cell Stem Cell. 2008;2(3):219–29.
68. Takaya T, Ono K, Kawamura T, Takanabe R, Kaichi S, Morimoto T, Wada H, Kita T, Shimatsu A, Hasegawa K. MicroRNA-1 and MicroRNA-133 in spontaneous myocardial differentiation of mouse embryonic stem cells. Circ J. 2009;73(8):1492–7.
69. Xu T, Wu J, Han P, Zhao Z, Song X. Circular RNA expression profiles and features in human tissues: a study using RNA-seq data. BMC Genomics. 2017;18(Suppl 6):680.
70. Werfel S, Nothjunge S, Schwarzmayr T, Strom TM, Meitinger T, Engelhardt S. Characterization of circular RNAs in human, mouse and rat hearts. J Mol Cell Cardiol. 2016;98:103–7.
71. Lei W, Feng T, Fang X, Yu Y, Yang J, Zhao ZA, Liu J, Shen Z, Deng W, Hu S. Signature of circular RNAs in human induced pluripotent stem cells and derived cardiomyocytes. Stem Cell Res Ther. 2018;9(1):56.
72. Du WW, Yang W, Chen Y, Wu ZK, Foster FS, Yang Z, Li X, Yang BB. Foxo3 circular RNA promotes cardiac senescence by modulating multiple factors associated with stress and senescence responses. Eur Heart J. 2017;38(18):1402–12.
73. Kelly RG, Buckingham ME, Moorman AF. Heart fields and cardiac morphogenesis. Cold Spring Harb Perspect Med. 2014;4(10):a015750.
74. Stennard FA, Harvey RP. T-box transcription factors and their roles in regulatory hierarchies in the developing heart. Development. 2005;132(22):4897–910.
75. Stennard FA, Costa MW, Lai D, Biben C, Furtado MB, Solloway MJ, McCulley DJ, Leimena C, Preis JI, Dunwoodie SL, Elliott DE, Prall OW, Black BL, Fatkin D, Harvey RP. Murine T-box transcription factor Tbx20 acts as a repressor during heart development, and is essential for adult heart integrity, function and adaptation. Development. 2005;132(10):2451–62.
76. Chen H, VanBuren V. A provisional gene regulatory atlas for mouse heart development. PLoS One. 2014;9(1):e83364.
77. Johnson EK, Matkovich SJ, Nerbonne JM. Regional differences in mRNA and lncRNA expression profiles in non-failing human atria and ventricles. Sci Rep. 2018;8(1):13919.
78. Zhang Q, Cheng Z, Yu Z, Zhu C, Qian L. Role of lncRNA uc.457 in the differentiation and maturation of cardiomyocytes. Mol Med Rep. 2019;19(6):4927–34.
79. Kakimoto Y, Tanaka M, Kamiguchi H, Hayashi H, Ochiai E, Osawa M. MicroRNA deep sequencing reveals chamber-specific miR-208 family expression patterns in the human heart. Int J Cardiol. 2016;211:43–8.
80. Deacon DC, Nevis KR, Cashman TJ, Zhou Y, Zhao L, Washko D, Guner-Ataman B, Burns CG, Burns CE. The miR-143-adducin3 pathway is essential for cardiac chamber morphogenesis. Development. 2010;137(11):1887–96.
81. Morton SU, Scherz PJ, Cordes KR, Ivey KN, Stainier DY, Srivastava D. microRNA-138 modulates cardiac patterning during embryonic development. Proc Natl Acad Sci U S A. 2008;105(46):17830–5.
82. Kolpa HJ, Peal DS, Lynch SN, Giokas AC, Ghatak S, Misra S, Norris RA, Macrae CA, Markwald RR, Ellinor P, Bischoff J, Milan DJ. miR-21 represses Pdcd4 during cardiac valvulogenesis. Development. 2013;140(10):2172–80.
83. Wamstad JA, Alexander JM, Truty RM, Shrikumar A, Li F, Eilertson KE, Ding H, Wylie JN, Pico AR, Capra JA, Erwin G, Kattman SJ, Keller GM, Srivastava D, Levine SS, Pollard KS, Holloway AK, Boyer LA, Bruneau BG. Dynamic and coordinated epigenetic regulation of developmental transitions in the cardiac lineage. Cell. 2012;151(1):206–20.
84. Zhang Y, Sun L, Xuan L, Pan Z, Hu X, Liu H, Bai Y, Jiao L, Li Z, Cui L, Wang X, Wang S, Yu T, Feng B, Guo Y, Liu Z, Meng W, Ren H, Zhu J, Zhao X, Yang C, Zhang Y, Xu C, Wang Z, Lu Y, Shan H, Yang B. Long non-coding RNA CCRR controls cardiac conduction via regulating intercellular coupling. Nat Commun. 2018;9(1):4176.
85. Li H, Jiang L, Yu Z, Han S, Liu X, Li M, Zhu C, Qiao L, Huang L. The role of a novel Long non-coding RNA TUC40- in Cardiomyocyte induction and maturation in P19 cells. Am J Med Sci. 2017;354(6):608–16.
86. Liu H, Hu Y, Yin J, Yan X, Chen W, Wang X, Han S, Yu Z, Li M. Effects of long non-coding RNA uc.245 on cardiomyocyte-like differentiation in P19 cells via FOG2. Gene. 2019;694:83–92.
87. Song G, Shen Y, Ruan Z, Li X, Chen Y, Yuan W, Ding X, Zhu L, Qian L. LncRNA-uc.167 influences cell proliferation, apoptosis and differentiation of P19 cells by regulating Mef2c. Gene. 2016;590(1):97–108.
88. Wu R, Xue P, Wan Y, Wang S, Gu M. LncRNA-uc.40 silence promotes P19 embryonic cells differentiation

to cardiomyocyte via the PBX1 gene. In Vitro Cell Dev Biol Anim. 2018;54(8):600–9.
89. Crist CG, Montarras D, Pallafacchina G, Rocancourt D, Cumano A, Conway SJ, Buckingham M. Muscle stem cell behavior is modified by microRNA-27 regulation of Pax3 expression. Proc Natl Acad Sci U S A. 2009;106(32):13383–7.
90. Hernandez-Torres F, Martinez-Fernandez S, Zuluaga S, Nebreda A, Porras A, Aranega AE, Navarro F. A role for p38alpha mitogen-activated protein kinase in embryonic cardiac differentiation. FEBS Lett. 2008;582(7):1025–31.
91. Chinchilla A, Lozano E, Daimi H, Esteban FJ, Crist C, Aranega AE, Franco D. MicroRNA profiling during mouse ventricular maturation: a role for miR-27 modulating Mef2c expression. Cardiovasc Res. 2011;89(1):98–108.
92. Nishi H, Ono K, Horie T, Nagao K, Kinoshita M, Kuwabara Y, Watanabe S, Takaya T, Tamaki Y, Takanabe-Mori R, Wada H, Hasegawa K, Iwanaga Y, Kawamura T, Kita T, Kimura T. MicroRNA-27a regulates beta cardiac myosin heavy chain gene expression by targeting thyroid hormone receptor beta1 in neonatal rat ventricular myocytes. Mol Cell Biol. 2011;31(4):744–55.
93. Miyasaka KY, Kida YS, Banjo T, Ueki Y, Nagayama K, Matsumoto T, Sato M, Ogura T. Heartbeat regulates cardiogenesis by suppressing retinoic acid signaling via expression of miR-143. Mech Dev. 2011;12(1–2):18–28.
94. Saxena A, Tabin CJ. miRNA-processing enzyme dicer is necessary for cardiac outflow tract alignment and chamber septation. Proc Natl Acad Sci U S A. 2010;107(1):87–91.
95. Callis TE, Pandya K, Seok HY, Tang RH, Tatsuguchi M, Huang ZP, Chen JF, Deng Z, Gunn B, Shumate J, Willis MS, Selzman CH, Wang DZ. MicroRNA-208a is a regulator of cardiac hypertrophy and conduction in mice. J Clin Invest. 2009;119(9):2772–86.
96. Duisters RF, Tijsen AJ, Schroen B, Leenders JJ, Lentink V, van der Made I, Herias V, van Leeuwen RE, Schellings MW, Barenbrug P, Maessen JG, Heymans S, Pinto YM, Creemers EE. miR-133 and miR-30 regulate connective tissue growth factor: implications for a role of microRNAs in myocardial matrix remodeling. Circ Res. 2009;104(2):170–8.. 176p following 178
97. Cao X, Wang J, Wang Z, Du J, Yuan X, Huang W, Meng J, Gu H, Nie Y, Ji B, Hu S, Zheng Z. MicroRNA profiling during rat ventricular maturation: a role for miR-29a in regulating cardiomyocyte cell cycle re-entry. FEBS Lett. 2013;587(10):1548–55.
98. Orr N, Arnaout R, Gula LJ, Spears DA, Leong-Sit P, Li Q, Tarhuni W, Reischauer S, Chauhan VS, Borkovich M, Uppal S, Adler A, Coughlin SR, Stainier DYR, Gollob MH. A mutation in the atrial-specific myosin light chain gene (MYL4) causes familial atrial fibrillation. Nat Commun. 2016;7:11303.
99. Khan MA, Reckman YJ, Aufiero S, van den Hoogenhof MM, van der Made I, Beqqali A, Koolbergen DR, Rasmussen TB, van der Velden J, Creemers EE, Pinto YM. RBM20 regulates circular RNA production from the Titin gene. Circ Res. 2016;119(9):996–1003.
100. Siede D, Rapti K, Gorska AA, Katus HA, Altmuller J, Boeckel JN, Meder B, Maack C, Volkers M, Muller OJ, Backs J, Dieterich C. Identification of circular RNAs with host gene-independent expression in human model systems for cardiac differentiation and disease. J Mol Cell Cardiol. 2017;109:48–56.
101. Aufiero S, Reckman YJ, Pinto YM, Creemers EE. Circular RNAs open a new chapter in cardiovascular biology. Nat Rev Cardiol. 2019;16(8):503–14.
102. Miyamoto K, Akiyama M, Tamura F, Isomi M, Yamakawa H, Sadahiro T, Muraoka N, Kojima H, Haginiwa S, Kurotsu S, Tani H, Wang L, Qian L, Inoue M, Ide Y, Kurokawa J, Yamamoto T, Seki T, Aeba R, Yamagishi H, Fukuda K, Ieda M. Direct in vivo reprogramming with Sendai virus vectors improves cardiac function after myocardial infarction. Cell Stem Cell. 2018;22(1):91–103.. e105
103. Sampaolesi M, Pozzo E, Duelen R. In the heart of the in vivo reprogramming. Stem Cell Investig. 2018;5:38.
104. Yang J, Meng X, Pan J, Jiang N, Zhou C, Wu Z, Gong Z. CRISPR/Cas9-mediated noncoding RNA editing in human cancers. RNA Biol. 2018;15(1):35–43.

Part IV

Non-coding RNAs and Cardiovascular Diseases

Noncoding RNAs and Heart Failure

12

Bihui Luo, Xiaojun Zeng, Peiying Liu, and Hua Zhu

Abstract

Heart failure (HF) is a leading cause of death worldwide and is still growing. Thus, it's critical to understand the molecular causes of HF and develop effecitive therapies to treat HF. Recently, scientists and clinicians identified that noncoding RNAs play important roles in pathogenesis of HF. Some of noncoding RNAs can serve as novel biomarkers for HF and some of them contribute to the progression of HF. In addition, noncoding RNAs can be related to well-known HF risk factors, such as hypertension, diabetes etc. In this review, we sought to summarize current knowledge about noncoding RNAs and noncoding RNAs mediated regulation of HF and its risk factors.

Keywords

Noncoding RNA · Heart failure · Regulation · Risk factors

B. Luo · X. Zeng · P. Liu
Department of Cardiology, Cardiovascular Research Center, The First Affiliated Hospital of Guangzhou Medical University, Guangzhou, Guangdong, China

H. Zhu (✉)
Department of Surgery, Davis Heart and Lung Research Institute, The Ohio State University Wexner Medical Center, Columbus, OH, USA
e-mail: Hua.Zhu@osumc.edu

1 Introduction

Accompanied with the development of genomic sequencing, the biology and functions of noncoding RNAs (ncRNAs), which were considered as genetic waste, have been gradually revealed. From human genome project, people have known that about 98% of human genome do not encode proteins [1], thus, the roles of ncRNAs, which are not translated into proteins, have drawn intensive attention and have been extensively studied since then. With great efforts from both basic and translational researchers, ncRNAs have been linked to human physiology and diseases, including HF [2].

Heart failure (HF) is a stage that heart is unable to pump enough blood to meet physical demand of human body. While there are some advances in treating HF, the current mortality of HF is still very high due to poor understanding of the cellular and molecular causes of HF, which is an unmet medical need worldwide [3]. Fortunately, recent studies have revealed that ncRNAs might contribute to pathologies of HF [4]. More importantly, modulation of ncRNA has been shown to ameliorate HF [4]. In addition, some specific circulating ncRNAs in peripheral blood have been shown to serve as novel biomarkers for HF [5, 6]. In this chapter, we will review the functions of ncRNAs in development of HF and summarize ncRNA biomarkers for HF (see summary of Fig. 12.1).

J. Xiao (ed.), *Non-coding RNAs in Cardiovascular Diseases*, Advances in Experimental Medicine and Biology 1229, https://doi.org/10.1007/978-981-15-1671-9_12

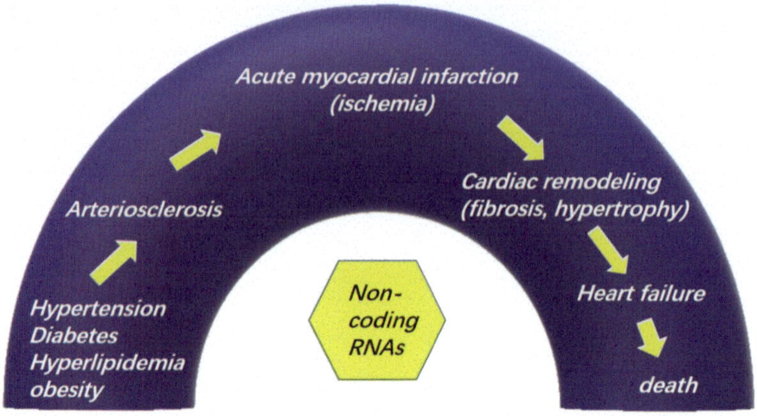

Fig. 12.1 Overview of noncoding RNAs in development of HF

1.1 Members of ncRNAs

To date, ncRNAs mainly refer to microRNA (miRNA), long-noncoding RNA (lncRNA), and circular RNA (circRNA). miRNAs, considered as small ncRNA as well, consist of less than 200 nucleotides while lncRNAs are usually more than 200 nucleotides and regarded as large ncRNA. miRNAs are relatively stable and easy to measure in both tissues and body fluids. Furthermore, miRNA have been proven as a reliable therapeutic agent to treat cardiovascular disease [7]. Based on their genomic location, lncRNAs are grouped into five subclasses: (1) sense, transcribed from the same strand of the nearest protein-coding gene,and can be exonic, intronic, or both; (2) antisense, transcribed from the opposite strand of the surrounding protein-coding gene; (3) intronic, totally transcribed from an intronic region of protein-coding gene with the same direction; (4) intergenic, located between two protein-coding genes; (5) bidirectional, share the same premotor with coding genes, but transcribed from the opposite direction. lncRNAs have been shown to play a role in cardiovascular disease, the dysregulation of lncRNAs are commonly linked to exacerbation of cardiovascular functions [8, 9]. Uniquely, with a 5′ to 3′-phosphodiester bond, circular RNA forms a circular structure. Besides, no 5′ or 3′ free terminus enables its superior stability in cells. Though less well-known than miRNA and lncRNA, circular RNAs have been emerging as a novel biomarker and therapeutic target for treatment of HF [10].

1.2 General Functions of ncRNAs

In canonical way, miRNAs suppress specific gene by binding to partial complemental to 3′-untranlational region (UTR) of mRNA [11]. Furthermore, scientists found that miRNAs can target other ncRNAs, like rRNAs, tRNAs, and even other miRNAs [12]. And miRNAs are able to modulate gene expression in transcription level [13] or suppress both transcription and translation [14]. Unlike miRNAs, the functions of lncRNAs vary. It is mainly classified into signal, decoy, guide, and scaffold aspects [15]. Later, researches demonstrate an unexpected mechanism of lncRNAs by acting as a molecular sponge to miRNAs [16]. Surprisingly, some lncRNAs were recently reported to encode small peptides [17]. Despite more and more researchers have proved important functional role of lncRNAs, our understanding about lncRNAs remains limited. Compared with miRNA and lncRNA, circRNAs are less known. It is believed that circRNA also works as miRNA sponge [18] and regulates the transcription [19]. But further studies are needed to unveil the functional role of this special molecules in our bodies.

1.3 Noncoding RNAs Therapies: Promising but Challenging

Considerable researches have shown miRNA is a potential therapeutic target in cardiovascular disease. However, targeting a single miRNA may result in altering multiple targets, which greatly limits its efficacy as a therapeutic agent [20]. LncRNAs mediate multiple functional regulations in heart. Unlike miRNAs, lncRNAs are less conserved, thus, it is difficult to study their potential functions in human bodies with animal models [21]. Taken together, while ncRNAs can contribute to progression of HF, it is still challenging to utilize them as therapeutic targets to treat HF.

2 Noncoding RNAs in Risk Factors for Heart Failure

2.1 Hypertension

Significantly, patients with high blood pressure more likely suffer from heart failure. Also, noncoding RNAs play roles in pathogenesis and progression of hypertension [22]. Researchers figure out that miRNAs contribute to hypertension by their effects on rein-angiotensin-aldosterone system (RAAS), endothelial cells and vascular smooth muscle cells (VSMCs) [22, 23]. And circulating microRNAs are considered as modulators, like miR-181a, and biomarkers, like miR-505, for hypertension [24]. In a profile of long noncoding RNAs, 235 long noncoding RNAs were found deregulation and the lncRNA-XR007793 participates in remodeling of VSMCs, thus results in hypertension [25]. Similarly, lncRNA GAS5 and lncRNA AK098656 take part in pathogenesis of hypertension by vascular remodeling via their effects on VSMCs [26, 27]. Besides, circular RNA is believed to take part in hypertension pathogenesis and couples of circular RNA profiles were carried to figure out those deregulated. For instance, Wu et al. reported 13 downregulated and 46 upregulated circRNAs in hypertension patients. Then they validated circRNA has-circ-0005870 was significantly downregulated in hypertensive patients and hypothesized a has-circ-0005870-miRNA-mRNA network with utilization of Gene Oncology and KEGG analysis [28]. Whereas, more specific mechanism of circular RNAs in hypertension remains to be told.

2.2 Diabetes

Considerable clues have implied diabetes a risk factor for cardiovascular disease, including heart failure [29]. At the meantime, noncoding RNAs act as regulators of diabetes. MicroRNAs modulate Beta cells development (like miR-106b and miR-222), insulin sensitivity (like miR-103 and miR-107), resistance (like miR-190b), production (like miR-124a), secretion and insulin signaling (like miR-128a) [30]. In addition, miRNAs are involved in diabetic complications, like diabetic retinopathy, diabetic nephropathy, diabetic microvascular kidney disease and diabetic wound healing, etc. [31]. LncRNA can modulate diabetic related metabolism through interact with miRNA. For example, lncRNA Gomafu, by sponging miR-139-5p, upregulates Foxo1 expression to accelerate hepatic insulin resistance [32]. Similarly, circular RNA Crd1as regulates insulin transcription and secretion by sponging miR-7 [33]. Furthermore, circular RNAs, for instance, circHIPK3 and ciRS-7/CDR1as, are involved in regulations of beta-cell activities under diabetic conditions [34].

2.3 Hyperlipidemia

As known, hyperlipidemia puts risk on the occurrence of heart failure [35]. Therefore, promising treatment for hyperlipidemia is in great need. Excitedly, the researches of noncoding RNA shed new lights on solutions to hyperlipidemia. Of note, inhibition of miR-33a/b raises plasma HDL and reduces VLDL triglyceride levels, which may provide a novel therapy for hyperlipidemia [36]. And microRNA-24 contributes to hepatic lipid accumulation and hyperlipidemia by repressing insulin-induced gene 1 [37]. MicroRNA -30c decreases lipid synthesis through both MTP (microsomal triglyceride transfer protein)-dependent and MTP-independent manners, thus, reduces hyperlipidemia [38]. At the same time, long noncoding RNA takes part in process of lipid metabolism. A liver-enriched long noncoding RNA, lncLSTR, enhances triglyceride clearance by modulating the bile acid pool [39]. The long non-coding RNA LeXis, behaves a mediator of a transcriptional regulation to cholesterol hemostasis by liver X receptors (LXRs) [40]. Unlike miRNA and lncRNA, there is still few researches to unveil the relation between circular RNA and hyperlipidemia and further recognition remains in infancy.

2.4 Obesity and Others

Plenty of clinical trials have proved that obesity causes rising risk to heart failure [41]. And noncoding RNAs influence the pathogenesis of obesity as well. Micro RNAs function as a stimulator or a repressor to the differentiation of adipocytes, which directly link to the development of obesity [42]. There are two kinds of adipose tissue in our body: white adipose tissue (WAT) which acts as largest energy storage, and brown adipose tissue (BAT) which consumes energy to produce enough heat in case of low body temperature. And modulation of WAT and BAT associates with process of obesity tightly [42]. Elevating the level of miR-34a is found to inhibit BAT formation then promote obesity happening. On the opposite, downregulation of miR-34a increases browning marker UCP1 and additional browning in brown fat [43]. It implies that inhibits the expression of miR-34a may be a new treatment for obesity. Similarly, miR-378 regulates BAT expansion and obesity resistance [44]. LncRNA is also a regulator of adipogenesis and controls the differentiation of preadipocytes [45]. For example, lncRNA Blnc1 is able to protect cold-induced thermogenesis and browning and impede obesity-associated brown fat whitening [46]. And lncRNA H19 was found inverse correlations with BMI in humans [47]. In addition, noncoding RNAs are involved in other risk factors for heart failure, like hyperuricemia and aging. It's reported that miR-34a suppresses the expression of human urate anion exthanger 1(URAT1) and decreases the excretion of uric acid [48]. And lncRNA is of potential to act as diagnostic and therapeutic targets to impede age associated pathologies and prolong lifespan [49].

2.5 Acute Myocardial Infarction-Induced HF

Acute myocardial infarction (AMI) refers to acute death of the myocardium because of sudden and lasting insufficient blood supply to the heart. The risk factors we mentioned above contributes to the development of atherosclerosis accumulatively. And the most common cause of AMI is the rupture of unstable atherosclerosis plaques in coronary, which lead to cardiac ischemia and damage [50]. Horribly, this is not the end. Following the AMI, heart failure which means not enough blood pumped to meet body's need happens.

2.5.1 Arteriosclerosis

In atherosclerosis, endothelial maladaptation to disturbed blood flow at bifurcations courses slight endothelial apoptosis and chronic inflammatory process. Besides, overloading subendothelial lipoprotein retention leads to macrophage failure [51].

From the very beginning, exosome-mediated miR-155 from smooth muscle cells to endothelial cells impairs the junctions and the integrity of endothelial cells, causing increasing endothelial permeability, and results in endothelial injury [52]. In endothelial maladaptation, miR-103 impedes endothelial cells proliferation and accelerate endothelial DNA damage by preventing lncRNA WDR59 interact with Notch1-inhibitor to interrupt Notch1-induced EC proliferation, rather than targeting at conventional protein-coding RNAs [53]. In endothelial inflammation, couples of noncoding RNAs are involved and nuclear factor-κB pathway is widely regulated in this process. MiR-103 mediated suppression of Krüppel-like factor 4 raises monocyte adhesion to ECs by promoting nuclear factor-κB-dependent endothelial C-X-C motif chemokine 1 expression [54]. Increasing miR-146a mediates the suppression of NF-κB–mediated inflammation by cellular apolipoprotein E [55]. Suppression of miR-499 expression upregulates programmed cell death 4 (PDCD4) expression and ameliorates endothelial inflammatory damage by inhibiting NF-κB/TNF-α signaling pathway [56]. In macrophage, miR-33 regulates its autophagy and reduce lipid droplet catabolism [57]. And miR-155 inhibits the transformation of macrophage into foam cells through activating cholesterol ester hydrolase (CEH) signaling pathway, then eases atherosclerosis [58].

Long noncoding RNA regulates the atherosclerosis circuit as well [59]. On the one hand, lncRNA plays a role in atherosclerosis-associated cell proliferation. LncRNA-p21, which is downregulated in a atherosclerosis plaques of an animal atherosclerosis model mice, increases p53 transcriptional activity by binding to a p53 repressor MDM2, therefore regulates p53-dependent cell proliferation [60] . Smooth muscle enriched long noncoding RNA (SMILR) is identified to be a driver of SMCs proliferation and upregulated in unstable atherosclerosis plaques in human samples [61]. Similarly, knockdown the long noncoding RNA-RNCR3, which is upregulated in cultured ECs and VSMSs with ox-LDL treated, inhibits the proliferation and migration of ECs and VSMCs by acting as a ceRNA to compete with miR-185-5p [62]. On the other hand, lncRNA is involved atherosclerosis-associated inflammation. Compared with control mice, researchers find MALAT1-deficient mice showed more severe plaque size and higher infiltration of inflammatory CD45 cells [63]. Another research discovers that MALAT1 is associated with immune system which mediates atherosclerosis. In parallel with the former research, the MALAT1-deficient mice show increased plaque area. Furthermore, massive deregulations of immune system happen. Serum levels of IFN γ, TNF, IL6 are increasing and macrophages in bone marrow cells and splenocytes of MALAT1-deficient mice are undergoing a series of immunological disturbance [64].

Tough less well known as microRNA and lncRNA, circular RNA shouldn't be ignored in regulation of atherosclerosis pathogenesis. Holdt et al. find that Circular RNA ANRIL increases p53 activation and induces nucleolar stress by targeting ribosomal RNA maturation and regulating pathways of atherogenesis, thus promotes apoptosis and inhibits proliferation, which slow down the process of atherosclerosis [65]. However, Song et al. gave opposite opinion about circRNA ANRIL. They found that atherosclerotic plaques and thrombi showed up in over-expressed circRNA ANRIL group while didn't in under-expressed circRNA ANRIL group. Furthermore, compared with model group, the levels of indicators pointed to atherosclerosis were decreased in low-expressed circRNA ANRIL group while the opposite outcome in over-expressed circRNA ANRIL group. So they claimed that high expression level of circRNA ANRIL may lead to atherogenesis [66]. The controversy remains to be further discussed and solved by more powerful researches data.

2.5.2 Ischemia

Usually, the coronary arteries can be restricted or totally blocked by the embolus caused by the unstable plaque in atherosclerosis, resulting in the insufficient blood supply for myocardium, which is termed cardiac ischemia.

In ischemic heart disease, cell death is caused by couples of reasons, such as lack of oxygen, insufficient adenosine triphosphate (ATP) and mitochondrial impairment, etc. [67] As known, mitochondria is a factory generated power, termed ATP, to meet body's physiological demand, which highlights the importance of mitochondrial function. As widespread regulators, microRNAs are involved in mitochondrial function in cardiac ischemia. Downregulation of miRNA-361 showed talent in reducing mitochondrial fission and apoptosis by clearing the repression of prohibitin1 (PHB1), resulting smaller myocardial infarction sizes after operation causing ischemia performing [68]. Hong et al. reported that miRNA-143 impaired mitochondrial membrane by downregulating the expression of protein kinase Cepsilon in both ischemia model in vivo and in vitro [69]. Apart from mitochondrial dysfunction, cardiomyocytes apoptosis, a kind of programmed cell death, is an important process in cardiac ischemia. Artificial modulation of the miRNA expression is able to improve the apoptotic cell death, thus increases cardiac function in ischemic heart disease. He et al. reported that suppression of miRNA-124 with AMO124 decreased the apoptotic cell death by targeting STAT3 protein in a mice model of MI and neonatal rat ventricular myocytes (NRVMs) treated with H2O2 as well. Besides, AMO124 is of ability to ameliorate mitochondrial dysfunction in NRVMs with H_2O_2 treatment [70]. Tang et al. observed that miRNA-150 regulated cardiomyocyte death in ischemic injury. They revealed that miRNA-150 directly repress the expression of the pro-apoptotic gene egr2, a zinc-binding transcription factor triggered by ischemia, and p2x7 (pro-inflammatory ATP receptor) during ischemic injury [71]. Interestingly, Huang et al. explored the effect of combination of miRNA-21 and miRNA-146a to cardiac function and apoptosis in a mice model of AMI. In this research, they found that it augmented the effect to decrease apoptosis under ischemia when combined miRNA-21 and miRNA-146a together, compared with each of them respectively [72].

Long noncoding RNA was little known in the onset of myocardial ischemia. To explore more lncRNAs with potential to regulate the development of cardiac ischemia, couples of researches were carried out. As a case, Saddic et al. measured the lncRNAs in left ventricular tissue in patients before and after cardiopulmonary bypass carrying ischemia insult. Then they obtained a list of deregulated lncRNAs which may point to regulators for cardiac ischemia. Furthermore, for the reason that lncRNAs tightly links with neighboring coding genes in co-expression, regulation and even functions, they figured out neighboring coding genes of these deregulated lncRNAs modulates the stress and immune response and mRNA co-expressed with them played roles in metabolism and heart physiology as well. Last but not least, they claimed differentially expressed lncRNAs with transcription factor binding sites enrichment were associated with ischemia injury [73]. They have showed us lncRNA is related to ischemic heart disease and metabolism, stress and immune response may be the field lncRNA interrupts in cardiac ischemia. However, specific mechanism lncRNA regulates ischemia process rely on other researches. Gong et al. reported that knockdown of lncRNA H19 promoted hypoxia-induced injury in H9c2 cells by up-regulating miR-139. And repression of Sox8, the target of H19, activates the PI3K/AKT/mTOR pathway and MAPK, then ameliorates hypoxia-induced cell injury. The H19-miR-139-Sox8-PI3K/AKT/mTOR and MAPK axis shows us alternative mechanism of lncRNA in cardiac ischemia [74]. Interestingly, they also observed the overexpression of H19 reversed the down-expression of SERCA2a which was induced by hypoxia and promoted contractility [74]. More specifically, targeting SERCA2a as H19 did, Zhang et al. reported that lncRNA ZFAS1 exacerbated contractile dysfunction in mouse models of myocardial infarction. According to the research, ZFAS1 was able to binding to SERCA2a protein and repress its expression so as to alter the transient of Ca^{2+}, which caused intracellular Ca^{2+} overload, then contributed to cardiac contractile dysfunction [75]. Modulation of ZFAS1 provides us a new potential therapy to battle with ischemia-induced heart failure by elevating contractile function.

A microarray expression profile of circular RNAs by *Wu* et al. showed differential expression of circular RNAs in myocardial tissue during AMI-induced HF, comparing with transcriptome profiles of hypertrophy one. And they found a handful of deregulated circular RNAs showed up in this process, which meant circular RNAs were involved in post-AMI regulation at least [76]. But how does circular work in cardiac ischemia? *Wang* et al. reported that a mitochondrial fission and apoptosis-related circular RNA MFACR regulated cardiomyocytes death. MFACR downregulated miR-652-3p, which suppressed the expression MTP18. And MTP18 increased mitochondrial fission and promoted cardiomyocyte apoptosis. Taking together, the MFACR-miRNA-652-3p-MTP18 axis is crucial to the regulation of mitochondrial fission and cardiomyocyte apoptosis in an ischemia/reperfusion model [77]. Li et al. found that a circular RNA NCX1, which was transcribed from the sodium/calcium exchanger 1 gene, acted as a miRNA-133a-3p sponge, thus weaken the effect of miRNA-133a-3p to suppress the expression pro-apoptotic gene cell death-inducing protein (CDIPI). As a result, less apoptosis and ischemic myocardial injury happen when knockdown the expression of circNCX1 [78]. This circRNA-miRNA interaction shows us a novel mechanism of circular RNA modulating manner in cardiac ischemia disease. However, specific signal pathway involved in circular RNA regulation is under to be unpacked.

Alteration of noncoding RNAs in risk factors of heart failure

	MiRNA [Refs.]	LncRNA [Refs.]	CircRNA [Refs.]
Hypertension	miR-181a [24] miR-505 [24]	lncRNA-XR007793 [25] lncRNA GAS5 [26] lncRNA AK098656 [27]	has-circ-0005870 [28]
Diabetes	miR-106b miR-222 miR-103 miR-107 [30] miR-190b miR-124a miR-128a	lncRNA Gomafu [32]	circHIPK3 [33, 34] ciRS-7/CDR1as [33]
Hyperlipidemia	miR-33a/b [36] microRNA-24 [37] MicroRNA-30c [38]	LncRNA LSTR [39] LncRNA LeXis [40]	–
Obesity	miR-34a [43] miR-378 [44]	lncRNA Blnc1 [46] lncRNA H19 [47]	–
Hyperuricemia	miR-34a [48]	–	–
Age	–	–	–
Genders	–	–	–
Arteriosclerosis	miR-155 [52] miR-103 [53, 54] miR-146a [55] miR-499 [56] miR-33 [57] miR-155 [79]	lncRNA-p21 [60] SMILR [61] RNCR3 [62] MALAT1 [63, 64]	ANRIL [65]
Ischemia	miRNA-361 [68] miRNA-143 [69] miRNA-124 [70] miRNA-150 [71] miRNA-21 [72] miRNA-146a [72]	H19 [74] ZFAS1 [75]	MFACR [77] NCX1 [78]

3 Noncoding RNAs as Pivotal Roles in HF Remodeling

The two most common modes of myocardial remodeling are cardiac hypertrophy and myocardial fibrosis in heart failure. In the compensatory phase of cardiac hypertrophy, the cardiomyocyte increases its size to enhance the contractile force against abnormal resistance and maintain the blood supply to meet the body's demand. If the pathological resistance persists, however, the increasing size of myocardial cells leads to an elevation in oxygen consumption, which results in a relatively insufficient blood supply from the coronary arteries, which causes the myocardial contractility to decrease and lack of blood supply to maintain normal pump function of heart. Myocardial fibrosis is characterized by excessive deposition of the extracellular matrix, which leads to a decrease in myocardial compliance. And the decreasing myocardial compliance causes reducing myocardial contractility and insufficient blood pumped to maintain the physiological needs. It is meaningful to slow down, even reverse these pathological processes in case of occurrence of heart failure. And researchers have found that noncoding RNAs are involved in cardiac remodeling and present a novel therapeutic strategy for heart failure [80].

3.1 Cardiac Hypertrophy

Cardiac hypertrophy is a maladaptation to overload pressure. At the very beginning, cardiomyocytes change into larger size to strengthen the contractibility so as to output enough blood volume to meet body's need against the unusual obstruction, which termed compensate phase. But cardiomyocytes will not be of ability to cope with long-term lasting overload pressure and insufficient blood supplied, then leads to heart failure, which we term it decompensate phase. In decompensate phase, though no enough blood supplement, cardiomyocytes still try to suit the abnormal pressure condition, resulting in pathological hypertrophy. Attenuating this maladaptation has been proved a promising therapeutic method and thus reduces heart failure suffering. Researchers found that noncoding RNAs were able to regulate the process of hypertrophy and modulation of specific noncoding RNAs showed satisfied outcome against hypertrophy [80].

Micro RNA can alter the genes expression that have been pointed to cardiac hypertrophy, thus ameliorate heart failure [81]. And miRNA can modulate hypertrophy through various of signal pathways. For instance, Tijsen et al. observed that miR-15 was a negative regulator to hypertrophy by inhibiting TGFβ signaling pathway [82]. Li et al. generated miR-199-sponge transgenic mice and figured out that the absence of endogenous miR-199 induced physiological cardiac hypertrophy [83]. Later, they showed more details about miR-199 in another research. They found that miR-199 acted as a negative regulator of cardiac autophagy by targeting GSKβ/mTOR complex signaling, then induced cardiac hypertrophy [84]. Sassi et al. reported that inhibition of miR-29 attenuated cardiac hypertrophy and improved cardiac function by abolishing activating effect of miR-29 on Wnt signal pathway [85]. Besides, miRNA can play as a mediator in modulation of cardiac hypertrophic pathogenesis. Huang et al. revealed that miR-18 acted as a mediator in regulation. In this process, P53 activation promoted heat shock factor 1(HSF1) expression and IGF-IIR-induced cardiomyocytes hypertrophy by downregulating miR-18 [86]. Right ventricular hypertrophy (RVH) is mainly caused by pulmonary arterial hypertension (PAH). So miRNA involved in PAH affects the pathogenesis of RVH indirectly [87]. Brock et al. reported that suppression of miR-20a with antagomiR-20a attenuated right ventricular hypertrophy by upregulating the expression bone morphogenetic protein receptor type 2(BMPR2), which is related with PAH occurrence [88]. Similarly, Baptista et al. observed that miR-424(322) upregulated BMPR2 pathway activity by targeting smad ubiquitination regulator factor1 (SMURF1) in right ventricular hypertrophic models. Besides, they revealed that the level of miR-424(322) was parallel to the severity of heart disease, which enabled miR-424(322) an novel prognostic biomarker [89].

Long noncoding RNA is an important regulator in cardiac hypertrophy development as well. Viereck et al. observed that a long noncoding RNA, selected by global lncRNA expression profiling in cardiac hypertrophy mice heart tissue and named Chast (cardiac hypertrophy-associated transcript) promoted cardiac hypertrophy. Overexpression and suppression of Chast induced cardiac hypertrophy and attenuated pressure overload-induced pathological hypertrophy respectively. In mechanism, Chast inhibited cardiomyocyte autophagy and led to hypertrophy by targeting Pleckstrin homology domain-containing protein family M member 1 [90]. And lncRNA can interact with miRNA in this regulation. Wang et al. firstly reported this novel hypertrophy regulating mechanism. They revealed that long noncoding RNA CHRF (cardiac hypertrophy related factor) functioned as an endogenous sponge of miR-489, which was found to be involved in cardiac hypertrophy pathogenesis. Furthermore, suppression of miR-489 target gene Myd88 attenuated hypertrophic response [91]. Taken together, they found a lncRNA-miRNA-miRNA target genes axis in cardiac hypertrophy regulation at first. Since then, this regulation pattern was reported in dozens of researches, like lncRNA XIST-miR-101-TLR2 axis [92], MIAT-miR-93-TLR4 (toll like receptor 4) axis [93] etc. Differently, *Liu* et al. observed that long noncoding RNA H19 and its encoded miR-675 cooperated in cardiac hypertrophy regulation. They found that H19 overexpression attenuated hypertrophy while H19 suppression promoted hypertrophy. Furthermore, inhibition of miR-675 abolished the inhibitory effect of H19 on hypertrophy. Next, they figured out that miR-675 targeted CaMKIIδ directly in regulation of cardiac hypertrophy [94]. Overall, they showed us a lncRNA together with its own encoding miRNA regulating the process of cardiac hypertrophy.

Compared with miRNA and lncRNA, Circular RNA is much less reported in cardiac hypertrophic regulation. However, scientists do find its role in this modulation process. Wang et al. reported that a heart-related circular RNA (HRCR) impeded cardiac hypertrophy. They found miR-233 was a positive regulator of cardiac hypertrophy while HRCR functioned as a miR-233 sponge. As a result, HRCR blocked adverse effect of miR-233 on myocardium by modulating ARC, a downstream target of miR-233 which mediated cardiac hypertrophy induction [95]. For limited recognition, there are still lots of challenges on the way to unveil the secret of circular RNA in cardiac hypertrophy pathogenesis.

3.2 Cardiac Fibrosis

Similarly, cardiac interstitial fibrosis leads to left ventricular dysfunction resulting in the occurrence of heart failure [96]. Abundant research has provided evidences for the cellular and molecular mechanisms behind these pathological changes and the pathways by which it renders an adverse effect on cardiac function [97].

In particular, Thum T's research shows that microRNA-21 (miR-21, also known as Mirn21) was involved in the regulation of the ERK-MAP kinase signaling pathway in cardiac fibroblasts, affecting global cardiac structure and function. MiR-21 levels are selectively up-regulated in the failing heart fibroblasts, enhancing ERK-MAP kinase activity through suppression of sprouty homologue 1 (Spry1). Therefore, in response to cardiac pressure overload in cardiac fibrosis, miR-21 is specifically enriched in cardiac fibroblasts facilitating fibroblast survival and growth factor secretion [98]. In Lorenzen's study, furthermore, miR-21 silencing in vivo prevented the development of Ang II-induced cardiac fibrosis [99]. Another well-studied miRNA involved in cardiac fibrosis is microRNA-101, which has been found to inhibit post-infarction myocardial fibrosis and improve left ventricular compliance through the FBJ osteosarcoma gene/transforming growth factor-1 pathway. Overexpression of miR-101a can respite interstitial fibrosis and the failure of cardiac function, demonstrating miR-101a therapeutic potential for cardiac disease associated with fibrosis [100]. Other cardiomyocyte-enriched miRNAs, such as miR-378 and miR-133a, are also involved in cardiac fibrosis. Among them, miR-378 is secreted by cardiomyocytes after mechanical stress and acts as an inhibitor of excessive myocardial fibrosis through a paracrine mechanism [101]. And overexpression of miR-133 in the heart can prevent fibrosis without affecting the degree of hypertrophy during left ventricular pressure overload [102] or in a mouse model of type 1 diabetes [103].

In addition to microRNA, many long noncoding RNAs were found to be involved in cardiac fibrosis with the advancement of bioinformatics analysis of microarray data [104]. For example, using an integrated genomic screen, Thum T's research group characterized Wisper (Wisp2 super-enhancer–associated RNA) as a cardiac fibroblast–enriched lncRNA regulating cardiac fibrosis after damage. Of note, ASO-mediated silencing of Wisper mitigated MI-induced fibrosis and cardiac dysfunction *in vivo*. Furthermore, its binding to TIA1-related proteins enables it to control the expression of profibrotic forms of lysine hydroxylase 2, which involves collagen cross-linking and matrix stabilization [105]. At the same time, the CF-rich lncRNA maternal expression gene 3 (MEG3) has also been found participating in the regulation of cardiac fibrosis. Researchers figure out that Meg3 regulated the matrix metalloproteinase-2 (MMP-2) production *in vitro*, and that GapmeR-mediated silencing of Meg3 in CFs resulted in Mmp-2 transcription decrease, which, in turn, depending on P53 activity both in the absence and in the presence of transforming growth factor-β I [106]. In addition to the above lncRNA, by using microarray data for bioinformatics analysis, the researchers also found lncRNA NONMMUT022555, named profibrotic lncRNA (PFL), and found that PFL is increased in the hearts of mice in response to myocardial infarction (MI) and in the fibrotic cardiac fibroblasts (CFs). Further studies indicate that overexpression of PFL promotes fibroblast-myofibroblast transformation and fibrosis in CFs by regulating let-7d. PFL acts as a competitive endogenous RNA (ceRNA) for let-7d, thereby reducing the expression and activity of let-7d, and inhibition of let-7d leads to fibrosis of CFs [107]. Collectively, a growing number of studies have revealed the key role of lncRNAs in the regulation of fibrosis in vitro and in vivo in CFs, identifying new roles in the development of cardiac fibrosis and potential new targets for preventing cardiac remodeling.

As other ncRNAs, Circular RNA also plays a role in the regulation of cardiac fibrosis [108]. For instance, CircRNA_010567 was found to be significantly up-regulated in the circRNA expression profiles of cardiac and cardiac fibroblasts (CF) in Ang II treated diabetic mice. Bioinformatics analysis pointed out that circRNA_010567, sponge miR-141 and miR-141 directly target TGF-β1. In addition, functional experiments showed that circRNA_010567 silencing up-regulated miR-141 and down-regulated TGF-β1 expression, and inhibited fibrosis-associated protein excision in CFs, including Col I, Col III and α-SMA [109]. Regrettably, little is known about the mechanistic function of circRNAs in the heart or vessels, which needs to be determined in future studies.

Noncoding RNAs involved in cardiac hypertrophy and fibrosis

	MiRNA	LncRNA	CircRNA
Hypertrophy	miR-15 [82] miR-199 [83] miR-29 [85] miR-18 [86] miR-20a [88] miR-424(322) [89]	Chast [90] CHRF [91] XIST [92] MIAT [93] H19 [94]	HRCR [95]
Fibrosis	miR-21 [98, 99] miR-101a [100] miR-378 [101] miR-133a [102, 103]	Wisper [105] MEG3 [106] PFL [107]	CircRNA_010567 [109]

4 Conclusion

Heart failure is a worldwide problem that threatens patients' lifespan. The cognition of noncoding RNA has shown us their expression patterns, regulation modes and roles in heart failure and heart failure related risk factors as well. And noncoding RNA provides a novel potential therapy, diagnostic implication and prognostic prediction. In human being research, some noncoding RNAs have proved to be potential biomarkers for heart, such as miRNA-19b, miRNA-148-3b, miRNA-409-3p, lncRNA LIPCAR etc. [110–112]. However, the sample amounts involved in these researches are limited and there is no multiple centers research yet. As a result, the conclusions they draw may ignore the existence of bias. As for noncoding RNA therapy in human, it still stays infancy. No matter technical safety nor ethical issue is a stumbling block at present.

Overall, identification of noncoding RNA in heart failure benefits the treatment for heart. And there is still a long way to go before universal clinical utilization against heart failure.

References

1. Kung JT, Colognori D, Lee JT. Long noncoding RNAs: past, present, and future. Genetics. 2013;193(3):651–69.
2. Sun M, Kraus WL. From discovery to function: the expanding roles of long noncoding RNAs in physiology and disease. Endocr Rev. 2015;36(1):25–64.
3. Braunwald E. The war against heart failure: the lancet lecture. Lancet (London, England). 2015;385(9970):812–24.
4. Lucas T, Bonauer A, Dimmeler S. RNA therapeutics in cardiovascular disease. Circ Res. 2018;123(2):205–20.
5. Dickinson BA, Semus HM, Montgomery RL, Stack C, Latimer PA, Lewton SM, Lynch JM, Hullinger TG, Seto AG, van Rooij E. Plasma microRNAs serve as biomarkers of therapeutic efficacy and disease progression in hypertension-induced heart failure. Eur J Heart Fail. 2013;15(6):650–9.
6. Xuan L, Sun L, Zhang Y, Huang Y, Hou Y, Li Q, Guo Y, Feng B, Cui L, Wang X, Wang Z, Tian Y, Yu B, Wang S, Xu C, Zhang M, Du Z, Lu Y, Yang BF. Circulating long non-coding RNAs NRON and MHRT as novel predictive biomarkers of heart failure. J Cell Mol Med. 2017;21(9):1803–14.
7. Barwari T, Joshi A, Mayr M. MicroRNAs in cardiovascular disease. J Am Coll Cardiol. 2016;68(23):2577–84.
8. Han P, Li W, Lin CH, Yang J, Shang C, Nuernberg ST, Jin KK, Xu W, Lin CY, Lin CJ, Xiong Y, Chien H, Zhou B, Ashley E, Bernstein D, Chen PS, Chen HV, Quertermous T, Chang CP. A long noncoding RNA protects the heart from pathological hypertrophy. Nature. 2014;514(7520):102–6.
9. Lorenzen JM, Thum T. Long noncoding RNAs in kidney and cardiovascular diseases. Nat Rev Nephrol. 2016;12(6):360–73.
10. Devaux Y, Creemers EE, Boon RA, Werfel S, Thum T, Engelhardt S, Dimmeler S, Squire I. Circular RNAs in heart failure. Eur J Heart Fail. 2017;19(6):701–9.
11. Ghildiyal M, Zamore PD. Small silencing RNAs: an expanding universe. Nat Rev Genet. 2009;10(2):94–108.
12. Helwak A, Kudla G, Dudnakova T, Tollervey D. Mapping the human miRNA interactome by CLASH reveals frequent noncanonical binding. Cell. 2013;153(3):654–65.
13. Pu M, Chen J, Tao Z, Miao L, Qi X, Wang Y, Ren J. Regulatory network of miRNA on its target: coordination between transcriptional and post-transcriptional regulation of gene expression. Cell Mol Life Sci. 2018;76(3):441–51.
14. Miao L, Yao H, Li C, Pu M, Yao X, Yang H, Qi X, Ren J, Wang Y. A dual inhibition: microRNA-552 suppresses both transcription and translation of cytochrome P450 2E1. Biochim Biophys Acta. 2016;1859(4):650–62.
15. Ma L, Bajic VB, Zhang Z. On the classification of long non-coding RNAs. RNA Biol. 2013;10(6):925–33.
16. Kallen AN, Zhou XB, Xu J, Qiao C, Ma J, Yan L, Lu L, Liu C, Yi JS, Zhang H, Min W, Bennett AM, Gregory RI, Ding Y, Huang Y. The imprinted H19 lncRNA antagonizes let-7 microRNAs. Mol Cell. 2013;52(1):101–12.
17. Rion N, Ruegg MA. LncRNA-encoded peptides: more than translational noise? Cell Res. 2017;27(5):604–5.
18. Hansen TB, Jensen TI, Clausen BH, Bramsen JB, Finsen B, Damgaard CK, Kjems J. Natural RNA circles function as efficient microRNA sponges. Nature. 2013;495(7441):384–8.
19. Li Z, Huang C, Bao C, Chen L, Lin M, Wang X, Zhong G, Yu B, Hu W, Dai L, Zhu P, Chang Z, Wu Q, Zhao Y, Jia Y, Xu P, Liu H, Shan G. Exon-intron circular RNAs regulate transcription in the nucleus. Nat Struct Mol Biol. 2015;22(3):256–64.
20. Bush EW, van Rooij E. miR-25 in heart failure. Circ Res. 2014;115(7):610–2.
21. Sallam T, Sandhu J, Tontonoz P. Long noncoding RNA discovery in cardiovascular disease: decoding form to function. Circ Res. 2018;122(1):155–66.
22. Leimena C, Qiu H. Non-coding RNA in the pathogenesis, progression and treatment of hypertension. Int J Mol Sci. 2018;19(4):927.
23. Bátkai S, Thum TJCHR. MicroRNAs in hypertension: mechanisms and therapeutic targets. Curr Hypertens Rep. 2012;14(1):79–87.
24. Romaine SP, Charchar FJ, Samani NJ, Tomaszewski M. Circulating microRNAs and hypertension–from new insights into blood pressure regulation to biomarkers of cardiovascular risk. Curr Opin Pharmacol. 2016;27:1–7.
25. Yao QP, Xie ZW, Wang KX, Zhang P, Han Y, Qi YX, Jiang ZL. Profiles of long noncoding RNAs in hypertensive rats: long noncoding RNA XR007793 regulates cyclic strain-induced proliferation and migration of vascular smooth muscle cells. J Hypertens. 2017;35(6):1195–203.
26. Wang YN, Shan K, Yao MD, Yao J, Wang JJ, Li X, Liu B, Zhang YY, Ji Y, Jiang Q, Yan B. Long noncoding RNA-GAS5: a novel regulator of hypertension-induced vascular remodeling. Hypertension (Dallas, Tex : 1979). 2016;68(3):736–48.
27. Jin L, Lin X, Yang L, Fan X, Wang W, Li S, Li J, Liu X, Bao M, Cui X, Yang J, Cui Q, Geng B, Cai J. AK098656, a novel vascular smooth muscle cell-dominant Long noncoding RNA, promotes hypertension. Hypertension (Dallas, Tex : 1979). 2018;71(2):262–72.
28. Wu N, Jin L, Cai J. Profiling and bioinformatics analyses reveal differential circular RNA expression in hypertensive patients. Clin Exp Hypertens (New York, NY : 1993). 2017;39(5):454–9.

29. Rawshani A, Rawshani A, Franzén S, Eliasson B, Svensson A-M, Miftaraj M, McGuire DK, Sattar N, Rosengren A, Gudbjörnsdottir S. Mortality and cardiovascular disease in type 1 and type 2 diabetes. N Engl J Med. 2017;376(15):1407–18.
30. Yaribeygi H, Katsiki N, Behnam B, Iranpanah H, Sahebkar A. MicroRNAs and type 2 diabetes mellitus: molecular mechanisms and the effect of antidiabetic drug treatment. Nat Metab. 2018;87:48–55.
31. Zhang Y, Sun X, Icli B, Feinberg MW. Emerging roles for MicroRNAs in diabetic microvascular disease: novel targets for therapy. Endocr Rev. 2017;38(2):145–68.
32. Yan C, Li J, Feng S, Li Y, Tan L. Long noncoding RNA Gomafu upregulates Foxo1 expression to promote hepatic insulin resistance by sponging miR-139-5p. Cell Death Dis. 2018;9:289.
33. Xu H, Guo S, Li W, Yu P. The circular RNA Cdr1as, via miR-7 and its targets, regulates insulin transcription and secretion in islet cells. Sci Rep. 2015;5:12453.
34. Stoll L, Sobel J, Rodriguez-Trejo A, Guay C, Lee K, Venø MT, Kjems J, Laybutt DR, Regazzi R. Circular RNAs as novel regulators of β-cell functions in normal and disease conditions. Mol metab. 2018;9:69–83.
35. Bozkurt B, Aguilar D, Deswal A, Dunbar SB, Francis GS, Horwich T, Jessup M, Kosiborod M, Pritchett AM, Ramasubbu K, Rosendorff C, Yancy C. Contributory risk and Management of Comorbidities of hypertension, obesity, diabetes mellitus, hyperlipidemia, and metabolic syndrome in chronic heart failure: a scientific statement from the American Heart Association. Circulation. 2016;134(23):e535–78.
36. Rayner KJ, Esau CC, Hussain FN, McDaniel AL, Marshall SM, van Gils JM, Ray TD, Sheedy FJ, Sheedy FJ, Goedeke L, Liu X, Khatsenko OG, Kaimal V, Lees CJ, Fernandez-Hernando C, Fisher EA, Temel RE, Moore KJ. Inhibition of miR-33a/b in non-human primates raises plasma HDL and lowers VLDL triglycerides. Nature. 2011;478:404–7.
37. Ng R, Wu H, Xiao H, Chen X, Willenbring H, Steer CJ, Song G. Inhibition of microRNA-24 expression in liver prevents hepatic lipid accumulation and hyperlipidemia. Hepatology. 2014;60(2):554–64.
38. Soh J, Iqbal J, Queiroz J, Fernandez-Hernando C, Hussain MM. MicroRNA-30c reduces hyperlipidemia and atherosclerosis in mice by decreasing lipid synthesis and lipoprotein secretion. Nat Med. 2013;19(7):892–900.
39. Li P, Ruan X, Yang L, Kiesewetter K, Zhao Y, Luo H, Chen Y, Gucek M, Zhu J, Cao H. A liver-enriched long non-coding RNA, lncLSTR, regulates systemic lipid metabolism in mice. Cell Metab. 2015;21(3):455–67.
40. Sallam T, Jones MC, Gilliland T, Zhang L, Wu X, Eskin A, Sandhu J, Casero D, Vallim TQA, Hong C, Katz M, Lee R, Whitelegge J, Tontonoz P. Feedback modulation of cholesterol metabolism by the lipid-responsive non-coding RNA LeXis. Nature. 2016;534(7605):124–8.
41. Rosengren A, Åberg M, Robertson J, Waern M, Schaufelberger M, Kuhn G, Åberg D, Schiöler L, Torén K. Body weight in adolescence and long-term risk of early heart failure in adulthood among men in Sweden. Eur Heart J. 2017;38(24):1926–33.
42. Arner P, Kulyté A. MicroRNA regulatory networks in human adipose tissue and obesity. Nat Rev Endocrinol. 2015;11:276.
43. Fu T, Seok S, Choi S, Huang Z, Suino-Powell K, Xu HE, Kemper B, Kemper JK. MicroRNA 34a inhibits beige and brown fat formation in obesity in part by suppressing adipocyte fibroblast growth factor 21 signaling and SIRT1 function. Mol Cell Biol. 2014;34(22):4130–42.
44. Pan D, Mao C, Quattrochi B, Friedline RH, Zhu LJ, Jung DY, Kim JK, Lewis B, Wang Y-X. MicroRNA-378 controls classical brown fat expansion to counteract obesity. Nat Prod Commun. 2014;5:4725.
45. Wei S, Du M, Jiang Z, Hausman GJ, Zhang L, Dodson MV. Long noncoding RNAs in regulating adipogenesis: new RNAs shed lights on obesity. Cell Mol Life Sci. 2016;73(10):2079–87.
46. Zhao X-Y, Li S, DelProposto JL, Liu T, Mi L, Porsche C, Peng X, Lumeng CN, Lin JD. The long noncoding RNA Blnc1 orchestrates homeostatic adipose tissue remodeling to preserve metabolic health. Mol Metab. 2018;14:60–70.
47. Schmidt E, Dhaouadi I, Gaziano I, Oliverio M, Klemm P, Awazawa M, Mitterer G, Fernandez-Rebollo E, Pradas-Juni M, Wagner W, Hammerschmidt P, Loureiro R, Kiefer C, Hansmeier NR, Khani S, Bergami M, Heine M, Ntini E, Frommolt P, Zentis P, Ørom UA, Heeren J, Blüher M, Bilban M, Kornfeld J-W. LincRNA H19 protects from dietary obesity by constraining expression of monoallelic genes in brown fat. Nat Prod Commun. 2018;9:3622.
48. Sun W-F, Zhu M-M, Li J, Zhang X-X, Liu Y-W, Wu X-R, Liu Z-G. Effects of Xie-Zhuo-Chu-Bi-Fang on miR-34a and URAT1 and their relationship in hyperuricemic mice. J Ethnopharmacol. 2015;161:163–9.
49. Kim J, Kim KM, Noh JH, Yoon J-H, Abdelmohsen K, Gorospe M. Long noncoding RNAs in diseases of aging. Biochim Biophys Acta. 2016;1859(1):209–21.
50. Reed GW, Rossi JE, Cannon CP. Acute myocardial infarction. Lancet (London, England). 2017;389(10065):197–210.
51. Schober A, Weber C. Mechanisms of MicroRNAs in atherosclerosis. Annu Rev Pathol. 2016;11(1):583–616.
52. Zheng B, Yin W-N, Suzuki T, Zhang X-H, Zhang Y, Song L-L, Jin L-S, Zhan H, Zhang H, Li J-S, Wen J-K. Exosome-mediated miR-155 transfer from smooth muscle cells to endothelial cells induces endothelial injury and promotes atherosclerosis. Mol Ther. 2017;25(6):1279–94.

53. Natarelli L, Geißler C, Csaba G, Wei Y, Zhu M, di Francesco A, Hartmann P, Zimmer R, Schober A. miR-103 promotes endothelial maladaptation by targeting lncWDR59. Nat Commun. 2018;9:2645.
54. Hartmann P, Zhou Z, Natarelli L, Wei Y, Nazari-Jahantigh M, Zhu M, Grommes J, Steffens S, Weber C, Schober A. Endothelial dicer promotes atherosclerosis and vascular inflammation by miRNA-103-mediated suppression of KLF4. Nat Prod Commun. 2016;7:10521.
55. Li K, Ching D, Luk FS, Raffai RL. Apolipoprotein E enhances microRNA-146a in monocytes and macrophages to suppress nuclear factor-κB-driven inflammation and atherosclerosis. Circ Res. 2015;117(1):e1–e11.
56. Zhang YH, He K, Shi G. Effects of MicroRNA-499 on the inflammatory damage of endothelial cells during coronary artery disease via the targeting of PDCD4 through the NF-Kβ/TNF-α signaling pathway. Cell Physiol Biochem. 2017;44(1):110–24.
57. Ouimet M, Ediriweera H, Afonso MS, Ramkhelawon B, Singaravelu R, Liao X, Bandler RC, Rahman K, Fisher EA, Rayner KJ, Pezacki JP, Tabas I, Moore KJ. microRNA-33 regulates macrophage autophagy in atherosclerosis. Arterioscler Thromb Vasc Biol. 2017;37(6):1058–67.
58. Zhang F, Zhao J, Sun D, Wei N. MiR-155 inhibits transformation of macrophages into foam cells via regulating CEH expression. Biomed Pharmacother. 2018;104:645–51.
59. Zhang Z, Salisbury D, Sallam T. Long noncoding RNAs in atherosclerosis: JACC review topic of the week. J Am Coll Cardiol. 2018;72(19):2380–90.
60. Wu G, Cai J, Han Y, Chen J, Huang Z-P, Chen C, Cai Y, Huang H, Yang Y, Liu Y, Xu Z, He D, Zhang X, Hu X, Pinello L, Zhong D, He F, Yuan G-C, Wang D-Z, Zeng C. LincRNA-p21 regulates neointima formation, vascular smooth muscle cell proliferation, apoptosis, and atherosclerosis by enhancing p53 activity. Circulation. 2014;130(17):1452–65.
61. Ballantyne MD, Pinel K, Dakin R, Vesey AT, Diver L, Mackenzie R, Garcia R, Welsh P, Sattar N, Hamilton G, Joshi N, Dweck MR, Miano JM, McBride MW, Newby DE, McDonald RA, Baker AH. Smooth muscle enriched Long noncoding RNA (SMILR) regulates cell proliferation. Circulation. 2016;133(21):2050–65.
62. Shan K, Jiang Q, Wang XQ, Wang YNZ, Yang H, Yao MD, Liu C, Li XM, Yao J, Liu B, Zhang YY, J Y, Yan B. Role of long non-coding RNA-RNCR3 in atherosclerosis-related vascular dysfunction. Cell Death Dis. 2016;7:e2248.
63. Cremer S, Michalik KM, Fischer A, Pfisterer L, Jaé N, Winter C, Boon RA, Muhly-Reinholz M, John D, Uchida S, Weber C, Poller W, Günther S, Braun T, Li DY, Maegdefessel L, Perisic LM, Hedin U, Soehnlein O, Zeiher A, Dimmeler S. Hematopoietic deficiency of the Long non-coding RNA MALAT1 promotes atherosclerosis and plaque inflammation. Circulation. 2019;139(10):1320–34.
64. Gast M, Rauch BH, Nakagawa S, Haghikia A, Jasina A, Haas J, Nath N, Jensen L, Stroux A, Böhm A, Friebel J, Rauch U, Skurk C, Blankenberg S, Zeller T, Prasanth KV, Meder B, Kuss A, Landmesser U, Poller W. Immune system-mediated atherosclerosis caused by deficiency of long non-coding RNA MALAT1 in ApoE−/−mice. Cardiovasc Res. 2018;115(2):302–14.. cvy202-cvy202
65. Holdt LM, Stahringer A, Sass K, Pichler G, Kulak NA, Wilfert W, Kohlmaier A, Herbst A, Northoff BH, Nicolaou A, Gäbel G, Beutner F, Scholz M, Thiery J, Musunuru K, Krohn K, Mann M, Teupser D. Circular non-coding RNA ANRIL modulates ribosomal RNA maturation and atherosclerosis in humans. Nat Prod Commun. 2016;7:12429.
66. Song CL, Wang JP, Xue X, Liu N, Zhang XH, Zhao Z, Liu JG, Zhang CP, Piao ZH, Liu Y, Yang YB. Effect of circular ANRIL on the inflammatory response of vascular endothelial cells in a rat model of coronary atherosclerosis. Cell Physiol Biochem. 2017;42(3):1202–12.
67. Greco S, Gaetano C, Martelli F. HypoxamiR regulation and function in ischemic cardiovascular diseases. Antioxid Redox Signal. 2014;21(8):1202–19.
68. Wang K, Liu CY, Zhang XJ, Feng C, Zhou LY, Zhao Y, Li PF. miR-361-regulated prohibitin inhibits mitochondrial fission and apoptosis and protects heart from ischemia injury. Cell Death Differ. 2015;22(6):1058–68.
69. Hong H, Tao T, Chen S, Liang C, Qiu Y, Zhou Y, Zhang R. MicroRNA-143 promotes cardiac ischemia-mediated mitochondrial impairment by the inhibition of protein kinase Cepsilon. Basic Res Cardiol. 2017;112(6):60.
70. He F, Liu H, Guo J, Yang D, Yu Y, Yu J, Yan X, Hu J, Du Z. Inhibition of MicroRNA-124 reduces Cardiomyocyte apoptosis following myocardial infarction via targeting STAT3. Cell Physiol Biochem. 2018;51(1):186–200.
71. Tang Y, Wang Y, Park KM, Hu Q, Teoh JP, Broskova Z, Ranganathan P, Jayakumar C, Li J, Su H, Tang Y, Ramesh G, Kim IM. MicroRNA-150 protects the mouse heart from ischaemic injury by regulating cell death. Cardiovasc Res. 2015;106(3):387–97.
72. Huang W, Tian SS, Hang PZ, Sun C, Guo J, Du ZM. Combination of microRNA-21 and microRNA-146a attenuates cardiac dysfunction and apoptosis during acute myocardial infarction in mice. Mol Ther Nucleic Acids. 2016;5:e296.
73. Saddic LA, Sigurdsson MI, Chang TW, Mazaika E, Heydarpour M, Shernan SK, Seidman CE, Seidman JG, Aranki SF, Body SC, Muehlschlegel JD. The Long noncoding RNA landscape of the ischemic human left ventricle. Circ Cardiovasc Genet. 2017;10(1)
74. Gong LC, Xu HM, Guo GL, Zhang T, Shi JW, Chang C. Long non-coding RNA H19 protects H9c2 cells against hypoxia-induced injury by targeting MicroRNA-139. Cell Physiol Biochem. 2017;44(3):857–69.

75. Zhang Y, Jiao L, Sun L, Li Y, Gao Y, Xu C, Shao Y, Li M, Li C, Lu Y, Pan Z, Xuan L, Zhang Y, Li Q, Yang R, Zhuang Y, Zhang Y, Yang B. LncRNA ZFAS1 as a SERCA2a inhibitor to cause intracellular ca(2+) overload and contractile dysfunction in a mouse model of myocardial infarction. Circ Res. 2018;122(10):1354–68.
76. Wu HJ, Zhang CY, Zhang S, Chang M, Wang HY. Microarray expression profile of circular RNAs in heart tissue of mice with myocardial infarction-induced heart failure. Cell Physiol Biochem. 2016;39(1):205–16.
77. Wang K, Gan TY, Li N, Liu CY, Zhou LY, Gao JN, Chen C, Yan KW, Ponnusamy M, Zhang YH, Li PF. Circular RNA mediates cardiomyocyte death via miRNA-dependent upregulation of MTP18 expression. Cell Death Differ. 2017;24(6):1111–20.
78. Li M, Ding W, Tariq MA, Chang W, Zhang X, Xu W, Hou L, Wang Y, Wang J. A circular transcript of ncx1 gene mediates ischemic myocardial injury by targeting miR-133a-3p. Theranostics. 2018;8(21):5855–69.
79. Zhang F, Zhao J, Sun D, Wei N. MiR-155 inhibits transformation of macrophages into foam cells via regulating CEH expression. Biomed Pharmacother. 2018;104:645–51.
80. Kumarswamy R, Thum T. Non-coding RNAs in cardiac remodeling and heart failure. Circ Res. 2013;113(6):676–89.
81. Sadiq S, Crowley TM, Charchar FJ, Sanigorski A, Lewandowski PA. MicroRNAs in a hypertrophic heart: from foetal life to adulthood. Biol Rev Camb Philos Soc. 2017;92(3):1314–31.
82. Tijsen AJ, van der Made I, van den Hoogenhof MM, Wijnen WJ, van Deel ED, de Groot NE, Alekseev S, Fluiter K, Schroen B, Goumans MJ, van der Velden J, Duncker DJ, Pinto YM, Creemers EE. The microRNA-15 family inhibits the TGFbeta-pathway in the heart. Cardiovasc Res. 2014;104(1):61–71.
83. Li Z, Liu L, Hou N, Song Y, An X, Zhang Y, Yang X, Wang J. miR-199-sponge transgenic mice develop physiological cardiac hypertrophy. Cardiovasc Res. 2016;110(2):258–67.
84. Li Z, Song Y, Liu L, Hou N, An X, Zhan D, Li Y, Zhou L, Li P, Yu L, Xia J, Zhang Y, Wang J, Yang X. miR-199a impairs autophagy and induces cardiac hypertrophy through mTOR activation. Cell Death Differ. 2017;24(7):1205–13.
85. Sassi Y, Avramopoulos P, Ramanujam D, Gruter L, Werfel S, Giosele S, Brunner AD, Esfandyari D, Papadopoulou AS, De Strooper B, Hubner N, Kumarswamy R, Thum T, Yin X, Mayr M, Laggerbauer B, Engelhardt S. Cardiac myocyte miR-29 promotes pathological remodeling of the heart by activating Wnt signaling. Nat Prod Commun. 2017;8(1):1614.
86. Huang CY, Pai PY, Kuo CH, Ho TJ, Lin JY, Lin DY, Tsai FJ, Padma VV, Kuo WW, Huang CY. p53-mediated miR-18 repression activates HSF2 for IGF-IIR-dependent myocyte hypertrophy in hypertension-induced heart failure. Cell Death Dis. 2017;8(8):e2990.
87. Batkai S, Bar C, Thum T. MicroRNAs in right ventricular remodelling. Cardiovasc Res. 2017;113(12):1433–40.
88. Brock M, Samillan VJ, Trenkmann M, Schwarzwald C, Ulrich S, Gay RE, Gassmann M, Ostergaard L, Gay S, Speich R, Huber LC. AntagomiR directed against miR-20a restores functional BMPR2 signalling and prevents vascular remodelling in hypoxia-induced pulmonary hypertension. Eur Heart J. 2014;35(45):3203–11.
89. Baptista R, Marques C, Catarino S, Enguita FJ, Costa MC, Matafome P, Zuzarte M, Castro G, Reis A, Monteiro P, Pego M, Pereira P, Girao H. MicroRNA-424(322) as a new marker of disease progression in pulmonary arterial hypertension and its role in right ventricular hypertrophy by targeting SMURF1. Cardiovasc Res. 2018;114(1):53–64.
90. Viereck J, Kumarswamy R, Foinquinos A, Xiao K, Avramopoulos P, Kunz M, Dittrich M, Maetzig T, Zimmer K, Remke J, Just A, Fendrich J, Scherf K, Bolesani E, Schambach A, Weidemann F, Zweigerdt R, de Windt LJ, Engelhardt S, Dandekar T, Batkai S, Thum T. Long noncoding RNA Chast promotes cardiac remodeling. Sci Transl Med. 2016;8(326):326ra322.
91. Wang K, Liu F, Zhou LY, Long B, Yuan SM, Wang Y, Liu CY, Sun T, Zhang XJ, Li PF. The long noncoding RNA CHRF regulates cardiac hypertrophy by targeting miR-489. Circ Res. 2014;114(9):1377–88.
92. Xiao L, Gu Y, Sun Y, Chen J, Wang X, Zhang Y, Gao L, Li L. The long noncoding RNA XIST regulates cardiac hypertrophy by targeting miR-101. J Cell Physiol. 2019;234(8):13680–92.
93. Li Y, Wang J, Sun L, Zhu S. LncRNA myocardial infarction-associated transcript (MIAT) contributed to cardiac hypertrophy by regulating TLR4 via miR-93. Eur J Pharmacol. 2018;818:508–17.
94. Liu L, An X, Li Z, Song Y, Li L, Zuo S, Liu N, Yang G, Wang H, Cheng X, Zhang Y, Yang X, Wang J. The H19 long noncoding RNA is a novel negative regulator of cardiomyocyte hypertrophy. Cardiovasc Res. 2016;111(1):56–65.
95. Wang K, Long B, Liu F, Wang JX, Liu CY, Zhao B, Zhou LY, Sun T, Wang M, Yu T, Gong Y, Liu J, Dong YH, Li N, Li PF. A circular RNA protects the heart from pathological hypertrophy and heart failure by targeting miR-223. Eur Heart J. 2016;37(33):2602–11.
96. Gonzalez A, Schelbert EB, Diez J, Butler J. Myocardial interstitial fibrosis in heart failure: biological and translational perspectives. J Am Coll Cardiol. 2018;71(15):1696–706.
97. Thum T. Noncoding RNAs and myocardial fibrosis. Nat Rev Drug Discov. 2014;11(11):655–63.
98. Thum T, Gross C, Fiedler J, Fischer T, Kissler S, Bussen M, Galuppo P, Just S, Rottbauer W, Frantz S, Castoldi M, Soutschek J, Koteliansky V, Rosenwald A, Basson MA, Licht JD, Pena JT, Rouhanifard SH,

Muckenthaler MU, Tuschl T, Martin GR, Bauersachs J, Engelhardt S. MicroRNA-21 contributes to myocardial disease by stimulating MAP kinase signalling in fibroblasts. Nature. 2008;456(7224):980–4.
99. Lorenzen JM, Schauerte C, Hubner A, Kolling M, Martino F, Scherf K, Batkai S, Zimmer K, Foinquinos A, Kaucsar T, Fiedler J, Kumarswamy R, Bang C, Hartmann D, Gupta SK, Kielstein J, Jungmann A, Katus HA, Weidemann F, Muller OJ, Haller H, Thum T. Osteopontin is indispensible for AP1-mediated angiotensin II-related miR-21 transcription during cardiac fibrosis. Eur Heart J. 2015;36(32):2184–96.
100. Pan Z, Sun X, Shan H, Wang N, Wang J, Ren J, Feng S, Xie L, Lu C, Yuan Y, Zhang Y, Wang Y, Lu Y, Yang B. MicroRNA-101 inhibited postinfarct cardiac fibrosis and improved left ventricular compliance via the FBJ osteosarcoma oncogene/transforming growth factor-beta1 pathway. Circulation. 2012;126(7):840–50.
101. Yuan J, Liu H, Gao W, Zhang L, Ye Y, Yuan L, Ding Z, Wu J, Kang L, Zhang X, Wang X, Zhang G, Gong H, Sun A, Yang X, Chen R, Cui Z, Ge J, Zou Y. MicroRNA-378 suppresses myocardial fibrosis through a paracrine mechanism at the early stage of cardiac hypertrophy following mechanical stress. Theranostics. 2018;8(9):2565–82.
102. Matkovich SJ, Wang W, Tu Y, Eschenbacher WH, Dorn LE, Condorelli G, Diwan A, Nerbonne JM, Dorn GW 2nd. MicroRNA-133a protects against myocardial fibrosis and modulates electrical repolarization without affecting hypertrophy in pressure-overloaded adult hearts. Circ Res. 2010;106(1):166–75.
103. Chen S, Puthanveetil P, Feng B, Matkovich SJ, Dorn GW 2nd, Chakrabarti S. Cardiac miR-133a overexpression prevents early cardiac fibrosis in diabetes. J Cell Mol Med. 2014;18(3):415–21.
104. Qu X, Song X, Yuan W, Shu Y, Wang Y, Zhao X, Gao M, Lu R, Luo S, Zhao W, Zhang Y, Sun L, Lu Y. Expression signature of lncRNAs and their potential roles in cardiac fibrosis of post-infarct mice. Biomater Sci Rep. 2016;36(3):e00337.
105. Micheletti R, Plaisance I, Abraham BJ, Sarre A, Ting CC, Alexanian M, Maric D, Maison D, Nemir M, Young RA, Schroen B, Gonzalez A, Ounzain S, Pedrazzini T. The long noncoding RNA Wisper controls cardiac fibrosis and remodeling. Sci Transl Med. 2017;9(395):eaai9118.
106. Piccoli MT, Gupta SK, Viereck J, Foinquinos A, Samolovac S, Kramer FL, Garg A, Remke J, Zimmer K, Batkai S, Thum T. Inhibition of the cardiac fibroblast-enriched lncRNA Meg3 prevents cardiac fibrosis and diastolic dysfunction. Circ Res. 2017;121(5):575–83.
107. Liang H, Pan Z, Zhao X, Liu L, Sun J, Su X, Xu C, Zhou Y, Zhao D, Xu B, Li X, Yang B, Lu Y, Shan H. LncRNA PFL contributes to cardiac fibrosis by acting as a competing endogenous RNA of let-7d. Theranostics. 2018;8(4):1180–94.
108. Devaux Y, Creemers EE, Boon RA, Werfel S, Thum T, Engelhardt S, Dimmeler S, Squire I, Cardiolinc N. Circular RNAs in heart failure. Eur J Heart Fail. 2017;19(6):701–9.
109. Zhou B, Yu JW. A novel identified circular RNA, circRNA_010567, promotes myocardial fibrosis via suppressing miR-141 by targeting TGF-beta1. Biochem Biophys Res Commun. 2017;487(4):769–75.
110. Beaumont J, Lopez B, Ravassa S, Hermida N, Jose GS, Gallego I, Valencia F, Gomez-Doblas JJ, de Teresa E, Diez J, Gonzalez A. MicroRNA-19b is a potential biomarker of increased myocardial collagen cross-linking in patients with aortic stenosis and heart failure. Sci Rep. 2017;7:40696.
111. Chen MC, Chang TH, Chang JP, Huang HD, Ho WC, Lin YS, Pan KL, Liu WH, Huang YK. Circulating miR-148b-3p and miR-409-3p as biomarkers for heart failure in patients with mitral regurgitation. Int J Cardiol. 2016;222:148–54.
112. Kumarswamy R, Bauters C, Volkmann I, Maury F, Fetisch J, Holzmann A, Lemesle G, de Groote P, Pinet F, Thum T. Circulating long noncoding RNA, LIPCAR, predicts survival in patients with heart failure. Circ Res. 2014;114(10):1569–75.

Non-coding RNAs and Pathological Cardiac Hypertrophy

13

Jianfeng He, Yanhong Luo, Junxia Song, Tao Tan, and Hua Zhu

Abstract

Cardiovascular disease (CVD) is a common disease which poses a serious threat to human health and it is characterized by high prevalence, high disability and high mortality. Myocardial hypertrophy (MH) is a common pathological process of various cardiovascular diseases and is considered as an independent risk factor for increased cardiovascular morbidity and mortality. Therefore, it is particularly important to understand its pathological mechanism and treatment. In recent years, it has been found that many non-coding RNAs (ncRNAs) play key regulatory roles in humans' various pathophysiological processes. Abnormal expression of ncRNAs in different types of cardiac cells is associated with pathological cardiac hypertrophy. Understanding the relationship between various ncRNAs and intercellular communication through extracellular vesicles (EV) can identify the key ncRNAs which are the accurate targets of precise therapy in this network of action, it also can potentially be a marker for clinical disease diagnosis, which will reflect the progress of the disease earlier and more accurately. There are many factors that regulate the occurrence and development of cardiac hypertrophy, ncRNAs are only a part of them. There are also mutual promotion or inhibition between ncRNAs and other molecules. It will be helpful for us to comprehend the mechanism of cardiac hypertrophy better and provide a sufficient theoretical basis for clinical diagnosis and treatment by defining these relationships.

Keywords

Myocardial hypertrophy · Non-coding RNA · Extracellular vesicles

1 Background

Normal myocardium consists of cardiomyocytes and non-cardiomyocytes. The cardiomyocytes account for only one-third in the number, but they assume the two-thirds of the function of the heart; the non-cardiac cells include cardiac fibroblasts, smooth muscle cells, macrophages and so on. Cardiac hypertrophy is classified into physiological hypertrophy and pathological hypertrophy. Physiological hypertrophy is a protective response. In order to adapt to the increase of work force under the action of various physiolog-

J. He · Y. Luo · J. Song
Children's Hospital Chongqing Medical University, Chongqing, People's Republic of China

T. Tan · H. Zhu (✉)
Department of Surgery, Davis Heart and Lung Research Institute, The Ohio State University Wexner Medical Center, Columbus, OH, USA
e-mail: Hua.Zhu@osumc.edu

J. Xiao (ed.), *Non-coding RNAs in Cardiovascular Diseases*, Advances in Experimental Medicine and Biology 1229, https://doi.org/10.1007/978-981-15-1671-9_13

ical factors, it increases the contraction to increase the myocardial reserve capacity, which is mainly shown as increased myocardial weight and myocardial cells hypertrophy along the horizontal axis of the cell, but it isn't accompanied by fibrosis and is usually reversible [1]. Pathological cardiac hypertrophy refers to an injurious reaction that occurs when the heart is overloaded, including long-term mechanical stimulation [2, 3] or endocrine factors change or metabolic disorders [4–6], which mainly due to an increase of myocardial cell volume, protein synthesis and sarcomere, and also due to the re-expression of embryonic genes and the proliferation of mesenchymal cells, the proliferation of collagen and other connective tissues. It eventually leads to myocardial structure disorder, reduced contractility, insufficient blood supply, myocardial contraction and diastole dysfunction, which prone to heart failure, arrhythmia, and even sudden death [7]. At present, pathological cardiac hypertrophy is considered to be one of the independent risk factors for increased cardiovascular morbidity and mortality [8]. Cardiac hypertrophy is common in clinical practice, and there is a high risk in the progression of the disease. Therefore, it is particularly important to understand its pathological mechanism and treatment. However, the pathogenesis of cardiac hypertrophy is complicated, and there is still no thorough research. The main mechanisms of cardiomyocyte involvement in cardiac hypertrophy are as follows: calcium regulation mechanism, metabolism-related regulation, gene expression regulation, and cell death process (such as apoptosis process and autophagy process) [9]. Pathological cardiac hypertrophy is usually accompanied by cardiomyocyte death and myocardial fibrosis, resulting in functional deficits in contraction and relaxation, which further progress to heart failure. Neurohormonal regulation, such as the adrenaline and renin-angiotensin system, is widely activated, with early protective effects, and later decompensation will result in irreversible cardiac dysfunction. Studies have confirmed that it can be achieved by activating NFAT, CaMKII, cGMP/PKG, MAPK, PI3/Akt and other pathways [10]. In recent years, studies have found that non-coding RNA plays an important role in the occurrence and development of cardiac hypertrophy.

Recent data show that less than 2% of the human genome encodes proteins, and most sequences can be transcribed but not encoded. These gene sequence transcripts cannot encode proteins are called as non-coding RNAs (ncRNAs). Until now, we have discovered many of the ncRNAs play roles in DNA replication, chromatin processing, transcription and post-transcriptional gene expression of other RNAs, genomic integrity, and the controlling stability of mRNA [11]. Different ncRNAs have been found to play a key role in regulating pathophysiological process. In different types and tissues of cardiomyocyte, abnormal expression of miRNAs and lncRNAs is associated with many cardiovascular diseases. Circular RNA (circRNA) is another RNA which is classic, diversity, endogenous and lack of research, it also regulate eukaryotic gene expression leading to cardiovascular disease. Below is a summary of the relationship between non-coding RNA and cardiac hypertrophy (Fig. 13.1).

2 MicroRNAs in Cardiac Hypertrophy

So far, there are about 2000 microRNAs (miRNAs) found in humans, and new microRNAs are constantly being discovered [12, 13]. MicroRNAs are endogenous small molecule non-coding RNAs, whose length is from 21 to 25 nucleotides. The sequence and hairpin structure of mature miRNAs are highly evolutionarily conserved among different species; gene clustering and space-time specificity [14, 15]; mature miRNAs expression is tissue-specific; the same miRNA can regulate multiple messenger RNAs at the same time, and a messenger RNA can also be regulated simultaneously by multiple miRNAs. These features are the functional basis for miRNAs to play important regulatory roles in the development of different organs at different stages of growth and development of organisms. There are two ways for microRNAs to silence the target mRNA expression: ① the single-stranded

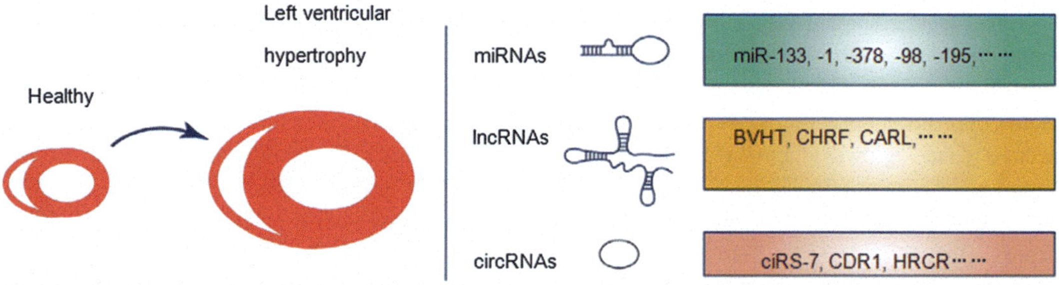

The Journal of Physiology

Fig. 13.1 Part of non-coding RNAs which is significantly associated with cardiac hypertrophy
Different types of non-coding RNAs are essential regulators for cellular function. The chronic stress of cardiomyocytes can induce hypertrophic growth, microRNAs, long non-coding RNAs (lncRNAs) and circular RNAs (circRNAs) interact with their respective targets to regulate specific cellular functions and induce pathological cell hypertrophic growth, which will eventually develop into heart failure

microRNA is complete complementary pairing to the specific sequence base of the 3′-non-coding region (3′-UTR) of the mRNA of the target protein, cleaving the messenger RNA;②The single-stranded microRNA is incomplete complementary pairing to the 3′-UTR specific sequence base of the mRNA of the target protein, restraining the translation of target mRNA without affecting the stability of messenger RNA. MicroRNAs participate in the regulation of multiple physiological and pathological activities by the above two methods. Studies have reported that the changes in microRNAs are closely related to the occurrence development of cardiac hypertrophy. The network of microRNAs regulating cardiac hypertrophy is very complicated. The role of MicroRNAs in cardiac hypertrophy ventricular remodeling is described below.

2.1 MicroRNAs That Inhibit Cardiac Hypertrophy

miR-1 is highly expressed in heart tissue and its absence can lead to cardiac malformations. Tracking the changes of miRNA expression levels timely, during the 14-day stress overload period, miR-1 was the only miRNA that was first discovered to be down-regulated. The specific overexpression of miR-1 in myocardium leads to inhibition of target genes such as Ras GTPase activating protein (RasGAP), cyclin-dependent kinase 9 (Cdk9), fibronectin and Ras homolog (Rheb), which means that the miR- 1 by acting on multiple target genes associated with cardiac hypertrophy can reduce cardiac hypertrophy, reduce fibrosis, reduce myocardial apoptosis and improve calcium signaling [16]. miR-1 reduces the expression of CaM and MEF2a at the level of post-transcriptional modification by binding to calmodulin (CaM) and 3″-UTR of MEF2a. In cardiomyocytes, NFATs and MEF2a can act together on GATA4, activating the transcription of hypertrophic genes. GATA4 mRNA 3′-UTR lacks a sequence which directly binds to miR-1, so it is speculated that miR-1 reduces the expression of GATA4 protein by direct action of MEF2a to act indirectly on GATA4, without altering the level of GATA4 mRNA [17]. In addition, the direct target of miR-1 acting on cardiomyocytes including insulin-like growth factor (IGF1) and IGF1-receptor (IGF1-R). IGF1 usually binds to IGF1-R to activate different pathways, such as PI3K-AKT and hence inhibitory FOXO3A. In turn, these factors in cardiomyocytes also directly affect the level of miR-1 expression [18]. In summary, the interaction of miR-1 with IGF1 plays a role in many processes of regulating cardiac function.

miR-133 is abundant in cardiomyocytes and markedly decreased on serious pathological hypertrophy. MiR-133 regulates extracellular matrix deposition via acting as a repressor of connective tissue growth factor (CTGF). During pathological cardiac remodeling CTGF is secreted by cardiomyocytes as well, although it is mostly expressed in fibroblasts [19]. In addition, miR-133 regulates cell proliferation, cytoskeletal formation and rearrangement of muscle fibers mainly by inhibiting the expression of its target gene RHOA (a GTP-GDP exchange protein gene), CDC42 (a signal transduction kinase gene) and NELF-A/WHSC2 (a nuclear factor gene involved in cardiac development) [20]. The nuclear factor-activated T (NFAT)-mediated hypertrophic signaling pathway plays an important role in cardiac hypertrophy caused by various stimuli. It has been confirmed that NFAT is a target gene of miRNA-133, and miRNA-133 can also participate in the regulation of cardiac hypertrophy by affecting the expression of NFAT. miR-133a inhibits the expression of NFAT3. NFAT3 has two regions in the 3-UTR that can bind to miR-133a. With over-expression of miR-133a, the expression of NFAT3 mRNA and protein were both reduced, and the cardiomyocyte hypertrophy was alleviated. It is suggested that miR-133a can protect the heart by inhibiting the CaN-NFATs signaling pathway [21]. Specific transgenic mice with miR-133 heart can maintain cardiac performance and decrease myocardial apoptosis and collagen deposition under overload stress, which is related to inhibition of, a target gene of miR-133,β1-adrenergic receptor kinase [22].

miR-378 is mainly expressed in cardiomyocytes. MiR-378 overexpression in neonatal rat cardiomyocytes can inhibit PE-stimulated cardiomyocyte hypertrophy; under the same conditions, the number of hypertrophic cardiomyocytes increased significantly after myocardial cells were transfected with anti-miR-378. In the myocardium, miR-378 can inhibit the expression of the following proteins: MAPK, insulin-like growth factor receptor 1 (IGF1R), growth factor receptor-bound protein 2(GRB2), kinase suppressor of ras 1 (KSP1). miR-378 inhibit cardiac hypertrophy by binding with the 3′-UTR of mRNA and regulating the expression of these four proteins at the post-transcriptional level [23]; in addition, miR-378 overexpression in primary cardiomyocytes inhibits PE-stimulated Ras activity, thus suppressing the activation of two major cell growth signaling pathways, PI3K-AKT and Raf1-MEK1-ERK 1/ 2, which act in the downstream of Ras signaling [24].

miR-9 reduces the expression of myocardin. Myocardin is a transcriptional cofactor, and various hypertrophic stimulating factors can up-regulate myocardin, which mediates cardiac hypertrophy signals. Overexpression of myocardin can induce cardiac hypertrophy. Myocardin is a member of the CaN-NFAT4 signaling pathway. Knockout of the myocardin gene can attenuate the amplification of surface area in NFAT4-induced myocardial cell. miR-9 can binds directly to the 3 UTR of myocardin mRNA, affecting the translation of myocardin protein to reduce cardiac hypertrophy [25].

miR-98/let-7i reduces cyclin D2 expression. AngII significantly up-regulates the expression of cyclin D2, which promotes AngII-induced cardiac hypertrophy. Up-regulation of miR-98/let-7i can significantly reduce the basal expression of cyclin D2. It partially inhibits AngII-induced cardiac hypertrophy by inhibiting the expression of cyclin D2 induced by AngII. The overexpression of miR-98/let-7i can significantly reduced the expression of atrial natriuretic peptide (ANP) mRNA and cardiomyocyte hypertrophy induced by AngII, suggesting that miR-98/let-7i can inhibit AngII-induced cardiac hypertrophy [26].

miR-26b reduces the expression of GATA4. GATA4 has a zinc finger structure that binds to a specific DNA. GATA4 regulates the expression of some genes in the myocardium by interacting with other transcription factors such as myocyte enhancer factor 2a (MEF2a), NFATs, and plasma response factor (SRF). miR-26b can regulate the occurrence of cardiac hypertrophy by acting on the 3′-UTR of GATA4 mRNA. Down-regulation of miR-26b can up-regulate GATA4 expression and cause cardiac hypertrophy induced by pressure overload; overexpression of miR-26b can inhibit cardiac hypertrophy [27].

In a mouse model with cardiac hypertrophy conducted by TAC and AngI1, miR-21-3p was found to effectively inhibit cardiac enlargement, inhibit cardiomyocyte hypertrophy and reduce the expression of cardiac hypertrophy marker protein. It was also detected that it can directly target the 3′-UTR of histone deacetylase 8(HDAC8) mRNA, and can also inhibit the expression of HDAC8. HDAC8 belongs to the class II of HDACs and is a group of proteases that promote cardiac hypertrophy [28].

Thioredoxin 1 (Trx1) produced by miR-98 can inhibit cardiac hypertrophy. Therefore, in a rodent model with cardiac hypertrophy induced by angiotensin II (AngII), the down-regulation of miR-98 accelerates the cardiac growth, which most likely due to the increased expression levels of its target gene cyclin D2. Trx1 acts as a negative feedback regulator of cardiac hypertrophy induced by Ang II [26].

The miR-30 family is significantly down-regulated in hypertrophic heart of mouse and cardiac biopsies from patients with left ventricular hypertrophy (LVH). MiR-30c regulates connective tissue growth factor (CTGF), and plays a role in myocardial matrix remodeling and participates in cardiac remodeling [19]. By culturing rat primary cardiomyocytes in vitro, the level of miR-30a in myocardial cells of cardiomyocyte hypertrophy induced by AngII were down-regulated. The overexpression of miR-30a in cardiomyocytes can attenuate myocardial autophagy and myocardial cell morphological hypertrophy induced by AngII; inhibiting the activity of miR-30a in myocardial cell can aggravate myocardial autophagy and morphological hypertrophy of cardiomyocytes induced by AngII [29].

The expression of miR-92b-3p was significantly decreased in the hypertrophic myocardium of rat induced by Ang-II perfusion and also decreased in the myocardium of patients with cardiac hypertrophy. miR-92b-3p can inhibit the expression of MEF2D at the post-transcriptional level. Enhancing the expression of miR-92b-3p or decreasing the level of MEF2D can consistently inhibit the cardiomyocytes hypertrophic phenotype in milk mouse induced by AngII. miR-92b-3p can inhibit cardiomyocyte hypertrophy [30].

2.2 MicroRNA That Promotes Cardiac Hypertrophy

miR-350 plays an important role in regulating the pathological process of cardiac hypertrophy, especially in the late stage of cardiac hypertrophy. The expression of miR-350 is increased in rats with myocardial hypertrophy induced by pressure overload. miR-350 inhibits protein synthesis of P38 and JNK at the post-transcriptional level, leading to dephosphorylation of NFAT4, promoting NFAT4 entry into the nucleus, and increasing transcription of ANP, brain natriuretic peptide (BNP) and α-actinin. Transfection of H9c2 cells with anti-miR-350 can reduce the level of intracellular miR-350 and inhibit the silencing effect of miR-350 on its target gene and reduce cardiac hypertrophy [31].

miR-206 increases in cardiac hypertrophy. Adenovirus transfectes mouse ventricular myocytes leading to the overexpression of miR-206, and 48 hours later, cardiomyocyte hypertrophy happens; mice with cardiac-specific overexpression of miR-206 is prone to catch cardiac hypertrophy; inhibition of miR-206 can reduce cardiac hypertrophy induced by stress. miR-206 inhibits the expression of forkhead box protein P1 (FOXP1). FOXP1 is an anti-cardiac-hypertrophy protein. Down-regulation of FOXP1 can significantly enlarge cardiomyocytes. Overexpression of FOXP1 attenuates cardiac hypertrophy induced by miR-206 [32].

MiR-195 was one of the first miRNAs which demonstrated to be up-regulated in pathological cardiac remodelling. Increased expression of miR-195 leads to cardiomyocytes growth disorganization followed by development of severe hypertrophy already at 6 weeks of age in mice [33]. The AMPK pathway is also involved in the regulation of cardiac hypertrophy. The MO25/Ste20 Related Adaptor (STRAD)/liver kinase B1 (LKB1) complexus is an important molecule of the AMPK pathway. miR-195 can target mouse protein-25 (MO25) to promote cardiac hypertrophy [34].

The overexpression of miR-208 induces cardiac hypertrophy by inhibiting the nuclear transfer factor SOX6 (Y-box 6 protein, SOX6). It shows that miR-208 is increased and SOX6 is decreased in hypertrophic cardiomyocytes induced by PE. After knocking out miR-208 in cardiomyocytes, SOX6 expression is increased, accompanied by decreased expression of ANP and α-actinin, and cardiomyocyte hypertrophy was inhibited [35].

miR-19a/b inhibits the expression of atroginl and Murfl. Atroginl and muscle ring finger protein (Murf1) are the two common E3 ligases in ubiquitination. Atroginl inhibits cardiac hypertrophy by inhibiting the expression of calcineurin and alpha-actinin. The overexpression of miR-19a/b in neonatal mouse cardiomyocytes can significantly induce cardiomyocyte hypertrophy. The miR-19a/b family directly inhibits the expression of atroginl and Murfl, increases the expression of CaN, and then activates the CaN-NFATs signaling pathway to promote cardiac hypertrophy [36].

miR-328 inhibits the expression of Serca2a. And the expression of ANP, BNP and β-myosin heavy chain (β-MHC) is significantly increased in mice with overexpressing miR-328 induced by pressure overload. Sarco/endoplasmic reticulum Ca2 + -ATPase 2a(ATP2a2 or Serca2a) is responsible for maintaining intracellular Ca2+ balance. The expression of miR-328 increased during cardiac hypertrophy. It can directly act on Serea2a to reduce its expression, and increase the intracellular Ca2+ concentration to activate CaN-NFATs signaling pathway, then promote cardiac hypertrophy [37].

miR-199a inhibits the expression of GSK313. Overexpression of miR-199a in neonatal rat can increase the size of cardiomyocytes; knocking out miR-199a reduces cardiomyocyte hypertrophy induced by isoproterenol. In mice with overexpressing miR-199a, miR-199a inhibits the expression of GSK3B by binding to the 3′-UTR terminus of GSK3B, which activates the PI3K-AKT-mTOR signaling pathway to attenuate autophagy and promote cardiac hypertrophy [38].

We also discover the up-regulation of MiR-499 in human and mouse hypertrophic hearts. Under cardiac stress overload, the expression of miR-499 is increased, leading to cardiac maladaptation and accelerates the transition to heart failure, via Akt and MAPK targeting the cardiac kinase and phosphatase pathways [39].

The up-regulated expression of the miR-212/132 family results in cardiac hypertrophy, heart failure, and death through regulation of their target gene FOXO3 and its subsequent alteration of calcineurin-NFAT signaling. Thus, in a genetic animal model or animals treated with antagomir, the reduction of miR-212/132 inhibits cardiac hypertrophic growth [40].

2.3 Controversial microRNA in Cardiac Hypertrophy

The role of miR-21 in cardiac hypertrophy is still controversial. Studies have shown that the expression of miRNA-21 in myocardial tissue under pressure load continues to increase [41]. In cardiomyocytes whose miRNA-21 gene is knocked out, cell proliferation and embryonic gene expression induced by factors that promote cardiac hypertrophy were both inhibited. MiRNA-21 may promote cardiomyocyte proliferation by regulating the expression of SPRY2 protein as the inhibitor of the mitogen-activated protein kinase MAPK [42]. However, in neonatal rat cardiomyocytes, inhibiting the expression of miR-21 can prevent cardiomyocyte hypertrophy caused by adrenal and angiotensin 2 [43]. Some studies show that, in the regulation of cardiac hypertrophy, miR-21 does not directly regulate the target but regulate it by an indirect mechanism [44].

3 Long Non-coding RNAs in Cardiac Hypertrophy

Long non-coding RNA (lncRNA) is a class of pseudogenes (about 200 nucleotides in length) that lose the function of protein coding. It belongs to the non-coding RNA family and its diversity and complexity in function is determined by its high heterogeneity in sequence structure [45]. By targeting promoters, enhancers and insulators as a cis- or trans- functional regulatory element, lncRNA is the central component to regulate and modify epigenetics, regulate alleles (genomic imprinting) and regulate transcription/transcriptional genes [46]. Studies have found that changes in lncRNA structure or expression levels can cause many diseases by affecting gene expressions and the regulatory of signaling pathways. More and more scholars have begun to study long-chain non-coding RNAs that affect myocardial function and value their pathophysiological effects in the heart [47].

3.1 Myosin Heavy Chain Associated RNA Transcripts (Mhrt)

Long non-coding RNA Mhrt is an antisense transcript of myosin heavy chain 7(Myh7) [48]. In mouse myocardium with Pre-overexpression of Mhrt and pathological stimulation, we find the progression of cardiac hypertrophy becomes slow, suggesting that Mhrt has a protective effect on the heart. During this process, Mhrt achieves it by inhibiting cardiac stress-activated chromatin remodeling factor (Brg1). First, Mhrt recognizes the target gene of Brg1 and represses its abnormal gene expression under pathological stimulation (inhibit the pathological conversion of α-MHC to β-MHC). At the same time, Mhrt inhibits chromatin remodeling by competitively inhibiting the combination of chromatinized NDA and Brg1, thereby inhibiting cardiac hypertrophy.

3.2 Chaer (Cardiac-Hypertrophy-Associated Epigenetic Regulator)

Chaer affects the function of the PRC2 sequence, rendering PRC2 unable to target its genomic locus, thereby inhibiting the methylation of histone H3 lysine 27 on the promoter region of genes associated with cardiac hypertrophy. Studies have shown that, by inhibiting the expression of Chaer in the heart, it can significantly reduce cardiac hypertrophy and myocardial dysfunction caused by stress stimulation. Chaer and PRC2 can be transiently induced to interact with each other under the stimulation of hormones, which is one of the prerequisites for epigenetic reprogramming and related pathological gene expression in the occurrence of cardiac hypertrophy [49].

3.3 Chast (Cardiac-Hypertrophy-Associated Transcript)

In a model of cardiac hypertrophy in the mouse with thoracic aortic coarctation, the expression of Chast in cardiomyocytes is specifically up-regulated. The expression of this lncRNA is rising in cardiac tissue derived from human aortic stenosis and cardiomyocytes derived from human embryonic stem cell under hypertrophic irritation. The overexpression of Chast in cell and animal models with cardiac hypertrophy is sufficient to induce cardiomyocyte hypertrophy, while the silence of Chast can prevent and reverse pathological cardiac remodeling induced by pressure overload. The mechanism is to activate Chast by NFST which is the factor of promoting hypertrophic transcrition, and up-regulate the expression of the Plekhm1 protein (Plekhm1, also known as platelet-leukocyte C kinase substrate) of the autophagy regulator protein family M member 1, then block the myocardium cell autophagy [50].

3.4 Cardiac Hypertrophy Related Factor (CHRF)

The expression of cardiac hypertrophy related factor (CHRF) is up-regulated in the mouse heart with transverse aortic coarctation and the human samples with heart failure, it is also extensively expressed in cardiovascular cells and has peculiar functions in cardiomyocytes. CHRF induces cardiomyocyte hypertrophy and apoptosis by acting as a sponge of miRNA-489. By chelating with miR-489, CHFR up-regulates its target gene, myeloid differentiation primary response gene (Myd88), and induces cardiac hypertrophy through NFkB pathway [51]. In addition, studies have found that CHRF inhibits the expression of miR-93 by direct interaction, and the inhibition of miR-93 attenuates the anti-hypertrophic response mediated by si-CHRF in Iso-treated cardiomyocytes. miR-93 blocks the hypertrophy induced by Iso, which can be reversed by exogenous overexpression of Akt3 [52]. Study finds that the persistent overexpression of Akt3 triggers systolic dysfunction and enhances the sensitivity to injury for heart, ultimately making adaptive hypertrophy evolve into maladaptive hypertrophy [53]. In summary, at least, CHRF promotes cardiac hypertrophy by partially modulating the miR-93 / Akt3 axis in Iso-induced cardiomyocytes. These studies connect the effects of long non-coding RNA, microRNA and its downstream target genes, inflammatory signaling pathways and so on, by the specific combination role of long non-coding RNA, which is the latest discovery of the mechanism of cardiac hypertrophy.

3.5 Long Non-coding RNA H19

It is up-regulated in the cardiac hypertrophy model of mouse with thoracic aortic coarctation, and the silence of H19 or microRNA-675 in primary cardiomyocytes of mouse can both lead to cardiomyocyte hypertrophy. The overexpression of microRNA-675 can reverse the cell hypertrophy induced by the knockdown of H19, but the overexpression of H19 and knockdown of microRNA-675 can not inhibit cardiomyocyte hypertrophy. Thus, it is confirmed that long non-coding RNA H19 can inhibit cardiac hypertrophy by regulating microRNA-675. And it is determined that Ca/calmodulin-dependent protein kinase IIδ (CaMKIIδ) is the direct target of microRNA-675, and partially mediating the effect of H19 on cardiomyocyte hypertrophy. It reveals a new function of H19-microRNA-675 axis targeting CaMKIIδ as a negative regulator of cardiac hypertrophy, which shows its potential therapeutic effects in heart disease [54].

3.6 Long Non-coding RNA ROR (Reprogramming Regulator)

Long non-coding RNA ROR, which is up-regulated during cardiac hypertrophy, is also involved in the occurrence and development of cardiac hypertrophy. ROR has been verified to regulate reprogramming and inhibit the damage from P53 to DNA. Its function is to promote the occurrence of cardiac hypertrophy by adsorbing microRNA-133 [55].

3.7 Long Non-coding RNA TINCR (Terminal Differentiation Inducing Non-coding RNA)

TINCR is down-regulated in a mouse model with aortic coarctation. While up-regulating TINCR can reduce cardiac hypertrophy. It was also found that primary cardiomyocyte hypertrophy caused by angiotensin II (Ang II) in blood culture was associated with the decreased expression of TINCR. TINCR can directly combine with EZH2 in cardiomyocytes, and EZH2 can directly combine with the promoter region of CaMKII, which mediates the modification of h3k27me3. So the knock-down of TINCR can reduce its combination with EZH2 and decrease the combination between CaMKII promoter and h3k27me3 in cardiomyocytes. Furthermore, the enhanced expression of TINCR can reduce the expression of CaMKII and attenuated cardiomyocyte hypertrophy induced by Ang II. TINCR can alleviate cardiac hypertrophy by epigenetic silencing of CaMKII, which may provide a new therapeutic strategy for cardiac hypertrophy [56].

3.8 Long Non-coding RNA HOX Transcript Antisense RNA (HOTAIR)

HOTAIR facilitates the pathogenic mechanism of cardiac hypertrophy mainly by functioning as a miRNA sponge to derepress the miRNA target mRNAs in the ceRNA regulatory network. It may serve as a ceRNA for miR-19 to modulate the dis-inhibition of its endogenous target phosphatase and tensin homolog (PTEN) and attenuate cardiac hypertrophy progress [57].

3.9 Long Non-coding RNA MIAT

LncRNA myocardial infarction-associated transcript (Miat), MIAT was upregulated while miR-93 was downregulated in cardiac hypertrophy induced by Ang-II, and the expressions of the hypertrophic markers including ANF and β-MHC were increased. Knockdown of MIAT inhibited AngII-induced cardiac hypertrophy by decreasing cell surface area and lowering the expressions of ANF and β-MHC. It has been varified that TLR4 as a target of miR-93, and MIAT acted as a ceRNA to up-regulate TLR4 expression by sponging miR-93 in cardiac hypertrophy. The over-expression of TLR4 facilitated AngII-induced cardiac hypertrophy through PI3K/Akt/mTOR pathway. Knockdown of MIAT inhibited AngII-induced cardiac hypertrophy by regulating miR-93/TLR4 axis. It clarifies a potential therapy target for cardiac hypertrophy [58]. In addition, it was identified that MIAT which was increased in AngII-induced cardiac hypertrophy was contributed to the pathological process of cardiac hypertrophy by sponging miR-150 [59].

4 Circular RNAs in Cardiac Hypertrophy

Circular RNAs (circRNAs) is a kind of special noncoding RNAs (ncRNAs). Unlike linear RNAs, circRNAs have a covalently closed circular structure and, lacking of both 5' and 3'polarity and a poli-A tail [60]. The current study suggests that circRNAs have stable structure and high conservation, and have tissue-specific and developmental stage-specific expression [61]. Studies have found that circRNAs have the following functions: the sponge of microRNAs [62, 63]; regulating cleavage or transcription [64, 65]; regulating gene expression by interacting with RNA binding proteins (RBPs) [66, 67]. Recently, they have been received many attentions in in many processes, including ageing, cancer, cardiovascular diseases and tissue development [60].

4.1 Heart-Related circRNA (HRCR)

As an endogenous sponge of miR-223, HRCR can inhibit cardiac hypertrophy by adsorbing miR-223 and inhibiting the action of miR-223. miR-223 can induce cardiac hypertrophy by modulating the apoptotic repressor with CARD domain (ARC). ARC can inhibit cardiac hypertrophy, which is high-expressive in myocardium and skeletal muscle cells. ARC is a downstream target of miR-223. And HRCR inhibits the activity of miR-223 by adsorbing miR-223, resulting in the increased expression of cytoskeleton-associated protein ARC which targeting gene activity in downstream increased, it is associated with mitigating cardiac hypertrophy induced by stress overload [62], a novel regulatory pathway consisting of HRCR, miR-223 and ARC. Regulating their levels provides promising therapeutic targets for the treatment of cardiac hypertrophy.

4.2 Circular RNA ciRS-7/CDR1as

ciRS-7/CDR1as has the binding sites of miR-7 up to 70 and can adsorb miR-7 to inhibit its biological function [62]. miR-7a inhibits cardiomyocyte apoptosis by inhibiting the expression of PARP (poly ADP-ribose polymerase) and transcription factor SP1; ciRS-7 inhibits the action of miR-7a by adsorbing it. The up-regulated PARP and SP1, which aggravates the apoptosis of myocardial cells after myocardial infarction, can be reversed by the overexpression of miR-7a and reduce cardiac hypertrophy [68].

4.3 Circular RNA circ-Foxo3

In the mouse model of cardiac hypertrophy stimulated by doxorubicin, the extremely high expression of circ-Foxo3 can aggravate myocardial lesions induced by doxorubicin, and the inhibition of circ-Foxo3 expression can inhibit aging of mouse embryonic fibroblasts, while the abnormally high expression of circ-Foxo3 can promote the aging of mouse embryonic fibroblasts. Circ-Foxo3, which is mainly distributed in the cytoplasm, takes effect by combining with the aging-related proteins ID-1, E2F1 and stress-related proteins FAK and HIF1α. The expression of ID-1, E2F1, FAK, and HIF1αis inhibited by the up-regulation of circ-Foxo3. The decreased expression of these anti-aging proteins can accelerate myocardial cell aging. However the down-regulation of circ-Foxo3 can inhibit cardiomyocyte and apoptosis again, and can reduce cardiac hypertrophy [69].

5 Other Non-coding RNAs in Cardiac Hypertrophy

A new class of small RNAs, tRFs (tRNA-derived fragments), are produced by stress-released ribonuclease cleaves mature tRNA into fragments. Study has been reported that lots of stress conditions can specifically induce tRNA cleavage [70]. Besides, tRFs could function as a paternal epigenetic factor in sperm, and mediate the intergenerational inheritance of paternal disease [71]. Other studies also revealed that tRFs could serve as small interfering RNA that modulated diverse biological processes [72]. In a model of typical cardiac hypertrophy induced by isoproterenol, the tRFs were extremely enriched (84%) in the hypertrophic heart. tRFs1 and tRFs2 overexpression would both increase cardiomyocytes area and elevation the expression of hypertrophic markers (ANF, BNP, and β-MHC) through target 3'UTR of Timp3. Besides, tRFs1, tRFs2, tRFs3, and tRFs4 were highly expressed in Hyp F0 sperm and in Hyp F1 offspring hearts. Compared to Con F1 offspring, Hyp F1 offspring had elevated expression levels of β-MHC and ANP genes, as well as increased cardiac fibrosis and apoptosis. These data revealed that tRFs are involved in regulating the response of myocardial hypertrophy. Also, tRFs might serve as novel epigenetic factors that contribute to the intergenerational inheritance of cardiac hypertrophy [73].

6 Intercellular Delivery of Non-coding RNA in Cardiac Hypertrophy

Different Cell types cross-talk with each other and create specific microenvironments to share resources that are essential to maintain homeostasis and respond to external stimuli. To gain deep views into the molecular mechanisms underlying pathological cardiac hypertrophy, the contribution of cell to cell communication in the heart related to this process must be taken into consideration. More researches have been focused on extracellular vesicles (EVs) that allow long-range cellular communication. EVs are secreted by cells and act as transport vehicles for a lot of small molecules like mRNA, miRNAs, lncRNAs, small amounts of DNA, as well as low molecular weight lipids and proteins [74, 75]. EVs can be classified in three different subgroups: microvesicles (MVs) (0.1–1 μm), exosomes (20–100 nm) and apoptotic bodies (ABs) (0.5–2 μm). All major cardiac cell types, including cardiomyocytes, endothelial cells and fibroblasts, can release exosomes to modulate recipient cellular functions under physiological and pathological conditions, and might hence be involved in the process of cardiomyocyte hypertrophy.

6.1 Cardiomyocytes and Endothelial Cells

In the heart, cardiomyocytes-derived exosomes can lead to different metabolic functions when taken in by different cells [76]. In the glucose deprivation conditions, both the number and the contents of cardiomyocytes secreted exosomes are markedly differing from the normal glucose conditions [77]. Cardiomyocytes can exchange the exosomes' content with the recipient cells and therefore affecting their angiogenesis. Besides, in starved conditions, on one side, a class of miRNAs which have pro-angiogenic effects are enriched in exosomes derived from starved conditions in ECs. On the other side, cardiomyocytes could also absorbed ECs secreted exosomes and subsequently affect their physiological functions and responsive mechanisms to stress. As in women suffered from peripartum cardiomyopathy (PPCM), the anti-angiogenic 16-kDa N-terminal prolactin fragment (16 K PRL) acts on ECs, inducing the release of miR-146a-enriched exosomes. These released exosomes could be absorbed by cardiomyocytes, and consequently, increased miR-146a will affect the physiological metabolism of cardiomyocytes, leading to the development of hypertrophy [78].

6.2 Cardiac Fibroblasts and Cardiomyocytes

Fibroblasts would secrete exosomes to induce the expression of angiotensin and its receptor (AT1R and AT2R) in cardiomyocytes while stimulated with angiotensin II. These could finally cause hypertrophic cell growth. Therefore, AT1R and AT2R antagonists or with exosome inhibitors could both attenuate this exosome-induced effect. Besides, fibroblasts can cross-talk with cardiomyocytes via paracrine effects. Specifically, release the exosomes which contain the passenger strand of miR-21 (miR-21∗) and absorbed by cardiomyocytes. In cardiomyocytes, miR-21∗ induces cardiac hypertrophy by down-regulating sorbin and SH3 domain containing 2 (SORBS2) or PDZ and LIM domain 5 (PDLIM5), both involved in regulation of cardiac muscle structure and function [79].

6.3 Immune Cells and Cardiomyocytes

Mir-155 has been demonstrated to modulate pathological cardiac hypertrophy, while miR-155 knockout mice could prevent mice hearts from this pathological process. It has been reported that this benefit effect are due to the decreased miR-155 level in macrophages rather than in cardiomyocytes [80]. miR-155-deficient macrophages could prevent this hypertrophic phenotype through a paracrine effect.

7 Perspective

Cardiovascular disease (CVD) is a common disease which poses a serious threat to human health and it is characterized by high prevalence, high disability and high mortality. It imposes a heavy burden on society and family. Myocardial hypertrophy (MH) is a common pathological process of various cardiovascular diseases and is considered to be an independent risk factor for increased cardiovascular morbidity and mortality. Therefore, understanding its pathological mechanism and treatment is particularly important. However, the pathogenesis of cardiac hypertrophy is complicated, and there is still no thorough research.

In recent years, ncRNAs have been reported to take important parts in pathophysiological processes, and abnormal expression of ncRNAs in different cardiac cell types being associated with many cardiovascular abnormalities. The types of ncRNAs involved in different kind of cardiovascular disease are not unique. Different cardiovascular diseases may also be regulated by the same ncRNAs. Extracellular vesicles (EV) secreted by cells play an important role in cell-to-cell communication. A more detailed understanding of the relationship between ncRNAs can help us find the key ncRNAs of this network of action, provide a target for precise treatment, and may also become a marker for clinical disease diagnosis, reflecting the progress of the disease earlier and more accurately. NcRNAs have promising therapeutic potential. Using antisense oligonucleotides to inhibit the ncRNAs may bring hope to the treatment of the disease, but currently the technical means are still immature, and there are still some problems left to be solved. There are many factors regulating the development of cardiac hypertrophy, and NcRNAs are only a part of them. There are also mutual promotions or inhibition between ncRNAs with other molecules. Defining these relationships will inspire us to understand the mechanism of cardiac hypertrophy better, and it also will be beneficial to provide a sufficient theoretical basis for clinical diagnosis and treatment.

Competing Financial Interests The authors declare no competing finicial interests

References

1. Oka T, Akazawa H, Naito AT, Komuro I. Angiogenesis and cardiac hypertrophy: maintenance of cardiac function and causative roles in heart failure. Circ Res. 2014;114(3):565–71.
2. Mohamed BA, Asif AR, Schnelle M, Qasim M, Khadjeh S, Lbik D, Schott P, Hasenfuss G, Toischer K. Proteomic analysis of short-term preload-induced eccentric cardiac hypertrophy. J Transl Med. 2016;14(1):149.
3. Maack C. The cardiac re-AKT-ion to chronic volume overload. Eur J Heart Fail. 2016;18(4):372–4.
4. Ferrario CM. Cardiac remodelling and RAS inhibition. Ther Adv Cardiovasc Dis. 2016;10(3):162–71.
5. Pires A, Martins P, Pereira AM, Silva PV, Marinho J, Marques M, Castela E, Sena C, Seica R. Insulin resistance, dyslipidemia and cardiovascular changes in a group of obese children. Arq Bras Cardiol. 2015;104(4):266–73.
6. Houstek J, Vrbacky M, Hejzlarova K, Zidek V, Landa V, Silhavy J, Simakova M, Mlejnek P, Kazdova L, Miksik I, Neckar J, Papousek F, Kolar F, Kurtz TW, Pravenec M. Effects of mtDNA in SHR-mtF344 versus SHR conplastic strains on reduced OXPHOS enzyme levels, insulin resistance, cardiac hypertrophy, and systolic dysfunction. Physiol Genomics. 2014;46(18):671–8.
7. Hou J, Kang YJ. Regression of pathological cardiac hypertrophy: signaling pathways and therapeutic targets. Aliment Pharmacol Ther. 2012;135(3):337–54.
8. Zakharov P, Dewarrat F, Caduff A, Talary MS. The effect of blood content on the optical and dielectric skin properties. Physiol Meas. 2011;32(1):131–49.
9. Tham YK, Bernardo BC, Ooi JY, Weeks KL, McMullen JR. Pathophysiology of cardiac hypertrophy and heart failure: signaling pathways and novel therapeutic targets. Arch Toxicol. 2015;89(9):1401–38.
10. Lyon RC, Zanella F, Omens JH, Sheikh F. Mechanotransduction in cardiac hypertrophy and failure. Circ Res. 2015;116(8):1462–76.
11. Ghildiyal M, Zamore PD. Small silencing RNAs: an expanding universe. Nat Rev Genet. 2009;10(2):94–108.
12. Condorelli G, Latronico MV, Cavarretta E. microRNAs in cardiovascular diseases: current knowledge and the road ahead. J Am Coll Cardiol. 2014;63(21):2177–87.
13. Braunwald E. The war against heart failure: the lancet lecture. Lancet. 2015;385(9970):812–24.
14. Suarez Y, Fernandez-Hernando C, Pober JS, Sessa WC. Dicer dependent microRNAs regulate gene expression and functions in human endothelial cells. Circ Res. 2007;100(8):1164–73.
15. Wang N, Zhou Z, Liao X, Zhang T. Role of microRNAs in cardiac hypertrophy and heart failure. IUBMB Life. 2009;61(6):566–71.
16. Karakikes I, Chaanine AH, Kang S, Mukete BN, Jeong D, Zhang S, Hajjar RJ, Lebeche D. Therapeutic cardiac-targeted delivery of miR-1 reverses pressure overload-induced cardiac hypertrophy and attenuates pathological remodeling. J Am Heart Assoc Cardiovasc Cerebrovasc Dis. 2013;2(2):e000078.
17. Ikeda S, He A, Kong SW, Lu J, Bejar R, Bodyak N, Lee KH, Ma Q, Kang PM, Golub TR, Pu WT. MicroRNA-1 negatively regulates expression of the hypertrophy-associated calmodulin and Mef2a genes. Mol Cell Biol. 2009;29(8):2193–204.
18. Elia L, Contu R, Quintavalle M, Varrone F, Chimenti C, Russo MA, Cimino V, De Marinis L, Frustaci A, Catalucci D, Condorelli G. Reciprocal regulation of microRNA-1 and insulin-like growth factor-1 signal transduction cascade in cardiac and skeletal muscle in physiological and pathological conditions. Circulation. 2009;120(23):2377–85.
19. Duisters RF, Tijsen AJ, Schroen B, Leenders JJ, Lentink V, van der Made I, Herias V, van Leeuwen RE, Schellings MW, Barenbrug P, Maessen JG, Heymans S, Pinto YM, Creemers EE. miR-133 and miR-30 regulate connective tissue growth factor: implications for a role of microRNAs in myocardial matrix remodeling. Circ Res. 2009;104(2):170–8.. 176p following 178
20. Care A, Catalucci D, Felicetti F, Bonci D, Addario A, Gallo P, Bang ML, Segnalini P, Gu Y, Dalton ND, Elia L, Latronico MV, Hoydal M, Autore C, Russo MA, Dorn GW 2nd, Ellingsen O, Ruiz-Lozano P, Peterson KL, Croce CM, Peschle C, Condorelli G. MicroRNA-133 controls cardiac hypertrophy. Nat Med. 2007;13(5):613–8.
21. Li Q, Lin X, Yang X, Chang J. NFATc4 is negatively regulated in miR-133a-mediated cardiomyocyte hypertrophic repression. Am J Phys Heart Circ Phys. 2010;298(5):H1340–7.
22. Castaldi A, Zaglia T, Di Mauro V, Carullo P, Viggiani G, Borile G, Di Stefano B, Schiattarella GG, Gualazzi

MG, Elia L, Stirparo GG, Colorito ML, Pironti G, Kunderfranco P, Esposito G, Bang ML, Mongillo M, Condorelli G, Catalucci D. MicroRNA-133 modulates the beta1-adrenergic receptor transduction cascade. Circ Res. 2014;115(2):273–83.
23. Ganesan J, Ramanujam D, Sassi Y, Ahles A, Jentzsch C, Werfel S, Leierseder S, Loyer X, Giacca M, Zentilin L, Thum T, Laggerbauer B, Engelhardt S. MiR-378 controls cardiac hypertrophy by combined repression of mitogen-activated protein kinase pathway factors. Circulation. 2013;127(21):2097–106.
24. Knezevic I, Patel A, Sundaresan NR, Gupta MP, Solaro RJ, Nagalingam RS, Gupta M. A novel cardiomyocyte-enriched microRNA, miR-378, targets insulin-like growth factor 1 receptor: implications in postnatal cardiac remodeling and cell survival. J Biol Chem. 2012;287(16):12913–26.
25. Wang K, Long B, Zhou J, Li PF. miR-9 and NFATc3 regulate myocardin in cardiac hypertrophy. J Biol Chem. 2010;285(16):11903–12.
26. Yang Y, Ago T, Zhai P, Abdellatif M, Sadoshima J. Thioredoxin 1 negatively regulates angiotensin II-induced cardiac hypertrophy through upregulation of miR-98/let-7. Circ Res. 2011;108(3):305–13.
27. Han M, Yang Z, Sayed D, He M, Gao S, Lin L, Yoon S, Abdellatif M. GATA4 expression is primarily regulated via a miR-26b-dependent post-transcriptional mechanism during cardiac hypertrophy. Cardiovasc Res. 2012;93(4):645–54.
28. Kee HJ, Kook H. Roles and targets of class I and IIa histone deacetylases in cardiac hypertrophy. J Biomed Biotechnol. 2011;2011:928326.
29. Li P, Hao Y, Pan FH, Zhang M, Ma JQ, Zhu DL. SGK1 inhibitor reverses hyperglycemia partly through decreasing glucose absorption. J Mol Endocrinol. 2016;56(4):301–9.
30. Hu ZQ, Luo JF, Yu XJ, Zhu JN, Huang L, Yang J, Fu YH, Li T, Xue YM, Feng YQ, Shan ZX. Targeting myocyte-specific enhancer factor 2D contributes to the suppression of cardiac hypertrophic growth by miR-92b-3p in mice. Oncotarget. 2017;8(54):92079–89.
31. Ge Y, Pan S, Guan D, Yin H, Fan Y, Liu J, Zhang S, Zhang H, Feng L, Wang Y, Xu R, Yin JQ. MicroRNA-350 induces pathological heart hypertrophy by repressing both p38 and JNK pathways. Biochim Biophys Acta, Mol Cell Res. 2013;1832(1):1–10.
32. Yang Y, Del Re DP, Nakano N, Sciarretta S, Zhai P, Park J, Sayed D, Shirakabe A, Matsushima S, Park Y, Tian B, Abdellatif M, Sadoshima J. miR-206 mediates YAP-induced cardiac hypertrophy and survival. Circ Res. 2015;117(10):891–904.
33. van Rooij E, Sutherland LB, Liu N, Williams AH, McAnally J, Gerard RD, Richardson JA, Olson EN. A signature pattern of stress-responsive microRNAs that can evoke cardiac hypertrophy and heart failure. Proc Natl Acad Sci U S A. 2006;103(48):18255–60.
34. Chen H, Untiveros GM, McKee LA, Perez J, Li J, Antin PB, Konhilas JP. Micro-RNA-195 and -451 regulate the LKB1/AMPK signaling axis by targeting MO25. PLoS One. 2012;7(7):e41574.
35. Huang X, Li Z, Bai B, Li X, Li Z. High expression of microRNA-208 is associated with cardiac hypertrophy via the negative regulation of the sex-determining region Y-box 6 protein. Exp Ther Med. 2015;10(3):921–6.
36. Song DW, Ryu JY, Kim JO, Kwon EJ, Kim DH. The miR-19a/b family positively regulates cardiomyocyte hypertrophy by targeting atrogin-1 and MuRF-1. Biochem J. 2014;457(1):151–62.
37. Li C, Li X, Gao X, Zhang R, Zhang Y, Liang H, Xu C, Du W, Zhang Y, Liu X, Ma N, Xu Z, Wang L, Chen X, Lu Y, Ju J, Yang B, Shan H. MicroRNA-328 as a regulator of cardiac hypertrophy. Int J Cardiol. 2014;173(2):268–76.
38. Xydous M, Prombona A, Sourlingas TG. Corrigendum to "the role of h3k4me3 and H3K9/14ac in the induction by dexamethasone of Per1 and Sgk1, two glucocorticoid early response genes that mediate the effects of acute stress in mammals" [Biochim Biophys Acta 1839 (2014) 866–872]. Biochimica et Biophysica Acta Gene Regul Mech. 2017;1860(3):392.
39. Matkovich SJ, Hu Y, Eschenbacher WH, Dorn LE, Dorn GW 2nd. Direct and indirect involvement of microRNA-499 in clinical and experimental cardiomyopathy. Circ Res. 2012;111(5):521–31.
40. Ucar A, Gupta SK, Fiedler J, Erikci E, Kardasinski M, Batkai S, Dangwal S, Kumarswamy R, Bang C, Holzmann A, Remke J, Caprio M, Jentzsch C, Engelhardt S, Geisendorf S, Glas C, Hofmann TG, Nessling M, Richter K, Schiffer M, Carrier L, Napp LC, Bauersachs J, Chowdhury K, Thum T. The miRNA-212/132 family regulates both cardiac hypertrophy and cardiomyocyte autophagy. Nat Commun. 2012;3:1078.
41. Thum T, Gross C, Fiedler J, Fischer T, Kissler S, Bussen M, Galuppo P, Just S, Rottbauer W, Frantz S, Castoldi M, Soutschek J, Koteliansky V, Rosenwald A, Basson MA, Licht JD, Pena JT, Rouhanifard SH, Muckenthaler MU, Tuschl T, Martin GR, Bauersachs J, Engelhardt S. MicroRNA-21 contributes to myocardial disease by stimulating MAP kinase signalling in fibroblasts. Nature. 2008;456(7224):980–4.
42. Cheng Y, Ji R, Yue J, Yang J, Liu X, Chen H, Dean DB, Zhang C. MicroRNAs are aberrantly expressed in hypertrophic heart: do they play a role in cardiac hypertrophy? Am J Pathol. 2007;170(6):1831–40.
43. Tatsuguchi M, Seok HY, Callis TE, Thomson JM, Chen JF, Newman M, Rojas M, Hammond SM, Wang DZ. Expression of microRNAs is dynamically regulated during cardiomyocyte hypertrophy. J Mol Cell Cardiol. 2007;42(6):1137–41.
44. Cheng Y, Zhang C. MicroRNA-21 in cardiovascular disease. J Cardiovasc Transl Res. 2010;3(3):251–5.
45. Xie M, Kong Y, Tan W, May H, Battiprolu PK, Pedrozo Z, Wang ZV, Morales C, Luo X, Cho G, Jiang N, Jessen ME, Warner JJ, Lavandero S, Gillette TG, Turer AT, Hill JA. Histone deacetylase inhibition blunts ischemia/reperfusion injury by inducing cardiomyocyte autophagy. Circulation. 2014;129(10):1139–51.

46. Nakagawa S. Lessons from reverse-genetic studies of lncRNAs. BBA-Biomembranes. 2016;1859(1):177–83.
47. Klattenhoff CA, Scheuermann JC, Surface LE, Bradley RK, Fields PA, Steinhauser ML, Ding H, Butty VL, Torrey L, Haas S, Abo R, Tabebordbar M, Lee RT, Burge CB, Boyer LA. Braveheart, a long noncoding RNA required for cardiovascular lineage commitment. Cell. 2013;152(3):570–83.
48. Han P, Li W, Lin CH, Yang J, Shang C, Nuernberg ST, Jin KK, Xu W, Lin CY, Lin CJ, Xiong Y, Chien H, Zhou B, Ashley E, Bernstein D, Chen PS, Chen HV, Quertermous T, Chang CP. A long noncoding RNA protects the heart from pathological hypertrophy. Nature. 2014;514(7520):102–6.
49. Wang Z, Zhang XJ, Ji YX, Zhang P, Deng KQ, Gong J, Ren S, Wang X, Chen I, Wang H, Gao C, Yokota T, Ang YS, Li S, Cass A, Vondriska TM, Li G, Deb A, Srivastava D, Yang HT, Xiao X, Li H, Wang Y. The long noncoding RNA Chaer defines an epigenetic checkpoint in cardiac hypertrophy. Nat Med. 2016;22(10):1131–9.
50. Viereck J, Kumarswamy R, Foinquinos A, Xiao K, Avramopoulos P, Kunz M, Dittrich M, Maetzig T, Zimmer K, Remke J, Just A, Fendrich J, Scherf K, Bolesani E, Schambach A, Weidemann F, Zweigerdt R, de Windt LJ, Engelhardt S, Dandekar T, Batkai S, Thum T. Long noncoding RNA Chast promotes cardiac remodeling. Sci Transl Med. 2016;8(326):326ra322.
51. Wang K, Liu F, Zhou LY, Long B, Yuan SM, Wang Y, Liu CY, Sun T, Zhang XJ, Li PF. The long noncoding RNA CHRF regulates cardiac hypertrophy by targeting miR-489. Circ Res. 2014;114(9):1377–88.
52. Wo Y, Guo J, Li P, Yang H, Wo J. Long non-coding RNA CHRF facilitates cardiac hypertrophy through regulating Akt3 via miR-93. Cardiovasc Pathol. 2018;35:29–36.
53. Taniyama Y, Ito M, Sato K, Kuester C, Veit K, Tremp G, Liao R, Colucci WS, Ivashchenko Y, Walsh K, Shiojima I. Akt3 overexpression in the heart results in progression from adaptive to maladaptive hypertrophy. J Mol Cell Cardiol. 2005;38(2):375–85.
54. Liu L, An X, Li Z, Song Y, Li L, Zuo S, Liu N, Yang G, Wang H, Cheng X, Zhang Y, Yang X, Wang J. The H19 long noncoding RNA is a novel negative regulator of cardiomyocyte hypertrophy. Cardiovasc Res. 2016;111(1):56–65.
55. Jiang F, Zhou X, Huang J. Long non-coding RNA-ROR mediates the reprogramming in cardiac hypertrophy. PLoS One. 2016;11(4):e0152767.
56. Shao M, Chen G, Lv F, Liu Y, Tian H, Tao R, Jiang R, Zhang W, Zhuo C. LncRNA TINCR attenuates cardiac hypertrophy by epigenetically silencing CaMKII. Oncotarget. 2017;8(29):47565–73.
57. Lai Y, He S, Ma L, Lin H, Ren B, Ma J, Zhu X, Zhuang S. HOTAIR functions as a competing endogenous RNA to regulate PTEN expression by inhibiting miR-19 in cardiac hypertrophy. Mol Cell Biochem. 2017;432(1–2):179–87.
58. Li Y, Wang J, Sun L, Zhu S. LncRNA myocardial infarction-associated transcript (MIAT) contributed to cardiac hypertrophy by regulating TLR4 via miR-93. Eur J Pharmacol. 2018;818:508–17.
59. Zhu XH, Yuan YX, Rao SL, Wang P. LncRNA MIAT enhances cardiac hypertrophy partly through sponging miR-150. Eur J Pharmacol. 2016;20(17):3653–60.
60. Qu S, Yang X, Li X, Wang J, Gao Y, Shang R, Sun W, Dou K, Li H. Circular RNA: a new star of noncoding RNAs. Cancer Lett. 2015;365(2):141–8.
61. Conn SJ, Pillman KA, Toubia J, Conn VM, Salmanidis M, Phillips CA, Roslan S, Schreiber AW, Gregory PA, Goodall GJ. The RNA binding protein quaking regulates formation of circRNAs. Cell. 2015;160(6):1125–34.
62. Hansen TB, Jensen TI, Clausen BH, Bramsen JB, Finsen B, Damgaard CK, Kjems J. Natural RNA circles function as efficient microRNA sponges. Nature. 2013;495(7441):384–8.
63. Li F, Zhang L, Li W, Deng J, Zheng J, An M, Lu J, Zhou Y. Circular RNA ITCH has inhibitory effect on ESCC by suppressing the Wnt/beta-catenin pathway. Oncotarget. 2015;6(8):6001–13.
64. Yang W, Du WW, Li X, Yee AJ, Yang BB. Foxo3 activity promoted by non-coding effects of circular RNA and Foxo3 pseudogene in the inhibition of tumor growth and angiogenesis. Oncogene. 2016;35(30):3919–31.
65. Wang K, Long B, Liu F, Wang JX, Liu CY, Zhao B, Zhou LY, Sun T, Wang M, Yu T, Gong Y, Liu J, Dong YH, Li N, Li PF. A circular RNA protects the heart from pathological hypertrophy and heart failure by targeting miR-223. Eur Heart J. 2016;37(33):2602–11.
66. Li Z, Huang C, Bao C, Chen L, Lin M, Wang X, Zhong G, Yu B, Hu W, Dai L, Zhu P, Chang Z, Wu Q, Zhao Y, Jia Y, Xu P, Liu H, Shan G. Exon-intron circular RNAs regulate transcription in the nucleus. Nat Struct Mol Biol. 2015;22(3):256–64.
67. Du WW, Yang W, Liu E, Yang Z, Dhaliwal P, Yang BB. Foxo3 circular RNA retards cell cycle progression via forming ternary complexes with p21 and CDK2. Nucleic Acids Res. 2016;44(6):2846–58.
68. Geng HH, Li R, Su YM, Xiao J, Pan M, Cai XX, Ji XP. The circular RNA Cdr1as promotes myocardial infarction by mediating the regulation of miR-7a on its target genes expression. PLoS One. 2016;11(3):e0151753.
69. Du WW, Yang W, Chen Y, Wu ZK, Foster FS, Yang Z, Li X, Yang BB. Foxo3 circular RNA promotes cardiac senescence by modulating multiple factors associated with stress and senescence responses. Eur Heart J. 2017;38(18):1402–12.
70. Selitsky SR, Baran-Gale J, Honda M, Yamane D, Masaki T, Fannin EE, Guerra B, Shirasaki T, Shimakami T, Kaneko S, Lanford RE, Lemon SM, Sethupathy P. Small tRNA-derived RNAs are increased and more abundant than microRNAs in chronic hepatitis B and C. Sci Rep. 2015;5:7675.
71. Chen Q, Yan M, Cao Z, Li X, Zhang Y, Shi J, Feng GH, Peng H, Zhang X, Zhang Y, Qian J, Duan E, Zhai

Q, Zhou Q. Sperm tsRNAs contribute to intergenerational inheritance of an acquired metabolic disorder. Science. 2016;351(6271):397–400.
72. Sobala A, Hutvagner G. Small RNAs derived from the 5′ end of tRNA can inhibit protein translation in human cells. RNA Biol. 2013;10(4):553–63.
73. Shen L, Gan M, Tan Z, Jiang D, Jiang Y, Li M, Wang J, Li X, Zhang S, Zhu L. A novel class of tRNA-derived small non-coding RNAs respond to myocardial hypertrophy and contribute to intergenerational inheritance. Biomolecules. 2018;8(3):54.
74. S ELA, Mager I, Breakefield XO, Wood MJ. Extracellular vesicles: biology and emerging therapeutic opportunities. Nat Rev Drug Discov. 2013;12(5):347–57.
75. Valadi H, Ekstrom K, Bossios A, Sjostrand M, Lee JJ, Lotvall JO. Exosome-mediated transfer of mRNAs and microRNAs is a novel mechanism of genetic exchange between cells. Nat Cell Biol. 2007;9(6):654–9.
76. Waldenstrom A, Genneback N, Hellman U, Ronquist G. Cardiomyocyte microvesicles contain DNA/RNA and convey biological messages to target cells. PLoS One. 2012;7(4):e34653.
77. Garcia NA, Ontoria-Oviedo I, Gonzalez-King H, Diez-Juan A, Sepulveda P. Glucose starvation in Cardiomyocytes enhances exosome secretion and promotes angiogenesis in endothelial cells. PLoS One. 2015;10(9):e0138849.
78. Halkein J, Tabruyn SP, Ricke-Hoch M, Haghikia A, Nguyen NQ, Scherr M, Castermans K, Malvaux L, Lambert V, Thiry M, Sliwa K, Noel A, Martial JA, Hilfiker-Kleiner D, Struman I. MicroRNA-146a is a therapeutic target and biomarker for peripartum cardiomyopathy. J Clin Investig. 2013;123(5):2143–54.
79. Bang C, Batkai S, Dangwal S, Gupta SK, Foinquinos A, Holzmann A, Just A, Remke J, Zimmer K, Zeug A, Ponimaskin E, Schmiedl A, Yin X, Mayr M, Halder R, Fischer A, Engelhardt S, Wei Y, Schober A, Fiedler J, Thum T. Cardiac fibroblast-derived microRNA passenger strand-enriched exosomes mediate cardiomyocyte hypertrophy. J Clin Investig. 2014;124(5):2136–46.
80. Heymans S, Corsten MF, Verhesen W, Carai P, van Leeuwen RE, Custers K, Peters T, Hazebroek M, Stoger L, Wijnands E, Janssen BJ, Creemers EE, Pinto YM, Grimm D, Schurmann N, Vigorito E, Thum T, Stassen F, Yin X, Mayr M, de Windt LJ, Lutgens E, Wouters K, de Winther MP, Zacchigna S, Giacca M, van Bilsen M, Papageorgiou AP, Schroen B. Macrophage microRNA-155 promotes cardiac hypertrophy and failure. Circulation. 2013;128(13):1420–32.

Non-coding RNAs and Cardiac Aging

14

Cuimei Zhao, Guoping Li, and Jin Li

Abstract

Aging is an important risk factor for cardiovascular diseases. Aging increasing the morbidity and mortality in cardiovascular disease patients. With the society is aging rapidly in the world, medical burden of aging-related cardiovascular diseases increasing drastically. Hence, it is urgent to explore the underlying mechanism and treatment of cardiac aging. Noncoding RNAs (ncRNAs, including microRNAs, long noncoding RNAs and circular RNAs) have been reported to be involved in many pathological processes, including cell proliferation, cell death differentiation, hypertrophy and aging in wide variety of cells and tissues. In this chapter, we will summarize the physiology and molecular mechanisms of cardiac aging. Then, the recent research advances of ncRNAs in cardiac aging will be provided. The lessons learned from ncRNAs and cardiac aging studies would bring new insights into the regulatory mechanisms ncRNAs as well as treatment of aging-related cardiovascular diseases.

Keywords

Cardiac ageing · miRNA · Long noncoding RNA · Circular RNA

C. Zhao
Department of Cardiology, Shanghai Tongji Hospital, Tongji University School of Medicine, Shanghai, China

G. Li
Cardiovascular Division, Massachusetts General Hospital, Harvard Medical School, Boston, MA, USA

J. Li (✉)
Cardiac Regeneration and Ageing Lab, Institute of Cardiovascular Sciences, School of Life Science, Shanghai University, Shanghai, China

1 Introduction

Aging is a main factor for cardiovascular diseases. It has been reported that the incidence of myocardial infarction, cardiac hypertrophy, atrial fibrillation and coronary arteriosclerosis were dramatically increased with aging [1–3]. Besides, myocardial structure and function changed with ageing always accompanied with pathological conditions, such as aortic stiffening, atrial enlargement, loss of myocytes, pathological hypertrophy and proliferation of cardiac fibroblasts [4]. Additionally, aged heart making it more sensitive to cardiovascular risk factors [5, 6]. Therefore, exploring the molecular mechanism of cardiac aging is helpful to prevent cardiovascular risk and reveal the occurrence of cardiovascular diseases.

Along with transcriptomics, next generation sequencing and bioinformatics development, the concept that proteins were the main regulators in

J. Xiao (ed.), *Non-coding RNAs in Cardiovascular Diseases*, Advances in Experimental Medicine and Biology 1229, https://doi.org/10.1007/978-981-15-1671-9_14

gene expression regulation has been updated in the past two decades. Only 2% of the transcribed genomic DNA can be translated into protein, mostly of the transcripts can't translatable, which were known as noncoding RNAs (ncRNAs). NcRNAs have been shown to be involved in almost all physiological and pathological processes of heart. In this chapter, we will summarize (1) the physiology and molecular mechanisms of cardiac aging, (2) the function of ncRNAs in cardiac aging.

2 Cardiac Ageing

Cardiac aging is a heterogeneous process which is characterized by damaged genomic DNA, shortened telomere length, altered epigenetic modifications, as well as accumulated senescent cells [7].With the growth of age, the performance of the heart gradually decline, thus, the structural and functional capacity of the heart would be impaired, which is the mainly inducing factor of cardiovascular disease in elderly. Cardiovascular disease is the major reason of death in the western world. Recent statistical study has reported a 171% increase in cardiovascular deaths among patients ages 65–85 [8]. The physiological changes of cardiac aging mainly include left ventricular hypertrophy, diastolic dysfunction, valve degeneration, increased cardiac fibrosis, increased prevalence of atrial fibrillation, and decreased maximum exercise ability [9]. Although the phenotype of heart aging can be well characterized, the study on the molecular mechanism of heart aging is just beginning. Here, we mainly focus on the physiological change and molecular mechanism of cardiac aging in view of the recent research progress, and provide new treatment opportunities for age-related cardiovascular diseases.

2.1 Physiology of Cardiac Aging

2.1.1 Ventricular Changes

Increased left ventricular thickness is an important factor for cardiovascular disease. According to the Framingham Heart Study and the Baltimore Longitudinal Study of aging, left ventricular wall thickness significantly increased with age in both men and women regardless of whether they previously had hypertension. Caused by decreased ventricular elasticity, fibrosis and delayed ventricular active diastole, left ventricular filling in early diastole may gradually weaken in elderly. Moreover, the decreased rate of calcium ATPase calcium reuptake in myocardial reticulum will further aggravate this damage. As a result, in order to maintain the filling of left ventricle with increase of age, atrial contraction gradually increases, leading to increased atrial pressure, which is not benefit to hypertrophy and increases the incidence of atrial fibrillation [1, 2, 10]. Studies have shown that, the ratio of early (E) and late (A) diastolic left ventricular filling decreased in elderly people [11, 12], which is clinically defined as cardiac diastolic dysfunction [13] In addition, cardiac aging also leads to a decrease in maximal heart rate and induces a range of cardiovascular diseases [14, 15].

2.1.2 Valvular Changes

Echocardiography revealed that 30–80% of the elderly had aortic valve sclerosis [16–18], mainly including aortic lobular calcification and aortic ring [19, 20]. Valve sclerosis are age-related valve lesions which include myxomatosis degeneration and collagen deposition. Elderly patients with cardiac hypertrophy, hyperlipidemia, hypertension, end-stage renal disease, and congenital bicuspid aortic valve have an increased risk of cardiovascular disease and mortality compared with their peers [21–24].

The prevalence of aortic stenosis increased with age. Fibrosis and valve calcification can lead to aortic stenosis [21]. In order to maintain adequate systolic function, left ventricular wall thickening enables effective pumping of blood, while excessive left ventricular wall thickening causes left ventricular dilatation, result in systolic function. In addition, with age, aortic valve insufficiency, blood flows from the aorta to the left ventricle, resulting in increased left ventricular volume, accounting for 13–16% of the elderly with aortic regurgitation [17].

Mitral annular calcification (MAC) is a degenerative disease involving the mitral annulus. MAC patients often suffer from a complications, such as hypertension, aortic stenosis, mitral valve prolapse, heart failure, atrial fibrillation, and so on [25, 26]. Besides, mitral regurgitation is another common abnormality in the elderly. Mitral regurgitation happens when the mitral valve does not seal tightly, causing blood to flow back to the heart, resulting in insufficient blood flow. Two major causes of mitral regurgitation are myxomatous degeneration and ischemic heart disease [27]. Changes in central ventricles and valves during cardiac aging result in cardiac functional impaired and more likely to development into heart failure [14]. Which makes the elderly heart more sensitive to risk factors, leading to cardiovascular mortality in the elderly population.

2.2 Molecular Mechanisms of Cardiac Aging

2.2.1 Nutrition and Growth Signaling

There are many cell signaling regulators involved in the process of heart failure, many of which are associated with cardiac hypertrophy. Insulin-like growth factor-1 (IGF-1) is an important signaling pathway participate in this process [30, 31], Normally, depression of IGF-1 level can lead to heart failure, which may be reduced if drugs are used to increase IGF-1 levels in the body [32–34]. At the same time, IGF-1 can weaken the oxidative stress response in the organ, making it less sensitive [28]. Therefore, IGF-1 pathway can be an effective target to ameliorate cardiac function [35, 36], Another important cell signaling regulator in the heart failure process is mTOR. Overexpression of eIF4E in this signaling pathway can lead to impairment in cardiac function. Therefore, the mTOR/eIF4E signaling pathway also a great influence on the aging process of the heart [29].

SIRTs are a conserved family of NAD^+-dependent deacetylases (class III histone deacetylases). Additional copies of the *Sirt* gene in fermentation were associated with increased longevity [29–31]. There are seven SIRTs subtypes in mammals, sirt1-7. Sir2 controls the extension of replication life under the effect of DR (decreased glucose) [32, 33]. Mice lacking SIRT1 showed shorter life span compared with peers. In addition, SIRTs also taken important regulatory role in mitochondria of cardiomyocytes. Sirt3 was reported expression decreases with age in people who have been sedentary for a long time, and can be increased after endurance training [34]. The low to medium expression of Sirt1 in the heart can reduce the age dependence of cardiac hypertrophy, cardiac dysfunction and aging markers. Besides, SIRT3 knockout showed signs of accelerated aging, including myocardial hypertrophy and accelerated fibrosis [35]. Increased SIRT3 expression was associated with longer human lifespan [36]. SIRTs are involved in nutritional signal transduction and epigenetic regulation of histone deacetylation and DNA expression directly related to cardiac aging. This is consistent with the growing recognition of the epigenetic modifications in aging [37] and cardiovascular disease [38]. DNA hypomethylation is link with cardiovascular disease risk [39].

2.2.2 Abnormal Mitochondrial Function

Studies have been suggested that the accumulation of mitochondrial reactive oxygen species (ROS) would cause damage of mitochondrial DNA and proteins, leading to dysregulation of cellular activity, organ dysfunction, and ultimately limiting health and lifespan [40]. Besides, ROS production in the heart increases significantly in age [41]. Mitochondrial ROS can lead to mitochondrial dysfunction and cardiomyopathy in the elderly [42, 43]. In addition, abnormal overexpressed catalase-targeted mitochondria is clearly detected in the aging heart of mice, which is the most direct evidence of mitochondrial oxidative damage leading to cardiac aging. Therefore, decreasing mitochondrial oxidative damage is one of the important strategies to prevent heart aging. Further studies have shown that peroxisome proliferator-activated receptor gamma coactivator 1α (PCG-1α) is a major molecule in regulating mitochondrial function. Overexpression of PCG-1α can ameliorate the function of mitochondrial in the myocardium. Thus, interfering PCG-1α expression might be an effective way to alleviate the occurrence of mitochondrial oxidation [44]. Knockout PCG-1α in mice, the mitochondrial gene expression was reduced but developed cardiac dysfunction [45]. In adult mice, PCG-1α overexpression was directly associated with cardiomyopathy [46].

Some studies have shown that mitochondrial dysfunction increases with age, which is associated with abnormal production of mtROS [42, 43, 47]. For example, reduced mitochondrial oxidative phosphorylation is associated with reduced activity of electron transport complexes I and IV, while compounds II, III, and V are relatively unaffected [48]. Damage to electron transport function may be result in increased electron leakage and mtROS generation. Mitochondrial energy dysfunction resulting from mitochondrial decoupling, decreased substrate availability [49] and increased mitochondrial DNA deletion have been demonstrated in human and experimental heart failure animals [50, 51].

2.2.3 Neurohormonal Regulation

Renin-angiotensin aldosterone system (RAAS) is an important system regulating hypertension and is associated with cardiovascular disease and age-related failing in cardiac function [52]. The concentration of Ang II in the heart significantly increased with age, and many structural, functional and molecules alterations consistent with the action of Ang II were found in the elderly heart [12, 53]. Inhibitor captopril or angiotensin receptor I inhibitor could reduce myocardial fibrosis and fibrosis-related arrhythmias in older mice [54]. And destroy angiotensin receptor type I would extend the lifespan [55]. RAAS is associated with tissue aging in a variety of tissues. Such as in kidneys, angiotensin blocking was beneficial for kidney aging [56].

Epinephrine have adverse effects on cardiovascular health. β-adrenergic signaling pathway is associated with aging, and adenylate cyclase 5 can significantly improve the effects of age-related cardiac dysfunction, and lifespan [57–59]. With increasing evidence supporting that the important role of epinephrine is mediated by mitochondrial ROS [60]. The increase of ROS plays an important role in β adrenalin. Although β-adrenergic antagonists are commonly used in heart disease [61], their effect on longevity has not been evaluated. To determine a safety and effective approach, these inhibitors are combined with other signaling pathways inhibitors for maximum positive effect.

Insulin-like growth factor (IGF) signaling is another important element of longevity. Lack of the insulin-like receptor extends the lifespan of mammals [62, 63], and could reduce the specific benefits of the IGF-1 signaling pathway for heart aging in mouse models [64, 65]. Unfortunately, the role of IGF-1 signaling in human heart aging is complex. IGF-1 levels significantly decreased with age, and in elderly patients without a history of heart disease, low serum IGF-1 levels are associated with an increased risk of heart failure [66]. In growth hormone therapy, IGF-1 pathway was proposed to be beneficial for heart failure patients [67]. Insulin activates a phosphorinosine-3-kinase (PI3K) signaling cascade that phosphorylates and activates AKT. Activated AKT is transferred into the nucleus, and then inhibit the transcription activity of FOXO by phosphorylation. In the heart, the FOXO family is link with oxidative stress [68], metabolic regulation [69], and apoptosis [70]. FOXO transcription factor has an anti-aging effect, therefore, inhibiting insulin signaling or overexpression of FOXO can prevent cardiac function from declining with ageing [65].

3 Noncoding RNAs (ncRNAs)

In the early of the molecular biology, RNA was divided into two groups: protein-coding RNAs and functional RNAs, such as ribosomal RNAs (rRNAs), small nuclear RNAs (snRNAs), small nucleolar RNAs (snoRNAs), and transfer RNAs (tRNAs). With the development of transcriptome, especially the innovation of RNA-sequencing, more and more ncRNAs have been discovered. The study of RNAs from protein-coding RNAs to ncRNAs. Many ncRNAs, demonstrated new regulatory function. Considering the complexity of such ncRNAs in structures, genomic orientation, function, cellular localization, or other emerging criteria, a simple and common ncRNAs classification was needed to be raised. The most well-accepted classification model was based on the length of RNA: (1) small RNAs, the transcripts are shorter than 200 nt, including microRNAs (miRNAs, miRs). (2) long noncoding RNAs (lncRNAs), the transcripts are longer than 200 nt. In addition, a class of special lncRNA, circular RNA (circRNA), which is covalently closed, single-stranded RNA molecules, recently obtained much attention. These ncRNAs display distinct temporal and spatial expression patterns, and almost involved in all biological processes [71]. As details of the impact of ncRNAs on molecular and cellular processes are becoming better understood, their roles in aging-associated physiologic processes and disease conditions are also starting to emerge. Some ncRNAs have a connection between cardiac aging (Fig. 14.1). The research of ncRNAs in aging-associated heart dysfunction provides new perspective in deeper insights into disease mechanisms and innovative therapeutic strategies.

4 MiRNAs in Cardiac Ageing

MiRNAs are single-stranded RNAs ~22 nt in length and found in both the intergenic and coding regions of the genome. The primary miRNAs (pri-miRNAs) are transcribed from both intronic and exonic regions by RNA polymerase II. Then the pri-miRNAs are processed to precursor miRNAs (pre-miRNAs) in nucleus by Drosha and DGCR8. The pre-miRNAs were stem-loop

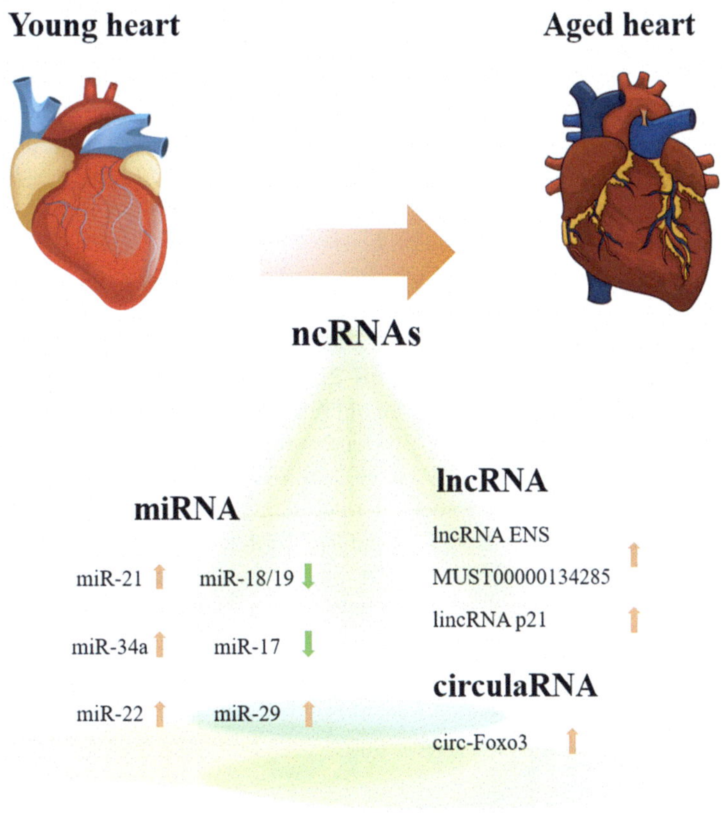

Fig. 14.1 Noncoding RNAs in cardiac ageing

structures with ~70 nt long. The pre-miRNAs exported to cytoplasm from nucleus with the assistance of exportin-5. In cytoplasm, the stem-loop structures cleaved by Dicer and turn into a mature miRNAs with ~22 nt length. Classically, miRNAs repress the expression of their target mRNA by binding to the specific untranslated regions (UTRs) based on complementary base pairing. The single stranded miRNA, associated with Ago, assembled into the RNA-induced silencing complex (RISC), miRNA–RISC complex induces translation inhibition and mRNA degradation, result in mediates post-transcriptional repression of a target mRNA. In this mode, miRNAs can regulate all physiological and pathological processes.

Some miRNA arrays or miRNA profiling were performed to identify the dysregulated miRNAs in the hearts of young and aged mice. 65 miRNAs changed over 1.5-fold in aged heart, among them, 34 miRNAs were up-regulated while 31 were down-regulated [72]. Addition, the expression of the miRNA machinery proteins Ago1 and Ago2 were also found to be increased with age, and synergistically induced miR-21 and miR-21∗ in ageing. MiR-21was involved in myocardial diseases [73]. MiR-21 was up-regulated in left ventricular myocardium, myocardial hypertrophy and failing human left ventricular myocardium. Also, miR-21 was enriched in fibroblasts, and increased in fibroblasts of failing heart, inhibiting ERK-MAP kinase pathway via inhibiting Spry1. Inhibiting miR-21 by antagomir in vivo could reduce fibrosis and attenuate cardiac dysfunction. Interestingly, miR-21 was also found to be increased in 15-month old mice compared with 2-month old mice [74]. Overexpression of miR-21 promoted Dox-induced cardiomyocytes, whereas miR-21 knockout mice demonstrated the ability of resist to Dox-induced cardiac alterations. Mechanistically, PTEN was a target gene of miR-21 involved in D-gal and Dox-induced cardiac senescence.

From another miRNA profiling, Reinier A. Boon found that miR-34a was up-regulated in ageing heart, and significantly correlated with age in human heart biopsies [75]. Inhibit the expression of miR-34a would prevent age-related and myocardial infarction-induced cardiomyocytes death and improve cardiac function. Pnuts was the target gene of miR-34a that mediated age-induced cardiac cell death and functional decline. miR-34a has also been reported to be involved in the repair and regeneration of myocardial infarction in neonatal mice, increasing the level of miR-34a could suppress the neonatal cardiomyocytes reentry into cell cycle and reduce the survival rate of neonatal cells [76]. Also, miR-34a has been reported to mediate a variety of myocardial injuries [77–80]. Some new therapies have been developed by inhibiting the expression of miR-34a, such as miRNA sponges and drug interventions [81, 82]. In addition, miR-22 was also found to be elevated in 19 months old mice [83]. Overexpression of miR-22 would induce cellular senescence and promote migratory activity of cardiac fibroblasts via inhibiting mimecan.

Accumulation of the extracellular matrix (ECM) are recognized as a key feature of cardiac ageing [84]. miR-17-92 cluster has been proved taken the crucial role in regulating matrix genes in ageing cell [85]. Among them, miR-18 and miR-19 were down-regulated in ageing induced heart failure and regulated the fibrosis in ageing cardiomyocytes through miR-18/19- CTGF/TSP-1 axis [86] MiR-17, another member of miR-17-92 cluster, was also reported to participate in cardiac ageing [87]. Unlike miR-18 and miR-19 mainly expressed in cardiomyocytes, miR-17 was expressed in ageing cardiac fibroblasts and inhibited the cellular senescence and apoptosis of fibroblasts via targeting par4. Furthermore, miR-17 transgenic mice suppressed mouse cardiac senescence. Additionally, TGFβ-Smad signaling is one of the prominent pathways both involved in fibrosis and senescence [88–91] TGFβ-Smad regulates expression of miR-29 (miR-29a, miR-29b and miR-29c), which mediated the reduction of H4K20me3 through targeting Suv4-20 h, leading to premature cellular senescence and cardiac dysfunction [92].

5 Long Noncoding RNAs in Cardiac Ageing

LncRNAs are defined as being ncRNA sequences of >200 nucleotides. LncRNAs are transcribed by RNA polymerase II or III, may be multi-exonic, 5′-capped, and poly-adenylated. According to their genomic location, lncRNAs have been classified into six categories, which is intergenic, intronic, bidirectional, enhancer, sense, and antisense lncRNAs. LncRNAs localized in the nucleus or cytoplasm where they may regulate gene expression at transcriptional or posttranscriptional levels, respectively. Briefly, when lncRNA located in nuclear, the regulated models of lncRNA acted as signal, decoy, guide, scaffold or enhancer [93]. While the cytoplasm-localized lncRNAs were usually mediates the stability the ribonucleoprotein complexes and mRNA, as well as sponge miRNAs [94]. Especially, some lncRNAs hold the ability to encode small peptides, such as LINC00961, LOC100507537 (NONMMUG026737 in mice) and LINC00948 (2310015B20Rik in mice) [95–97]. LncRNAs extensively participates in physiological processes such as cell proliferation, hypertrophy and metabolic regulation. The dysfunction of lncRNA is closely related to the occurrence of tumors and other diseases [98–102]. Specifically, SAL-RNA1, H19 and lncRNA Chronos involved in regulating senescence [103–105]. However, there are few studies on lncRNA in cardiac aging have been reported.

Detected by lncRNA/mRNA microarray, a total of 1957 lncRNAs and 984 mRNAs were found to be uniquely differentially expressed between young and aged heart tissue. Among then, lncRNA (ENSMUST00000134285) was increasing in aged heart as well as aged cardiac-myocytes. Overexpression of lncRNA (ENSMUST00000134285) significantly reduced cardiomyocyte apoptotic. LncRNA (ENSMUST00000134285) was co-expressed with MAPK11 and promoted MAPK11 via miR-760 [106]. Besides, lincRNA-p21 was investigated in Dox-induced cardiomyocytes senescence. Knockdown of lincRNA-p21 was significantly increased the cellular viability and decreased the cell cardiomyocytes senescence via regulation of senescence-related genes p53 and p16. Furthermore, the pro-senescent effect of lincRNA-p21 via Wnt/β-catenin signaling pathway [107].

6 Circular RNAs in Cardiac Ageing

Circular RNAs (circRNAs) is a special type of lncRNAs. They are generated from either intron or exon. Its specialty lies in forming a loop without 5′-3′ polarity or polyadenylated tail through back splicing of the 5′ and 3′ ends after transcribed from genomic DNA. The regulation mechanisms of circRNAs have been revealed by increasing studies. Such as miRNA sponges, binds to RNA binding proteins (RBPs), competes with canonical pre-mRNA splicing in gene regulation, and translated [108]. CircRNAs have been identified as crucial regulators of diverse cellular processes [109]. Only one circRNA was reported to involved in cardiac senescence so far [110]. Circ-Foxo3 was found to be up-regulated in old heart patients, older mice and H_2O_2 treated primary cardiomyocytes. In Dox-induced cardiomyopathy, in vivo overexpression of circ-Foxo3 could worsen the heart function, myocardial hypertrophy and myocardial fibrosis, whereas repressed circ-Foxo3 would reverse that. Also, in vitro, circ-Foxo3 overexpress could worsen cellular senescence independent of linear Foxo3. Specifically, circ-Foxo3 could bind to senescence-related proteins ID1 and E2F1, and stress-related proteins HIF1a and FAK in cytoplasm. Result in its associated proteins arrest in cytoplasm and abolished the transcriptional regulation, and induced cellular senescence in heart.

7 Conclusion

With elderly population in the world increases, ageing-related diseases are attracting more and more attention. Aging increases the risk of cardiovascular disease, thus there is an urgent need to reveal the underlying mechanisms of cardiac ageing. As we discussed here, some ncRNAs have been reported to involved in cardiac ageing. However, the researches focus on cardiac ageing obviously fewer and more efforts definitely need to be taken. Besides, the circulating ncRNA (miRNAs, lncRNAs and circRNAs) have been proposed to serve as biomarkers in many diseases. Unfortunately, there is no research on cardiac ageing so far. Further studies taken into this aspect should be of great interests. In conclusion, ncRNAs have been demonstrated to be excellent therapeutic targets in many diseases, and more depth and extensive investigations in cardiac ageing should be of great significant.

Acknowledgements This work was supported by the grants from Shanghai Health and Family Planning Commissio (20154Y0026 to Cuimei Zhao), and National Natural Science Foundation of China (81600228 to Cuimei Zhao).

Competing Financial Interests The authors declare no competing financial interests.

References

1. Lakatta EG. Arterial and cardiac aging: major shareholders in cardiovascular disease enterprises: part III: cellular and molecular clues to heart and arterial aging. Circulation. 2003;107(3):490–7.
2. Lakatta EG, Levy D. Arterial and cardiac aging: major shareholders in cardiovascular disease enterprises: part II: the aging heart in health: links to heart disease. Circulation. 2003;107(2):346–54.
3. Shih H, Lee B, Lee RJ, Boyle AJ. The aging heart and post-infarction left ventricular remodeling. J Am Coll Cardiol. 2011;57(1):9–17.
4. Horn MA. Cardiac physiology of aging: extracellular considerations. Compr Physiol. 2015;5(3):1069–121.
5. Benjamin EJ, Muntner P, Alonso A, Bittencourt MS, Callaway CW, Carson AP, Chamberlain AM, Chang AR, Cheng S, Das SR. Heart disease and stroke statistics—2019 update: a report from the American Heart Association. Circulation: CIR. 2018;139(10):e56–e528. https://doi.org/10.1161/CIR.0000000000000659.
6. Dai DF, Chen T, Johnson SC, Szeto H, Rabinovitch PS. Cardiac aging: from molecular mechanisms to significance in human health and disease. Antioxid Redox Signal. 2012;16(12):1492–526.
7. Lopez-Otin C, Blasco MA, Partridge L, Serrano M, Kroemer G. The hallmarks of aging. Cell. 2013;153(6):1194–217.
8. Go AS, Mozaffarian D, Roger VL, Benjamin EJ, Berry JD, Blaha MJ, Dai S, Ford ES, Fox CS, Franco S, Fullerton HJ, Gillespie C, Hailpern SM, Heit JA, Howard VJ, Huffman MD, Judd SE, Kissela BM, Kittner SJ, Lackland DT, Lichtman JH, Lisabeth LD, Mackey RH, Magid DJ, Marcus GM, Marelli A, Matchar DB, DK MG, Mohler ER 3rd, Moy CS, Mussolino ME, Neumar RW, Nichol G, Pandey DK, Paynter NP, Reeves MJ, Sorlie PD, Stein J, Towfighi A, Turan TN, Virani SS, Wong ND, Woo D, Turner MB, American Heart Association Statistics C, Stroke Statistics S. Heart disease and stroke statistics--2014 update: a report from the American Heart Association. Circulation. 2014;129(3):e28–e292.
9. Batacan RB Jr, Duncan MJ, Dalbo VJ, Buitrago GL, Fenning AS. Effect of different intensities of physical activity on cardiometabolic markers and vascular and cardiac function in adult rats fed with a high-fat high-carbohydrate diet. J Sport Health Sci. 2018;7(1):109–19.
10. Lakatta EG, Levy D. Arterial and cardiac aging: major shareholders in cardiovascular disease enterprises: part I: aging arteries: a "set up" for vascular disease. Circulation. 2003;107(1):139–46.
11. Dai DF, Rabinovitch PS. Cardiac aging in mice and humans: the role of mitochondrial oxidative stress. Trends Cardiovasc Med. 2009;19(7):213–20.
12. Dai DF, Santana LF, Vermulst M, Tomazela DM, Emond MJ, MacCoss MJ, Gollahon K, Martin GM, Loeb LA, Ladiges WC, Rabinovitch PS. Overexpression of catalase targeted to mitochondria attenuates murine cardiac aging. Circulation. 2009;119(21):2789–97.
13. Bursi F, Weston SA, Redfield MM, Jacobsen SJ, Pakhomov S, Nkomo VT, Meverden RA, Roger VL. Systolic and diastolic heart failure in the community. JAMA J Am Med Assoc. 2006;296(18):2209–16.
14. Correia LC, Lakatta EG, O'Connor FC, Becker LC, Clulow J, Townsend S, Gerstenblith G, Fleg JL. Attenuated cardiovascular reserve during prolonged submaximal cycle exercise in healthy older subjects. J Am Coll Cardiol. 2002;40(7):1290–7.
15. Fleg JL, O'Connor F, Gerstenblith G, Becker LC, Clulow J, Schulman SP, Lakatta EG. Impact of age on the cardiovascular response to dynamic upright exercise in healthy men and women. J Appl Physiol. (1985. 1995;78(3):890–900.
16. Karavidas A, Lazaros G, Tsiachris D, Pyrgakis V. Aging and the cardiovascular system. Hell J Cardiol. 2010;51(5):421–7.
17. Nassimiha D, Aronow WS, Ahn C, Goldman ME. Association of coronary risk factors with progression of valvular aortic stenosis in older persons. Am J Cardiol. 2001;87(11):1313–4.
18. Stewart BF, Siscovick D, Lind BK, Gardin JM, Gottdiener JS, Smith VE, Kitzman DW, Otto

CM. Clinical factors associated with calcific aortic valve disease. Cardiovascular Health Study. J Am Coll Cardiol. 1997;29(3):630–4.
19. Freeman RV, Otto CM. Spectrum of calcific aortic valve disease: pathogenesis, disease progression, and treatment strategies. Circulation. 2005;111(24):3316–26.
20. Otto CM, Lind BK, Kitzman DW, Gersh BJ, Siscovick DS. Association of aortic-valve sclerosis with cardiovascular mortality and morbidity in the elderly. N Engl J Med. 1999;341(3):142–7.
21. Olsen MH, Wachtell K, Bella JN, Gerdts E, Palmieri V, Nieminen MS, Smith G, Ibsen H, Devereux RB, substudy L. Aortic valve sclerosis relates to cardiovascular events in patients with hypertension (a LIFE substudy). Am J Cardiol. 2005;95(1):132–6.
22. Aronow WS, Ahn C, Shirani J, Kronzon I. Comparison of frequency of new coronary events in older subjects with and without valvular aortic sclerosis. Am J Cardiol. 1999;83(4):599–600.. A598
23. Palacios OM, Carmona JJ, Michan S, Chen KY, Manabe Y, Ward JL 3rd, Goodyear LJ, Tong Q. Diet and exercise signals regulate SIRT3 and activate AMPK and PGC-1alpha in skeletal muscle. Aging (Albany NY). 2009;1(9):771–83.
24. Otto CM. Why is aortic sclerosis associated with adverse clinical outcomes? J Am Coll Cardiol. 2004;43(2):176–8.
25. Fulkerson PK, Beaver BM, Auseon JC, Graber HL. Calcification of the mitral annulus: etiology, clinical associations, complications and therapy. Am J Med. 1979;66(6):967–77.
26. Kastman EK, Willette AA, Coe CL, Bendlin BB, Kosmatka KJ, McLaren DG, Xu G, Canu E, Field AS, Alexander AL, Voytko ML, Beasley TM, Colman RJ, Weindruch RH, Johnson SC. A calorie-restricted diet decreases brain iron accumulation and preserves motor performance in old rhesus monkeys. J Neurosci. 2010;30(23):7940–7.
27. Jebara VA, Dervanian P, Acar C, Grare P, Mihaileanu S, Chauvaud S, Fabiani JN, Deloche A, Carpentier A. Mitral valve repair using Carpentier techniques in patients more than 70 years old. Early and late results. Circulation. 1992;86(5 Suppl):II53–9.
28. Nedic O, Sunderic M, Miljus G, Valdevit Z, Jakovljevic V, Glibetic M, Vucic V. Preparatory training attenuates drastic response of the insulin-like growth factor binding protein 1 at the point of maximal oxygen consumption in handball players. J Sport Health Sci. 2017;6(3):372–7.
29. Bass TM, Weinkove D, Houthoofd K, Gems D, Partridge L. Effects of resveratrol on lifespan in Drosophila melanogaster and Caenorhabditis elegans. Mech Ageing Dev. 2007;128(10):546–52.
30. Baur JA, Sinclair DA. Therapeutic potential of resveratrol: the in vivo evidence. Nat Rev Drug Discov. 2006;5(6):493–506.
31. Kusama S, Ueda R, Suda T, Nishihara S, Matsuura ET. Involvement of Drosophila Sir2-like genes in the regulation of life span. Genes Genet Syst. 2006;81(5):341–8.
32. Anderson RM, Bitterman KJ, Wood JG, Medvedik O, Sinclair DA. Nicotinamide and PNC1 govern lifespan extension by calorie restriction in Saccharomyces cerevisiae. Nature. 2003;423(6936):181–5.
33. Lin J, Wu H, Tarr PT, Zhang CY, Wu Z, Boss O, Michael LF, Puigserver P, Isotani E, Olson EN, Lowell BB, Bassel-Duby R, Spiegelman BM. Transcriptional co-activator PGC-1 alpha drives the formation of slow-twitch muscle fibres. Nature. 2002;418(6899):797–801.
34. Lanza IR, Short DK, Short KR, Raghavakaimal S, Basu R, Joyner MJ, McConnell JP, Nair KS. Endurance exercise as a countermeasure for aging. Diabetes. 2008;57(11):2933–42.
35. Hafner AV, Dai J, Gomes AP, Xiao CY, Palmeira CM, Rosenzweig A, Sinclair DA. Regulation of the mPTP by SIRT3-mediated deacetylation of CypD at lysine 166 suppresses age-related cardiac hypertrophy. Aging (Albany NY). 2010;2(12):914–23.
36. Bellizzi D, Rose G, Cavalcante P, Covello G, Dato S, De Rango F, Greco V, Maggiolini M, Feraco E, Mari V, Franceschi C, Passarino G, De Benedictis G. A novel VNTR enhancer within the SIRT3 gene, a human homologue of SIR2, is associated with survival at oldest ages. Genomics. 2005;85(2):258–63.
37. Gravina S, Vijg J. Epigenetic factors in aging and longevity. Pflugers Archiv-Eur J Physiol. 2010;459(2):247–58.
38. Gluckman PD, Hanson MA, Buklijas T, Low FM, Beedle AS. Epigenetic mechanisms that underpin metabolic and cardiovascular diseases. Nat Rev Endocrinol. 2009;5(7):401–8.
39. Baccarelli A, Wright R, Bollati V, Litonjua A, Zanobetti A, Tarantini L, Sparrow D, Vokonas P, Schwartz J. Ischemic heart disease and stroke in relation to blood DNA methylation. Epidemiology. 2010;21(6):819–28.
40. Baysa A, Fedorov A, Kondratov K, Ruusalepp A, Minasian S, Galagudza M, Popov M, Kurapeev D, Yakovlev A, Valen G, Kostareva A, Vaage J, Stenslokken KO. Release of mitochondrial and nuclear DNA during on-pump heart surgery: kinetics and relation to extracellular vesicles. J Cardiovasc Transl Res. 2019;12(3):184–92.
41. Judge S, Jang YM, Smith A, Hagen T, Leeuwenburgh C. Age-associated increases in oxidative stress and antioxidant enzyme activities in cardiac interfibrillar mitochondria: implications for the mitochondrial theory of aging. FASEB J. 2005;19(3):419–21.
42. Terzioglu M, Larsson NG. Mitochondrial dysfunction in mammalian ageing. Novartis Found Symp. 2007;287:197–208; discussion 208-113.
43. Trifunovic A, Larsson NG. Mitochondrial dysfunction as a cause of ageing. J Intern Med. 2008;263(2):167–78.
44. Wenz T. Mitochondria and PGC-1alpha in aging and age-associated diseases. J Aging Res. 2011;2011:810619.

45. Arany Z, He H, Lin J, Hoyer K, Handschin C, Toka O, Ahmad F, Matsui T, Chin S, Wu PH, Rybkin II, Shelton JM, Manieri M, Cinti S, Schoen FJ, Bassel-Duby R, Rosenzweig A, Ingwall JS, Spiegelman BM. Transcriptional coactivator PGC-1 alpha controls the energy state and contractile function of cardiac muscle. Cell Metab. 2005;1(4):259–71.
46. Russell LK, Mansfield CM, Lehman JJ, Kovacs A, Courtois M, Saffitz JE, Medeiros DM, Valencik ML, McDonald JA, Kelly DP. Cardiac-specific induction of the transcriptional coactivator peroxisome proliferator-activated receptor gamma coactivator-1alpha promotes mitochondrial biogenesis and reversible cardiomyopathy in a developmental stage-dependent manner. Circ Res. 2004;94(4):525–33.
47. Mammucari C, Rizzuto R. Signaling pathways in mitochondrial dysfunction and aging. Mech Ageing Dev. 2010;131(7–8):536–43.
48. Navarro A, Boveris A. The mitochondrial energy transduction system and the aging process. Am J Phys Cell Phys. 2007;292(2):C670–86.
49. Murray AJ, Anderson RE, Watson GC, Radda GK, Clarke K. Uncoupling proteins in human heart. Lancet. 2004;364(9447):1786–8.
50. Dai DF, Johnson SC, Villarin JJ, Chin MT, Nieves-Cintron M, Chen T, Marcinek DJ, Dorn GW 2nd, Kang YJ, Prolla TA, Santana LF, Rabinovitch PS. Mitochondrial oxidative stress mediates angiotensin II-induced cardiac hypertrophy and Galphaq overexpression-induced heart failure. Circ Res. 2011;108(7):837–46.
51. Ventura-Clapier R, Garnier A, Veksler V. Transcriptional control of mitochondrial biogenesis: the central role of PGC-1alpha. Cardiovasc Res. 2008;79(2):208–17.
52. Tran N, Asad Z, Elkholey K, Scherlag BJ, Po SS, Stavrakis S. Autonomic neuromodulation acutely ameliorates left ventricular strain in humans. J Cardiovasc Transl Res. 2019;12(3):221–30.
53. Groban L, Pailes NA, Bennett CD, Carter CS, Chappell MC, Kitzman DW, Sonntag WE. Growth hormone replacement attenuates diastolic dysfunction and cardiac angiotensin II expression in senescent rats. J Gerontol Ser A-Biol Sci Med Sci. 2006;61(1):28–35.
54. Stein M, Boulaksil M, Jansen JA, Herold E, Noorman M, Joles JA, van Veen TA, Houtman MJ, Engelen MA, Hauer RN, de Bakker JM, van Rijen HV. Reduction of fibrosis-related arrhythmias by chronic renin-angiotensin-aldosterone system inhibitors in an aged mouse model. Am J Phys Heart Circ Phys. 2010;299(2):H310–21.
55. Benigni A, Corna D, Zoja C, Sonzogni A, Latini R, Salio M, Conti S, Rottoli D, Longaretti L, Cassis P, Morigi M, Coffman TM, Remuzzi G. Disruption of the Ang II type 1 receptor promotes longevity in mice. J Clin Investig. 2009;119(3):524–30.
56. Inserra F, Basso N, Ferder M, Userpater M, Stella I, Paglia N, Inserra P, Tenembaum D, Ferder L. Changes seen in the aging kidney and the effect of blocking the renin-angiotensin system. Ther Adv Cardiovasc Dis. 2009;3(5):341–6.
57. Okumura S, Takagi G, Kawabe J, Yang G, Lee MC, Hong C, Liu J, Vatner DE, Sadoshima J, Vatner SF, Ishikawa Y. Disruption of type 5 adenylyl cyclase gene preserves cardiac function against pressure overload. Proc Natl Acad Sci U S A. 2003;100(17):9986–90.
58. Okumura S, Vatner DE, Kurotani R, Bai Y, Gao S, Yuan Z, Iwatsubo K, Ulucan C, Kawabe J, Ghosh K, Vatner SF, Ishikawa Y. Disruption of type 5 adenylyl cyclase enhances desensitization of cyclic adenosine monophosphate signal and increases Akt signal with chronic catecholamine stress. Circulation. 2007;116(16):1776–83.
59. Yan L, Vatner DE, O'Connor JP, Ivessa A, Ge H, Chen W, Hirotani S, Ishikawa Y, Sadoshima J, Vatner SF. Type 5 adenylyl cyclase disruption increases longevity and protects against stress. Cell. 2007;130(2):247–58.
60. Remondino A, Kwon SH, Communal C, Pimentel DR, Sawyer DB, Singh K, Colucci WS. Beta-adrenergic receptor-stimulated apoptosis in cardiac myocytes is mediated by reactive oxygen species/c-Jun NH2-terminal kinase-dependent activation of the mitochondrial pathway. Circ Res. 2003;92(2):136–8.
61. Ellison KE, Gandhi G. Optimising the use of beta-adrenoceptor antagonists in coronary artery disease. Drugs. 2005;65(6):787–97.
62. Apfeld J, Kenyon C. Cell nonautonomy of C. elegans daf-2 function in the regulation of diapause and life span. Cell. 1998;95(2):199–210.
63. Dorman JB, Albinder B, Shroyer T, Kenyon C. The age-1 and daf-2 genes function in a common pathway to control the lifespan of Caenorhabditis elegans. Genetics. 1995;141(4):1399–406.
64. Li Q, Ceylan-Isik AF, Li J, Ren J. Deficiency of insulin-like growth factor 1 reduces sensitivity to aging-associated cardiomyocyte dysfunction. Rejuvenation Res. 2008;11(4):725–33.
65. Wessells RJ, Fitzgerald E, Cypser JR, Tatar M, Bodmer R. Insulin regulation of heart function in aging fruit flies. Nat Genet. 2004;36(12):1275–81.
66. Vasan RS, Sullivan LM, D'Agostino RB, Roubenoff R, Harris T, Sawyer DB, Levy D, Wilson PW. Serum insulin-like growth factor I and risk for heart failure in elderly individuals without a previous myocardial infarction: the Framingham Heart Study. Ann Intern Med. 2003;139(8):642–8.
67. Broglio F, Fubini A, Morello M, Arvat E, Aimaretti G, Gianotti L, Boghen MF, Deghenghi R, Mangiardi L, Ghigo E. Activity of GH/IGF-I axis in patients with dilated cardiomyopathy. Clin Endocrinol. 1999;50(4):417–30.
68. Kops GJ, Dansen TB, Polderman PE, Saarloos I, Wirtz KW, Coffer PJ, Huang TT, Bos JL, Medema RH, Burgering BM. Forkhead transcription factor FOXO3a protects quiescent cells from oxidative stress. Nature. 2002;419(6904):316–21.

69. Puigserver P, Rhee J, Donovan J, Walkey CJ, Yoon JC, Oriente F, Kitamura Y, Altomonte J, Dong H, Accili D, Spiegelman BM. Insulin-regulated hepatic gluconeogenesis through FOXO1-PGC-1alpha interaction. Nature. 2003;423(6939):550–5.
70. Stahl M, Dijkers PF, Kops GJ, Lens SM, Coffer PJ, Burgering BM, Medema RH. The forkhead transcription factor FoxO regulates transcription of p27Kip1 and Bim in response to IL-2. J Immunol. 2002;168(10):5024–31.
71. Wang L, Lv Y, Li G, Xiao J. MicroRNAs in heart and circulation during physical exercise. J Sport Health Sci. 2018;7(4):433–41.
72. Zhang X, Azhar G, Wei JY. The expression of microRNA and microRNA clusters in the aging heart. PLoS One. 2012;7(4):e34688.
73. Thum T, Gross C, Fiedler J, Fischer T, Kissler S, Bussen M, Galuppo P, Just S, Rottbauer W, Frantz S, Castoldi M, Soutschek J, Koteliansky V, Rosenwald A, Basson MA, Licht JD, Pena JT, Rouhanifard SH, Muckenthaler MU, Tuschl T, Martin GR, Bauersachs J, Engelhardt S. MicroRNA-21 contributes to myocardial disease by stimulating MAP kinase signalling in fibroblasts. Nature. 2008;456(7224):980–4.
74. Bei Y, Wu X, Cretoiu D, Shi J, Zhou Q, Lin S, Wang H, Cheng Y, Zhang H, Xiao J, Li X. miR-21 suppression prevents cardiac alterations induced by d-galactose and doxorubicin. J Mol Cell Cardiol. 2018;115:130–41.
75. Boon RA, Iekushi K, Lechner S, Seeger T, Fischer A, Heydt S, Kaluza D, Treguer K, Carmona G, Bonauer A, Horrevoets AJ, Didier N, Girmatsion Z, Biliczki P, Ehrlich JR, Katus HA, Muller OJ, Potente M, Zeiher AM, Hermeking H, Dimmeler S. MicroRNA-34a regulates cardiac ageing and function. Nature. 2013;495(7439):107–10.
76. Yang Y, Cheng HW, Qiu Y, Dupee D, Noonan M, Lin YD, Fisch S, Unno K, Sereti KI, Liao R. MicroRNA-34a plays a key role in cardiac repair and regeneration following myocardial infarction. Circ Res. 2015;117(5):450–9.
77. Wu KH, Xiao QR, Yang Y, Xu JL, Zhang F, Liu CM, Zhang ZM, Lu YQ, Huang NP. MicroRNA-34a modulates the Notch signaling pathway in mice with congenital heart disease and its role in heart development. J Mol Cell Cardiol. 2018;114:300–8.
78. Fan F, Sun A, Zhao H, Liu X, Zhang W, Jin X, Wang C, Ma X, Shen C, Zou Y, Hu K, Ge J. MicroRNA-34a promotes cardiomyocyte apoptosis post myocardial infarction through down-regulating aldehyde dehydrogenase 2. Curr Pharm Biotechnol. 2013;19(27):4865–73.
79. Fu BC, Lang JL, Zhang DY, Sun L, Chen W, Liu W, Liu KY, Ma CY, Jiang SL, Li RK, Tian H. Suppression of miR-34a expression in the myocardium protects against ischemia-reperfusion injury through SIRT1 protective pathway. Stem Cells Dev. 2017;26(17):1270–82.
80. Piegari E, Russo R, Cappetta D, Esposito G, Urbanek K, Dell'Aversana C, Altucci L, Berrino L, Rossi F, De Angelis A. MicroRNA-34a regulates doxorubicin-induced cardiotoxicity in rat. Oncotarget. 2016;7(38):62312–26.
81. Bernardo BC, Gregorevic P, Ritchie RH, McMullen JR. Generation of microRNA-34 sponges and tough decoys for the heart: developments and challenges. Front Pharmacol. 2018;9:1090.
82. Bernardo BC, Gao XM, Winbanks CE, Boey EJ, Tham YK, Kiriazis H, Gregorevic P, Obad S, Kauppinen S, Du XJ, Lin RC, McMullen JR. Therapeutic inhibition of the miR-34 family attenuates pathological cardiac remodeling and improves heart function. Proc Natl Acad Sci U S A. 2012;109(43):17615–20.
83. Jazbutyte V, Fiedler J, Kneitz S, Galuppo P, Just A, Holzmann A, Bauersachs J, Thum T. MicroRNA-22 increases senescence and activates cardiac fibroblasts in the aging heart. Age (Dordr). 2013;35(3):747–62.
84. Boyle AJ, Shih H, Hwang J, Ye J, Lee B, Zhang Y, Kwon D, Jun K, Zheng D, Sievers R, Angeli F, Yeghiazarians Y, Lee R. Cardiomyopathy of aging in the mammalian heart is characterized by myocardial hypertrophy, fibrosis and a predisposition towards cardiomyocyte apoptosis and autophagy. Exp Gerontol. 2011;46(7):549–59.
85. Shan SW, Lee DY, Deng Z, Shatseva T, Jeyapalan Z, Du WW, Zhang Y, Xuan JW, Yee SP, Siragam V, Yang BB. MicroRNA MiR-17 retards tissue growth and represses fibronectin expression. Nat Cell Biol. 2009;11(8):1031–8.
86. van Almen GC, Verhesen W, van Leeuwen RE, van de Vrie M, Eurlings C, Schellings MW, Swinnen M, Cleutjens JP, van Zandvoort MA, Heymans S, Schroen B. MicroRNA-18 and microRNA-19 regulate CTGF and TSP-1 expression in age-related heart failure. Aging Cell. 2011;10(5):769–79.
87. Du WW, Li X, Li T, Li H, Khorshidi A, Liu F, Yang BB. The microRNA miR-17-3p inhibits mouse cardiac fibroblast senescence by targeting Par4. J Cell Sci. 2015;128(2):293–304.
88. Munoz-Espin D, Canamero M, Maraver A, Gomez-Lopez G, Contreras J, Murillo-Cuesta S, Rodriguez-Baeza A, Varela-Nieto I, Ruberte J, Collado M, Serrano M. Programmed cell senescence during mammalian embryonic development. Cell. 2013;155(5):1104–18.
89. Lighthouse JK, Small EM. Transcriptional control of cardiac fibroblast plasticity. J Mol Cell Cardiol. 2016;91:52–60.
90. Yao Z, Yang S, He W, Li L, Xu R, Zhang X, Li H, Zhan R, Sun W, Tan J, Zhou J, Luo G, Wu J. P311 promotes renal fibrosis via TGFbeta1/Smad signaling. Sci Rep. 2015;5:17032.
91. Tao L, Bei Y, Chen P, Lei Z, Fu S, Zhang H, Xu J, Che L, Chen X, Sluijter JP, Das S, Cretoiu D, Xu B, Zhong J, Xiao J, Li X. Crucial role of miR-433 in regulating cardiac fibrosis. Theranostics. 2016;6(12):2068–83.
92. Lyu G, Guan Y, Zhang C, Zong L, Sun L, Huang X, Huang L, Zhang L, Tian XL, Zhou Z, Tao

W. TGF-beta signaling alters H4K20me3 status via miR-29 and contributes to cellular senescence and cardiac aging. Nat Commun. 2018;9(1):2560.
93. Bar C, Chatterjee S, Thum T. Long noncoding RNAs in cardiovascular pathology, diagnosis, and therapy. Circulation. 2016;134(19):1484–99.
94. Chen X, Sun Y, Cai R, Wang G, Shu X, Pang W. Long noncoding RNA: multiple players in gene expression. BMB Rep. 2018;51(6):280–9.
95. Matsumoto A, Pasut A, Matsumoto M, Yamashita R, Fung J, Monteleone E, Saghatelian A, Nakayama KI, Clohessy JG, Pandolfi PP. mTORC1 and muscle regeneration are regulated by the LINC00961-encoded SPAR polypeptide. Nature. 2017;541(7636):228–32.
96. Nelson BR, Makarewich CA, Anderson DM, Winders BR, Troupes CD, Wu F, Reese AL, McAnally JR, Chen X, Kavalali ET, Cannon SC, Houser SR, Bassel-Duby R, Olson EN. A peptide encoded by a transcript annotated as long noncoding RNA enhances SERCA activity in muscle. Science. 2016;351(6270):271–5.
97. Anderson DM, Anderson KM, Chang CL, Makarewich CA, Nelson BR, McAnally JR, Kasaragod P, Shelton JM, Liou J, Bassel-Duby R, Olson EN. A micropeptide encoded by a putative long noncoding RNA regulates muscle performance. Cell. 2015;160(4):595–606.
98. Lorenzen JM, Thum T. Long noncoding RNAs in kidney and cardiovascular diseases. Nat Rev Nephrol. 2016;12(6):360–73.
99. Uchida S, Dimmeler S. Long noncoding RNAs in cardiovascular diseases. Circ Res. 2015;116(4):737–50.
100. Evans JR, Feng FY, Chinnaiyan AM. The bright side of dark matter: lncRNAs in cancer. J Clin Investig. 2016;126(8):2775–82.
101. Bartonicek N, Maag JL, Dinger ME. Long noncoding RNAs in cancer: mechanisms of action and technological advancements. Mol Cancer. 2016;15(1):43.
102. Devaux Y, Zangrando J, Schroen B, Creemers EE, Pedrazzini T, Chang CP, Dorn GW 2nd, Thum T, Heymans S, Cardiolinc N. Long noncoding RNAs in cardiac development and ageing. Nat Rev Cardiol. 2015;12(7):415–25.
103. Abdelmohsen K, Panda A, Kang MJ, Xu J, Selimyan R, Yoon JH, Martindale JL, De S, Wood WH 3rd, Becker KG, Gorospe M. Senescence-associated lncRNAs: senescence-associated long noncoding RNAs. Aging Cell. 2013;12(5):890–900.
104. Wang G, Lunardi A, Zhang J, Chen Z, Ala U, Webster KA, Tay Y, Gonzalez-Billalabeitia E, Egia A, Shaffer DR, Carver B, Liu XS, Taulli R, Kuo WP, Nardella C, Signoretti S, Cordon-Cardo C, Gerald WL, Pandolfi PP. Zbtb7a suppresses prostate cancer through repression of a Sox9-dependent pathway for cellular senescence bypass and tumor invasion. Nat Genet. 2013;45(7):739–46.
105. Neppl RL, Wu CL, Walsh K. lncRNA Chronos is an aging-induced inhibitor of muscle hypertrophy. J Cell Biol. 2017;216(11):3497–507.
106. Chun Yang X, Hui Zhao D, Bond Lau W, Qiang Liu K, Yu Tian J, Chao Cheng Z, Liang Ma X, Hua Liu J, Fan Q. lncRNA ENSMUST00000134285 increases MAPK11 activity, regulating aging-related myocardial apoptosis. J Gerontol Ser A-Biol Sci Med Sci. 2018;73(8):1010–7.
107. Xie Z, Xia W, Hou M. Long intergenic noncoding RNAp21 mediates cardiac senescence via the Wnt/betacatenin signaling pathway in doxorubicin-induced cardiotoxicity. Mol Med Rep. 2018;17(2):2695–704.
108. Zhang Z, Xie Q, He D, Ling Y, Li Y, Li J, Zhang H. Circular RNA: new star, new hope in cancer. BMC Cancer. 2018;18(1):834.
109. Hsiao KY, Sun HS, Tsai SJ. Circular RNA – new member of noncoding RNA with novel functions. Exp Biol Med. 2017;242(11):1136–41.
110. Du WW, Yang W, Chen Y, Wu ZK, Foster FS, Yang Z, Li X, Yang BB. Foxo3 circular RNA promotes cardiac senescence by modulating multiple factors associated with stress and senescence responses. Eur Heart J. 2017;38(18):1402–12.

Non-coding RNAs and Ischemic Cardiovascular Diseases

15

Tarik Smani, Isabel Mayoral-Gonzalez, Isabel Galeano-Otero, Isabel Gallardo-Castillo, Juan A. Rosado, Antonio Ordoñez, and Abdelkrim Hmadcha

Abstract

The Ischemic Heart Disease (IHD) is considered a clinical condition characterized by myocardial ischemia causing an imbalance between myocardial blood supply and demand, leading to morbidity and mortality across the worldwide. Prompt diagnostic and prognostic represents key factors for the treatment and reduction of the mortality rate. Therefore, one of the newest frontiers in cardiovascular research is related to non-coding RNAs (ncRNAs), which prompted a huge interest in exploring ncRNAs candidates for utilization as potential therapeutic targets for diagnostic and prognostic and/or biomarkers in IHD. However, there are undoubtedly many more functional ncRNAs yet to be discovered and characterized. Here we will discuss our current knowledge and we will provide insight on the roles and effects elicited by some ncRNAs related to IHD.

Keywords

RNAs · Non-coding RNAs · Ischemia and reperfusion · Cardioprotection

T. Smani (✉)
Department of Medical Physiology and Biophysics, Institute of Biomedicine of Seville (IBiS), University of Seville, Seville, Spain

CIBERCV, Madrid, Spain
e-mail: tasmani@us.es

I. Mayoral-Gonzalez
Department of Medical Physiology and Biophysics, Institute of Biomedicine of Seville (IBiS), University of Seville, Seville, Spain

Department of Surgery, University of Seville, Seville, Spain

I. Galeano-Otero
Department of Medical Physiology and Biophysics, Institute of Biomedicine of Seville (IBiS), University of Seville, Seville, Spain

I. Gallardo-Castillo
Department of Stomatology, School of Dentistry, University of Seville, Seville, Spain

J. A. Rosado
Department of Physiology (Cell Physiology Research Group), University of Extremadura, Cáceres, Spain

A. Ordoñez
Department of Medical Physiology and Biophysics, Institute of Biomedicine of Seville (IBiS), University of Seville, Seville, Spain

CIBERDEM, University of Pablo de Olavide-University of Seville-CSIC, ISCIII, Seville, Madrid, Spain

Department of Surgery, University of Seville, Seville, Spain

A. Hmadcha (✉)
Department of Generation and Cell Therapy, Andalusian Center for Molecular Biology and Regenerative Medicine (CABIMER), Seville, Spain
e-mail: khmadcha@upo.es

J. Xiao (ed.), *Non-coding RNAs in Cardiovascular Diseases*, Advances in Experimental Medicine and Biology 1229, https://doi.org/10.1007/978-981-15-1671-9_15

Abbreviations

AGO	Argonaute
AMI	acute myocardial infarct
BNIP3	Bcl2 interacting protein 3
CVD	Cardiovascular Disease
DGCR8	DiGeorge critical Region 8
ENCODE	Encyclopedia of DNA elements
GLP-1	glucagon like peptide 1
HGNC	Hugo Gene Nomenclature Committee
H/R	hypoxia/reoxygenation
IHD	Ischemia Heart Disease
lncRNAs	long non-coding RNAs
miRISC	miRNA-induced silencing complex
miRNAs	microRNAs
ncRNAs	non-coding RNAs
NRF	necrosis related factor
PARP	peroxisome proliferator activated receptor
PDCD4	programme cell death 4
piRNAs	piwi-interacting RNAs
pri-miRNA	primary-miRNAs
ROS	reactive oxygen species
siRNA	silencing RNAs
SIRT1	sirtuin-1
snoRNAs	small nucleolar RNAs
STEMI	ST Elevation myocardial infarct

1 Introduction

Ischemic Heart Disease (IHD) is the leading death cause in the western countries, which happens when the heart became unable to pump blood properly due to myocardial damage provoked by ischemia. Ischemia is mainly caused by the interruption of heart blood flow, which leads to heart infarcts [1–3]. During short ischemia and despite of the decrease in oxygen supply, there is a reversible loss of cardiac contractile function. However, when ischemia is sustained for a prolonged period, there is an irreversible cardiac muscle damage resulting in adverse cardiac remodeling [1]. Remodeling is primarily achieved by myocardial fibrosis resulting in decreased cardiac function, impairment of cardiac conduction system and at last arrhythmia. Actually, prompt and rapid myocardial reperfusion reduces significantly myocardial infarct size and improves clinical outcome [4]. Paradoxically, the subsequent reperfusion also activates various injury responses and tissue lesions. This phenomenon is known as Ischemia and Reperfusion (I/R) injury [4]. The absence of oxygen and nutrients during ischemia causes metabolic and biochemical changes. Furthermore, reperfusion provokes calcium overload, oxidative stress, mitochondrial dysfunction and activation of apoptotic and autophagy pathways, which worsen the cardiac remodeling [5–7].

Current therapeutic strategies applied in the treatment of myocardial infarction have effectively lowered early mortality from IHD. However, significant number of myocardial infarcted patients still suffers from the adverse left ventricular remodeling and further heart failure progression. For this reason, a better understanding of the pathophysiology of IHD and novel therapeutic strategies to provide more effective monitoring of disease progression are eagerly needed. Non-coding RNAs (ncRNAs) represent one of the increasing areas in the cardiovascular research field [8, 9]. There are different types of ncRNAs according to their sequences length: silencing RNA (siRNAs), small nucleolar RNAs (snoRNAs), microRNAs (miRNAs), long non-coding RNAs (lncRNAs), and the latest Piwi-interacting RNA (pi-RNAs) [10, 11].

There are increasing amount of studies of ncRNAs in recent years explained by the amount of biological functions and pathologies where ncRNAs seem involved [12–14]. In heart, ncRNAs regulate a plethora of cellular processes, including cardiomyocyte apoptosis, necrosis and fibrosis [15, 16]. They have been related to different Cardiovascular Diseases (CVD) processes such as atherosclerosis, I/R injury and myocardial infarction. ncRNAs are also examined as sensitive biomarkers for IHD that will allow early prognostic of patients with high risks of post-infarction remodeling and malfunction of the left ventricle [9, 17]. Currently, an extensive list of cardiovascular ncRNAs as well as mRNA targets have been reported. In this review, we will discuss the most relevant ncRNAs involved in I/R and cardioprotection.

2 Classification, Synthesis and Regulation of Non-coding RNAs

Until 1970s, central dogma of molecular biology established RNA as an intermediate in the process of protein translation from genes encoded in DNA [18]. Later on, this idea was challenged due to new discoveries of RNA molecules and the publication of the result of the International Human Genome Sequencing Consortium [19–21]. This consortium stated that approximately 98% of human genome contained non-protein coding sequences. Initially, these non-coding sequences were qualified as "DNA junk". With the recent emergence of high-throughput technologies and the establishment of new consortiums, like the Encyclopedia of DNA Elements (ENCODE), transcripts generated from these DNA were re-valued and given the importance that they deserved [22, 23]. Nowadays, these transcripts are named ncRNAs [24]. ncRNAs are divided into short non-coding (sncRNAs; <200 nt), including miRNAs, piRNAs, siRNAs as well as snoRNAs and lncRNA (200 nt–100 kb) [10, 11].

2.1 Long Non-coding RNAs

LncRNAs covers a heterogeneous group involved principally in the regulation of transcription at different levels. LncRNAs are transcripts which own a range of nucleotide from 200 nt to over 100 kb [10, 25]. Currently, 392 human lncRNAs are registered and published in the HUGO-Gene Nomenclature Committee (HGNC) (https://www.genenames.org/cgi-bin/genefamilies/set/788) and NONCODE collection of lncRNAs includes a number of 96,308 human lncRNAs gene loci and 172,216 human lncRNAs transcripts (http://www.noncode.org/analysis.php) [11].

LncRNAs can be grouped attending to different criteria, such as their sequence, structure, function, metabolism or interaction with genes and other DNA elements [26]. Nevertheless, a single and acceptable classification remains needed [27]. The most used classification is based on their localization with regard to protein-coding genes. Thus, there are *sense* lncRNAs, *antisense* lncRNAs, *intronic* lncRNAs, *intergenic* lncRNAs and *enhancer* lncRNAs [28]. Briefly, *sense* lncRNAs are located within exons; *antisense* lncRNAs are synthesized from the antisense DNA strand of protein exons; *intronic* lncRNAs are produced from protein intron; *intergenic* lncRNAs are positioned between protein-coding genes; and *enhancer* lncRNAs, transcripts from enhancer regions of protein-coding genes which can be mono or bidirectional [25, 29–31]. Conversely, in reference to their mechanism of action, lncRNAs can act as: *signals* enabling transcription control like a transcription factor, *decoys* that bind with effector to prevent their access and action, *guides* to ribonucleoprotein/chromatin complexes to locate target genes, *scaffolds* to generate a ribonucleoprotein complex acting as an adapter, and *enhancers* to build loops that connect enhancer and promoters regions [28, 32]. Furthermore, lncRNAs can also act as a regulator of alternative splicing in three ways. Concisely, lncRNAs interact directly with splicing factors, create a RNA-RNA complex with other pre-mRNA and/or interfere with chromatin remodeling [33]. Likewise, lncRNAs modulate post-transcriptional expression through translation control or altering mRNA stability [34, 35].

In relation to others ncRNAs, lncRNAs can be precursor of sncRNAs such as siRNAs or can control expression and action of miRNAs [32]. Interestingly, circular lncRNAs have been described as "sponges" able to sequestrate miRNAs [36, 37].

2.2 Small Non-coding RNAs

2.2.1 miRNAs

Huge number of studies made special attention to miRNAs within the ncRNAs, due to their high stability and the possibility to quantify easily in biological fluids. Nowadays, more than 2600 human mature miRNAs are known (http://www.mirbase.org/cgi-bin/query.pl?terms=hsa). miRNAs are molecules of sncRNAs (18–25 nt) vastly conserved, which participate in genetic regulation [22, 38, 39]. Generally, transcription of miRNA to primary-miRNAs (pri-miRNAs) is carried out by RNA polymerase II [40, 41]. There are two pathways to complete miRNAs biogenesis: *canonical*, the most typical pathway, and *non-canonical*. The pri-miRNA is next endonucleolytically cleaved by the nuclear microprocessor complex formed by the RNase III enzyme Drosha and the DiGeorge critical region 8 (DGCR8) protein Exportin 5/RanGTP complex is the responsible to transport the pre-miRNA to the cytoplasm and then other RNase III, Dicer, cleaves the terminal loop and generates a mature miRNA duplex. Once associated with the Argonaute (AGO) family of proteins, this duplex of RNA removes the passenger strand. Hence, AGO with mature miRNA guide strand conforming miRNA-Induced Silencing Complex (miRISC) [41, 42]. Non-canonical pathways are less characterized; they do not use one of the RNases (DROSHA or DICER) to reach the miRISC construction and use alternative ways and molecules. Interestingly, through this pathway "mirtrons", pre-miRNAs created from introns of mRNA during splicing are generated [43, 44]. Generally, miRNAs have a guide role within RISC in RNA silencing 3′UTR level, whereas, other seed matches region have been described [45].

2.2.2 siRNAs

siRNAs are 19–24 nt widely used in gene silencing studies, including therapeutic purposes [46–48]. This kind of sncRNAs were characterized due to their highly stable double strand of RNA and a perfect complementarity with the target mRNA [49]. siRNAs are transcribed by RNase III, and the rest of the biogenesis is roughly similar to miRNAs biogenesis. Thus, siRNAs conducted the silencing post-transcriptional process through RISC complex too. Interestingly, in the same way as miRNAs, there are evidences suggesting that siRNAs actively participate in epigenetic modifications [50, 51]. Therefore, siRNAs are considered as valuable experimental tools [52]. However, their clinical use still remain limited because of the low efficacy of their delivery to tissue [53].

2.2.3 piRNAs

piRNAs are special sncRNAs with a 26–31 nt of length able to bind with a kind of argonaute proteins, Piwi. The association of Piwi and Piwi-like proteins with piRNAs generates a complex which participates in gene's expression at epigenetic and post-transcriptional level, mainly in germline and gonadal somatic cells [54–56]. piRNAs are single strand sncRNAs with 2′-O-methylation at the 3′end [56]. According to the meiotic phase where piRNAs acts, there are two different subclusters called pachytene and pre-pachytene piRNA cluster. Currently, scientists hypothesize, but still with no consensus, about the piRNAs biogenesis. Two main ways comprise primary and secondary amplification cycle, known as "ping-pong cycle" [57]. What is clear is that piRNAs biology is more complex than other ncRNAs, and more studies are necessary to elucidate these emerging tools of genes' expression.

3 Non-coding RNAs in Ischemia and Reperfusion

Relevant advances have been made in determining the role of ncRNAs in cellular process associated with ischemia. Earlier, most research focus on the role of miRNAs in ischemic responses. Only in recent years and thanks to the advances in OMICs technologies (genomics, transcriptomics, proteomics, metabolomics, and beyond), there is an increasing interest on studying the others ncRNAs. Here, we will highlight role of miRNAs and lncRNAs in responses to I/R, as well as in strategies of cardioprotection.

3.1 Role of miRNAs

miRNAs control many processes in the infarcted heart, such as cardiomyocyte cell death and proliferation, neovascularization and progenitor-cell-mediated repair [25, 58]. Initial attentions have been given to describe the role of miRNA in cellular processes associated with ischemia and/or revascularization in patients undergoing percutaneous coronary intervention and in vitro and in vivo, using animal models of Acute Myocardial Infarcts (AMI) [59, 60]. During the AMI, miRNAs can be up- or down-regulated, having either a pathological or protective role because they are involved in genes' regulation, inflammation, stress responses, angiogenesis or apoptosis [3, 61–63]. Independent reports suggested a protective role of miRNAs, whereas others demonstrated deleterious effects of miRNAs dysregulation in AMI and I/R [3, 64–68].

Since the number of miRNAs related to ischemia and/or reperfusion is substantially increasing, here we will describe the role of only few of them on cell-death and survival.

3.1.1 miRNAs and Cardiomyocytes Survival

Earlier studies highlighted the role of miRNAs in cardiomyocytes survival and the regulation of apoptosis, necrosis or autophagy after considerable duration of ischemia. Gain- and loss-of-function studies were conducted in vivo and in vitro to demonstrate that miRNAs may promote or impair cardiomyocyte survival by regulation of caspases, Bcl-2 family or p53, among other apoptotic signaling pathways [58, 69].

Plenty of miRNAs families have been related to anti-apoptosis effects and cell survival during cardiac I/R as illustrated in Fig. 15.1, such as miR-1, miR-21, miR-24, miR-125, miR-133 or miR-98 [3, 70–78] as illustrated in Fig. 15.1. Using experimental model of AMI and I/R previous studies indicated that miR-21 has anti-apoptotic action regulating the called Programmed Cell Death 4 (PDCD4) [70], PTEN/Akt signaling pathway [71] or via Akt and the Bcl2/Bax pathway [72]. miR-1 and miR-133a mimics also attenuate apoptosis by the inhibition of caspase 9. In contrast pre-treatment of rat hearts with antimiR-133a increases caspase-9 and the apoptosis rate induced by I/R. Other reports demonstrated that miR-24 and miR-214 suppress cardiomyocyte apoptosis by Bim-1 repression, and attenuate infarct size in mouse model of AMI [74, 75]. A recent report suggested that miR-214 mimic suppresses the expression and translocation of Bim1 from cytosol to mitochondria and induces Bad phosphorylation, involving PTEN suppression in H9c2 cardiac cell line under I/R [75]. Similarly, miR-93 inhibits cardiomyocyte I/R-mediated apoptosis by targeting PI3K/Akt/PTEN signaling in H9c2 [79]. miR-98 also attenuates apoptosis-induced by I/R in H9c2, by inhibiting of Bcl-2, Bax and caspase-3 among others apoptotic genes [77]. Recently, we demonstrated that the transfection of neonatal cardiac myocyte with miR-125a-3p mimics inhibits the expression of BRCA1 [3].

In contrast, other reports revealed that miRNAs might promote pro-apoptotic action and cell death in ischemic condition as shown in Fig. 15.1. Actually, significant upregulation of miR-15 was

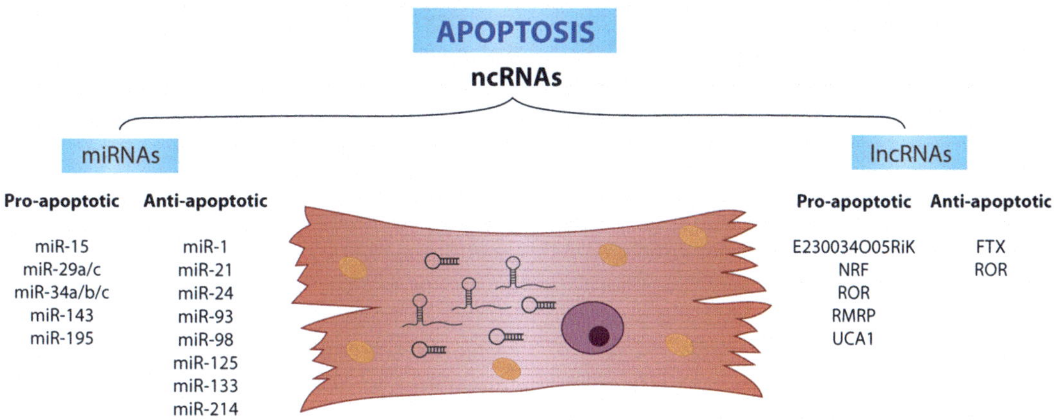

Fig. 15.1 Scheme showing a list of miRNAs and lncRNAs with confirmed pro- and anti-apoptotic effects in cardiac myocyte under ischemia and/or reperfusion

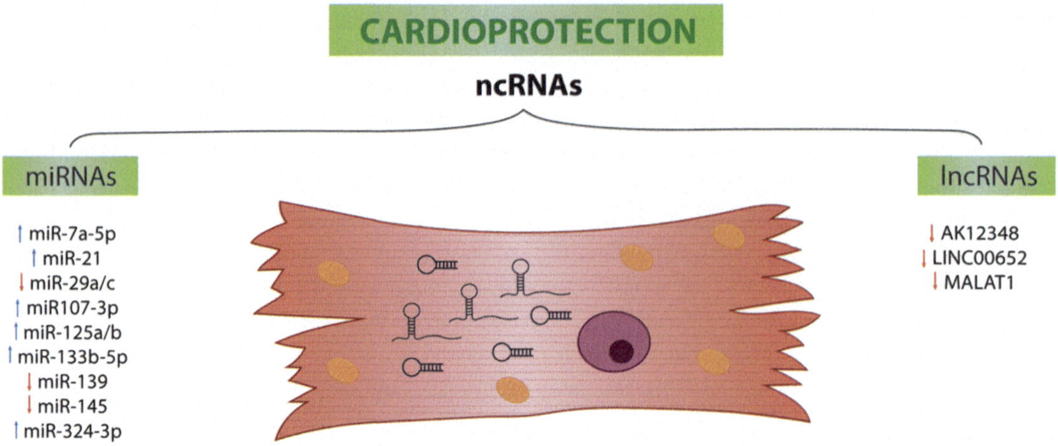

Fig. 15.2 Scheme indicating miRNAs and lncRNAs involved in cardioprotection against ischemia and reperfusion injury

observed in the infarcted zone of porcine and mice cardiac tissue in response to ischemic injury, which was associated with cell-death through Bcl-2 activation [80, 81]. Similarly, miR-195 that is related to the miR-15 family, contributes to apoptosis by its downregulation of NAD-dependent protein deacetylase sirtuin-1 (SIRT1) [82]. Another study described that the inhibition of miR-143 with antagomir prevents its pro-apoptotic effects by caspase-3 inhibition and LDH release [83]. miR-29a and miR-29c also negatively regulate cardiac cell survival under I/R, because they increase the expression of Mcl-1, an anti-apoptotic Bcl-2 family member [84]. Indeed, miR-29a or miR-29c downregulation with antagomiRs significantly reduce myocardial infarct size and apoptosis in hearts subjected to I/R injury [84]. Likewise, significant upregulation of miR-34 family (miR-34a, miR-34b, and miR-34c), was observed after AMI. miR-34 family are regulated by cellular tumor antigen p53, and contribute to cardiomyocyte cell death. In fact, the inhibition of the three miR-34 in vivo using antimiRs or antagomiRs improves cardiomyocyte survival after AMI and preserves cardiac contractile function [85, 86].

Altogether, these independent studies demonstrated that gain- and loss-of-functions of some miRNAs may play a pivital role in AMI-mediated cardiac malfunction and cell death.

3.1.2 miRNAs and Cardioprotection

Compelling evidence confirmed the important role of miRNAs under different strategies of cardioprotection as summarized in Fig. 15.2. In fact, several miRNAs are released in patients with AMI after coronary reperfusion with percutaneous coronary intervention, namely miR-1, miR-133a, miR-133b, and miR-499-5p [87]. Interestingly, a protocol using remote ischemic-preconditioning to attenuate myocardial I/R injury releases up to 26 miRNAs in blood sample of anaesthetized patients undergoing coronary artery bypass surgery [88].

Moreover, anesthetic and pain drugs have confirmed cardioprotective effects [11, 89, 90], involving miRNAs activation (90). For example, isoflurane protects mouse and rat hearts from I/R injury by miR-21 activation, involving Akt/nitric oxide synthase pathway [91] and PDCD4 respectively [92]. Fentanyl, a synthetic opiates, also reduces injury evoked by Hypoxia/Reoxygenation (H/R), a simulated in vitro protocol of I/R, through the inhibition of miR-145-5p and Bcl-2 Interacting Protein 3 (BNIP3) [93]. Others studies demonstrated that the administration of the δ-opioid receptor agonist in rats, under normoxic conditions, increases cardiac expression of miR-107-3p, miR-141-3p, and miR-350-5p, while it rises miR-7a/b, miR-107-3p, miR-200b-5p, miR-376a-3p, and miR134-5p levels under hypoxic conditions [94]. Although, the exact contribution of these miRNAs and their targets to cardioprotection have not been examined. Nevertheless, another study demonstrated that the activation of δ-opioid receptor mediated-cardioprotection modifies the expression of 39 miRNAs, while it decreases cell death and LDH levels in isolated cardiomyocytes subjected to H/R (93). This study demonstrated an upregulation of miR-7a-5p which inhibits I/R-induced apoptosis by negatively regulating the expression of PARP (Peroxisome Proliferator-Activated Receptor) [95], and miR-107-3p that regulates HIF-1β stimulation od endothelial progenitor cells differentiation [95]. Other group suggested that miR-133b-5p has a preponderant role in morphine signaling and cardioprotection by targeting Fas gene [96]. Recently, the upregulation of miR-133b-5p was demonstrated to contribute to preconditioning mediated cardioprotection in cardiomyocytes, associated with inhibition of caspase-8 and caspase-3 apoptotic signaling [97].

Others stimuli also changes the expression of miRNA under I/R. For example, pioglitazone, an agonist of PPAR-gamma, protects against myocardial I/R injury by miR-29a and miR-29c downregulation [84]. Recently, we showed that the addition of urocortin at the onset of reperfusion protects the heart from I/R injuries and dysregulates the expression of several miRNAs, such as miR-125a-3p, miR-139 and miR-324-3p [3]. We demonstrated that mimics of miR-125a-3p, miR-324-3p and miR-139-3p modify the expression of genes involved in cell death and apoptosis (BRCA1, BIM, STAT2), in cAMP and Ca^{2+} signaling (PDE4a, CASQ1), in cell stress (NFAT5, XBP1, MAP 3K12) and in metabolism (CPT2, FoxO1, MTRF1, TAZ). Interestingly, a recent study described that circadian rhythm is involved in ischemia preconditioning through the upregulation of the light elicited-circadian rhythm protein Period 2 (Per2). This study identified miR-21 as cardioprotective downstream target of Per2 [98].

Recently, a study belonging to the discussions of the European Union-CARDIOPROTECTION COST Action, confirmed that the concentration of numerous ncRNAs molecules is altered by ischemia, I/R, conditioning stimuli and medications to conclude that miR-21 and miR-125b are highly relevant for cardioprotection [99].

3.2 Role of LncRNAs in Ischemia and Reperfusion

3.2.1 LncRNAs and Cardiomyocytes Survival

LncRNAs play different roles in cellular physiology. Concretely, they participate in immune responses, chemotaxis, cell death and/or in the production of Reactive Oxygen Species (ROS) in I/R [100–103]. Actually, an aberrant expression of lncRNAs was observed at early stages of reperfusion in a mouse model of I/R, where the microarray analysis of sample taken from the infracted zone shows differential expression of 151 lncRNAs as compare to sham [100]. Using quantitative-PCR the upregulation of five lncRNAs was confirmed in the infarcted zone, namely; uc007prv.1, AK080112, ENSMUST00000170410, AK156124 and ENSMUST00000166777. Using gene ontology and pathways analyses, authors revealed several target genes for theses lncRNAs, related with immune responses, cytokine activity, NOD-like receptor and chemokine signaling pathways, which have been linked to I/R injury [100].

Recent studies demonstrated that lncRNAs might interact with miRNAs to modulate cell death. For instance, lncRNA Necrosis-Related Factor (NRF) inhibits the expression of miR-873 which blocks RIPK1 and RIPK3, involved in I/R--induced myocardial necrosis [104]. Meanwhile, lncRNA FTX regulates cardiomyocyte apoptosis in I/R animal models, through modulation of the Bcl2l2 expression, which is mediated by miR-29b-1-5 [105]. A recent research demonstrated that the upregulation of lncRNA RMRP exacerbates H/R injury by downregulation of miR-206 and subsequently upregulation of ATG3 in H9c2. In contrast, suppression of RMPR improves cardiac function and inhibited apoptosis after H/R [106]. Other studies also demonstrated the contribution of lncRNAs to apoptosis (Fig. 15.1). For instance, UCA1 stimulates p27 protein and caspase3 in I/R rat model [107] as well as ROR, which aggravates H/R-induced myocardial injury through the stimulation of ROS production and apoptosis in H9c2 cells [101]. Indeed, ROR increases the expression of Bax, cytochrome C, Smac/Diablo, cleaved-caspase-3 and cleaved-caspase-9 expressions, but it also decreases Bcl-2 expression in H9c2 under H/R [101]. Finally, lncRNA E230034O05Rik is considered as effective modulator of autophagy since it repressed autolysosome formation under H/R in in H9c2 [108]. In fact, silencing of this lncRNA markedly decreased autophagy and increased H9c2 myocytes viability during H/R [108].

3.2.2 LncRNAs and Cardioprotection

The role of lncRNAs in cardioprotection has been barely explored. Nevertheless, recent studies suggested that they could be valuable therapeutic target in myocardial I/R (Fig. 15.2). For example, knockdown of lncRNA AK12348 prevents I/R-induced LDH release and inhibits PARP and caspase-3 [109]. Similarly, MALAT1 was suggested as a key mediator of cardioprotective effects of fentanyl against I/R injury. MALAT1 inhibition prevents LDH release and apoptosis, involving miR-145 and BNIP3 axis [93]. Furthermore, suppression of the lncRNA LINC00652 restores sevoflurane-induced cardioprotection. Moreover, its silencing reduces I/R injury and alleviates inflammatory damage by targeting the receptor of Glucagon-Like Peptide-1 (GLP-1), a protein with known anti-oxidative effect on various tissues [110].

4 ncRNAs as Biomarkers for Ischemic CVD

Great interest has arisen toward the potential use of ncRNAs as promising novel biomarkers for the diagnosis and/or prognosis of CVD. Researchers made special emphasis on miRNAs because of their high stability against circulating RNases, their easy detection in human samples obtained through minimal invasive methods (e.g. serum), their specific expression pattern in the disease and their long expectance and easy quantification by quantitative PCR [39, 111–114]. Precisely, it has been demonstrated that ncRNAs participate actively in the pathophysiology of ischemic CVD [60, 113, 115, 116].

Increasing data are confirming that changes in the expression of miRNAs were observed in plasma of patients with AMI [117–119]. Recently, a pilot study examined and compared the expression profile of circulating miRNAs in patients with normal coronary artery, unstable angina and with ST elevation myocardial infarct (STEMI). This study identified 38 miRNAs whose expression level is consistently changed in unstable angina and STEMI patients compared with control patients. This fact indicates dynamic changes of miRNAs expression with the pathogenesis and progression of coronary artery disease [119]. Bioinformatic analysis suggests that target genes of these miRNAs are involved in various biological processes including angiogenesis, inflammation, proliferation, migration and apoptosis [119]. Another study suggested that miRNA-1254 fairly predicts ventricular remodeling at 6 months after STEMI [120]. Similarly, the analysis of circulating miRNAs in patients with an acute coronary syndrome determined that 3 miRNAs (miR-26b-5p, miR-320a and miR-660-5p) are significantly and differentially expressed in patients with Major Cardiovascular Event (MACE), defined as cardiac death or recurrent myocardial infarction, within 1 year of follow-up. These data suggest that these three miRNAs may reflect the activation of molecular pathways that will improve the clinical outcome after STEMI [121].

In the case of lncRNAs, information is limited comparing to miRNAs, however the number of lncRNAs associated with diagnosis and/or prognosis of ischemic CVD keep increasing [122–124]. Precisely, changes in the expression of MYHEART, HIF1A-AS2, KCNQ1OT, MALAT1, LIPCAR and UCA1 were proposed as warning sign for the diagnosis of STEMI [125, 126]. Actually, LIPCAR is considered a potential biomarker of STEMI, which could predict the severity and progression of coronary artery disease [126]. Interestingly, another study analyzed the expression of lncRNAs in peripheral blood mononuclear cells to evaluate their role as diagnostic biomarkers to differentiate between STEMI and non-STEMI patients. This study identified 58 lncRNAs and confirmed by qRT-PCR that ENST00000508020.2, LNC_002011, LNC_000303, LNC_000898, ENST00000573866.2 and ENST00000562710.1 are abnormally expressed in mononuclear cells of STEMI compared with non-STEMI participants [127]. Future studies will be helpful to understand whether lncRNAs may serve as a potential noninvasive diagnostic for AMI.

5 Conclusions and Perspectives

ncRNAs have emerged in recent years as key factors in a multitude of pathways across several diseases including CVD and specially IHD. Clinicians are in pursuit of a reliable ncRNAs marker similar to the widely used cardiac troponin, to evaluate the extent of AMI injury. Whereas, it remains challenging to understand which of them are important and how their implication and effect is completely achieved.

We recommend to take in consideration:

- New bioinformatic tools to predict the ncRNAs-IHD associated. Certainly, they will be helpful in identifying biological functions of ncRNAs in disease prevention, diagnosis and management.
- Specific ncRNAs-disease associated (and/or -disease severity associated), to be used as novel diagnosis biomarkers.
- For cardioprotection purpose; specific and reliable method to deliver possible therapeutic ncRNAs to the heart during ischemia, or during primary percutaneous coronary intervention to modulate gene's expression in the infarcted heart.
- It can be envisaged that deep understanding of ncRNAs identification, characterization and regulation in cardiovascular health and disease will yield novel therapeutic interventions tailored to the development of patients' disease.FundingThis work was supported by Spanish Ministry of Economy and Competitiveness [BFU2016–74932-C2]; Institute of Carlos III [PI15/00203; PI16/00259; CB16/11/00431]; the Andalusia Government [PI-0313-2016]. This study was co-financed by FEDER Funds.

References

1. Pfeffer MA, Braunwald E. Ventricular remodeling after myocardial infarction. Experimental observations and clinical implications. Circulation. 1990;81(4):1161–72.
2. Thiele H, Akin I, Sandri M. PCI strategies in patients with acute myocardial infarction and cardiogenic shock. N Engl J Med. 2017;377(25):2419–32.
3. Díaz I, Calderón-Sánchez E, del Toro R, Ávila-Médina J, de Rojas-de Pedro ES, Domínguez-Rodríguez A, Rosado JA, Hmadcha A, Ordóñez A, Smani T. miR-125a, miR-139 and miR-324 contribute to Urocortin protection against myocardial ischemia-reperfusion injury. Sci Rep. 2017;7:8898.
4. Hausenloy DJ, Garcia-Dorado D, Bøtker HE, et al. Novel targets and future strategies for acute cardioprotection: position paper of the European Society of Cardiology Working Group on Cellular Biology of the Heart. Cardiovasc Res. 2017;113(6):564–85.
5. Manuscript A, Diseases N. NIH Public. Access. 2014;36:1–17.
6. Ruiz-Meana M, García-Dorado D. Fisiopatología del daño miocárdico por isquemia-reperfusión: nuevas oportunidades terapéuticas en el infarto agudo de miocardio. Rev Esp Cardiol. 2009;62(2):199–209.
7. Dhalla NS, Saini HK, Tappia PS, Sethi R, Mengi SA, Gupta SK. Potential role and mechanisms of subcellular remodeling in cardiac dysfunction due to ischemic heart disease. J Cardiovasc Med (Hagerstown). 2007;8(4):238–50.
8. Giral H, Landmesser U, Kratzer A. Into the wild: GWAS exploration of non-coding RNAs. Front Cardiovasc Med. 2018;5:181.
9. Hobuß L, Bär C, Thum T. Long non-coding RNAs: at the heart of cardiac dysfunction? Front Physiol. 2019;10:30.
10. Bhat SA, Ahmad SM, Mumtaz PT, Malik AA, Dar MA, Urwat U, Shah RA, Ganai NA. Long non-coding RNAs: mechanism of action and functional utility. Non-coding RNA Res. 2016;1(1):43–50.
11. Melo Z, Ishida C, de la Paz Goldaraz M, Rojo R, Echavarria R. Novel roles of non-coding RNAs in opioid signaling and cardioprotection. Non-coding RNA. 2018;4(3):22.
12. Yang L, Cai Y, Zhang D, Sun J, Xu C, Zhao W, Jiang W, Pan C. miR-195/miR-497 regulate *CD274* expression of immune regulatory ligands in triple-negative breast Cancer. J Breast Cancer. 2018;21(4):371.

13. Heo MJ, Yun J, Kim SG. Role of non-coding RNAs in liver disease progression to hepatocellular carcinoma. Arch Pharm Res. 2019;42(1):48–62.
14. Chen J-B, Zhu Y-W, Guo X, et al. Microarray expression profiles analysis revealed lncRNA OXCT1-AS1 promoted bladder cancer cell aggressiveness via miR-455-5p/JAK1 signaling. J Cell Physiol. 2019;234(8):13592–601.
15. Guo Y, Luo F, Liu Q, Xu D. Regulatory non-coding RNAs in acute myocardial infarction. J Cell Mol Med. 2017;21(5):1013–23.
16. Das A, Samidurai A, Salloum FN. Deciphering non-coding RNAs in cardiovascular health and disease. Front Cardiovasc Med. 2018;5:73.
17. Wang S-S, Wu L-J, Li J-J-H, Xiao H-B, He Y, Yan Y-X. A meta-analysis of dysregulated miRNAs in coronary heart disease. Life Sci. 2018;215:170–81.
18. CRICK F. Central dogma of molecular biology. Nature. 1970;227:561–3.
19. Reinhart BJ, Slack FJ, Basson M, Pasquinelli AE, Bettinger JC, Rougvie AE, Horvitz HR, Ruvkun G. The 21-nucleotide let-7 RNA regulates developmental timing in Caenorhabditis elegans. Nature. 2000;403(6772):901–6.
20. Human Genome Sequencing Consortium I. Finishing the euchromatic sequence of the human genome. Nature. 2004;431(7011):931–45.
21. Mattick JS. The state of long non-coding RNA biology. Non-coding RNA. 2018;4(3):17.
22. He L, Hannon GJ. Erratum: MicroRNAs: small RNAs with a big role in gene regulation. Nat Rev Genet. 2004;5:522–31.
23. Niu D-K, Jiang L. Can ENCODE tell us how much junk DNA we carry in our genome? Biochem Biophys Res Commun. 2013;430(4):1340–3.
24. Brosnan CA, Voinnet O. The long and the short of noncoding RNAs. Curr Opin Cell Biol. 2009;21(3):416–25.
25. Boon RA. Non-coding RNAs in cardiovascular health and disease. Front Cardiovasc Med. 2018;5:71.
26. Bolha L, Ravnik-Glavač M, Glavač D. Long non-coding RNAs as biomarkers in Cancer. Dis Markers. 2017;2017:1–14.
27. St Laurent G, Wahlestedt C, Kapranov P. The landscape of long noncoding RNA classification. Trends Genet. 2015;31(5):239–51.
28. Dhanoa JK, Sethi RS, Verma R, Arora JS, Mukhopadhyay CS. Long non-coding RNA: its evolutionary relics and biological implications in mammals: a review. J Anim Sci Technol. 2018;60:25.
29. Ma L, Bajic VB, Zhang Z. On the classification of long non-coding RNAs. RNA Biol. 2013;10(6):925–33.
30. Hangauer MJ, Vaughn IW, McManus MT. Pervasive transcription of the human genome produces thousands of previously unidentified Long intergenic noncoding RNAs. PLoS Genet. 2013;9(6):e1003569.
31. Kim T-K, Hemberg M, Gray JM. Enhancer RNAs: a class of long noncoding RNAs synthesized at enhancers. Cold Spring Harb Perspect Biol. 2015;7(1):a018622.
32. Goyal N, Kesharwani D, Datta M. Lnc-ing non-coding RNAs with metabolism and diabetes: roles of lncRNAs. Cell Mol Life Sci. 2018;75(10):1827–37.
33. Romero-Barrios N, Legascue MF, Benhamed M, Ariel F, Crespi M. Survey and summary splicing regulation by long noncoding RNAs. Nucleic Acids Res. 2018;46(5):2169–84.
34. Geisler S, Coller J. RNA in unexpected places: long non-coding RNA functions in diverse cellular contexts. Nat Rev Mol Cell Biol. 2013;14(11):699–712.
35. Gong C, Maquat LE. lncRNAs transactivate STAU1-mediated mRNA decay by duplexing with 3′ UTRs via Alu elements. Nature. 2011;470(7333):284–8.
36. Memczak S, Jens M, Elefsinioti A, et al. Circular RNAs are a large class of animal RNAs with regulatory potency. Nature. 2013;495(7441):333–8.
37. Hansen TB, Jensen TI, Clausen BH, Bramsen JB, Finsen B, Damgaard CK, Kjems J. Natural RNA circles function as efficient microRNA sponges. Nature. 2013;495(7441):384–8.
38. Pasquinelli AE. MicroRNAs: heralds of the noncoding RNA revolution. RNA. 2015;21(4):709–10.
39. De Gonzalo-Calvo D, Iglesias-Gutié Rrez E, Llorente-Corté V. Epigenetic biomarkers and cardiovascular disease: circulating microRNAs. Rev Esp Cardiol (Engl Ed). 2017;70(9):763–9.
40. Lee Y, Kim M, Han J, Yeom K-H, Lee S, Baek SH, Kim VN. MicroRNA genes are transcribed by RNA polymerase II. EMBO J. 2004;23(20):4051–60.
41. Ha M, Kim VN. Regulation of microRNA biogenesis. Nat Rev Mol Cell Biol. 2014;15(8):509–24.
42. Kawamata T, Tomari Y. Making RISC. Trends Biochem Sci. 2010;35(7):368–76.
43. Denli AM, Tops BBJ, Plasterk RHA, Ketting RF, Hannon GJ. Processing of primary microRNAs by the microprocessor complex. Nature. 2004;432(7014):231–5.
44. O'Brien J, Hayder H, Zayed Y, Peng C. Overview of microRNA biogenesis, mechanisms of actions, and circulation. Front Endocrinol (Lausanne). 2018;9:402.
45. Xu W, San Lucas A, Wang Z, Liu Y. Identifying microRNA targets in different gene regions. BMC Bioinformatics. 2014;15:S4.
46. Karimizadeh E, Motamed N, Mahmoudi M, Jafarinejad-Farsangi S, Jamshidi A, Faridani H, Gharibdoost F. Attenuation of fibrosis with selective inhibition of c-Abl by siRNA in systemic sclerosis dermal fibroblasts. Arch Dermatol Res. 2015;307(2):135–42.
47. Suzuki K, Yokoyama J, Kawauchi Y, et al. Phase 1 clinical study of siRNA targeting carbohydrate sulphotransferase 15 in Crohn's disease patients with active mucosal lesions. J Crohns Colitis. 2017;11(2):221–8.
48. Fitzgerald K, White S, Borodovsky A, et al. A highly durable RNAi therapeutic inhibitor of PCSK9. N Engl J Med. 2017;376(1):41–51.

49. Elbashir SM, Harborth J, Lendeckel W, Yalcin A, Weber K, Tuschl T. Duplexes of 21-nucleotide RNAs mediate RNA interference in cultured mammalian cells. Nature. 2001;411(6836):494–8.
50. Holoch D, Moazed D. RNA-mediated epigenetic regulation of gene expression. Nat Rev Genet. 2015;16(2):71–84.
51. Wei J-W, Huang K, Yang C, Kang C-S. Non-coding RNAs as regulators in epigenetics. Oncol Rep. 2017;37(1):3–9.
52. Morris KV, Mattick JS. The rise of regulatory RNA. Nat Rev Genet. 2014;15(6):423–37.
53. Dana H, Chalbatani GM, Mahmoodzadeh H, et al. Molecular mechanisms and biological functions of siRNA. Int J Biomed Sci. 2017;13(2):48–57.
54. Cox DN, Chao A, Baker J, Chang L, Qiao D, Lin H. A novel class of evolutionarily conserved genes defined by piwi are essential for stem cell self-renewal. Genes Dev. 1998;12:3715–27.
55. Kuramochi-Miyagawa S, Kimura T, Ijiri TW, et al. Mili, a mammalian member of piwi family gene, is essential for spermatogenesis. Development. 2004;131:839–49.
56. Weng W, Li H, Goel A. Piwi-interacting RNAs (piRNAs) and cancer: emerging biological concepts and potential clinical implications. Biochim Biophys Acta Rev Cancer. 2018; https://doi.org/10.1016/J.BBCAN.2018.12.005.
57. Czech B, Hannon GJ. One loop to rule them all: the ping-pong cycle and piRNA-guided silencing. Trends Biochem Sci. 2016;41:324–37.
58. Boon RA, Dimmeler S. MicroRNAs in myocardial infarction. Nat Rev Cardiol. 2015;12:135–42.
59. Eltzschig HK, Eckle T. Ischemia and reperfusion—from mechanism to translation. Nat Med. 2011;17:1391–401.
60. Su Q, Ye Z, Sun Y, Yang H, Li L. Relationship between circulating miRNA-30e and no-reflow phenomenon in S.TEMI patients undergoing primary coronary intervention. Scand J Clin Lab Investig. 2018;78:318–24.
61. Arif M, Pandey R, Alam P, Jiang S, Sadayappan S, Paul A, Ahmed RPH. MicroRNA-210-mediated proliferation, survival, and angiogenesis promote cardiac repair post myocardial infarction in rodents. J Mol Med. 2017;95:1369–85.
62. Yang T, Cao C, Yang J, Liu T, Lei XG, Zhang Z, Xu S. miR-200a-5p regulates myocardial necroptosis induced by Se deficiency via targeting RNF11. Redox Biol. 2018;15:159–69.
63. Shao H, Yang L, Wang L, Tang B, Wang J, Li Q. MicroRNA-34a protects myocardial cells against ischemia–reperfusion injury through inhibiting autophagy via regulating TNFα expression. Biochem Cell Biol. 2018;96:349–54.
64. Fan ZX, Yang J. The role of micrornas in regulating myocardial ischemia reperfusion injury. Saudi Med J. 2015;36:787–93.
65. Lorenzen JM, Batkai S, Thum T. Regulation of cardiac and renal ischemia-reperfusion injury by microRNAs. Free Radic Biol Med. 2013;64:78–84.
66. Condorelli G, Latronico MVG, Cavarretta E. microRNAs in cardiovascular diseases. J Am Coll Cardiol. 2014;63:2177–87.
67. Weiss JB, Eisenhardt SU, Stark GB, Bode C, Moser M, Grundmann S. MicroRNAs in ischemia-reperfusion injury. Am J Cardiovasc Dis. 2012;2:237–47.
68. Zhu H, Fan GC. Role of microRNAs in the reperfused myocardium towards post-infarct remodelling. Cardiovasc Res. 2012;94:284–92.
69. Sun T, Dong Y-H, Du W, Shi C-Y, Wang K, Tariq M-A, Wang J-X, Li P-F. The role of MicroRNAs in myocardial infarction: from molecular mechanism to clinical application. Int J Mol Sci. 2017;18(4):e745.
70. Cheng Y, Zhu P, Yang J, Liu X, Dong S, Wang X, Chun B, Zhuang J, Zhang C. Ischaemic preconditioning-regulated miR-21 protects heart against ischaemia/reperfusion injury via anti-apoptosis through its target PDCD4. Cardiovasc Res. 2010;87:431–9.
71. Tu Y, Wan L, Fan Y, Wang K, Bu L, Huang T, Cheng Z, Shen B. Ischemic postconditioning-mediated miRNA-21 protects against cardiac ischemia/reperfusion injury via PTEN/Akt pathway. PLoS One. 2013;8:e75872.
72. Ma N, Bai J, Zhang W, Luo H, Zhang X, Liu D, Qiao C. Trimetazidine protects against cardiac ischemia/reperfusion injury via effects on cardiac miRNA-21 expression, Akt and the Bcl-2/Bax pathway. Mol Med Rep. 2016;14(5):4216–22.
73. Xu X, Kriegel AJ, Jiao X, Liu H, Bai X, Olson J, Liang M, Ding X. miR-21 in ischemia/reperfusion injury: a double-edged sword? Physiol Genomics. 2014;46(21):789–97.
74. Qian L, Van Laake LW, Huang Y, Liu S, Wendland MF, Srivastava D. miR-24 inhibits apoptosis and represses Bim in mouse cardiomyocytes. J Exp Med. 2011;208(3):549–60.
75. Wang X, Ha T, Hu Y, Lu C, Liu L, Zhang X, Kao R, Kalbfleisch J, Williams D, Li C. MicroRNA-214 protects against hypoxia/reoxygenation induced cell damage and myocardial ischemia/reperfusion injury via suppression of PTEN and Bim1 expression. Oncotarget. 2016;7(52):86926–36.
76. Tan H, Qi J, Fan B-Y, Zhang J, Su F-F, Wang H-T. MicroRNA-24-3p attenuates myocardial ischemia/reperfusion injury by suppressing RIPK1 expression in mice. Cell Physiol Biochem. 2018;51(1):46–62.
77. Zhai CL, Tang GM, Qian G, Hu HL, Wang SJ, Yin D, Zhang S. MicroRNA-98 attenuates cardiac ischemia-reperfusion injury through inhibiting DAPK1 expression. IUBMB Life. 2018;71(2):166–76.
78. He B, Xiao J, Ren A-J, Zhang Y-F, Zhang H, Chen M, Xie B, Gao X-G, Wang Y-W. Role of miR-1 and miR-133a in myocardial ischemic postconditioning. J Biomed Sci. 2011;18:22.

79. Ke Z-P, Xu P, Shi Y, Gao A-M. MicroRNA-93 inhibits ischemia-reperfusion induced cardiomyocyte apoptosis by targeting PTEN. Oncotarget. 2016;7(20):28796–805.
80. Hullinger TG, Montgomery RL, Seto AG, et al. Inhibition of miR-15 protects against cardiac ischemic injury. Circ Res. 2012;110(1):71–81.
81. Cimmino A, Calin GA, Fabbri M, et al. miR-15 and miR-16 induce apoptosis by targeting BCL2. Proc Natl Acad Sci. 2005;102(39):13944–9.
82. Zhu H, Yang Y, Wang Y, Li J, Schiller PW, Peng T. MicroRNA-195 promotes palmitate-induced apoptosis in cardiomyocytes by down-regulating Sirt1. Cardiovasc Res. 2011;92(1):75–84.
83. Hong H, Tao T, Chen S, Liang C, Qiu Y, Zhou Y, Zhang R. MicroRNA-143 promotes cardiac ischemia-mediated mitochondrial impairment by the inhibition of protein kinase Cepsilon. Basic Res Cardiol. 2017;112(60):60.
84. Ye Y, Hu Z, Lin Y, Zhang C, Perez-Polo JR. Downregulation of microRNA-29 by antisense inhibitors and a PPAR-γ agonist protects against myocardial ischaemia–reperfusion injury. Cardiovasc Res. 2010;87(3):535–44.
85. Bernardo BC, Gao X-M, Winbanks CE, et al. Therapeutic inhibition of the miR-34 family attenuates pathological cardiac remodeling and improves heart function. Proc Natl Acad Sci U S A. 2012;109(43):17615–20.
86. Boon RA, Iekushi K, Lechner S, et al. MicroRNA-34a regulates cardiac ageing and function. Nature. 2013;495(7439):107–10.
87. D'Alessandra Y, Devanna P, Limana F, et al. Circulating microRNAs are new and sensitive biomarkers of myocardial infarction. Eur Heart J. 2010;31(22):2765–73.
88. Frey UH, Klaassen M, Ochsenfarth C, et al. Remote ischaemic preconditioning increases serum extracellular vesicle concentrations with altered micro-RNA signature in CABG patients. Acta Anaesthesiol Scand. 2018;63(4):483–92.
89. Lang X-E, Wang X, Jin J-H. Mechanisms of cardioprotection by isoflurane against I/R injury. Front Biosci (Landmark Ed). 2013;18:387–93.
90. Tanaka K, Kersten JR, Riess ML. Opioid-induced cardioprotection. Curr Pharm Des. 2014;20:5696–705.
91. Qiao S, Olson JM, Paterson M, et al. MicroRNA-21 mediates isoflurane-induced cardioprotection against ischemia-reperfusion injury via Akt/nitric oxide synthase/mitochondrial permeability transition pore pathway. Anesthesiology. 2015;123(4):786–98.
92. Olson JM, Yan Y, Bai X, Ge Z-D, Liang M, Kriegel AJ, Twaroski DM, Bosnjak ZJ. Up-regulation of microRNA-21 mediates isoflurane-induced protection of cardiomyocytes. Anesthesiology. 2015;122(4):795–805.
93. Zhao Z, Hao W, Meng Q, Du X, Lei S, Xia Z. Long non-coding RNA MALAT1 functions as a mediator in cardioprotective effects of fentanyl in myocardial ischemia-reperfusion injury. Cell Biol Int. 2017;41(1):62–70.
94. Zhi F, Xue L, Shao N, Deng D, Kang X, Chao D, Xu Y, Wang R, Yang Y, Xia Y. δ-opioid receptor activation and microRNA expression in the rat heart under prolonged hypoxia. Cell Physiol Biochem. 2016;39:1118–28.
95. Meng S, Cao J, Wang L, Zhou Q, Li Y, Shen C, Zhang X, Wang C. MicroRNA 107 partly inhibits endothelial progenitor cells differentiation via HIF-1β. PLoS One. 2012;7(7):e40323.
96. He S-F, Zhu H-J, Han Z-Y, Wu H, Jin S-Y, Irwin MG, Zhang Y. MicroRNA-133b-5p is involved in cardioprotection of morphine preconditioning in rat cardiomyocytes by targeting Fas. Can J Cardiol. 2016;32(8):996–1007.
97. Pan Y, Han Z, He S, Yang W, Cheng J, Zhang Y, Chen Z. miR-133b-5p contributes to hypoxic preconditioning-mediated cardioprotection by inhibiting the activation of caspase-8 and caspase-3 in cardiomyocytes. Mol Med Rep. 2018;17(5):7097–104.
98. Oyama Y, Bartman CM, Gile J, Eckle T. Circadian microRNAs in cardioprotection. Curr Pharm Des. 2017;23(25):3723–30.
99. Davidson SM, Andreadou I, Barile L, et al. Circulating blood cells and extracellular vesicles in acute cardioprotection. Cardiovasc Res. 2018;115(7):1156–66.
100. Liu Y, Li G, Lu H, Li W, Li X, Liu H, Li X, Li T, Yu B. Expression profiling and ontology analysis of long noncoding RNAs in post-ischemic heart and their implied roles in ischemia/reperfusion injury. Gene. 2014;543(1):15–21.
101. Zhang W, Li Y, Wang P. Long non-coding RNA-ROR aggravates myocardial ischemia/reperfusion injury. Braz J Med Biol Res. 2018;51(6):e6555.
102. Wu X, Zhu H, Zhu S, Hao M, Li Q. lncRNA expression character associated with ischemic reperfusion injury. Mol Med Rep. 2017;16:3745–52.
103. S yang Y, Tang L, hua ZS. Long noncoding RNAs: new players in ischaemia-reperfusion injury. Heart Lung Circ. 2018;27(3):322–32.
104. Wang K, Liu F, Liu C-Y, et al. The long noncoding RNA NRF regulates programmed necrosis and myocardial injury during ischemia and reperfusion by targeting miR-873. Cell Death Differ. 2016;23(8):1394–405.
105. Long B, Li N, Xu X-X, Li X-X, Xu X-J, Guo D, Zhang D, Wu Z-H, Zhang S-Y. Long noncoding RNA FTX regulates cardiomyocyte apoptosis by targeting miR-29b-1-5p and Bcl2l2. Biochem Biophys Res Commun. 2018;495(1):312–8.
106. Kong F, Jin J, Lv X, Han Y, Liang X, Gao Y, Duan X. Long noncoding RNA RMRP upregulation aggravates myocardial ischemia-reperfusion injury by sponging miR-206 to target ATG3 expression. Biomed Pharmacother. 2019;109:716–25.
107. Liu Y, Zhou D, Li G, Ming X, Y feng T, Tian J, Lu H, Yu B. Long non coding RNA-UCA1 contributes to cardiomyocyte apoptosis by suppres-

sion of p27 expression. Cell Physiol Biochem. 2015;35(5):1986–98.

108. Huang Z, Ye B, Wang Z, Han J, Lin L, Shan P, Cai X, Huang W. Inhibition of LncRNA-HRIM increases cell viability by regulating autophagy levels during hypoxia/reoxygenation in myocytes. Cell Physiol Biochem. 2018;46(4):1341–51.
109. Zheng C, Wu Z, Tian L, et al. Long noncoding RNA AK123483 is involved in the regulation of myocardial ischaemia-reperfusion injury by targeting PARP and caspase-3. Heart Lung Circ. 2018;27(5):e51–8.
110. Zhang S-B, Liu T-J, Pu G-H, Li B-Y, Gao X-Z, Han X-L. Suppression of long non-coding RNA LINC00652 restores sevoflurane-induced cardioprotection against myocardial ischemia-reperfusion injury by targeting GLP-1R through the cAMP/PKA pathway in mice. Cell Physio Biochem. 2018;49(4):1476–91.
111. Xu Y, Huang R, Gu J, Jiang W. Identification of long non-coding RNAs as novel biomarker and potential therapeutic target for atrial fibrillation in old adults. Oncotarget. 2016;7(10):10803–11.
112. Backes C, Meese E, Keller A. Specific miRNA disease biomarkers in blood, serum and plasma: challenges and prospects. Mol Diagn Ther. 2016;20(6):509–18.
113. Vierek J, Thum T. Circulating noncoding RNAs as biomarkers of cardiovascular disease and injury. Circ Res. 2013;120(2):381–99.
114. Busch A, Eken SM, Maegdefessel L. Prospective and therapeutic screening value of non-coding RNA as biomarkers in cardiovascular disease. Ann Transl Med. 2016;4(12):236.
115. Liu X, Dong Y, Chen S, Zhang G, Zhang M, Gong Y, Li X. Circulating microRNA-146a and microRNA-21 predict left ventricular remodeling after ST-elevation myocardial infarction. Cardiology. 2015;132(4):233–41.
116. Vegter EL, Ovchinnikova ES, van Veldhuisen DJ, Jaarsma T, Berezikov E, van der Meer P, Voors AA. Low circulating microRNA levels in heart failure patients are associated with atherosclerotic disease and cardiovascular-related rehospitalizations. Clin Res Cardiol. 2017;106(8):598–609.
117. Wang G-K, Zhu J-Q, Zhang J-T, Li Q, Li Y, He J, Qin Y-W, Jing Q. Circulating microRNA: a novel potential biomarker for early diagnosis of acute myocardial infarction in humans. Eur Heart J. 2010;31:659–66.
118. Gidlöf O, Andersson P, van der Pals J, Götberg M, Erlinge D. Cardiospecific microRNA plasma levels correlate with troponin and cardiac function in patients with ST elevation myocardial infarction, are selectively dependent on renal elimination, and can be detected in urine samples. Cardiology. 2011;118(4):217–26.
119. Zhong Z, Hou J, Zhang Q, Zhong W, Li B, Li C, Liu Z, Yang M, Zhao P. Circulating microRNA expression profiling and bioinformatics analysis of dysregulated microRNAs of patients with coronary artery disease. Medicine (Baltimore). 2018;97(27):e11428.
120. de Gonzalo-Calvo D, Cediel G, Bär C, et al. Circulating miR-1254 predicts ventricular remodeling in patients with ST-segment-elevation myocardial infarction: a cardiovascular magnetic resonance study. Sci Rep. 2018;8:15115.
121. Jakob P, Kacprowski T, Briand-Schumacher S, et al. Profiling and validation of circulating microRNAs for cardiovascular events in patients presenting with ST-segment elevation myocardial infarction. Eur Heart J. 2016;38(7):511–5.
122. Hu H, Wu J, Li D, Zhou J, Yu H, Ma L. Knockdown of lncRNA MALAT1 attenuates acute myocardial infarction through miR-320-Pten axis. Biomed Pharmacother. 2018;106:738–46.
123. Yan Y, Zhang B, Liu N, Qi C, Xiao Y, Tian X, Li T, Liu B. Circulating long noncoding RNA UCA1 as a novel biomarker of acute myocardial infarction. Biomed Res Int. 2016;2016:8079372.
124. Greco S, Zaccagnini G, Perfetti A, et al. Long noncoding RNA dysregulation in ischemic heart failure. J Transl Med. 2016;14(1):183.
125. Sun C, Jiang H, Sun Z, Gui Y, Xia H. Identification of long non-coding RNAs biomarkers for early diagnosis of myocardial infarction from the dysregulated coding-non-coding co-expression network. Oncotarget. 2016;7(45):73541–51.
126. Li MB, Wang L-FA, Yang X-CC, Xu LA, Li W-MDE, Xia KB, Zhang D-PC, Wu R-NC, Gan Corresponding Author T, Yang X-C. Circulating long noncoding RNA LIPCAR acts as a novel biomarker in patients with ST-segment elevation myocardial infarction. Med Sci Monit. 2018;24:5064–70.
127. Zhong Z, Hou J, Zhang Q, Li B, Li C, Liu Z, Yang M, Zhong W, Zhao P. Differential expression of circulating long non-coding RNAs in patients with acute myocardial infarction. Medicine (Baltimore). 2018;97(51):e13066.

Non-coding RNAs and Coronary Artery Disease

16

Alejandro Cardona-Monzonís, José Luis García-Giménez, Salvador Mena-Mollá, Helios Pareja-Galeano, Fernando de la Guía-Galipienso, Giuseppe Lippi, Federico V. Pallardó, and Fabian Sanchis-Gomar

Abstract

Coronary artery disease (CAD) is the leading death cause worldwide. Non-coding RNA (ncRNA) are key regulators of genetic expression and thus can affect directly or indirectly the development and progression of different diseases. ncRNA can be classified in several types depending on the length or structure, as long non-coding RNA (lncRNA), microRNA (miRNA) and circularRNA (circRNA), among others. These types of RNA are present within cells or in circulation, and for this reason they have been used as biomarkers of different diseases, therefore revolutionizing precision medicine. Recent research studied the capability of circulating ncRNA to inform about CAD presence and predict the outcome of the disease. In this chapter we present a list of the miRNA, lncRNA and circRNA which are potential biomarkers of CAD.

Keywords

Coronary artery disease (CAD) · miRNA · lncRNA · circRNA · Biomarker

1 Introduction

Coronary artery disease (CAD), also known as coronary heart disease (CHD), is currently the major cause of death worldwide [1, 2] *accounting for* almost 110 million affected people in 2015 [3] and generating nearly 7.6 million deaths [2].

CAD has a complex etiology, which begins with chronic inflammation and endothelial injuries in coronary arteries. Afterwards, atherosclerotic plaques are formed in the intima of coronary arteries [4], where they can reduce or even block the blood supply to the heart, in turn leading to

A. Cardona-Monzonís · J. L. García-Giménez
F. V. Pallardó
Center for Biomedical Network Research-Instituto de Salud Carlos III. Department of Physiology, School of Medicine, University of Valencia and INCLIVA Biomedical Research Institute, Valencia, Spain

S. Mena-Mollá
Department of Physiology, School of Medicine, University of Valencia, Valencia, Spain

H. Pareja-Galeano
Universidad Europea de Madrid, Madrid, Spain

F. de la Guía-Galipienso
Department of Cardiology, Hospital de la Marina Baixa, Alicante, Spain

G. Lippi
Section of Clinical Biochemistry, University of Verona, Verona, Italy

F. Sanchis-Gomar (✉)
Department of Physiology, Faculty of Medicine, University of Valencia and INCLIVA Biomedical Research Institute, Valencia, Spain
e-mail: fabian.sanchis@uv.es

J. Xiao (ed.), *Non-coding RNAs in Cardiovascular Diseases*, Advances in Experimental Medicine and Biology 1229, https://doi.org/10.1007/978-981-15-1671-9_16

myocardial ischemia due to the decreased blood flow through the lumen or breakdown of atherosclerotic plaques and complete occlusion of coronary arteries with superimposed thrombosis. All these events can finally lead to the onset of unstable angina, acute myocardial infarction (AMI) or sudden coronary death, which are the major clinical manifestations of CAD [5].

There are several molecular processes underlying CAD and atherosclerotic plaque formation. An excess of oxidized low-density lipoproteins (ox-LDL) or proinflammatory molecules trigger the recruitment of monocytes at sites of endothelial dysfunction caused by oxidative stress. Molecular signaling favors monocytes to adhere to endothelium and to transendothelial migration into intima, which would enhance chronic inflammation. In the intima, monocytes are engulfed with oxidized fat, which leads to their transformation into foam cells, and promoting the large deposition of lipids and cell debris [6, 7]. In the process of atherosclerotic plaque formation vascular smooth muscle cells migrate from the tunica media to intima. These cells can proliferate and produce extracellular matrix components, thus generating a fibrous cap which ultimately covers the plaque. This plaque can remain stable or undergo a necrotic process, culminating in possible breakdown of the plaque and thrombosis [8]. In summary, several cell types and processes can be affected and participate in the development of this disease, sharing an interaction in the artery wall: endothelial cells dysfunction, macrophage activation, vascular smooth muscle cells migration, deposition of lipids and fibrosis [9].

Is it widely accepted that the development of CAD is determined by genetics and epigenetics also plays an important role. The most important risk factors for CAD are high blood pressure, hypercholesterolemia, diabetes, smoking, sedentary life, poor diet, obesity, depression and excessive alcohol intake [10].

Because CAD is a starting point for other cardiovascular diseases such as AMI, biomarkers for early diagnosis and prognostication play an essential role to prevent progression. Currently, the most common biomarkers in CAD are inflammatory proteins, being C-reactive protein (CRP) the best studied [11]. Moreover, PPBP (pro-platelet basic protein) and DEFA1/DEFA3 (α-defensin) are correlated with CAD development [12]. Therefore, these biomarkers are occasionally used in CAD.

Noncoding RNAs (ncRNAs) are major components of the human transcriptome accounting for the majority of RNA transcribed by human genes, including microRNA (miRNAs), long noncoding RNA (lncRNA) and circular RNA (circRNA), among others. These ncRNAs play important roles regulating, either directly or indirectly, key biological processes in cells, and so contributing to the development and progression of human diseases [13]. Beyond their regulatory role in many molecular pathways, ncRNAs can also act controlling the expression of other ncRNAs, such is the case of the potential of lncRNAs and circRNAs to sequester miRNAs, therefore acting as miRNA sponges [14]. There is cumulative evidence that these ncRNAs are largely implicated in cardiovascular disorders [15]. In recent years, the study of non-coding RNA has help to unravel the comprehension of these molecular mechanisms, so ncRNAs such as miRNAs, lncRNAs and circRNAs have emerged as important regulators for CAD development and candidate biomarkers for diagnosis and prognostication (see Fig. 16.1).

2 miRNAs

miRNAs are a class of conserved, short (18–24 nt), non-coding RNAs, with the potential of regulating gene expression at the posttranscriptional level in different biological networks. Importantly, miRNAs have demonstrated the potential to be used as biomarkers [16]. The miRNA mechanism of genetic regulation is based in the pairing of bases of miRNA and 3′-UTR (3′ untranslated region) of target mRNA, although it has been also described that some miRNA are able to bind to translated regions and to 5′-UTR regions [17]. Firstly, miRNAs were considered to be only able to dysregulate gene expression by inhibiting target mRNA translation or enhancing target mRNA degradation, but some cases have

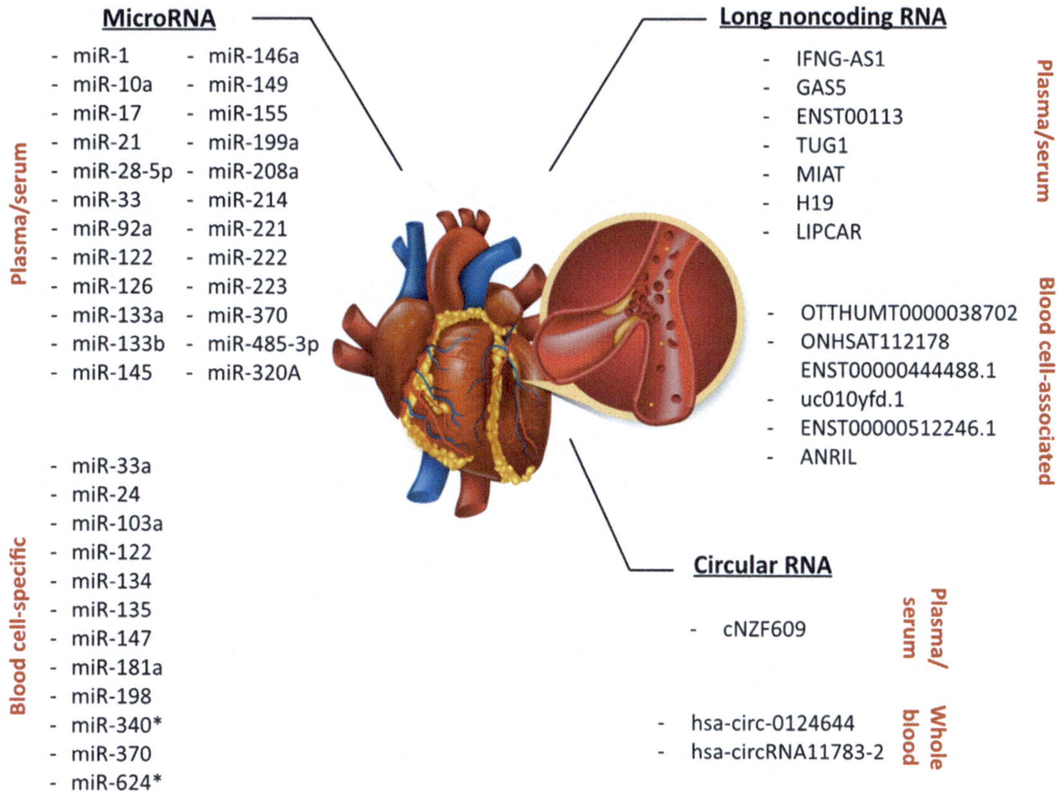

Fig. 16.1 Circulating and blood cell-associated Long non-coding RNA (lncRNA), microRNA (miRNA), and circular RNA (circRNA) associated with atherogenesis and coronary artery disease

been described where miRNA are capable of enhancing target mRNA translation [18]. Each miRNA can bind to multiple target mRNA, and a mRNA can be regulated by multiple miRNA [19], in a complex network of interactions. As occur for other diseases, miRNAs are the most studied ncRNA in CAD.

2.1 Circulating miRNAs

2.1.1 Plasma and Serum miRNAs

In recent years, a large number of studies has been published showing a correlation between levels of circulating miRNA and presence of CAD. These results prompted the researchers to propose circulating miRNAs as promising biomarkers for diagnostics and prognosis of this disease. Fichtlscherer et al. [20] studied circulating miRNA by using a microRNA profiling of 8 healthy subjects and 8 CAD patients. After evaluation of miRNA profiling, the authors confirmed the results obtained in an independent cohort of 36 patients with CAD and 17 healthy volunteers. They found that circulating levels of cardiac, muscle-enriched microRNAs miR-133 and miR-208a were upregulated. Conversely, miR-126, miR-17, miR-92a (miR-17/92a cluster, associated with endothelial cells), miR-145 (associated with vascular smooth cells) and miR-155 (participating in inflammation) were decreased in CAD patients compared to healthy subjects. The results obtained by Fichtlscherer and collaborators seem contradictory, because an up-regulation of circulating levels of miRNA related with these processes in CAD patients would be expected as consequence of enhancement of inflammation and vascular remodeling during CAD. However, the authors hypothesize that this unexpected reduction in the levels of circulating miRNAs could be a consequence of sequestration of circulating miRNA into atherosclerotic lesions instead of remaining into the circulation [20]. This hypothesis become relevant as some studies showed that miRNA can be transported by apoptotic bodies to atherosclerotic lesion [21].

In another study, Faccini et al. [22] compared 69 CAD patients and 32 healthy controls and obtained results similar to those described by Fichtlscherer et al. (i.e., downregulation of circulating miR-155 and miR-145 in CAD patients compared with control subjects). They also found that let-7c was also downregulated in CAD patients [22]. Interestingly, a research by Gao et al. compared circulating miRNA in 167 CAD patients and 28 controls, confirmed the association between low circulating levels of miR-145 and CAD, but also found a strong correlation between miR-145 and CAD severity [23]. Regarding miR-133, other studies found similar results. In the work of Wang et al. based on three different cohorts (13 AMI patients, 176 with angina pectoris and 127 control subjects), concluded that miR-133 can be used as a potential biomarker to identify and evaluate the severity of lesions in CAD patients, since miR-133 levels were efficient predictors of acute myocardial infarction or coronary stenosis. Importantly, miR-133 was more strongly correlated with CAD than other traditional biomarkers, such as cardiac troponins [24]. Similar to the results reported by Fichstslcherer et al. [20], two additional studies observed upregulated miR-208a levels in patients with CAD. Zhang et al. found an association between miR-208a and CAD severity in a study based on 290 CHD patients and 110 healthy subjects [25]. On the other hand, Liu et al. [26] performed another study in a cohort of 95 CAD patients and 50 healthy controls, and found that miR-208a and miR-370 were upregulated. Notably, the combination of both circulating miRNA showed the best performance for diagnosing CAD [26]. It is noteworthy to mention here that miR-208a is expressed in heart (a tissue strongly vulnerable to CAD) whilst miR-370 interplays with lipid metabolism, since its misregulation leads to hyperlipidemia, one of the major risk factors of CAD.

Some studies have also unveiled differences in miRNA levels depending on type of CAD patients. D'Alessandra et al. performed a study to assess differences in plasma miRNA profile between control and CAD patients. Interestingly, two groups of CAD patients were compared, the former including 34 subjects with stable angina (SA) and the latter 19 subjects with unstable angina (UA). The miRNA profile was then compared with those obtained in another cohort of 20 healthy controls. Interestingly, miR-1, miR-122, miR-126, miR-133a, miR-133b, and miR-199a were found to be upregulated in both UA and SA patients, and the combination of cardiac-enriched miR-1, endothelial-enriched miR-126, and miR-485-3p allowed discriminating between CAD-SA patients and control subjects. In addition, the combination of miR-1, miR-126 and miR-133a has the potential of differentiating CAD-UA patients from control subjects [27]. Regarding, UA diagnosis miR-28-5p was found to be a feasible biomarker, since this miRNA was increased in UA patients compared to control subjects [28].

From the previous works which analyzed circulating miRNAs profiles in CAD patients, it can be concluded that miR-145, miR-155, miR-133a and miR-208a are the circulating miRNA most strongly associated with CAD. However, other relevant studies proposed other circulating miRNA which can be related with CAD. This is for example the case of upregulated miR-149 [29], miR-223 [30], miR-33 [31], miR-320A [32], miR-122 and miR-370 [33], and downregulated miR-214 [34], miR-10a [35], and miR-126 [36].

Several other studies revealed that miRNA become biomarkers of atherosclerosis development. For instance, miR-221 and miR-222 were found to be downregulated in atherosclerotic patients compared to controls in a study performed by Yilmaz et al. in serum samples of 89 CAD patients and 93 subjects without atherosclerosis [37].

Some miRNA can reflect atherosclerosis in some pathologies. For example, some circulating miRNA can be useful to detect atherosclerosis in patients with hypertension, including miR-92a [38], and upregulated miR-21 [39]. In the case of subclinical hypothyroidism, circulating miR-146a was also found to correlate with CAD severity [40].

2.1.2 Blood Cell-Specific miRNAs

As previously discussed, subclinical inflammation is one of the main features associated to CAD [8]. miRNAs participate in the regulation of immune cells during disease progression [41]. For this reason, it seems reasonable to analyze those miRNAs more strongly related to inflammation, or those controlling the differentiation and function of immune cells, for finally using these molecules as CAD biomarkers. Hoekstra et al. [42] studied miRNA signatures of peripheral blood mononuclear cells (PBMCs) from CAD patients and controls. The authors found that miR-135a was fivefold higher and miR-147 was fourfold lower in CAD patients compared to ostensibly healthy people, whilst the ratio miR-135a/miR-147 was also 19-fold higher in CAD patients [42]. Interestingly, these two miRNAs are part of the pathway of Wnt/Cadherin. In addition, miR-134, miR-198, and miR-370 were upregulated in PBMCs of UA-CAD compared to SA-CAD patients, and this may represent a promising perspective for discriminating unstable from stable CAD [42].

miRNA signatures have been also explored in monocytes. In this regard, miR-181a was found to be downregulated in patients with CAD and obesity [43]. Notably, obesity is one of the leading risk factors of CAD. Dong et al. [44] studied 161 CAD patients and 149 healthy controls, and identified a panel of 4 miRNA (miR-24, miR-33a, miR-103a, and miR-122) in PBMCs that were upregulated in CAD patients and correlated with blood lipid concentration.

Platelets are also responsible of CAD progression, as they participate in atherosclerotic plaque development and in thrombus formation after the plaque disruption [45]. A study performed by Sondermeijer et al. [46], including two different cohorts, found that miR-340* and miR-624* were upregulated in platelets of CAD patients compared to healthy controls. Nevertheless, the function of these miRNA remains still uncertain.

3 Long Non-coding RNAs

Long non-coding RNA (lncRNA) are a heterogeneous group of transcripts, ranging from 200 to over 10,000 nucleotides. This type of ncRNA has the largest proportion of non-coding transcriptome [47]. However, many of these lncRNA are functional and are involved in physiological and pathological processes through epigenetics and transcriptional or post-transcriptional regulatory mechanisms [48].

3.1 Circulating lncRNAs

3.1.1 Plasma and Serum lncRNAs

LncRNAs are thought to regulate a wide array of pathways related to inflammation. Local or systemic inflammation plays an important role in the development of atherosclerotic plaques characteristic of CAD [49]. Some researchers found a correlation between the amounts of circulating lncRNAs and proinflammatory mediators. A reliable example is the case-control study (comprising 102 CAD patients and 89 controls) of Xu et al. in which lncRNA IFNG-AS1 was found to be significantly upregulated in CAD patients. This lncRNA was also positively associated with proinflammatory cytokines such as TNF-α, and IL-6, whilst negatively correlated with IL-10. These findings would suggest that the presence of this lncRNA in plasma reflect a proinflammatory state in CAD patients [50].

Pro-inflammatory responses can be activated by several pathways. One of these key mechanisms is regulated by the mammalian target of rapamycin (mTOR). Gao et al. [51] found that the activation of mTOR pathway initiates the monocytes pro-inflammatory response in patients with CAD, thus contributing to disease progression. The lncRNA GAS5 was found to be downregulated in plasma of CAD patients in a study including 30 CAD patients and 30 healthy controls [52]. Similar results were found in other study performed by Li and collaborators [53]. The lncRNA GAS5 can be transported within exomes, with the ability to regulate macrophage and vascular cells apoptosis [54]. Although many studies were focused on the identification of the relationship of circulating lncRNAs levels with cytokine expression, in this study the authors explored the association with mTOR pathway, and lncRNA GAS5 was found to regulate mTOR responses [55], thus pointing out its role mediating an indirect activation of pro-inflammatory responses. This event acquire major relevance since the knockdown of lncRNA GAS5 leads to increasing activation of mTOR pathway through phosphorylation of mTOR. However, a inhibition of mTOR does not seemingly affect lncRNA GAS5 levels, which would lead us to conclude that lncRNA GAS5 plays a role as upstream regulator of mTOR pathway and participate in CAD development [52]. Notably, the fact that lncRNA GAS5 can modulate indirectly mTOR pro-inflammatory responses remains to be definitely elucidated.

There are other key molecular upstream pathways involved in atherosclerotic development and CAD progression. This is the case of PI3K/Akt/mTOR, which signal transduction can be modulated by the lncRNA ENST00113. This lncRNA is upregulated in serum of atherosclerotic patients compared to healthy subjects. In vitro experiments performed in HUVEC and VSMCs (Vascular smooth muscle cells) demonstrated that lncRNA ENST00113 has the ability to control PI3K/Akt/mTOR axis, so promoting cell proliferation, cell survival and migration of many cellular types implicated in atherosclerosis and CAD development [56]. LncRNA TUG1 was found to be upregulated in serum of atherosclerotic patients as well as in a model of mice atherosclerotic plaques. It was hence hypothesized that lncRNA TUG1 may alter the proliferation VSMCs by affecting PTEN function, a phosphatase that inhibits PI3K/Akt pathway [57].

Other study performed by Zhong et al. identified other relevant lncRNA, called lncRNA MIAT, which was found to be upregulated in the serum of patients with atherosclerosis compared to controls. When assessing its functional role, lncRNA MIAT, enhanced the proliferation and prevent apoptosis in a cellular model of atherosclerosis treated with ox-LDL by regulating miR-181b and STAT3 activities [58].

Zhang et al. [59] proposed lncRNA H19 and LIPCAR as biomarkers for CAD. In this study, the authors investigated the circulating levels of eight lncRNA related with atherosclerosis (THRIL, LincRNA-Cox2, LIPCAR, LincRNA-p21, HULC, SLC26A4-AS1, APOA1-AS, and H19) in 480 subjects. Both lncRNA H19 and LIPCAR were significantly increased in CAD patients. Interestingly, this two lncRNA were also increased with CAD patients with heart failure compared to patients with normal cardiac function. Moreover, this study showed that all lncRNAs associated to atherosclerosis are not characteristic of CAD [59]. Another study showed that lncRNA H19 overexpression may promote atherosclerosis by activation of MAPK and NF-Kβ inflammatory signaling pathways [60]. Other studies were successful to demonstrate that cardiac lncRNA H19 was increased in ischemic end-stage failing hearts [61] and that LIPCAR had the ability to predict survival in patients with heart failure [62].

3.1.2 Blood Cell-Specific lncRNAs

Some studies showed that circulating PBMCs play a pivotal role in development of CAD by migrating into arterial wall and increasing the size of atherosclerotic lesions [63]. Therefore, the study of transcriptional differences in PBMCs' lncRNAs can be useful to garner information about their role as possible biomarkers of CAD.

Cai et al. studied expression levels of lncRNA transcribed in PBMCs in 15 CAD patients and 15 healthy subjects. Up to 86 lncRNAs were found to be differentially expressed in CAD patients; 3 of these lncRNAs were then validated in a larger cohort. In an ensuing study based on a much larger cohort, lncRNA OTTHUMT0000038702 (renamed as CoroMarker) was found to be the most upregulated lncRNA in PBMCs. Interestingly, CoroMarker upregulation was an independent risk factor of CAD and its expression was not associated with other risk factors or with CAD. The design of a CoroMarker siRNA demonstrated that this strategy was effective to lower the concentration of some proinflammatory cytokines (such as IL-1b, IL-6 and TNF-a) in cell culture medium of a human leukemia monocyte THP-1 cells, thus suggesting that this lncRNA plays an important role regulating proinflammatory cytokine expression [64]. lncRNA OTTHUMT0000038702 was also found in plasma of CAD patients, thus supporting its potential role as cardiovascular biomarker due to its relative stability, high sensitivity and specificity. Interestingly, the stability of this lncRNA in plasma was found to be due to the fact that it is incorporated within extracellular vesicles, probably released from monocytes [65].

The same group of authors identified another monocyte lncRNA (ONHSAT112178, also called LncPPARδ) as possible candidate biomarker for CAD using a similar strategy. This lncRNA regulates the expression of neighboring protein-coding genes such as peroxisome proliferator-activated receptor-δ (PPARδ), adipose differentiation-related protein (ADRP), and angiopoietin-like 4 (ANGPTL4), which are involved in the pathogenesis of CAD. In contrast with CoroMarker, the authors found differences in LncPPARδ according to the sex of the subjects, as well as depending on other variables such as hypertension, tobacco and alcohol intake. This evidence leads the authors to conclude that LncPPARδ, combined with other risk factors, can be a useful biomarker for CAD, with the ability to differentiate CAD patients from healthy subjects [66].

Other lncRNAs from PBMCs such as lncRNA ENST00000444488.1 and lncRNA uc010yfd.1 are also putative candidate biomarkers of CAD. In a study performed by Li et al. [67], in which PBMCs-associated lncRNA expression in 93 CAD patients and 48 healthy controls was compared, the authors identified up to 1210 lncRNA with differential expression between groups. Afterwards, the authors validated up to 7 of them in a larger cohort, and found that lncRNA ENST00000444488.1 and lncRNA uc010yfd.1 were the most specific biomarkers for diagnosing CAD. Interestingly, lncRNA ENST00000444488.1 also contributed to the diagnosis of AMI. The functional significance of these findings remains unclear, but the knock-out of these lncRNAs downregulate the synthesis of pro-inflammatory cytokines and near genes, so relating with the chronic vascular inflammation of CAD [67].

In other studies, focused on involvement of lncRNAs in CAD, the presence of circulating lncRNAs from blood cells in peripheral whole blood was explored. Li et al. [68] reported differential expression of 31 lncRNAs of peripheral blood from 6 CAD patients and 6 healthy subjects. The authors studied the most differentially expressed lncRNA in a larger cohort with similar results, thus identifying upregulation of lncRNA ENST00000512246.1 (renamed "Upperhand"). The authors concluded that "Upperhand" is a potential diagnostic biomarker of CAD, although further research is needed for validating their potential value as CAD biomarkers in other independent studies [68].

Taken together, albeit these studies provide valuable information on the use of either PBMCs lncRNAs or circulating lncRNAs for diagnosing CAD they also have some limitations, mainly related to the relatively small sample cohorts and the limitation to some specific patient cohorts (e.g., Chinese populations). It shall hence be necessary to design additional validation studies for lncRNAs as candidate biomarkers of CAD.

ANRIL, one of the most studied lncRNA, has been recently associated with CAD and Type 2 diabetes susceptibility and ink4/arf locus SNP on human chromosome 9p21.3 [69, 70]. ANRIL is expressed in tissues and cell types affected by atherosclerosis [70]. Likewise, ANRIL polymorphisms such as rs2383207, rs4977574, rs1333040, rs1333049, rs2383206 in east Asians, and rs2383207, rs10757274, and rs1075727 have been also associated with CAD [71–73], therefore analysis of the presence of these polymorphisms at the ANRIL gene would provide a biomarker of CAD. Regarding the function of this lncRNA, previous studies have shown that ANRIL increased miR-181b expression through inhibiting endothelial cell activation which ultimately induced vascular inflammation [74]. Guo et al. reported the connection between ANRIL, miR-181b and NF-κB to control CAD related-cellular proliferation and apoptosis as well as the release of inflammatory mediators such as cytokines IL-6, IL-8, TNF-α, NF-κB, the inducible nitric oxide synthase (iNOS), the adhesion molecules ICAM1, VCAM1 and the inducible pro-inflammatory cycloxigenase-2 (COX2) [75]. The DQ485454 ANRIL transcript is downregulated in endothelial cells of CAD patients. Moreover, the deficiency of this transcript leads to an increased monocyte adhesion to endothelial cells, transendothelial monocyte migration, and endothelial cell migration [76].

4 CircularRNAs

Circular RNAs (circRNA) are single stranded RNAs that form a covalently closed loop without free terminals. Circular RNAs (circRNAs) are abundant and stable RNAs formed by back-splicing events. During last few years a large number of studies have been planned to assess their functions. CircRNAs can act as miRNA sponges since they possess binding sites for miRNA, so that they can finally modulate gene expression of miRNA targets [77, 78]. Moreover, they can serve as RNA binding protein sponges [79] and scaffolds for assembly of other components [80], as well as they enhance splicing and transcription [81]. Finally, they can also be translated, in a limited number of cases [82].

4.1 Plasma and Serum circRNAs

Recent studies showed that circRNA levels found in plasma and serum are substantially modified in CAD. In a study performed by Pan et al. [83], comparing plasma samples between CAD patients and controls, 24 differentially expressed circRNAs were found (18 up-regulated and 6 down-regulated). Moreover, they compared plasma miRNAs levels in an independent population of 648 CAD patients and 284 healthy subjects, and found 9 CAD-related miRNA, 3 of which were downregulated in CAD subjects (miR-221, miR-155, and miR-130a) [83]. Interestingly, some of these circRNA can bind to miRNA, with an effect known as miRNA sponge. Using miRanda database tool a competing endogenous RNA network was constructed for hsa-miR-130a-3p, a miRNA whose downregulation is related with endothelial progenitor cell dysfunction, one of the early steps of atherosclerotic plaques formation [84, 85]. The network was composed of mRNA of TRPM3 and nine of the circRNA earlier identified by Pan and co-workers [83]. The down-regulation of hsa-miR-130a-3p resulted in the up-regulation of TREMP3 expression, a gene which regulates proliferation and contractility of VSMCs in co-ordination with cholesterol [86].

cNZF609 is other example of circRNA acting as miRNA sponge and dysregulated in patients with CAD, diabetes and hypertension. In CAD, cNZF609 is downregulated, and therefore miR-615-5p is upregulated. The authors conclude that cZNF609 regulates vascular dysfunction through a signaling network which is composed of cZNF609, miR-615-5p, and MEF2A, the mRNA targeted by miR-615-5p [87, 88].

4.2 Whole Blood-Associated circRNAs

Zhao et al. compared the levels of circRNA in whole blood from 12 CAD patients and 12 controls, discovering up to 22 differentially expressed circRNA (12 upregulated and 10 downregulated). Five upregulated circRNAs (hsa-circ-0082081, hsa-circ-0113854, hsa-circ-0124644, hsa-circ-0098964, and hsa-circ-5974-1) were identified as candidate biomarkers, and were validated in 30 CAD patients and 30 controls. hsa-circ-0124644 was found to be the circRNA with the highest diagnostic performance (area under the curve, 0.769), displaying a sensitivity of 0.86 and a specificity of 0.62, respectively. Its diagnostic value was then validated in a larger cohort of 115 controls and 137 CAD patients. The diagnostic performance was hence re-evaluated by adjusting data for CAD risk factors, yielding to an area under the curve of 0.804, a sensitivity of 0.76 and a specificity of 0.70, respectively. The authors concluded that this circRNA could be potentially used as a diagnostic biomarker for CAD [89]. Interestingly, the area under the curve was recalculated combining hsa_circ_0124644, has-circ-0098964 and other risk factors. With this further strategy, the area under the curve increased to 0.843, whist the sensitivity was 0.83 and the specificity 0.70. The previous findings suggest that the analysis of blood circRNA is a feasible strategy to identify new biomarkers for CAD diagnostics [89].

Li et al. performed a similar research studying circular RNA from 6 control individuals, 6 CAD patients, 6 diabetes mellitus patients and 6 CAD and diabetes mellitus patients [90]. Interestingly 40 circRNA were found to be differentially expressed (13 upregulated and 27 downregulated. A further analysis of data revealed that hsa-circRNA11783-2 (downregulated) is the circRNA more closely related to both CAD and type 2 diabetes mellitus.

It is noteworthy that since these circRNA have been found in whole blood, it is not possible to know whether they are cell-free circulating ncRNA or they are blood cell-associated circRNAs. Other concern regarding circRNAs is that most studies were performed using cohorts with low sample size.

5 Conclusions

Further studies are needed to establish the diagnostic value of circulating ncRNAs in CAD, as well as for establishing the settings where ncRNAs may provide the most useful information for screening, diagnosis and prognostication of patients with AMI, either alone or in combination with cardiac troponins [91]. Specifically, there is still a low number of studies assessing circulating circRNA levels and its possible role in CAD, although we predict that in the coming years the research in this type of ncRNAs will increase exponentially as occurred for miRNAs and lncRNAs.

Nevertheless, growing evidence seemingly attests that the measurement of ncRNAs may be a reliable and suitable alternative to other conventional cardiac biomarkers once technical issues, reference values, appropriate setting within diagnostic algorithms, and time course of ncRNAs release from affected tissues will be definitely clarified [92]. Finally, it is only a matter of time that silencing or mimicking agents of miRNAs such as antagomirs (also named also known as anti-miRs or blockmirs) or agomirs will be evaluated to treat certain CVD.

Acknowledgements Fabian Sanchis-Gomar is supported by a postdoctoral contract granted by *"Subprograma Atracció de Talent - Contractes Postdoctorals de la Universitat de València."*

References

1. GBD Mortality and Causes of Death Collaborators. Global, regional, and national age-sex specific all-cause and cause-specific mortality for 240 causes of death, 1990–2013: a systematic analysis for the Global Burden of Disease Study 2013. Lancet. 2015;385(9963):117–71.
2. GBD Mortality and Causes of Death Collaborators. Global, regional, and national life expectancy, all-cause mortality, and cause-specific mortality for 249 causes of death, 1980-2015: a systematic analysis for the Global Burden of Disease Study 2015. Lancet. 2016;388(10053):1459–544.
3. Global Burden of Disease Study, Disease and Injury Incidence, Prevalence Collaborators. Global, regional, and national incidence, prevalence, and years lived with disability for 310 diseases and injuries, 1990-2015: a systematic analysis for the Global Burden of Disease Study 2015. Lancet. 2016;388(10053):1545–602.
4. Silverthorn DU, Johnson BR, Ober WC, Ober CE, Silverthorn AC. Human physiology: an integrated approach. 7th ed. San Francisco: Pearson; 2016.
5. Wong ND. Epidemiological studies of CHD and the evolution of preventive cardiology. Nat Rev Cardiol. 2014;11(5):276–89.
6. Matsuzawa Y, Lerman A. Endothelial dysfunction and coronary artery disease: assessment, prognosis, and treatment. Coron Artery Dis. 2014;25(8):713–24.
7. Lessner SM, Prado HL, Waller EK, Galis ZS. Atherosclerotic lesions grow through recruitment and proliferation of circulating monocytes in a murine model. Am J Surg Pathol. 2002;160(6):2145–55.
8. Libby P, Ridker PM, Hansson GK. Progress and challenges in translating the biology of atherosclerosis. Nature. 2011;473(7347):317–25.
9. Nabel EG, Braunwald E. A tale of coronary artery disease and myocardial infarction. N Engl J Med. 2012;366(1):54–63.
10. Mendis S, Puska P, Norrving B, World Health Organization, World Heart Federation, World Stroke Organization. Global atlas on cardiovascular disease prevention and control. Geneva: World Health

Organization in collaboration with the World Heart Federation and the World Stroke Organization; 2011.
11. Deodhar SD. C-reactive protein: the best laboratory indicator available for monitoring disease activity. Cleve Clin J Med. 1989;56(2):126–30.
12. Maneerat Y, Prasongsukarn K, Benjathummarak S, Dechkhajorn W. PPBP and DEFA1/DEFA3 genes in hyperlipidaemia as feasible synergistic inflammatory biomarkers for coronary heart disease. Lipids Health Dis. 2017;16(1):80.
13. Beermann J, Piccoli MT, Viereck J, Thum T. Non-coding RNAs in development and disease: background, mechanisms, and therapeutic approaches. Physiol Rev. 2016;96(4):1297–325.
14. Militello G, Weirick T, John D, Doring C, Dimmeler S, Uchida S. Screening and validation of lncRNAs and circRNAs as miRNA sponges. Brief Bioinform. 2017;18(5):780–8.
15. Adams V. Assessment of micro ribonucleic acids after exercise: is this the future to detect coronary artery disease at its early stage? Eur J Prev Cardiol. 2019;26(4):346–7.
16. Ikeda S, Kong SW, Lu J, Bisping E, Zhang H, Allen PD, Golub TR, Pieske B, Pu WT. Altered microRNA expression in human heart disease. Physiol Genomics. 2007;31(3):367–73.
17. Lytle JR, Yario TA, Steitz JA. Target mRNAs are repressed as efficiently by microRNA-binding sites in the 5′ UTR as in the 3′ UTR. Proc Natl Acad Sci U S A. 2007;104(23):9667–72.
18. Vasudevan S, Tong Y, Steitz JA. Switching from repression to activation: microRNAs can up-regulate translation. Science. 2007;318(5858):1931–4.
19. Bartel DP. MicroRNAs: genomics, biogenesis, mechanism, and function. Cell. 2004;116(2):281–97.
20. Fichtlscherer S, De Rosa S, Fox H, Schwietz T, Fischer A, Liebetrau C, Weber M, Hamm CW, Roxe T, Muller-Ardogan M, Bonauer A, Zeiher AM, Dimmeler S. Circulating microRNAs in patients with coronary artery disease. Circ Res. 2010;107(5):677–84.
21. Zernecke A, Bidzhekov K, Noels H, Shagdarsuren E, Gan L, Denecke B, Hristov M, Koppel T, Jahantigh MN, Lutgens E, Wang S, Olson EN, Schober A, Weber C. Delivery of microRNA-126 by apoptotic bodies induces CXCL12-dependent vascular protection. Sci Signal. 2009;2(100):ra81.
22. Faccini J, Ruidavets JB, Cordelier P, Martins F, Maoret JJ, Bongard V, Ferrieres J, Roncalli J, Elbaz M, Vindis C. Circulating miR-155, miR-145 and let-7c as diagnostic biomarkers of the coronary artery disease. Sci Rep. 2017;7:42916.
23. Gao H, Guddeti RR, Matsuzawa Y, Liu LP, Su LX, Guo D, Nie SP, Du J, Zhang M. Plasma levels of microRNA-145 are associated with severity of coronary artery disease. PLoS One. 2015;10(5):e0123477.
24. Wang F, Long G, Zhao C, Li H, Chaugai S, Wang Y, Chen C, Wang DW. Plasma microRNA-133a is a new marker for both acute myocardial infarction and underlying coronary artery stenosis. J Transl Med. 2013;11:222.
25. Zhang Y, Li HH, Yang R, Yang BJ, Gao ZY. Association between circulating microRNA-208a and severity of coronary heart disease. Scand J Clin Lab Investig. 2017;77(5):379–84.
26. Liu H, Yang N, Fei Z, Qiu J, Ma D, Liu X, Cai G, Li S. Analysis of plasma miR-208a and miR-370 expression levels for early diagnosis of coronary artery disease. Biomed Rep. 2016;5(3):332–6.
27. D'Alessandra Y, Carena MC, Spazzafumo L, Martinelli F, Bassetti B, Devanna P, Rubino M, Marenzi G, Colombo GI, Achilli F, Maggiolini S, Capogrossi MC, Pompilio G. Diagnostic potential of plasmatic MicroRNA signatures in stable and unstable angina. PLoS One. 2013;8(11):e80345.
28. Liu J, Liu Y, Sun YN, Li S, Liu XQ, Li J, Li CM, Tian W, Zhou YT, Shang XM. miR-28-5p involved in LXR-ABCA1 pathway is increased in the plasma of unstable angina patients. Heart Lung Circ. 2015;24(7):724–30.
29. Wu C, Gong Y, Sun A, Zhang Y, Zhang C, Zhang W, Zhao G, Zou Y, Ge J. The human MTHFR rs4846049 polymorphism increases coronary heart disease risk through modifying miRNA binding. Nutr Metab Cardiovasc Dis. 2013;23(7):693–8.
30. Guo JF, Zhang Y, Zheng QX, Zhang Y, Zhou HH, Cui LM. Association between elevated plasma microRNA-223 content and severity of coronary heart disease. Scand J Clin Lab Investig. 2018;78(5):373–8.
31. Reddy LL, Shah SA, Ponde CK, Rajani RM, Ashavaid TF. Circulating miRNA-33: a potential biomarker in patients with coronary artery Disease (CAD). Biomarkers. 2018;24:1–27.
32. Chen C, Wang Y, Yang S, Li H, Zhao G, Wang F, Yang L, Wang DW. MiR-320a contributes to atherogenesis by augmenting multiple risk factors and down-regulating SRF. J Cell Mol Med. 2015;19(5):970–85.
33. Gao W, He HW, Wang ZM, Zhao H, Lian XQ, Wang YS, Zhu J, Yan JJ, Zhang DG, Yang ZJ, Wang LS. Plasma levels of lipometabolism-related miR-122 and miR-370 are increased in patients with hyperlipidemia and associated with coronary artery disease. Lipids Health Dis. 2012;11:55.
34. Lu HQ, Liang C, He ZQ, Fan M, Wu ZG. Circulating miR-214 is associated with the severity of coronary artery disease. J Geriatr Cardiol. 2013;10(1):34–8.
35. Luo L, Chen B, Li S, Wei X, Liu T, Huang Y, Lin X. Plasma miR-10a: a potential biomarker for coronary artery disease. Dis Markers. 2016;2016:3841927.
36. Wang X, Lian Y, Wen X, Guo J, Wang Z, Jiang S, Hu Y. Expression of miR-126 and its potential function in coronary artery disease. Afr Health Sci. 2017;17(2):474–80.
37. Yilmaz SG, Isbir S, Kunt AT, Isbir T. Circulating microRNAs as novel biomarkers for atherosclerosis. In Vivo. 2018;32(3):561–5.
38. Huang Y, Tang S, Ji-Yan C, Huang C, Li J, Cai AP, Feng YQ. Circulating miR-92a expression level in patients with essential hypertension: a potential marker of atherosclerosis. J Hum Hypertens. 2017;31(3):200–5.

39. Cengiz M, Yavuzer S, Kilickiran Avci B, Yuruyen M, Yavuzer H, Dikici SA, Karatas OF, Ozen M, Uzun H, Ongen Z. Circulating miR-21 and eNOS in subclinical atherosclerosis in patients with hypertension. Clin Exp Hypertens. 2015;37(8):643–9.
40. Quan X, Ji Y, Zhang C, Guo X, Zhang Y, Jia S, Ma W, Fan Y, Wang C. Circulating MiR-146a may be a potential biomarker of coronary heart disease in patients with subclinical hypothyroidism. Cell Physiol Biochem. 2018;45(1):226–36.
41. Tili E, Michaille JJ, Calin GA. Expression and function of micro-RNAs in immune cells during normal or disease state. Int J Med Sci. 2008;5(2):73–9.
42. Hoekstra M, van der Lans CA, Halvorsen B, Gullestad L, Kuiper J, Aukrust P, van Berkel TJ, Biessen EA. The peripheral blood mononuclear cell microRNA signature of coronary artery disease. Biochem Biophys Res Commun. 2010;394(3):792–7.
43. Hulsmans M, Sinnaeve P, Van der Schueren B, Mathieu C, Janssens S, Holvoet P. Decreased miR-181a expression in monocytes of obese patients is associated with the occurrence of metabolic syndrome and coronary artery disease. J Clin Endocrinol Metab. 2012;97(7):E1213–8.
44. Dong J, Liang YZ, Zhang J, Wu LJ, Wang S, Hua Q, Yan YX. Potential role of lipometabolism-related microRNAs in peripheral blood mononuclear cells as biomarkers for coronary artery disease. J Atheroscler Thromb. 2017;24(4):430–41.
45. Lippi G, Franchini M, Targher G. Arterial thrombus formation in cardiovascular disease. Nat Rev Cardiol. 2011;8(9):502–12.
46. Sondermeijer BM, Bakker A, Halliani A, de Ronde MW, Marquart AA, Tijsen AJ, Mulders TA, Kok MG, Battjes S, Maiwald S, Sivapalaratnam S, Trip MD, Moerland PD, Meijers JC, Creemers EE, Pinto-Sietsma SJ. Platelets in patients with premature coronary artery disease exhibit upregulation of miRNA340* and miRNA624*. PLoS One. 2011;6(10):e25946.
47. Diamantopoulos MA, Tsiakanikas P, Scorilas A. Non-coding RNAs: the riddle of the transcriptome and their perspectives in cancer. Ann Transl Med. 2018;6(12):241.
48. Schmitz SU, Grote P, Herrmann BG. Mechanisms of long noncoding RNA function in development and disease. Cell Mol Life Sci. 2016;73(13):2491–509.
49. Warnatsch A, Ioannou M, Wang Q, Papayannopoulos V. Inflammation. Neutrophil extracellular traps license macrophages for cytokine production in atherosclerosis. Science. 2015;349(6245):316–20.
50. Xu Y, Shao B. Circulating lncRNA IFNG-AS1 expression correlates with increased disease risk, higher disease severity and elevated inflammation in patients with coronary artery disease. J Clin Lab Anal. 2018;32(7):e22452.
51. Gao S, Liu W, Zhuo X, Wang L, Wang G, Sun T, Zhao Z, Liu J, Tian Y, Zhou J, Yuan Z, Wu Y. The activation of mTOR is required for monocyte pro-inflammatory response in patients with coronary artery disease. Clin Sci. 2015;128(8):517–26.
52. Yin Q, Wu A, Liu M. Plasma long non-coding RNA (lncRNA) GAS5 is a new biomarker for coronary artery disease. Med Sci Monit. 2017;23:6042–8.
53. Li X, Hou L, Cheng Z, Zhou S, Qi J, Cheng J. Overexpression of GAS5 inhibits abnormal activation of Wnt/beta-catenin signaling pathway in myocardial tissues of rats with coronary artery disease. J Cell Physiol. 2018;234(7):11348–59.
54. Chen L, Yang W, Guo Y, Chen W, Zheng P, Zeng J, Tong W. Exosomal lncRNA GAS5 regulates the apoptosis of macrophages and vascular endothelial cells in atherosclerosis. PLoS One. 2017;12(9):e0185406.
55. Xue D, Zhou C, Lu H, Xu R, Xu X, He X. LncRNA GAS5 inhibits proliferation and progression of prostate cancer by targeting miR-103 through AKT/mTOR signaling pathway. Tumor Biol. 2016;13:3151–8.
56. Yao X, Yan C, Zhang L, Li Y, Wan Q. LncRNA ENST00113 promotes proliferation, survival, and migration by activating PI3K/Akt/mTOR signaling pathway in atherosclerosis. Med Tumor Biol (Baltimore). 2018;97(16):e0473.
57. Li FP, Lin DQ, Gao LY. LncRNA TUG1 promotes proliferation of vascular smooth muscle cell and atherosclerosis through regulating miRNA-21/PTEN axis. Eur Rev Med Pharmacol Sci. 2018;22(21):7439–47.
58. Zhong X, Ma X, Zhang L, Li Y, Li Y, He R. MIAT promotes proliferation and hinders apoptosis by modulating miR-181b/STAT3 axis in ox-LDL-induced atherosclerosis cell models. Biomed Pharmacother. 2018;97:1078–85.
59. Zhang Z, Gao W, Long QQ, Zhang J, Li YF, Liu DC, Yan JJ, Yang ZJ, Wang LS. Increased plasma levels of lncRNA H19 and LIPCAR are associated with increased risk of coronary artery disease in a Chinese population. Sci Rep. 2017;7(1):7491.
60. Pan JX. LncRNA H19 promotes atherosclerosis by regulating MAPK and NF-kB signaling pathway. Eur Rev Med Pharmacol Sci. 2017;21(2):322–8.
61. Greco S, Zaccagnini G, Perfetti A, Fuschi P, Valaperta R, Voellenkle C, Castelvecchio S, Gaetano C, Finato N, Beltrami AP, Menicanti L, Martelli F. Long noncoding RNA dysregulation in ischemic heart failure. J Transl Med. 2016;14(1):183.
62. Kumarswamy R, Bauters C, Volkmann I, Maury F, Fetisch J, Holzmann A, Lemesle G, de Groote P, Pinet F, Thum T. Circulating long noncoding RNA, LIPCAR, predicts survival in patients with heart failure. Circ Res. 2014;114(10):1569–75.
63. Wang L, Qu P, Zhao J, Chang Y. NLRP3 and downstream cytokine expression elevated in the monocytes of patients with coronary artery disease. Arch Med Sci. 2014;10(4):791–800.
64. Cai Y, Yang Y, Chen X, Wu G, Zhang X, Liu Y, Yu J, Wang X, Fu J, Li C, Jose PA, Zeng C, Zhou L. Circulating 'lncRNA OTTHUMT00000387022' from monocytes as a novel biomarker for coronary artery disease. Cardiovasc Res. 2016;112(3):714–24.

65. Yang Y, Cai Y, Wu G, Chen X, Liu Y, Wang X, Yu J, Li C, Chen X, Jose PA, Zhou L, Zeng C. Plasma long non-coding RNA, CoroMarker, a novel biomarker for diagnosis of coronary artery disease. Clin Sci. 2015;129(8):675–85.
66. Cai Y, Yang Y, Chen X, He D, Zhang X, Wen X, Hu J, Fu C, Qiu D, Jose PA, Zeng C, Zhou L. Circulating "LncPPARdelta" from monocytes as a novel biomarker for coronary artery diseases. Medicine (Baltimore). 2016;95(6):e2360.
67. Li L, Wang L, Li H, Han X, Chen S, Yang B, Hu Z, Zhu H, Cai C, Chen J, Li X, Huang J, Gu D. Characterization of LncRNA expression profile and identification of novel LncRNA biomarkers to diagnose coronary artery disease. Atherosclerosis. 2018;275:359–67.
68. Li X, Zhao Z, Gao C, Rao L, Hao P, Jian D, Li W, Tang H, Li M. Identification of a peripheral blood long non-coding RNA (Upperhand) as a potential diagnostic marker of coronary artery disease. Int J Cardiol. 2018;25(3):393–402.
69. Broadbent HM, Peden JF, Lorkowski S, Goel A, Ongen H, Green F, Clarke R, Collins R, Franzosi MG, Tognoni G, Seedorf U, Rust S, Eriksson P, Hamsten A, Farrall M, Watkins H, PROCARDIS Consortium. Susceptibility to coronary artery disease and diabetes is encoded by distinct, tightly linked SNPs in the ANRIL locus on chromosome 9p. Hum Mol Genet. 2008;17(6):806–14.
70. Congrains A, Kamide K, Oguro R, Yasuda O, Miyata K, Yamamoto E, Kawai T, Kusunoki H, Yamamoto H, Takeya Y, Yamamoto K, Onishi M, Sugimoto K, Katsuya T, Awata N, Ikebe K, Gondo Y, Oike Y, Ohishi M, Rakugi H. Genetic variants at the 9p21 locus contribute to atherosclerosis through modulation of ANRIL and CDKN2A/B. Atherosclerosis. 2012;220(2):449–55.
71. Wang P, Dong P, Yang X. ANRIL rs2383207 polymorphism and coronary artery disease (CAD) risk: a meta-analysis with observational studies. Mol Biol Cell (Noisy-le-grand). 2016;62(12):6–10.
72. Xu B, Fang Z, He S, Wang J, Yang X. ANRIL polymorphism rs4977574 is associated with increased risk of coronary artery disease in Asian populations: a meta-analysis of 12,005 subjects. Medicine (Baltimore). 2018;97(39):e12641.
73. Xie Y, Zhao D, Dong P, Wang H, Li D, Lai L. Effects of ANRIL polymorphisms on the likelihood of coronary artery disease: a meta-analysis. J Cell Biochem. 2019;120(4):6113–9.
74. Sun X, He S, Wara AKM, Icli B, Shvartz E, Tesmenitsky Y, Belkin N, Li D, Blackwell TS, Sukhova GK, Croce K, Feinberg MW. Systemic delivery of microRNA-181b inhibits nuclear factor-kappaB activation, vascular inflammation, and atherosclerosis in apolipoprotein E-deficient mice. Circ Res. 2014;114(1):32–40.
75. Guo F, Tang C, Li Y, Liu Y, Lv P, Wang W, Mu Y. The interplay of LncRNA ANRIL and miR-181b on the inflammation-relevant coronary artery disease through mediating NF-kappaB signalling pathway. J Cell Mol Med. 2018;22(10):5062–75.
76. Cho H, Shen GQ, Wang X, Wang F, Archacki S, Li Y, Yu G, Chakrabarti S, Chen Q, Wang QK. Long noncoding RNA ANRIL regulates endothelial cell activities associated with coronary artery disease by up-regulating CLIP1, EZR, and LYVE1 genes. J Biol Chem. 2019;294(22):8715.
77. Hansen TB, Jensen TI, Clausen BH, Bramsen JB, Finsen B, Damgaard CK, Kjems J. Natural RNA circles function as efficient microRNA sponges. Nature. 2013;495(7441):384–8.
78. Memczak S, Jens M, Elefsinioti A, Torti F, Krueger J, Rybak A, Maier L, Mackowiak SD, Gregersen LH, Munschauer M, Loewer A, Ziebold U, Landthaler M, Kocks C, le Noble F, Rajewsky N. Circular RNAs are a large class of animal RNAs with regulatory potency. Nature. 2013;495(7441):333–8.
79. Ashwal-Fluss R, Meyer M, Pamudurti NR, Ivanov A, Bartok O, Hanan M, Evantal N, Memczak S, Rajewsky N, Kadener S. circRNA biogenesis competes with pre-mRNA splicing. Mol Cell. 2014;56(1):55–66.
80. Zeng Y, Du WW, Wu Y, Yang Z, Awan FM, Li X, Yang W, Zhang C, Yang Q, Yee A, Chen Y, Yang F, Sun H, Huang R, Yee AJ, Li RK, Wu Z, Backx PH, Yang BB. A circular RNA binds to and activates AKT phosphorylation and nuclear localization reducing apoptosis and enhancing cardiac repair. Theranostics. 2017;7(16):3842–55.
81. Li Z, Huang C, Bao C, Chen L, Lin M, Wang X, Zhong G, Yu B, Hu W, Dai L, Zhu P, Chang Z, Wu Q, Zhao Y, Jia Y, Xu P, Liu H, Shan G. Exon-intron circular RNAs regulate transcription in the nucleus. Nat Struct Mol Biol. 2015;22(3):256–64.
82. Wilusz JE. A 360 degrees view of circular RNAs: from biogenesis to functions. Wiley Interdiscip Rev-RNA. 2018;9(4):e1478.
83. Pan RY, Liu P, Zhou HT, Sun WX, Song J, Shu J, Cui GJ, Yang ZJ, Jia EZ. Circular RNAs promote TRPM3 expression by inhibiting hsa-miR-130a-3p in coronary artery disease patients. Oncotarget. 2017;8(36):60280–90.
84. de Gonzalo-Calvo D, Cenarro A, Garlaschelli K, Pellegatta F, Vilades D, Nasarre L, Camino-Lopez S, Crespo J, Carreras F, Leta R, Catapano AL, Norata GD, Civeira F, Llorente-Cortes V. Translating the microRNA signature of microvesicles derived from human coronary artery smooth muscle cells in patients with familial hypercholesterolemia and coronary artery disease. J Mol Cell Cardiol. 2017;106:55–67.
85. Zhang Q, Kandic I, Kutryk MJ. Dysregulation of angiogenesis-related microRNAs in endothelial progenitor cells from patients with coronary artery disease. Biochem Biophys Res Commun. 2011;405(1):42–6.
86. Naylor J, Li J, Milligan CJ, Zeng F, Sukumar P, Hou B, Sedo A, Yuldasheva N, Majeed Y, Beri D, Jiang S,

Seymour VA, McKeown L, Kumar B, Harteneck C, O'Regan D, Wheatcroft SB, Kearney MT, Jones C, Porter KE, Beech DJ. Pregnenolone sulphate- and cholesterol-regulated TRPM3 channels coupled to vascular smooth muscle secretion and contraction. Circ Res. 2010;106(9):1507–15.
87. Liu C, Yao MD, Li CP, Shan K, Yang H, Wang JJ, Liu B, Li XM, Yao J, Jiang Q, Yan B. Silencing of circular RNA-ZNF609 ameliorates vascular endothelial dysfunction. Theranostics. 2017;7(11):2863–77.
88. Boeckel JN, Jae N, Heumuller AW, Chen W, Boon RA, Stellos K, Zeiher AM, John D, Uchida S, Dimmeler S. Identification and characterization of hypoxia-regulated endothelial circular RNA. Circ Res. 2015;117(10):884–90.
89. Zhao Z, Li X, Gao C, Jian D, Hao P, Rao L, Li M. Peripheral blood circular RNA hsa_circ_0124644 can be used as a diagnostic biomarker of coronary artery disease. Sci Rep. 2017;7:39918.
90. Li X, Zhao Z, Jian D, Li W, Tang H, Li M. Hsa-circRNA11783-2 in peripheral blood is correlated with coronary artery disease and type 2 diabetes mellitus. Diab Vasc Dis Res. 2017;14(6):510–5.
91. Lippi G, Mattiuzzi C, Cervellin G. Circulating microRNAs (miRs) for diagnosing acute myocardial infarction: meta-analysis of available studies. Int J Cardiol. 2013;167(1):277–8.
92. Lippi G, Mattiuzzi C, Cervellin G. MicroRNAs for diagnosing myocardial infarction. Advantages and limitations. Int J Cardiol. 2013;168(5):4849–50.

Non-coding RNAs and Cardiac Arrhythmias

17

Filip Šustr, Zdeněk Stárek, Miroslav Souček, and Jan Novák

Abstract

Cardiac arrhythmias represent wide and heterogenic group of disturbances in the cardiac rhythm. Pathophysiology of individual arrhythmias is highly complex and dysfunction in ion channels/currents involved in generation or spreading of action potential is usually documented. Non-coding RNAs (ncRNAs) represent highly variable group of molecules regulating the heart expression program, including regulation of the expression of individual ion channels and intercellular connection proteins, e.g. connexins.

Within this chapter, we will describe basic electrophysiological properties of the myocardium. We will focus on action potential generation and spreading in pacemaker and non-pacemaker cells, including description of individual ion channels (natrium, potassium and calcium) and their ncRNA-mediated regulation. Most of the studies have so far focused on microRNAs, thus, their regulatory function will be described into greater detail. Clinical consequences of altered ncRNA regulatory function will also be described together with potential future directions of the research in the field.

Keywords

MicroRNA · Non-coding RNA · Connexin 43 · CACNA1C · Ion channels · Arrhythmia

1 Introduction

Cardiac arrhythmias represent wide and heterogenic group of disturbances in the cardiac rhythm and they arise as a result of plentiful functional and structural changes of the myocardium (e.g. changes in the ion channels expression or distribution, calcium handling abnormalities, cardiac fibrosis, ischemia etc.) [1]. Based on the location of the arrhythmic focus, they can be divided into supraventricular and ventricular; based on their rate, we can distinguish fast tachyarrhythmias and slow bradyarrhythmias. The most common supraventricular arrhythmia affecting up to 1% of

F. Šustr · M. Souček
Second Department of Internal Medicine of St. Anne's University Hospital in Brno and Faculty of Medicine, Masaryk University, Brno, Czech Republic

Z. Stárek
First Department of Internal Medicine and Cardioangiology of St. Anne's University Hospital in Brno and Faculty of Medicine, Masaryk University, Brno, Czech Republic

J. Novák (✉)
Second Department of Internal Medicine of St. Anne's University Hospital in Brno and Faculty of Medicine, Masaryk University, Brno, Czech Republic

CEITEC – Central European Institute for Technology, Masaryk University, Brno, Czech Republic
e-mail: jan.novak@fnusa.cz

J. Xiao (ed.), *Non-coding RNAs in Cardiovascular Diseases*, Advances in Experimental Medicine and Biology 1229, https://doi.org/10.1007/978-981-15-1671-9_17

general population and up to 8% of elderly population (age > 80 years) is atrial fibrillation (AF) – presence of AF significantly affect patients quality of life, increases the risk of embolic events (such as stroke) and thus substantially contributes to morbidity and mortality [2]. Ventricular arrhythmias are generally less common; however, their presence significantly increases the risk of sudden cardiac death [3].

Non-coding RNAs (ncRNAs), as a huge and heterogenic group of molecules, intracellularly regulate gene expression and orchestrate numerous processes occurring in our body, extracellularly they represent novel means of intercellular communication. Extracellular RNAs can easily be identified in the bodily fluids and as such they represent clinically relevant and intriguing group of novel diagnostic or prognostic biomarkers [4].

Within this chapter, we will mainly focus on the role of ncRNAs, especially microRNAs (miRNAs, miRs), in the regulation of cardiac automaticity and conductance and its pathophysiological and potentially clinical consequences.

2 Cardiac Electrophysiology in a "Nutshell"

Myocardial cells (cardiomyocytes) maintain cardiac function by precise orchestration of the electrical activation (including generation of action potentials in pacemaker cells and conduction of these potentials among other cardiomyocytes, i.e. non-pacemaker cells) and mechanical contractions (including signal transduction from activated cellular membranes to cardiomyocytes contractile apparatus). All of these processes include series of events orchestrated by four main groups of ion channels – natrium (Na^+), potassium (K^+), calcium (Ca^{2+}) and chloride (Cl^-). Generally Na^+ and Ca^{2+} ions are entering cardiomyocytes (via several types of ion channels) resulting in the rise of their resting membrane potential from negative to more positive values, which is called depolarization, subsequently resulting in the initiation of the action potential. Various intercellular proteins, mainly connexins, are responsible for spreading the generated potential from pacemaker cells to non-pacemaker cells and generally among individual cardiomyocytes. Efflux of K^+ ions then results in return of the action potential to the resting membrane potential. Ca^{2+} ions further regulate excitation-contraction coupling and generation of the muscle contraction [5, 6]. All processes described above are summarized in the Fig. 17.1 separately for pacemaker cells (A) and non-pacemaker cells (B).

3 Non-coding RNAs in the Regulation of Cardiac Automaticity and Conductance

3.1 Regulation of Cardiac Automaticity

Common sign of the cardiac pacemaker cells is the expression of f-channels for Na^+ ions [7]. After previous action potential is ended, Na^+ ions slowly influx into the cells through this channel causing spontaneous depolarization, which then opens T-type Ca^{2+} channels resulting in action potential development (Fig. 17.2).

HCN (hyperpolarization-activated cyclic nucleotide-gated) protein isoforms create for f-channels in the pacemaker cells. HCN4 is predominantly expressed in pacemaker cells, and its levels are known to be reduced in AF [8]. HCN4 posttranscriptional regulation is partially mediated by cardio-specific miRNAs, i.e. miR-1 and miR-133 [9]. During ageing it was shown that miR-1 and miR-133 levels decrease while levels of HCN2 and HCN4 increase which may partially contribute to development of age-dependent atrial fibrillation [10]. Vice versa, endurance training increases miR-1, which explains the downregulation of HCN4 which partly explains resting heart rate adaptation [11]. Another miRNA shown to be associated with HCN4 function was miR-423-5p, which was also upregulated during endurance training and knockdown of miR-423-5p with anti-miR-423-5p reversed training-induced bradycardia via rescue of HCN4

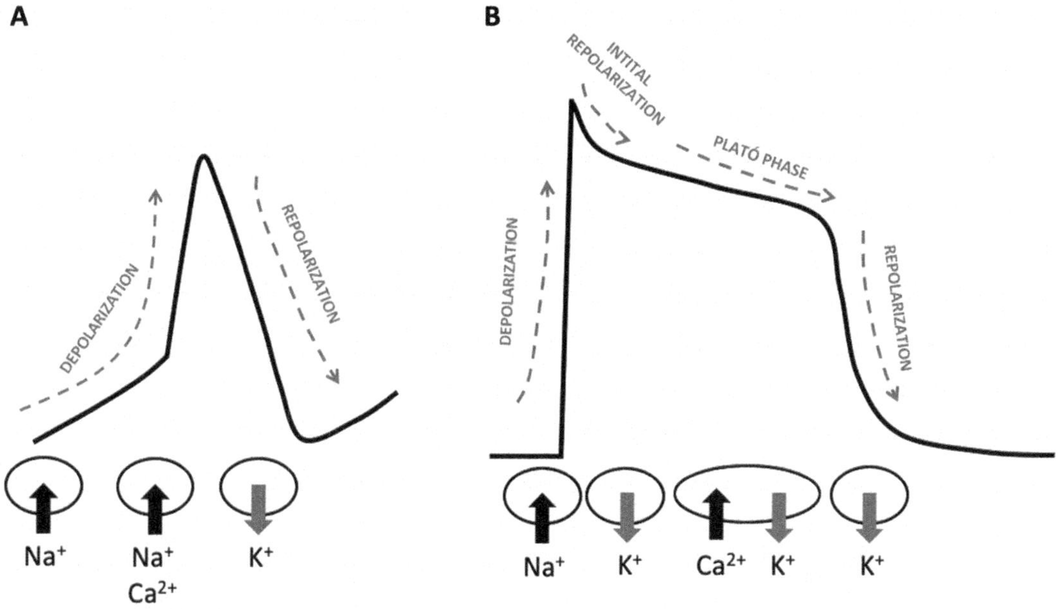

Fig. 17.1 Simplified action potential of pacemaker and non-pacemaker cardiomyocytes
(**A**) Action potential in pacemaker cells. After previous action potential is ended, Na^+ ions slowly enter pacemaker cells, causing their membrane potential to slowly increase from the resting membrane potential. This is further promoted by Ca^{2+} influx leading to action potential generation. K^+ efflux then returns membrane potential back to negative values, which again opens Na^+ channel resulting in Na^+ influx into cells.
(**B**) Action potential of non-pacemaker cells. At rest, non-pacemaker cells present with very negative resting membrane potential. After stimulation, rapid influx of Na^+ ions induce fast depolarization followed by initial transient repolarization by K^+ efflux. After this short period, both influx of Ca^{2+} and efflux of K^+ occur, resulting in plató phase of the action potential. At the end of the plató phase, K^+ efflux is more prominent resulting in repolarization and return of the membrane potential back to its negative resting values.

[12]. Lastly, HCN2 isoform levels were also shown to be regulated by miRNAs, as multi-targeted anti-miRNA anti-sense inhibitors (anti-miR-1/anti-miR-133) caused their increase [13].

All in all, these studies show that miR-1 and miR-133 are post-transcriptional regulators of HCN4 and HCN2 and their alterations correspond with the changes in the resting heart rate or with the occurrence of AF.

3.2 Regulation of Na^+ Channels Involved in Depolarization

Cardiac action potential is initiated by a fast-activating and fast-inactivating sodium current (I_{Na}) that is generated by the Na^+ channel composing of α- and one or more β-subunits [14]. SCN5A/Nav1.5 gene encodes for the α-subunit of this channels and its mutations are associated with several arrhythmogenic syndromes, e.g. Long QT syndrome, Brugada syndrome etc. [6]. In the whole genome network analysis, SCN5A was one of the targets identified to be highly regulated by miRNAs, together with CACNA1C and connexin 43 [15] (Fig. 17.2). In the study by Daimi et al. using HL-1 cardiomyocytes and luciferase assays they showed that SCN5A is directly (miR-98, miR-106, miR-200, and miR-219) and indirectly (miR-125 and miR-153) regulated by several miRNAs. Out of these miRNAs, miR-219 was shown to increases the sodium current in vitro and to abolish QRS prolongation induced by flecainide intoxication in mice [16]. Study by Poon et al. further focused on miR-200c and showed progressive down-regulation of this miRNA both during cardiac development and differentiation of human embryonic stem cells

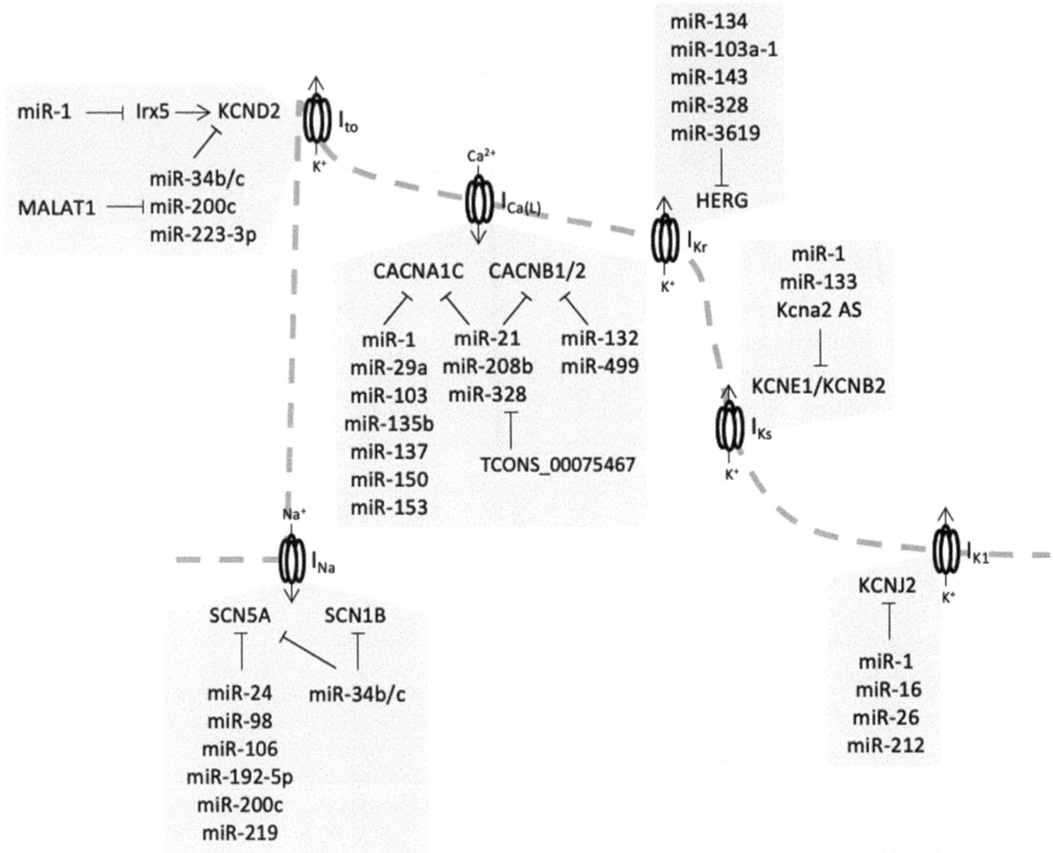

Fig. 17.2 Non-coding RNA regulation of individual ion channels in the non-pacemaker cardiomyocytes
Grey dashed line in the background of the figure schematically represents changes in the non-pacemaker cardiomyocytes action potential. Individual ion currents are visualized accordingly to approximate time corresponding with ion channels opening. Grey boxes linked to individual genes summarizes which ncRNAs are involved in their post-transcriptional regulation. Further explanation is provided in the text.

(hESCs) to cardiomyocytes – miR-200c knockdown or overexpression was associated with changes in SCN5A levels, together with the levels of K^+ and Ca^{2+} channels (as mentioned further) [17]. Zhao et al. proved that 3′-untranslated region (UTR) of human SCN5A is targeted by miR-192-5p causing its downregulation [18]. Recently, Zhang et al. showed that common single nucleotide polymorphism in SCN5A (rs1805126) alters miR-24 binding and that minor allele associates with decreased cardiac SCN5A expression [19]. This associated with decreased ejection fraction and increased mortality, but not increased occurrence of ventricular tachyarrhythmias, in homozygous subjects for the minor allele with heart failure [19]. Lastly, miR-34b/c was shown to target SCN5A and even SCN1B (gene encoding for β-subunit), and expression of miR-34 was shown to be mediated by KChIP2 (Potassium Channel Interacting Protein), through interaction with genetic elements; as long as KChIP2 reduced expression is consistently observed in numerous cardiac pathologies, KChIP2 may represent interesting therapeutic target for treating arrhythmogenesis in cardiovascular diseases [20].

3.3 Regulation of Ca^{2+} Handling (Depolarization and Contractility)

3.3.1 L-Type Ca^{2+} Currents

Voltage gated Cav1 channels mediate L-type Ca^{2+} currents through the heart. Cav1.3 channels are dominantly expressed in the sinoatrial node, atria and atrioventricular node and are responsible mainly for action potential generation, while Cav1.2 channels are expressed through the heart and regulate action potential duration and excitation-contraction coupling [21]. Cav1.2 channel comprise of α-subunit (encoded by CACNA1C gene) and β-subunit (encoded by CACNB1/2 genes), and their mutations are known to be associated with sudden infant death syndrome [21, 22].

One of the first attempts to prove association of miRNAs with Ca^{2+} channels and AF was made by Lu et al. [23] They performed transcriptomics profiling of the left atrial samples from canine model of AF and of human atrial samples from AF patients with rheumatic heart disease. They identified 3 miRNAs to be upregulated (miR-223, miR-328, and miR-664) and another 3 to be downregulated (miR-101, miR-320, and miR-499). Computational prediction showed miR-328 to regulate both CACNA1C and CACNB1 and forced expression of miR-328 in both murine and canine experiments enhanced AF vulnerability, diminished L-type Ca^{2+} current, and shortened atrial action potential duration [23]. Moreover, it was recently shown that long non-coding RNA, TCONS_00075467, serves as a sponge for miR-328 and thus regulates CACNA1C expression, which further underlines importance of miR-328 and Ca^{2+} handling in AF pathogenesis [24].

Wang et al. further identified miR-155 as a direct regulator of CACNA1C expression and their team also showed that miR-155, miR-142-3p, miR-19b, miR-223, miR-146b-5p, miR-486-5p, miR-301b, miR-193b, miR-519b were upregulated and miR-193a-5p was downregulated in the left atrial appendages from patients with AF compared to those without AF [25, 26]. Other miRNAs, miR-21 and miR-208b, were also shown to be increased in patients with chronic AF, leading to both CACNA1C and CACNB2 downregulation [27, 28], in the latter case, miR-208b was also shown to target SERCA, thus further affecting Ca^{2+} handling in cardiomyocytes [28]. In the setting of cardiac arrhythmias, miR-29a was another miRNA found to target CACNA1C [29] and similarly, miR-499 was shown to regulate CACNB2 expression [30]. In the mice long-term exposed to isoproterenol, levels of miR-21 and miR-132 were significantly increased while levels of CACNB2 were significantly decreased, decreasing arrhythmias susceptibility [31].

Apart from the arrhythmias, CACNA1C regulation was also studied in numerous diseases and tissues. In the cardiac hypertrophy model, miR-135b was significantly downregulated which led to the upregulation of CACNA1C [32], showing potential involvement of CACNA1C in the regulation of cardiomyocyte hypertrophy. In the myotonic dystrophy, it was shown that expression of miR-1 in the heart is lost, which leads to the overexpression of GJA1 gene (i.e. expression of connexin 43) and CACNA1C in the heart of affected individuals and partially explains cardiac dysfunction that is known to occur in these patients [33]. In the psychiatric patients, CACNA1C is known to be associated with bipolar disorder and Genome-Wide Association Study (GWAS) study performed by Schizophrenia Psychiatric GWAS Consortium identified miR-137 gene polymorphism to be associated with schizophrenia [34] and subsequent study by Kwon et al. confirmed CACNA1C as one of the targets for miR-137 using luciferase assays [35]. In the osteoblasts, where Cav1.2 is one of the important transductor of mechanical stimuli, miR-103 was shown to regulate CACNA1C expression [36]. Interestingly, miR-153, which is an intronic miRNA embedded in the islet antigen (IA) genes (IA-2 and IA-2β), was shown to regulate CACNA1C and thus regulate insulin and dopamine secretion [37].

Taken together data about CACNA1C and CACNB2 indicates that these proteins are highly regulated by various ncRNAs and they thus represent potential targets for the personalized therapy of individual arrhythmias.

3.3.2 SERCA Regulation

Besides Ca^{2+} channels, many other proteins are involved in Ca^{2+} handling in cardiomyocytes. These are represented but not limited to transmembrane calcium ATPase – SERCA. Compared to L-type Ca^{2+} channels, SERCA is mostly studied in the models of cardiac hypertrophy, which will be described into more detail in the corresponding chapter of this book.

Similarly to CACNA1C, SERCA-2A is also a target of miR-328, which was studied in several models of cardiac hypertrophy [38] and by miR-208b, as shown in the HL-1 atrial myocytes in the context of chronic AF [25]. Resistance training was shown to increase levels of miR-214 and decrease levels of SERCA [39], while endurance training in Wistar rats after myocardial infarction caused opposite effect, i.e. decrease in miR-214 levels [40]. Other miRNAs, like miR-25 or miR-22 were shown to regulate Ca^{2+} levels, partially and probably indirectly via SERCA in failing hearts [41, 42]. miR-29 was shown to be upregulated by the hypoxia-inducible factor-1 (HIF-1) which, in turn, inhibited SERCA2 expression and reduced cardiac contractility [43].

3.4 Regulation of K^+ Channels Involved in Repolarization

After depolarization generally driven by Na^+ and Ca^{2+} channels, plató phase and depolarization occur. During plató phase, delicate balance between inward and outward currents is established, while during repolarization, mostly outward efflux of K^+ ions occurs that is driven by the series of K^+ currents. These K^+ currents include:

- I_{to} (transition outward K^+ current).
- I_{Kr} (rapid delayed rectifier K+ current).
- I_{Ks} (slow delayed rectifier K+ current).
- I_{K1} (inward rectifier current).

and others.

Early studies in the field of ncRNAs in arrhythmogenesis performed in 2007 focused mainly on miR-1 and regulation of K^+ channels expression. Zhou et al. performed targeted deletion of miR-1-2 in murine model which led to the 50% lethality mainly due to ventricular septal defects and further to sudden death of approximately half of the surviving animals, due to conduction blockade [20]. Transcription factor Irx5 was identified as miR-1 target and KCND2, which encodes for Kv4.2 subunit of K^+ channel responsible for I_{to}, was found to be downregulated. Yang et al. showed that miR-1 is overexpressed in individuals with coronary artery disease and that it promotes arrhythmogenesis in murine model of myocardial infarction mainly by targeting KCNJ2 (which encodes the channel subunit Kir2.1, that is responsible for I_{K1} current) and GJA1 (which encodes connexin 43 that is responsible for action potential spreading over the myocardium as described further) [44]. Both of these studies hallmark dysregulation of miR-1 under various pathological conditions and link it to the arrhythmogenesis. Further studies were then performed focusing on individual K^+ currents, their underlying ion channels expression and other miRNAs, as described further.

3.4.1 I_{to} (Transition Outward K^+ Current)

Besides miR-1, KCND2 (i.e. I_{to} K^+ current) is also regulated by miR-223-3p as studied in the murine model of myocardial infarction [45] and miR-34 as studied in neonatal rat ventricular myocytes and human derived cardiomyocytes [20]. Expression of miR-223-3p was significantly upregulated, while protein level of Kv4.2 and I_{to} density were significantly downregulated in the infarcted myocardium and direct intramuscular injection of anti-miR-223-3p into the ischemic myocardium decreased the propensity of ischemic arrhythmias [45]. miR-34 levels were upregulated by KChIP silencing, which then caused KCND2 depletion. Inhibition of miR-34b/c then restores cellular excitability and limited the occurrence of conduction block and reentry [20].

Last but not the least, I_{to} is regulated by miR-200c [17] together with long non-coding RNA (lncRNA) Metastasis Associated Lung Adenocarcinoma Transcript 1 (MALAT1) [46]. MALAT1 acts as a competing endogenous RNA for miR-200c. Binding of miR-200c to MALAT1 leads to upregulation in the expression of high-mobility group box 1 (HMGB1) and downregulation in cardiac I_{to}.

3.4.2 I_{Kr} (Rapid Delayed Rectifier K^+ Current)

Changes in the I_{Kr} current/Kv11.1 channel that is encoded by ether-a-go-go-related gene (hERG) are known to be associated with long QT syndrome and life-threatening arrhythmias such as torsade de pointes [47]. hERG was shown to be targeted by several miRNAs in the recent study by Lien et al. [48] – using dual-luciferase reporter assay they showed that miR-134, miR-103a-1, miR-143, and miR-3619 directly regulates hERG expression and by patch-clamping they proved that miR-103a-1 decreased the maximum current and tail current amplitudes of the I_{Kr}. Interestingly, miR-328, mentioned previously in the context of atrial fibrillation and CACNA1C and SERCA regulation, was shown to have binding site in the 3'UTR of the hERG mRNA – in the in vitro study, administration of arsenic trioxide inhibited breast cancer cell growth at least partly via miR-328/hERG pathway [49]. Future electrophysiological studies are needed to determine, whether miR-328 dysregulation may have functional impact in the settings of AF or other arrhythmias by altering atrial K^+ currents changes.

3.4.3 I_{K1} (Inwardly Rectifying K^+ Channel)

In 2009, Girmatsion et al. described decreased levels of miR-1 in atrial tissues from patients with AF. This decrease was associated with increased I_{K1} density and corresponding increase in Kir2.1 protein expression [50]. Similarly, tachypacing of human atrial slices further decreased miR-1 levels and increased expression of Kir2.1 protein indicating potential primary role of atrial rate in miR-1 down-regulation [50]. Similarly, miR-26 levels were also decreased in atrial samples from animals and patients with AF and this downregulation was accompanied by upregulation of Kir2.1 protein [51]. Furthermore, in the canine model of chronic heart failure induced by ventricular tachypacing, miR-26a was also found to be downregulated in heart fibroblasts, while I_{K1} current and KCNJ2 expression were upregulated [52]. miR-26a knockdown was sufficient to mimic the effect of ventricular tachypacing on I_{K1} dysregulation. All of the studies are indicative that loss of specific miRNAs (miR-1, miR-26) may promote AF development partly by Kir2.1 upregulation.

Further miRNAs that were shown to regulate KCNJ2 expression are miR-212 [53] and miR-16 [54]. Regulation by miR-16 was studied in the settings of myocardial infarction related arrhythmias – miR-16 expression was increased in infarct border which led to decrease in I_{K1}/Kir2.1 level and this decrease was reversible by valsartan administration via NF-κB pathway [54].

3.4.4 I_{Ks} (Slow Delayed Rectifier K^+ Current)

I_{Ks} is another K+ current critical for the late phase repolarization that is known to be associated with long QT syndrome and severe ventricular arrhythmias [55]. In the rabbit model of diabetes (induced by alloxan administration), I_{Ks} density was significantly reduced and QT interval prolonged. This may be partly due to miR-1/133 upregulation in response to hyperglycemia [56]. In the rabbit right atrium tachypacing model, KCNE1 and KCNB2, which encodes for the I_{Ks} channel subunits, were also confirmed as miR-1 targets, and knockdown of miR-1 by anti-miR-1 inhibitor alleviated the downregulation of KCNE1 and KCNB2, the shortening of atrial effective refractory period and the increase in the I_{Ks} [57]. Besides miRNAs, lncRNA, Kcna2 Antisense RNA (KCNA2 AS) was shown to regulate I_{Ks} in rat model of chronic heart failure – ventricular levels of KCNA2 AS expression is increased in rats with heart failure, which contributes to reduced I_{Ks} and prolonged action potential duration [58].

3.4.5 Other K+ Channels

There are many other diverse K^+ channels that may be involved in arrhythmogenesis. Among them, small-conductance calcium-activated potassium channel 3 (SK3) encoded by KCNN3 gene is known to be associated with AF [59]. In the atria of the AF patients, SK3 protein expression was shown to be downregulated by 46% whilst miR-499 was upregulated by 2.33-fold. Luciferase assay confirmed miR-499 binding to KCNN3, thus linking it to the AF pathophysiology [59]. Another K^+ channel, acetylcholine-sensitive inward-rectifier K^+ current (I_KAch), was also shown to be downregulated in atria from the AF patients and levels of miR-30d were accordingly increased – transfection of the miR-30 precursor to the cultured cardiomyocytes significantly decreased I_KAch [60].

3.5 Regulation of Action Potential Intercellular Spreading

Discrete cardiomyocytes are functionally interconnected by a variety of molecules, one of them being connexins at the sites of the gap junctions. Connexins are transmembrane proteins that connect individual cardiomyocytes together thus enabling intercellular action potential spreading and generally intercellular cardiomyocytes communication. Connexin 40 (Cx40) is dominantly expressed in the atria and the conduction system, whereas Connexin 43 (Cx43) is highly expressed in the ventricles. Cx43 levels are also increased in rat female cardiomyocytes compared to male cardiomyocytes, and miR-1 levels corresponds with this expression pattern, which may partly contribute to the resistance of female hearts to arrhythmias [61]. After menopause, miR-23a regulation of Cx43 may also partly explain the loss of this cardioprotective effect – estrogen decrease is known to increase the incidence of arrhythmias in women and Wang et al. showed that estrogen decrease also increases levels of miR-23a, which decreases levels of Cx43 causing gap junction remodeling [62]. Estrogen supplementation or suppressing miR-23a by transfection of miR-23a specific inhibitory oligonucleotide reversed these effects.

In the context of non-coding RNAs, Cx43 was even shown to act as a miRNA transfer tool – Kim et al. showed that mesenchymal stem cells are able to transfer miR-210 to host cardiomyocytes via Cx43, thus improving their survival under hypoxic conditions [63].

Due to Cx43 numerous functions it is thus not surprising, that extensive miRNA analysis showed that Cx43 is under more intensive miRNA regulation compared with the other gap junction proteins and ion channels [15]. As mentioned above, miR-1 is a regulator of Cx43 and this was shown already in 2007 [44] and was further directly or indirectly confirmed by numerous others. In the rat model of myocardial infarction, miR-1 expression was repeatedly shown to be increased [64, 65]. Hearts of the transgenic mice overexpressing miR-1 were more susceptible to the development of atrioventricular block after the induction of myocardial infarction [65]. This was partly due to alterations in Cx43 expression, partly due to alteration of L-type Ca^{2+} channel and I_{K1} function. Liu and colleagues used anti-miR-1 oligonucleotide to prevent arrhythmias in ischemic heart and indeed, down-regulation of miR-1 by this anti-sense oligonucleotide caused Kir2.1 and Cx43 protein expression increase, which relieved ischemic arrhythmias in diseased animals [66]. Similarly, administration of propranolol in the rat model of myocardial infarction caused miR-1 downregulation, thus resulting in decline in arrhythmicity of the infarcted myocardium, probably via β-receptor cAMP – protein kinase A signaling pathway that suppressed its expression via serum response factor (SRF) – one of the transcription factors involved in miR-1 expression regulation [64].

Correspondingly to the myocardial infarction models, in the rat model of viral myocarditis, miR-1 expression was also shown to be increased leading to Cx43 decrease, thus making heart more vulnerable to arrhythmias [67].

On the contrary to myocardial infarction and viral myocarditis, miR-1 downregulation was proved to occur in the hypertrophied rat hearts, which increased levels of Cx43 and led to the development of ventricular tachyarrhythmias [68]. Similar effect was observed on the rat hearts exposed to the irradiation [69] and more importantly, in humans, expression of miR-1 was reduced by approx. 86% in the tissue samples from patients with AF [50]. Delicate regulation of miR-1 levels is thus necessary to prevent various arrhythmias in the heart as they may be triggered by both too low or too high levels if this miRNA.

Besides miR-1, Cx43 is regulated by other miRNAs and lncRNAs. Regulation by miR-133 was shown in zebrafish, where it also corresponded with regeneration and proliferation – if miR-133 is absent, cardiomyocytes tended to proliferate and Cx43 expression was increased [70]. Regulation by miR-19a/b, one of the miR-17-92 cluster, was shown using murine model – conditional overexpression of miR-17-92 in cardiac and smooth muscle tissues led to increased arrhythmia inducibility [71]. α-myosin heavy chain (α-MHC)-miR-130a transgenic mice demonstrated both atrial and ventricular arrhythmias – sustained ventricular tachycardia started to appear 6 weeks after induction of overexpression of miR-130a, Cx43 levels steadily decreased from 2nd to 10th week, when it reached up to 90% reduction [72]. Recently, long non-coding RNA CCRR (cardiac conduction regulatory RNA) was described to improve cardiac conduction by blocking endocytic trafficking of Cx43 [73] and exome-chip meta-analysis identified ADAM metallopeptidase with thrombospondin type 1 motif 6 (ADAMTS6) to be associated with cardiac conduction – loss-of function analysis in mice demonstrated its relation to Cx43 expression [74].

Atrial connexin – Cx40 – was shown to be regulated by miR-208a [75] and miR-27b [64]. Regulation of Cx40 by miR-208a is just a piece of highly interconnected regulatory network of cardiac hypertrophy, contractility and arrhythmogenesis – miR-208a is encoded by the intron of the Myh6 gene (encoding for cardiac α-MHC), while its isomiR, miR-208b, is encoded in the intron of Myh7 gene (encoding for cardiac β-MHC) [75]. Regulation of Cx40 by miR-27b is connected with the expression changes induced by high fat diet. Mice fed with high fat died showed prolonged P wave duration, increased inducibility of sustained atrial tachycardia and reduced atrial conduction velocity. miR-27b expression was up-regulated in these mice which corresponded with Cx40 decrease and contributed to the described conductance defects [76].

4 Clinical Utility of Circulating Non-coding RNAs in Arrhythmology

Circulating ncRNAs are present in body fluids, e.g. plasma, urine, or even saliva, where they participate in intercellular communication. Their levels are not stochastic as they reflect changes occurring within the organism. Due to their high stability, they can be repeatedly and reproducibly measured and as such, they can be used either as novel diagnostic or prognostics biomarkers.

Most of the studies focusing on circulating RNAs performed so far focuses on the utilization of circulating miRNAs in the settings of AF. Various miRNAs were shown to be increased (e.g. miR-103a, miR-107, miR-320d, miR-486, and let-7b [77]) or decreased (e.g. miR-21 [78], miR-29b [79], miR-150 [78, 80], miR-328 [81]) in plasmatic samples from patients with AF, compared to healthy controls or patients with other supraventricular arrhythmias. Levels of some miRNAs even differed between paroxysmal and persistent AF (e.g. miR-21, miR-150 [78, 80]) and interestingly, when comparing patients with new-onset AF with well-controlled AF, levels of other miRNAs were altered (e.g. miR-133b, miR-328 and miR-499 were reported to be increased [82]) indicating dynamic changes occur in plasmatic miRNA levels as AF progresses. Catheter ablation was also shown to restore altered miRNA levels (e.g. miR-21, miR-150 [78], miR-409-3p and miR-432 [83]), generally returning them to values closer to healthy individuals.

More details about the roles of non-coding RNA in atrial fibrillation and about circulating RNAs in general, can be found in the corresponding chapters of this book.

5 Conclusions and Future Directions

Regulation of cardiac conductance and arrhythmogenicity is highly complex and ncRNAs affect it in numerous ways and at various levels (transcriptional or post-transcriptional regulation of gene expression, intracellular protein trafficking etc.). Most of the studies have so far focused on miRNAs, however, more and more studies are coming out focusing of other ncRNA groups, thus deepening our knowledge and unveiling novel previously unappreciated links.

Muscle specific miRNAs, such as miR-1, miR-133 or miR-208, affect expression of main ion channels and connexins, thus significantly affecting arrhythmogenic potential of the myocardium. These miRNAs have plentiful other targets regulating also other critical processes occurring in the myocardium (e.g. cardiac hypertrophy, fibrosis, ischemia etc.) and they seem to act as "master regulators" of heart expression program. Other aforementioned miRNAs seem to act more like a "fine tuners" of ion channels and connexins gene expression. However, most of the studies have so far focused on individual miRNAs or individual miRNA targets and to improve our understanding of the of role of non-coding RNAs in arrhythmicity, more complex studies focusing on more targets at one time are needed.

Moreover, ion channels and connexins are not only involved in the regulation of cardiac action potential, but also neural action potentials or intercellular communication in cancer and other cells – various studies were thus performed in neural or cancer cell lines (or in patients with neurological diseases or cancer) identifying possible novel links between non-coding RNAs and their targets – functional and electrophysiological validation of these results on the myocardium is thus needed.

Better understanding of the regulation and interplay between non-coding RNAs and their targets may then result in the discovery of novel diagnostic or predictive biomarkers or in the development of novel treatment strategies.

Acknowledgements This work was written at Masaryk university as part of the project "Differential diagnostics and prognostic stratification in internal diseases #3 (DIDIPRON 3)" number MUNI/A/1475/2018 with the support of the Specific University Research Grant, as provided by the Ministry of Education, Youth and Sports of the Czech Republic in the year 2018 and it was also carried out under the project CEITEC 2020 (LQ1601) with financial support from the Ministry of Education, Youth and Sports of the Czech Republic under the National Sustainability Programme II.

Competing Financial Interests The authors declare no competing financial interests.

References

1. Fu D-G. Cardiac arrhythmias: diagnosis, symptoms, and treatments. Cell Biochem Biophys. 2015;73(2):291–6.
2. Anderson JL, Halperin JL, Albert NM, Bozkurt B, Brindis RG, Curtis LH, DeMets D, Guyton RA, Hochman JS, Kovacs RJ, Ohman EM, Pressler SJ, Sellke FW, Shen W-K, Wann LS, Curtis AB, Ellenbogen KA, Estes NAM, Ezekowitz MD, Jackman WM, January CT, Lowe JE, Page RL, Slotwiner DJ, Stevenson WG, Tracy CM, Fuster V, Rydén LE, Cannom DS, Crijns HJ, Curtis AB, Ellenbogen KA, Le Heuzey J-Y, Kay GN, Olsson SB, Prystowsky EN, Tamargo JL, Wann S. Management of patients with atrial fibrillation (compilation of 2006 ACCF/AHA/ESC and 2011 ACCF/AHA/HRS recommendations): a report of the American College of Cardiology/American Heart Association Task Force on Practice Guidelines. J Am Coll Cardiol. 2013;61(18):1935–44.
3. Martin CA, Matthews GDK, Huang CL-H. Sudden cardiac death and inherited channelopathy: the basic electrophysiology of the myocyte and myocardium in ion channel disease. Heart. 2012;98(7):536–43.
4. Novák J, Kružliak P, Bienertová-Vašků J, Slabý O, Novák M. MicroRNA-206: a promising theranostic marker. Theranostics. 2014;4(2):119–33.
5. Garcia-Elias A, Benito B. Ion channel disorders and sudden cardiac death. Int J Mol Sci. 2018;19(3):692.
6. Kim GH. MicroRNA regulation of cardiac conduction and arrhythmias. Transl Res. 2013;161:381–92.
7. Mangoni ME, Nargeot J. Genesis and regulation of the heart automaticity. Physiol Rev. 2008;88(3):919–82.
8. Stillitano F, Lonardo G, Giunti G, Del Lungo M, Coppini R, Spinelli V, Sartiani L, Poggesi C, Mugelli A, Cerbai E. Chronic atrial fibrillation alters the functional properties of if in the human atrium. J Cardiovasc Electrophysiol. 2013;24(12):1391–400.
9. Suffredini S, Stillitano F, Comini L, Bouly M, Brogioni S, Ceconi C, Ferrari R, Mugelli A, Cerbai E. Long-term treatment with ivabradine in post-

myocardial infarcted rats counteracts f-channel overexpression. Br J Pharmacol. 2012;165(5):1457–66.
10. Li Y-D, Hong Y-F, Yusufuaji Y, Tang B-P, Zhou X-H, Xu G-J, Li J-X, Sun L, Zhang J-H, Xin Q, Xiong J, Ji Y-T, Zhang Y. Altered expression of hyperpolarization-activated cyclic nucleotide-gated channels and microRNA-1 and -133 in patients with age-associated atrial fibrillation. Mol Med Rep. 2015;12(3):3243–8.
11. D'Souza A, Bucchi A, Johnsen AB, Logantha SJRJ, Monfredi O, Yanni J, Prehar S, Hart G, Cartwright E, Wisloff U, Dobryznski H, DiFrancesco D, Morris GM, Boyett MR. Exercise training reduces resting heart rate via downregulation of the funny channel HCN4. Nat Commun. 2014;5:3775.
12. D'Souza A, Pearman CM, Wang Y, Nakao S, Logantha SJRJ, Cox C, Bennett H, Zhang Y, Johnsen AB, Linscheid N, Poulsen PC, Elliott J, Coulson J, McPhee J, Robertson A, da Costa Martins PA, Kitmitto A, Wisløff U, Cartwright EJ, Monfredi O, Lundby A, Dobrzynski H, Oceandy D, Morris GM, Boyett MR. Targeting miR-423-5p reverses exercise training-induced HCN4 channel Remodeling and sinus bradycardia. Circ Res. 2017;121(9):1058–68.
13. Lu Y, Xiao J, Lin H, Bai Y, Luo X, Wang Z, Yang B. A single anti-microRNA antisense oligodeoxyribonucleotide (AMO) targeting multiple microRNAs offers an improved approach for microRNA interference. Nucleic Acids Res. 2009;37(3):e24.
14. Catterall WA. From ionic currents to molecular mechanisms: the structure and function of voltage-gated sodium channels. Neuron. 2000;26(1):13–25.
15. Zhou R, Hang P, Zhu W, Su Z, Liang H, Du Z. Whole genome network analysis of ion channels and connexins in myocardial infarction. Cell Physiol Biochem. 2011;27(3–4):299–304.
16. Daimi H, Lozano-Velasco E, Haj Khelil A, Chibani JBE, Barana A, Amorós I, González de la Fuente M, Caballero R, Aranega A, Franco D. Regulation of SCN5A by microRNAs: miR-219 modulates SCN5A transcript expression and the effects of flecainide intoxication in mice. Heart Rhythm. 2015;12(6):1333–42.
17. Poon EN-Y, Hao B, Guan D, Jun Li M, Lu J, Yang Y, Wu B, Wu SC-M, Webb SE, Liang Y, Miller AL, Yao X, Wang J, Yan B, Boheler KR. Integrated transcriptomic and regulatory network analyses identify microRNA-200c as a novel repressor of human pluripotent stem cell-derived cardiomyocyte differentiation and maturation. Cardiovasc Res. 2018;114(6):894–906.
18. Zhao Y, Huang Y, Li W, Wang Z, Zhan S, Zhou M, Yao Y, Zeng Z, Hou Y, Chen Q, Tu X, Wang QK, Huang Z. Post-transcriptional regulation of cardiac sodium channel gene SCN5A expression and function by miR-192-5p. Biochim Biophys Acta. 2015;1852(10):2024–34.
19. Zhang X, Yoon J-Y, Morley M, McLendon JM, Mapuskar KA, Gutmann R, Mehdi H, Bloom HL, Dudley SC, Ellinor PT, Shalaby AA, Weiss R, Tang WHW, Moravec CS, Singh M, Taylor AL, Yancy CW, Feldman AM, McNamara DM, Irani K, Spitz DR, Breheny P, Margulies KB, London B, Boudreau RL. A common variant alters SCN5A-miR-24 interaction and associates with heart failure mortality. J Clin Investig. 2018;128(3):1154–63.
20. Nassal DM, Wan X, Liu H, Maleski D, Ramirez-Navarro A, Moravec CS, Ficker E, Laurita KR, Deschênes I. KChIP2 is a core transcriptional regulator of cardiac excitability. eLife. 2017;6:e17304.
21. Klugbauer N, Welling A, Specht V, Seisenberger C, Hofmann F. L-type Ca2+ channels of the embryonic mouse heart. Eur J Pharmacol. 2002;447(2–3):279–84.
22. Sutphin BS, Boczek NJ, Barajas-Martínez H, Hu D, Ye D, Tester DJ, Antzelevitch C, Ackerman MJ. Molecular and functional characterization of rare CACNA1C variants in sudden unexplained death in the young. Congenit Heart Dis. 2016;11(6):683–92.
23. Lu Y, Zhang Y, Wang N, Pan Z, Gao X, Zhang F, Zhang Y, Shan H, Luo X, Bai Y, Sun L, Song W, Xu C, Wang Z, Yang B. MicroRNA-328 contributes to adverse electrical remodeling in atrial fibrillation. Circulation. 2010;122(23):2378–87.
24. Li Z, Wang X, Wang W, Du J, Wei J, Zhang Y, Wang J, Hou Y. Altered long non-coding RNA expression profile in rabbit atria with atrial fibrillation: TCONS_00075467 modulates atrial electrical remodeling by sponging miR-328 to regulate CACNA1C. J Mol Cell Cardiol. 2017;108:73–85.
25. Wang J, Meng X, Han J, Li Y, Luo T, Wang J, Xin M, Xi J. Differential expressions of miRNAs in patients with nonvalvular atrial fibrillation. Zhonghua Yi Xue Za Zhi. 2012;92(26):1816–9.
26. Wang J, Song S, Xie C, Han J, Li Y, Shi J, Xin M, Wang J, Luo T, Meng X, Yang B. MicroRNA profiling in the left atrium in patients with non-valvular paroxysmal atrial fibrillation. BMC Cardiovasc Disord. 2015;15:97.
27. Barana A, Matamoros M, Dolz-Gaitón P, Pérez-Hernández M, Amorós I, Núñez M, Sacristán S, Pedraz Á, Pinto Á, Fernández-Avilés F, Tamargo J, Delpón E, Caballero R. Chronic atrial fibrillation increases microRNA-21 in human atrial myocytes decreasing L-type calcium current. Circ Arrhythm Electrophysiol. 2014;7(5):861–8.
28. Cañón S, Caballero R, Herraiz-Martínez A, Pérez-Hernández M, López B, Atienza F, Jalife J, Hove-Madsen L, Delpón E, Bernad A. miR-208b upregulation interferes with calcium handling in HL-1 atrial myocytes: implications in human chronic atrial fibrillation. J Mol Cell Cardiol. 2016;99:162–73.
29. Zhao Y, Yuan Y, Qiu C. Underexpression of CACNA1C caused by overexpression of microRNA-29a underlies the pathogenesis of atrial fibrillation. Medical science monitor: international medical journal experimental. Clin Res. 2016;22:2175–81.
30. Ling T-Y, Wang X-L, Chai Q, Lu T, Stulak JM, Joyce LD, Daly RC, Greason KL, Wu L-Q, Shen W-K, Cha Y-M, Lee H-C. Regulation of cardiac CACNB2 by

microRNA-499: potential role in atrial fibrillation. BBA Clinical. 2017;7:78–84.
31. Carrillo ED, Escobar Y, González G, Hernández A, Galindo JM, García MC, Sánchez JA. Posttranscriptional regulation of the β2-subunit of cardiac L-type Ca^{2+} channels by MicroRNAs during long-term exposure to isoproterenol in rats. J Cardiovasc Pharmacol. 2011;58(5):470–8.
32. Chu Q, Li A, Chen X, Qin Y, Sun X, Li Y, Yue E, Wang C, Ding X, Yan Y, Zahra SM, Wang S, Jiang Y, Bai Y, Yang B. Overexpression of miR-135b attenuates pathological cardiac hypertrophy by targeting CACNA1C. Int J Cardiol. 2018;269:235–41.
33. Rau F, Freyermuth F, Fugier C, Villemin J-P, Fischer M-C, Jost B, Dembele D, Gourdon G, Nicole A, Duboc D, Wahbi K, Day JW, Fujimura H, Takahashi MP, Auboeuf D, Dreumont N, Furling D, Charlet-Berguerand N. Misregulation of miR-1 processing is associated with heart defects in myotonic dystrophy. Nat Struct Mol Biol. 2011;18(7):840–5.
34. Schizophrenia Psychiatric Genome-Wide Association Study (GWAS) Consortium. Genome-wide association study identifies five new schizophrenia loci. Nat Genet. 2011;43(10):969–76.
35. Kwon E, Wang W, Tsai L-H. Validation of schizophrenia-associated genes CSMD1, C10orf26, CACNA1C and TCF4 as miR-137 targets. Mol Psychiatry. 2013;18(1):11–2.
36. Sun Z, Cao X, Zhang Z, Hu Z, Zhang L, Wang H, Zhou H, Li D, Zhang S, Xie M. Simulated microgravity inhibits L-type calcium channel currents partially by the up-regulation of miR-103 in MC3T3-E1 osteoblasts. Sci Rep. 2015;5:8077.
37. Xu H, Abuhatzira L, Carmona GN, Vadrevu S, Satin LS, Notkins AL. The Ia-2β intronic miRNA, miR-153, is a negative regulator of insulin and dopamine secretion through its effect on the Cacna1c gene in mice. Diabetologia. 2015;58(10):2298–306.
38. Li C, Li X, Gao X, Zhang R, Zhang Y, Liang H, Xu C, Du W, Zhang Y, Liu X, Ma N, Xu Z, Wang L, Chen X, Lu Y, Ju J, Yang B, Shan H. MicroRNA-328 as a regulator of cardiac hypertrophy. Int J Cardiol. 2014;173(2):268–76.
39. Melo SFS, Barauna VG, Júnior MAC, Bozi LHM, Drummond LR, Natali AJ, de Oliveira EM. Resistance training regulates cardiac function through modulation of miRNA-214. Int J Mol Sci. 2015;16(4):6855–67.
40. Melo SFS, Barauna VG, Neves VJ, Fernandes T, Lara L d S, Mazzotti DR, Oliveira EM. Exercise training restores the cardiac microRNA-1 and -214 levels regulating Ca2+ handling after myocardial infarction. BMC Cardiovasc Disord. 2015;15:166.
41. Gurha P, Abreu-Goodger C, Wang T, Ramirez MO, Drumond AL, van Dongen S, Chen Y, Bartonicek N, Enright AJ, Lee B, Kelm RJ, Reddy AK, Taffet GE, Bradley A, Wehrens XH, Entman ML, Rodriguez A. Targeted deletion of microRNA-22 promotes stress-induced cardiac dilation and contractile dysfunction. Circulation. 2012;125(22):2751–61.
42. Wahlquist C, Jeong D, Rojas-Muñoz A, Kho C, Lee A, Mitsuyama S, van Mil A, Park WJ, Sluijter JPG, Doevendans PAF, Hajjar RJ, Mercola M. Inhibition of miR-25 improves cardiac contractility in the failing heart. Nature. 2014;508(7497):531–5.
43. Williams AL, Walton CB, MacCannell KA, Avelar A, Shohet RV. HIF-1 regulation of miR-29c impairs SERCA2 expression and cardiac contractility. Am J Physiol Heart Circ Physiol. 2019;316(3):H554–65.
44. Yang B, Lin H, Xiao J, Lu Y, Luo X, Li B, Zhang Y, Xu C, Bai Y, Wang H, Chen G, Wang Z. The muscle-specific microRNA miR-1 regulates cardiac arrhythmogenic potential by targeting GJA1 and KCNJ2. Nat Med. 2007;13(4):486–91.
45. Liu X, Zhang Y, Du W, Liang H, He H, Zhang L, Pan Z, Li X, Xu C, Zhou Y, Wang L, Qian M, Liu T, Yin H, Lu Y, Yang B, Shan H. MiR-223-3p as a novel MicroRNA regulator of expression of voltage-gated K+ channel Kv4.2 in acute myocardial infarction. Cellular physiology and biochemistry international journal of Exprimental cellular physiology and biochemistry. Pharmacology. 2016;39(1):102–14.
46. Zhu P, Yang M, Ren H, Shen G, Chen J, Zhang J, Liu J, Sun C. Long noncoding RNA MALAT1 downregulates cardiac transient outward potassium current by regulating miR-200c/HMGB1 pathway. J Cell Biochem. 2018;119(12):10239–49.
47. Vandenberg JI, Perry MD, Perrin MJ, Mann SA, Ke Y, Hill AP. hERG K(+) channels: structure, function, and clinical significance. Physiol Rev. 2012;92(3):1393–478.
48. Lian J, Guo J, Huang X, Yang XI, Huang G, Mao H, Sun HH, Ba Y, Zhou J. miRNAs Regulate hERG. J Cardiovasc Electrophysiol. 2016;27(12):1472–82.
49. Wang Y, Wang L, Yin C, An B, Hao Y, Wei T, Li L, Song G. Arsenic trioxide inhibits breast cancer cell growth via microRNA-328/hERG pathway in MCF-7 cells. Mol Med Rep. 2015;12(1):1233–8.
50. Girmatsion Z, Biliczki P, Bonauer A, Wimmer-Greinecker G, Scherer M, Moritz A, Bukowska A, Goette A, Nattel S, Hohnloser SH, Ehrlich JR. Changes in microRNA-1 expression and IK1 up-regulation in human atrial fibrillation. Heart Rhythm. 2009;6(12):1802–9.
51. Luo X, Pan Z, Shan H, Xiao J, Sun X, Wang N, Lin H, Xiao L, Maguy A, Qi X-Y, Li Y, Gao X, Dong D, Zhang Y, Bai Y, Ai J, Sun L, Lu H, Luo X-Y, Wang Z, Lu Y, Yang B, Nattel S. MicroRNA-26 governs profibrillatory inward-rectifier potassium current changes in atrial fibrillation. J Clin Investig. 2013;123(5):1939–51.
52. Qi X-Y, Huang H, Ordog B, Luo X, Naud P, Sun Y, Wu C-T, Dawson K, Tadevosyan A, Chen Y, Harada M, Dobrev D, Nattel S. Fibroblast inward-rectifier potassium current upregulation in profibrillatory atrial remodeling. Circ Res. 2015;116(5):836–45.
53. Goldoni D, Yarham JM, McGahon MK, O'Connor A, Guduric-Fuchs J, Edgar K, McDonald DM, Simpson DA, Collins A. A novel dual-fluorescence strategy

for functionally validating microRNA targets in 3′ untranslated regions: regulation of the inward rectifier potassium channel K(ir)2.1 by miR-212. Biochem J. 2012;448:103–13.
54. Li X, Hu H, Wang Y, Xue M, Li X, Cheng W, Xuan Y, Yin J, Yang N, Yan S. Valsartan ameliorates KIR2.1 in rats with myocardial infarction via the NF-κB-miR-16 pathway. Gene. 2016;590(2):201–9.
55. Liu Z, Du L, Li M. Update on the slow delayed rectifier potassium current (I(Ks)): role in modulating cardiac function. Curr Med Chem. 2012;19(9):1405–20.
56. Li Y, Yang C-M, Xi Y, Wu G, Shelat H, Gao S, Cheng J, Geng Y-J. MicroRNA-1/133 targeted dysfunction of potassium channels KCNE1 and KCNQ1 in human cardiac progenitor cells with simulated hyperglycemia. Int J Cardiol. 2013;167(3):1076–8.
57. Jia X, Zheng S, Xie X, Zhang Y, Wang W, Wang Z, Zhang Y, Wang J, Gao M, Hou Y. MicroRNA-1 accelerates the shortening of atrial effective refractory period by regulating KCNE1 and KCNB2 expression: an atrial tachypacing rabbit model. PLoS One. 2013;8(12):e85639.
58. Long Q-Q, Wang H, Gao W, Fan Y, Li Y-F, Ma Y, Yang Y, Shi H-J, Chen B-R, Meng H-Y, Wang Q-M, Wang F, Wang Z-M, Wang L-S. Long noncoding RNA Kcna2 antisense RNA contributes to ventricular arrhythmias via silencing Kcna2 in rats with congestive heart failure. J Am Heart Assoc. 2017;6(12):e005965.
59. Ling T-Y, Wang X-L, Chai Q, Lau T-W, Koestler CM, Park SJ, Daly RC, Greason KL, Jen J, Wu L-Q, Shen W-F, Shen W-K, Cha Y-M, Lee H-C. Regulation of the SK3 channel by microRNA-499--potential role in atrial fibrillation. Heart rhythm official journal of heart rhythm. Society. 2013;10(7):1001–9.
60. Morishima M, Iwata E, Nakada C, Tsukamoto Y, Takanari H, Miyamoto S, Moriyama M, Ono K. Atrial fibrillation-mediated Upregulation of miR-30d regulates myocardial electrical Remodeling of the G-protein-gated K(+) channel, IK.ACh. Circulation journal Offical journal of the Japanese circulation. Society. 2016;80(6):1346–55.
61. Stauffer BL, Sobus RD, Sucharov CC. Sex differences in cardiomyocyte connexin43 expression. J Cardiovasc Pharmacol. 2011;58(1):32–9.
62. Wang N, Sun L-Y, Zhang S-C, Wei R, Xie F, Liu J, Yan Y, Duan M-J, Sun L-L, Sun Y-H, Niu H-F, Zhang R, Ai J. MicroRNA-23a participates in estrogen deficiency induced gap junction remodeling of rats by targeting GJA1. Int J Biol Sci. 2015;11(4):390–403.
63. Kim HW, Jiang S, Ashraf M, Haider KH. Stem cell-based delivery of Hypoxamir-210 to the infarcted heart: implications on stem cell survival and preservation of infarcted heart function. J Mol Med Berlin Germany. 2012;90(9):997–1010.
64. Lu Y, Zhang Y, Shan H, Pan Z, Li X, Li B, Xu C, Zhang B, Zhang F, Dong D, Song W, Qiao G, Yang B. MicroRNA-1 downregulation by propranolol in a rat model of myocardial infarction: a new mechanism for ischaemic cardioprotection. Cardiovasc Res. 2009;84(3):434–41.
65. Zhang Y, Sun L, Zhang Y, Liang H, Li X, Cai R, Wang L, Du W, Zhang R, Li J, Wang Z, Ma N, Wang X, Du Z, Yang B, Gao X, Shan H. Overexpression of microRNA-1 causes atrioventricular block in rodents. Int J Biol Sci. 2013;9(5):455–62.
66. Liu M, Li M, Sun S, Li B, Du D, Sun J, Cao F, Li H, Jia F, Wang T, Chang N, Yu H, Wang Q, Peng H. The use of antibody modified liposomes loaded with AMO-1 to deliver oligonucleotides to ischemic myocardium for arrhythmia therapy. Biomaterials. 2014;35(11):3697–707.
67. Xu H-F, Ding Y-J, Shen Y-W, Xue A-M, Xu H-M, Luo C-L, Li B-X, Liu Y-L, Zhao Z-Q. MicroRNA- 1 represses Cx43 expression in viral myocarditis. Mol Cell Biochem. 2012;362(1–2):141–8.
68. Curcio A, Torella D, Iaconetti C, Pasceri E, Sabatino J, Sorrentino S, Giampà S, Micieli M, Polimeni A, Henning BJ, Leone A, Catalucci D, Ellison GM, Condorelli G, Indolfi C. MicroRNA-1 downregulation increases connexin 43 displacement and induces ventricular tachyarrhythmias in rodent hypertrophic hearts. PLoS One. 2013;8(7):e70158.
69. Viczenczova C, Szeiffova Bacova B, Egan Benova T, Kura B, Yin C, Weismann P, Kukreja R, Slezak J, Tribulova N. Myocardial connexin-43 and PKC signalling are involved in adaptation of the heart to irradiation-induced injury: implication of miR-1 and miR-21. Gen Physiol Biophys. 2016;35(2):215–22.
70. Yin VP, Lepilina A, Smith A, Poss KD. Regulation of zebrafish heart regeneration by miR-133. Dev Biol. 2012;365(2):319–27.
71. Danielson LS, Park DS, Rotllan N, Chamorro-Jorganes A, Guijarro MV, Fernandez-Hernando C, Fishman GI, Phoon CKL, Hernando E. Cardiovascular dysregulation of miR-17-92 causes a lethal hypertrophic cardiomyopathy and arrhythmogenesis. FASEB J. 2013;27(4):1460–7.
72. Osbourne A, Calway T, Broman M, McSharry S, Earley J, Kim GH. Downregulation of connexin43 by microRNA-130a in cardiomyocytes results in cardiac arrhythmias. J Mol Cell Cardiol. 2014;74:53–63.
73. Zhang Y, Sun L, Xuan L, Pan Z, Hu X, Liu H, Bai Y, Jiao L, Li Z, Cui L, Wang X, Wang S, Yu T, Feng B, Guo Y, Liu Z, Meng W, Ren H, Zhu J, Zhao X, Yang C, Zhang Y, Xu C, Wang Z, Lu Y, Shan H, Yang B. Long non-coding RNA CCRR controls cardiac conduction via regulating intercellular coupling. Nat Commun. 2018;9:4176.
74. Prins BP, Mead TJ, Brody JA, Sveinbjornsson G, Ntalla I, Bihlmeyer NA, van den Berg M, Bork-Jensen J, Cappellani S, Van Duijvenboden S, Klena NT, Gabriel GC, Liu X, Gulec C, Grarup N, Haessler J, Hall LM, Iorio A, Isaacs A, Li-Gao R, Lin H, Liu C-T, Lyytikäinen L-P, Marten J, Mei H, Müller-Nurasyid M, Orini M, Padmanabhan S, Radmanesh F, Ramirez J, Robino A, Schwartz M, van Setten J, Smith AV, Verweij N, Warren HR, Weiss S, Alonso A, Arnar DO, Bots ML, de Boer RA, Dominiczak AF, Eijgelsheim M, Ellinor PT, Guo X, Felix SB, Harris TB, Hayward C, Heckbert SR, Huang PL, Jukema

JW, Kähönen M, Kors JA, Lambiase PD, Launer LJ, Li M, Linneberg A, Nelson CP, Pedersen O, Perez M, Peters A, Polasek O, Psaty BM, Raitakari OT, Rice KM, Rotter JI, Sinner MF, Soliman EZ, Spector TD, Strauch K, Thorsteinsdottir U, Tinker A, Trompet S, Uitterlinden A, Vaartjes I, van der Meer P, Völker U, Völzke H, Waldenberger M, Wilson JG, Xie Z, Asselbergs FW, Dörr M, van Duijn CM, Gasparini P, Gudbjartsson DF, Gudnason V, Hansen T, Kääb S, Kanters JK, Kooperberg C, Lehtimäki T, Lin HJ, Lubitz SA, Mook-Kanamori DO, Conti FJ, Newton-Cheh CH, Rosand J, Rudan I, Samani NJ, Sinagra G, Smith BH, Holm H, Stricker BH, Ulivi S, Sotoodehnia N, Apte SS, van der Harst P, Stefansson K, Munroe PB, Arking DE, Lo CW, Jamshidi Y. Exome-chip meta-analysis identifies novel loci associated with cardiac conduction, including ADAMTS6. Genome Biol. 2018;19:87.

75. Callis TE, Pandya K, Seok HY, Tang R-H, Tatsuguchi M, Huang Z-P, Chen J-F, Deng Z, Gunn B, Shumate J, Willis MS, Selzman CH, Wang D-Z. MicroRNA-208a is a regulator of cardiac hypertrophy and conduction in mice. J Clin Investig. 2009;119(9):2772–86.
76. Takahashi K, Sasano T, Sugiyama K, Kurokawa J, Tamura N, Soejima Y, Sawabe M, Isobe M, Furukawa T. High-fat diet increases vulnerability to atrial arrhythmia by conduction disturbance via miR-27b. J Mol Cell Cardiol. 2016;90:38–46.
77. Mun D, Kim H, Kang J-Y, Park H, Park H, Lee S-H, Yun N, Joung B. Expression of miRNAs in circulating exosomes derived from patients with persistent atrial fibrillation. FASEB J. 2019;33(5):5979–89.
78. McManus DD, Tanriverdi K, Lin H, Esa N, Kinno M, Mandapati D, Tam S, Okike ON, Ellinor PT, Keaney JF, Donahue JK, Benjamin EJ, Freedman JE. Plasma microRNAs are associated with atrial fibrillation and change after catheter ablation (the miRhythm study). Heart Rhythm. 2015;12(1):3–10.
79. Dawson K, Wakili R, Ordög B, Clauss S, Chen Y, Iwasaki Y, Voigt N, Qi XY, Sinner MF, Dobrev D, Kääb S, Nattel S. MicroRNA29: a mechanistic contributor and potential biomarker in atrial fibrillation. Circulation. 2013;127(14):1466–75.. 1475e1–28
80. Liu Z, Zhou C, Liu Y, Wang S, Ye P, Miao X, Xia J. The expression levels of plasma micoRNAs in atrial fibrillation patients. PLoS One. 2012;7(9):e44906.
81. McManus DD, Lin H, Tanriverdi K, Quercio M, Yin X, Larson MG, Ellinor PT, Levy D, Freedman JE, Benjamin EJ. Relations between circulating microRNAs and atrial fibrillation: data from the Framingham offspring study. Heart rhythm Offical journal of the heart rhythm. Society. 2014;11(4):663–9.
82. da Silva AMG, de Araújo JNG, de Oliveira KM, Novaes AEM, Lopes MB, de Sousa JCV, Filho AA de A, Luchessi AD, de Rezende AA, Hirata MH, Silbiger VN. Circulating miRNAs in acute new-onset atrial fibrillation and their target mRNA network. J Cardiovasc Electrophysiol. 2018;29(8):1159–66.
83. Liu T, Zhong S, Rao F, Xue Y, Qi Z, Wu S. Catheter ablation restores decreased plasma miR-409-3p and miR-432 in atrial fibrillation patients. Eur Eur Pacing Arrhythm Card Electrophysiol J Work Groups Card Pacing Arrhythm Card Cell Electrophysiol Eur Soc Cardiol. 2015;18(1):92–9.

Non-coding RNA and Cardiac Electrophysiological Disorders

18

Jan A. Kleeberger, Philipp J. Tomsits, Stefan Kääb, and Sebastian Clauss

Abstract

Cardiac arrhythmias are common diseases affecting millions of people worldwide. A broad and diverse array of arrhythmias exists, ranging from harmless ones such as sinus arrhythmia to fatal disorders such as ventricular fibrillation. The underlying pathophysiology of arrhythmogenesis is complex and still not fully understood. Since their discovery, non-coding RNAs (ncRNAs) and especially microRNAs (miRNAs) came into the spotlight of arrhythmia research as it has been shown that they play an important role in regulating normal development of the cardiac conduction system and are involved in remodeling processes leading to arrhythmias. This chapter will give a brief overview on basic electrophysiologic concepts and will summarize the current knowledge on ncRNAs and their role in arrhythmogenesis.

Keywords

Non-coding RNA · Cardiac electrophysiology · Arrhythmia · Arrhythmogenesis · Remodeling · Reentry · Conduction

1 Background

Cardiac arrhythmias are common resulting in significant morbidity and mortality. Especially ventricular arrhythmias are a major cause for cardiovascular death in the context of ischemic heart failure (HF) or myocardial infarction [1].

A vast variety of structural changes (e.g. fibrosis, dilatation or inflammation) as well as changes in ion channel function or expression, alterations of the calcium homeostasis or neurohormonal dysregulation can lead to the onset and perpetuation of arrhythmias [1]. Those mechanisms are called 'proarrhythmic remodeling' and are induced by various triggers such as ischemia or pressure overload. On a cellular level these remodeling processes are regulated by numerous mediators such as non-coding RNAs. Non-coding RNAs (ncRNAs) are small RNA molecules that are not translated into proteins [2]. They are able to regulate gene expression on different levels

Authors Jan A. Kleeberger and Philipp J. Tomsits have equally contributed to this chapter.

This chapter will summarize the research progress on non-coding RNAs and their role in cardiac electrophysiology other than atrial fibrillation that will be discussed in the following chapter.

J. A. Kleeberger · P. J. Tomsits · S. Kääb · S. Clauss (✉)
Department of Medicine I, University Hospital Munich, Ludwig-Maximilians University Munich (LMU), Munich, Germany

German Center for Cardiovascular Research (DZHK), Partner Site Munich, Munich Heart Alliance, Munich, Germany
e-mail: Sebastian.clauss@med.uni-muenchen.de

J. Xiao (ed.), *Non-coding RNAs in Cardiovascular Diseases*, Advances in Experimental Medicine and Biology 1229, https://doi.org/10.1007/978-981-15-1671-9_18

like transcriptional modulation (e.g. by inhibiting expression of enhancers/repressors), epigenetic targeting (e.g. by affecting expression of enzymes involved in histone formation) or post transcriptional regulation (e.g. by mediating degradation of already transcribed target genes) [3]. When it comes to cardiac arrhythmias, research has focused on microRNAs (miRNAs) rather than other non-coding RNAs since they have been demonstrated as key regulators in electrical and structural remodeling of the heart [4, 5]. The underlying electrophysiological alterations leading to cardiac arrhythmias are various and often categorized as disorders of impulse formation or impulse conduction caused by complex processes summarized under the term proarrhythmic 'remodeling' consisting of structural and electrical remodeling [6, 7].

In recognition of the evidence currently available, this chapter will focus on microRNAs and give an outlook to other ncRNAs if there is evidence available.

1.1 Basics of Cardiac Conduction

In order to maintain sinus rhythm cardiac conduction system cells and the working myocardium are strictly orchestrated and require a perfect coordination of excitation, conduction, refractoriness and electromechanical coupling [1]. Any change in this fragile equilibrium may cause the occurrence of arrhythmias.

Under physiologic conditions a characteristic sequence of voltage changes driven by de- and repolarizing currents leads to the generation of the cardiac action potential. Cardiomyocytes normally display a resting membrane potential of −80 mV [7]. The electrical activity relies on different ion currents through various transmembrane-proteins – the so-called ion channels. Among them are Na^+, Ca^{2+}, and K^+ channels which contribute to the cardiac action potential by opening and closing at different time points [1]. The cardiac action potential is divided into different phases: first, the initial rapid depolarization driven mainly by voltage gated sodium channels; second, a long plateau phase driven mainly by an equilibrium between calcium and potassium currents; third, the repolarization driven by inward potassium currents, and fourth, the resting period when the cardiomyocyte comes back to its resting membrane potential [1, 8, 9].

A physiologic heartbeat begins with a spontaneous depolarization in a small atrial area, the so called sinus node. The sinus node myocytes are specialized and vary from other myocytes by their spontaneous depolarizations driven by a sodium current. After excitation of the atria the impulse reaches the atrioventricular node which electrically separates the atria from the ventricles. It then continues through the his bundle which divides into two branches, the left and the right bundle branch. These branches then taper out producing countless Purkinje fibers which finally reach the myocytes of the ventricles, distributing the electrical excitation among all myocytes.

1.2 Common Proarrhythmogenic Changes

Common changes favoring arrhythmia affect each part of physiologic excitation starting with the impulse formation. The ability of the sinus node (or other subsidiary pacemaker cells) to spontaneously generate electrical impulses is called 'automaticity'. Alterations of the gene expression in the sinus node, for example in heart failure, may lead to an enhanced automaticity that in turn may result in sinus tachycardia. Under normal conditions impulse formation takes place within the sinus node. If cells outside the sinus node reach their threshold potential before they are reached by a sinus impulse, so called ectopy occurs that may potentially lead to arrhythmias [7]. The most important mechanisms underlying ectopy are early and delayed afterdepolarisations due to imbalances in the calcium homeostasis [10]. Especially early afterdepolarisations are common in ventricular myocardium and are associated with ventricular arrhythmias such as long QT syndrome [11].

Another major cause for cardiac arrhythmias are changes favoring atrial or ventricular reentry by affecting the impulse conduction. Physiologically, a refractory period follows each excitation, making the cardiomyocyte resistant to premature electrical impulses and guaranteeing that only physiologic impulses from the sinus node can cause depolarizations. The cardiac refractoriness ultimately depends on the action potential duration (APD), meaning that all changes to APD may favor arrhythmias. Changes leading to slowed electrical conduction or a shortened refractory period can lead to a situation where a premature electrical impulse reaches cardiomyocytes that are already excitable (e.g. because the physiologic impulse from the sinus node is slow and has not reached the cardiomyocyte yet or the cardiomyocyte's repolarization is fastened) and will be conducted (which makes the cardiomyocytes refractory against physiologic impulses from the sinus node) establishing a 'reentry' circuit that can lead to atrial or ventricular (tachy-)arrhythmias [10]. Conduction velocity mainly depends on sodium channels, gap junctions and cardiac tissue structure [10]. For example in heart failure changes to cardiac ultrastructure like fibrosis favor reentry by altering conduction velocity [12].

Ion channel dysfunctions resulting from altered ion channel gene expression or function (so called channelopathies) following various triggers such as ischemia or genetic mutations often underly the phenomena described above [13].

2 MicroRNAs Described in Cardiac Arrhythmia

This section will provide a brief overview on miRNAs involved in cardiac arrhythmogenesis, purposely excluding atrial fibrillation, which will be discussed in Chap. 19. Figure 18.1 illustrates the interaction between miRNAs and their target genes, and Table 18.1 provides an overview of the miRNAs described in this section.

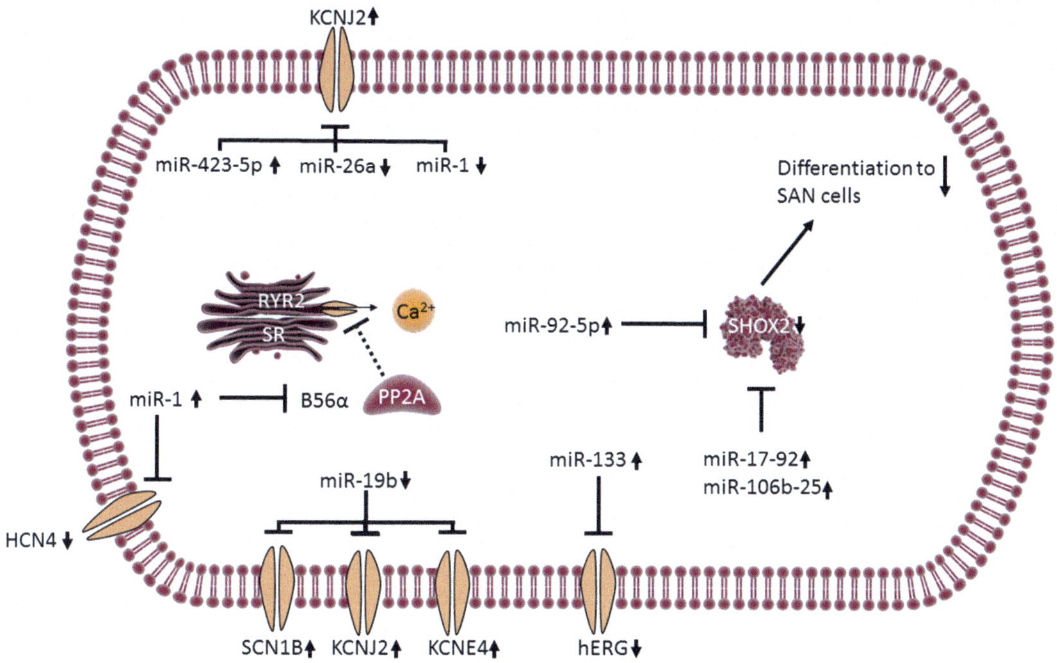

Fig. 18.1 Regulation of miRNAs involved in arrhythmogenesis and their respective targets

Table 18.1 Overview of microRNAs involved in the genesis of arrhythmias

Non-coding RNA	Regulation in disease	Mechanism	Species	Entity	References
miR-1	Downregulated	Upregulation of Kir2.1 potassium channel	Rat	SSS	[36]
miR-1	Upregulated	Downregulation of *HCN4*	Mouse	Sinus bradycardia	[16]
miR-19b	Downregulated	Upregulation of various sodium- and potassium channels; prolongation of APD	Zebrafish	AV- Block	[19]
miR-26a	Downregulated	Upregulation of *KCNJ2*	Dog	Heart failure	[22]
miR-30	Downregulated	CTGF mediated induction of fibrosis	Rat	Heart failure	[21]
miR-92b-5p	Upregulated	Repression of *SHOX2*	Mouse Human	SSS	[25]
miR-133	Upregulated	Repression of hERG (reduced potassium current I_{Kr})	Dog	Myocardial fibrosis	[20]
miR-17-92 & miR-106b-25	Downregulated	Alteration in cardiomyocyte differentiation	Mouse	SSS	[24]
miR-423-5p	Upregulated	Downregulation of *HCN4*	Mouse	Sinus bradycardia	[37]

2.1 miR-1

The first link between cardiac arrhythmias and miRNA was made by Yang et al. in 2007. They were able to show a dysregulation of miR-1 (overexpression) in a rat model of acute myocardial infarction leading to altered Ca^{2+} handling and thus, arrhythmias. Elimination of miR-1 was able to rescue the phenotype [14]. Further investigation revealed two miR-1 target genes: *GJA1*, which encodes connexin 43 (Cx43) that is one of the major gap junctions mediating the electrical conduction from cell to cell and *KCNJ2*, which encodes the potassium channel subunit Kir2.1 that is critical for establishing the resting membrane potential. Repression of these two proteins by miR-1 leads to a slowed conduction and a more depolarized resting membrane potential (seen as QRS complex widening and increased resting membrane potential in this model) thus potentially favoring cardiac arrhythmias [14]. A further role for miR-1 in cardiac arrhythmogenesis has been described by Terentyev et al. in 2009. They showed an increase in the amplitude of inward calcium current leading to increased excitation, elevated diastolic calcium leak from the sarcoplasmatic reticulum and reduced sarcoplasmatic reticulum calcium content, all potentially favoring arrhythmias in general [15]. The miRNA represses the Protein phosphatase 2 (*PP2A*) in this mode of action. These data were all not linked to a particular arrhythmia and describe general effects of miR-1 on the myocardial electrophysiology. Interestingly, miR-1 was also found to have an inhibitory effect on the expression of *HCN4* resulting in sinus bradycardia as an adaption to exercise training [16]. Fittingly, miR-1 was described to be upregulated in the blood of Marathon runners after running a marathon [17]. This miRNAs expression level also correlated with the diameter of the left atrium in elite runners, suggesting a potential use as a biomarker for atrial remodeling [18].

2.2 miR-19b

There is also some data available on the influence of miR-19b on the action potential duration (APD) in zebrafish. This miRNA exhibits an inhibitory effect on the expression of various sodium and potassium channels, thus prolonging the APD. Zebrafish lacking miR-19b presented bradycardia due to AV block with concomitant loss of contractile function [19].

2.3 miR-133

miR-133 has been shown to affect the QT interval. Shan and colleagues were able to demonstrate that upregulation of miR-133 in a dog tachypacing model led to decreased protein levels of hERG (a potassium channel subunit of the delayed rectifier potassium current I_{Kr}) and subsequently to prolonged QTc interval and increased mortality rates. The effect could be rescued by blocking miR-133 with an antisense inhibitor, thus proving a role for miR-133 in long QT syndrome [20].

2.4 miR-30

In a transgenic rat model of hypertension-induced heart failure downregulation of miR-30 has been shown to be associated with increased fibrosis via CTGF mediated induction of extracellular matrix protein expression [21]. This may lead to a proarrhythmogenic substrate, a link to a specific arrhythmia, however, was not demonstrated in this study.

2.5 miR-26a

In a dog model of chronic heart failure induced by atrial tachypacing miR-26 was significantly downregulated followed by an upregulation of its target gene *KCNJ2* and consecutive action potential shortening favoring reentry [22]. The authors linked this miRNA to atrial arrhythmias.

2.6 miR-17-92 and miR-106b-25

Sick sinus syndrome marks an important entity regarding both healthcare costs as well as patient morbidity since it is responsible for the vast majority of pacemaker implantations [23]. Recent studies have shown miR-17-92 and miR-106b-25 to be involved in the pathogenesis of sick sinus syndrome [24]. Regulated by *Pitx2* – a transcription factor – they directly target genes (*Shox2* and *Tbx3*) involved in the differentiation of cardiomyocytes into cells forming the sinus node (so called nodal cells). If those miRNAs are knocked out, the threshold for pacing induced atrial fibrillation in mice decreases significantly [24]. The same researchers were able to show that cardiac specific knockout of miR-17-92 alongside with haplotype insufficiency of miR-106b-25 leads to sinus node dysfunction and second degree atrioventricular block in mice [24].

2.7 miR-92b-5p

Strikingly, miR-92b-5p was found to act inhibitory in the same pathway as miR-17-92 and miR-106b-25 in mice and is dysregulated in the blood of patients with atrial fibrillation [25]. Mechanistically, a variant (c.*28 T > C) in the 3'UTR of the gene *Shox2* creates a functional binding site for this miRNA in patients with early onset atrial fibrillation. These results were validated in phenotypic rescue experiments in zebrafish. This group could also show that the expression of *Shox2* is significantly reduced in the right atrial appendages of atrial fibrillation patients.

2.8 miR-423-5p

The hearts of athletes react to repeated endurance training with an adaptive contractile and electrophysiological remodeling leading to sinus bradycardia. For instance, miR-423-5p was recently shown to be pivotal in the processes leading to sinus bradycardia by targeting *HCN4*, an ion channel responsible for the so called funny current in the sinus node [37]. Fittingly, knockdown of miR-423-5p reversed this training-induced bradycardia via normalization of HCN4 expression levels and establishing a regular funny current. Since these effects were elucidated in swim-trained mice, a similar mechanism in human athletes remains only speculative.

3 Long Non-coding RNAs Involved in the Development of Cardiac Arrhythmia

Since other ncRNAs, such as long non-coding RNAs (lncRNAs), only recently shifted into the spotlight of cardiovascular research there is only limited data available on their role in cardiac arrhythmogenesis. This section will provide a brief look into lncRNAs demonstrated as mediators in cardiac arrhythmias. Several lncRNAs have been described in cardiovascular disease (for example AK048451 (CHRF), myocardial infarction associated transcript (MIAT) or AK017121 (CARL)) which lead to cardiac hypertrophy, or interfere with cardiac apoptosis in ischemia/reperfusion injuries [26]. These are processes possibly triggering arrhythmias, and there are already some studies available proofing a link between lncRNA dysregulation and various arrhythmias. Table 18.2 shows a summary of the lncRNAs mentioned in this section.

3.1 Kcnq1ot1

Long QT syndrome can be caused by mutations in the gene *KCNQ1* [27]. Recent data has shown that the expression of *KCNQ1* can be inversely repressed in cis by Kcnq1ot1, a lncRNA produced from the introns of its gene. It has been shown that KCnq1ot1 loses its imprinting throughout the process of cardiac development leading to transcription, which then affects the expression of *KCNQ1* in differentiated cardiomyocytes rather than during early heart development [28, 29].

3.2 Cardiac Conduction Regulatory RNA (CCRR)

The remodeling processes in heart failure (HF) can lead to an enhanced arrhythmogenicity of the myocardium. Only recently, Zhang et al. established CCRR as an antiarrhythmic lncRNA in both mice and humans with HF. This lncRNA acts via preventing the degradation of Cx43, thus improving cardiac conduction. Knockdown of CCRR lead to a destruction of intercalated discs and gap junctions resulting in electrical conduction slowing, an effect similar to adverse cardiac remodeling seen in HF [30].

3.3 ZFAS1

As described above, calcium handling is one of the key factors in electromechanical coupling, with any disturbance potentially causing arrhythmias. ZFAS1 is a lncRNA reported to directly inhibit SERCA by suppressing its ATPase function, impairing cardiac contractility and favoring arrhythmias [31].

3.4 GAS5

The lncRNA GAS5 has been described to interact with miR-21 leading to hampered activation of cardiac fibroblasts via miR-21 upregulation in TGF-beta1 activated cardiac fibroblasts and subsequent lowered levels of *COL1A1*, *alpha-SMA* and *PTEN*. This indicates a role for GAS5 in the development of cardiac fibrosis, one major structural contributor to cardiac arrhythmias [32].

3.5 Kcna2 Antisense RNA (Kcna2 AS)

HF often triggers ventricular arrhythmias. Underlying mechanisms include APD prolongation due to decreased potassium currents (e.g. I_{Ks}). This was shown to be regulated by Kcna2, which in turn can be repressed by Kcna2 AS. In rats with congestive HF, the ventricular Kcna2 AS expression increases and the animals present a higher incidence of ventricular arrhythmias because of a prolonged APD [33].

3.6 TCONS_00075467

Knockout of TCONS_00075467 in rabbits lead to a shortened atrial effective refractory period

Table 18.2 Overview of lncRNAs involved in the genesis of arrhythmias

Non-coding RNA	Regulation in disease	Mechanism	Species	Entity	References
Kcnq1ot1	Upregulated	Downregulation of *KCNQ1*	Human	Long QT- Syndrome	[27–29]
Cardiac conduction regulatory RNA (CCRR)	Downregulated	Destruction of intercalated discs and gap junctions	Mouse	Heart failure	[30]
Kcna2 antisense RNA (Kcna2 AS)	Upregulated	Reduced IKs and prolongation of APD	Rat	Heart failure/ventricular Arrhythmias	[33]
Metastasis-associated lung adenocarcinoma transcript 1 (MALAT1)	Upregulated	Downregulation of I_{to}	Rat	Myocardial ischemia	[35]
GAS5	Downregulated	Increased fibrosis	Rat	Heart failure	[32]
TCONS_00075467	Downregulated	Shortened APD, lowered L-type Ca^{2+} current density	Rabbit	Heart failure	[34]
ZFAS1	Upregulated	Direct SERCA2a-inhibition	Mouse	Myocardial ischemia	[31]

(AERP), shortened action potential as well as lowered L-type calcium current density through sponging miR-328 in atrial myocytes favoring arrhythmia [34].

3.7 Metastasis-Associated Lung Adenocarcinoma Transcript 1 (MALAT1)

MALAT1 is highly abundant in the heart after myocardial ischemia. Downregulation of this transcript induces an increased expression level of Kv4.2 and Kv4.3, transient outward potassium current (I_{to}) and peak current density [35]. This suggests a potential link to cardiac arrhythmias, which needs to be elucidated by other studies.

4 Summary

To put it in a nutshell, a growing body of evidence suggests that microRNAs are crucial factors regulating both normal cardiac electrophysiology and the occurrence of arrhythmias. Mechanistically, an altered microRNA expression mostly triggers a different pattern of ion channels changing the electrophysiological properties of the cardiomyocytes. The role of other non-coding RNAs, such as lncRNAs, in arrythmogenesis are still more elusive today. Some lncRNAs could directly be linked to tachyarrhythmias, while there is no evidence on an involvement of lncRNAs in the genesis of bradyarrhythmias. In addition, no evidence could be found for an entanglement of other classes of non-coding RNAs in arrhythmogenesis yet.

All in all, non-coding RNAs are involved in the pathophysiology of arrhythmias and might therefore serve as targets for the development of innovative novel drugs that may allow to treat cardiac arrhythmias in a causal fashion in the future.

Competing Financial Interests The authors declare no competing financial interests.

References

1. Kim GH. MicroRNA regulation of cardiac conduction and arrhythmias. Transl Res. 2013;161(5):381–92.
2. Galasso M, Sana ME, Volinia S. Non-coding RNAs: a key to future personalized molecular therapy? Genome Med. 2010;2(2):12.
3. Papasaikas P, Valcarcel J. The spliceosome: the ultimate RNA chaperone and sculptor. Trends Biochem Sci. 2016;41(1):33–45.
4. Wakili R, Clauss S, Kaab S. Molecular mechanisms of atrial fibrillation: potential role of microRNAs as new therapeutic targets and potential biomarkers. Herz. 2012;37(2):166–71.
5. Wang Z, Luo X, Lu Y, Yang B. miRNAs at the heart of the matter. J Mol Med. 2008;86(7):771–83.
6. Liao C, Gui Y, Guo Y, Xu D. The regulatory function of microRNA-1 in arrhythmias. Mol BioSyst. 2016;12(2):328–33.
7. Clauss S, Sinner MF, Kaab S, Wakili R. The role of MicroRNAs in antiarrhythmic therapy for atrial fibrillation. Arrhythmia Electrophysiol Rev. 2015;4(3):146–55.
8. Benjamin EJ, Rice KM, Arking DE, Pfeufer A, van Noord C, Smith AV, Schnabel RB, Bis JC, Boerwinkle E, Sinner MF, Dehghan A, Lubitz SA, D'Agostino RB Sr, Lumley T, Ehret GB, Heeringa J, Aspelund T, Newton-Cheh C, Larson MG, Marciante KD, Soliman EZ, Rivadeneira F, Wang TJ, Eiriksdottir G, Levy D, Psaty BM, Li M, Chamberlain AM, Hofman A, Vasan RS, Harris TB, Rotter JI, Kao WHL, Agarwal SK, Stricker BHC, Wang K, Launer LJ, Smith NL, Chakravarti A, Uitterlinden AG, Wolf PA, Sotoodehnia N, Kottgen A, van Duijn CM, Meitinger T, Mueller M, Perz S, Steinbeck G, Wichmann HE, Lunetta KL, Heckbert SR, Gudnason V, Alonso A, Kaab S, Ellinor PT, Witteman JCM. Variants in ZFHX3 are associated with atrial fibrillation in individuals of European ancestry. Nat Genet. 2009;41(8):879–81.
9. Wang Z. The role of microRNA in cardiac excitability. J Cardiovasc Pharmacol. 2010;56(5):460–70.
10. Nattel S, Burstein B, Dobrev D. Atrial remodeling and atrial fibrillation: mechanisms and implications. Circ Arrhythm Electrophysiol. 2008;1(1):62–73.
11. Nattel S, Quantz MA. Pharmacological response of quinidine induced early afterdepolarisations in canine cardiac Purkinje fibres: insights into underlying ionic mechanisms. Cardiovasc Res. 1988;22(11):808–17.
12. Boixel C, Fontaine V, Rucker-Martin C, Milliez P, Louedec L, Michel JB, Jacob MP, Hatem SN. Fibrosis of the left atria during progression of heart failure is associated with increased matrix metalloproteinases in the rat. J Am Coll Cardiol. 2003;42(2):336–44.
13. Martin CA, Matthews GD, Huang CL. Sudden cardiac death and inherited channelopathy: the basic electrophysiology of the myocyte and myocardium in ion channel disease. Heart. 2012;98(7):536–43.

14. Yang B, Lin H, Xiao J, Lu Y, Luo X, Li B, Zhang Y, Xu C, Bai Y, Wang H, Chen G, Wang Z. The muscle-specific microRNA miR-1 regulates cardiac arrhythmogenic potential by targeting GJA1 and KCNJ2. Nat Med. 2007;13(4):486–91.
15. Terentyev D, Belevych AE, Terentyeva R, Martin MM, Malana GE, Kuhn DE, Abdellatif M, Feldman DS, Elton TS, Gyorke S. miR-1 overexpression enhances ca(2+) release and promotes cardiac arrhythmogenesis by targeting PP2A regulatory subunit B56alpha and causing CaMKII-dependent hyperphosphorylation of RyR2. Circ Res. 2009;104(4):514–21.
16. D'Souza A, Bucchi A, Johnsen AB, Logantha SJ, Monfredi O, Yanni J, Prehar S, Hart G, Cartwright E, Wisloff U, Dobryznski H, DiFrancesco D, Morris GM, Boyett MR. Exercise training reduces resting heart rate via downregulation of the funny channel HCN4. Nat Commun. 2014;5:3775.
17. Ling Xiao AH, Nickel T, Clauss S. microRNA-mediated cardiac remodeling in athletes. RNA & DISEASE. 2016
18. Clauss S, Wakili R, Hildebrand B, Kaab S, Hoster E, Klier I, Martens E, Hanley A, Hanssen H, Halle M, Nickel T. MicroRNAs as biomarkers for acute atrial Remodeling in Marathon runners (the miRathon study--a sub-study of the Munich Marathon study). PLoS One. 2016;11(2):e0148599.
19. Benz A, Kossack M, Auth D, Seyler C, Zitron E, Juergensen L, Katus HA, Hassel D. miR-19b regulates ventricular action potential duration in zebrafish. Sci Rep. 2016;6:36033.
20. Shan H, Zhang Y, Lu Y, Zhang Y, Pan Z, Cai B, Wang N, Li X, Feng T, Hong Y, Yang B. Downregulation of miR-133 and miR-590 contributes to nicotine-induced atrial remodelling in canines. Cardiovasc Res. 2009;83(3):465–72.
21. Duisters RF, Tijsen AJ, Schroen B, Leenders JJ, Lentink V, van der Made I, Herias V, van Leeuwen RE, Schellings MW, Barenbrug P, Maessen JG, Heymans S, Pinto YM, Creemers EE. miR-133 and miR-30 regulate connective tissue growth factor: implications for a role of microRNAs in myocardial matrix remodeling. Circ Res. 2009;104(2):170–8.
22. Luo X, Pan Z, Shan H, Xiao J, Sun X, Wang N, Lin H, Xiao L, Maguy A, Qi X-Y, Li Y, Gao X, Dong D, Zhang Y, Bai Y, Ai J, Sun L, Lu H, Luo X-Y, Wang Z, Lu Y, Yang B, Nattel S. MicroRNA-26 governs profibrillatory inward-rectifier potassium current changes in atrial fibrillation. J Clin Invest. 2013;123(5):1939–51.
23. Monfredi O, Boyett MR. Sick sinus syndrome and atrial fibrillation in older persons – a view from the sinoatrial nodal myocyte. J Mol Cell Cardiol. 2015;83:88–100.
24. Wang J, Bai Y, Li N, Ye W, Zhang M, Greene SB, Tao Y, Chen Y, Wehrens XH, Martin JF. Pitx2-microRNA pathway that delimits sinoatrial node development and inhibits predisposition to atrial fibrillation. Proc Natl Acad Sci U S A. 2014;111(25):9181–6.
25. Hoffmann S, Clauss S, Berger IM, Weiss B, Montalbano A, Roth R, Bucher M, Klier I, Wakili R, Seitz H, Schulze-Bahr E, Katus HA, Flachsbart F, Nebel A, Guenther SP, Bagaev E, Rottbauer W, Kaab S, Just S, Rappold GA. Coding and non-coding variants in the SHOX2 gene in patients with early-onset atrial fibrillation. Basic Res Cardiol. 2016;111(3):36.
26. Huang Y. The novel regulatory role of lncRNA-miRNA-mRNA axis in cardiovascular diseases. J Cell Mol Med. 2018;22(12):5768–75.
27. Andrsova I, Novotny T, Kadlecova J, Bittnerova A, Vit P, Florianova A, Sisakova M, Gaillyova R, Manouskova L, Spinar J. Clinical characteristics of 30 Czech families with long QT syndrome and KCNQ1 and KCNH2 gene mutations: importance of exercise testing. J Electrocardiol. 2012;45(6):746–51.
28. Korostowski L, Sedlak N, Engel N. The Kcnq1ot1 long non-coding RNA affects chromatin conformation and expression of Kcnq1, but does not regulate its imprinting in the developing heart. PLoS Genet. 2012;8(9):e1002956.
29. Coto E, Calvo D, Reguero JR, Moris C, Rubin JM, Diaz-Corte C, Gil-Pena H, Alosno B, Iglesias S, Gomez J. Differential methylation of lncRNA KCNQ1OT1 promoter polymorphism was associated with symptomatic cardiac long QT. Epigenomics. 2017;9(8):1049–57.
30. Zhang Y, Sun L, Xuan L, Pan Z, Hu X, Liu H, Bai Y, Jiao L, Li Z, Cui L, Wang X, Wang S, Yu T, Feng B, Guo Y, Liu Z, Meng W, Ren H, Zhu J, Zhao X, Yang C, Zhang Y, Xu C, Wang Z, Lu Y, Shan H, Yang B. Long non-coding RNA CCRR controls cardiac conduction via regulating intercellular coupling. Nat Commun. 2018;9(1):4176.
31. Zhang Y, Jiao L, Sun L, Li Y, Gao Y, Xu C, Shao Y, Li M, Li C, Lu Y, Pan Z, Xuan L, Zhang Y, Li Q, Yang R, Zhuang Y, Zhang Y, Yang B. LncRNA ZFAS1 as a SERCA2a inhibitor to cause intracellular ca($^{2+}$) overload and contractile dysfunction in a mouse model of myocardial infarction. Circ Res. 2018;122(10):1354–68.
32. Tao H, Zhang JG, Qin RH, Dai C, Shi P, Yang JJ, Deng ZY, Shi KH. LncRNA GAS5 controls cardiac fibroblast activation and fibrosis by targeting miR-21 via PTEN/MMP-2 signaling pathway. Toxicology. 2017;386:11–8.
33. Long QQ, Wang H, Gao W, Fan Y, Li YF, Ma Y, Yang Y, Shi HJ, Chen BR, Meng HY, Wang QM, Wang F, Wang ZM, Wang LS. Long noncoding RNA Kcna2 antisense RNA contributes to ventricular arrhythmias via silencing Kcna2 in rats with congestive heart failure. J Am Heart Assoc. 2017;6(12):e005965.
34. Li Z, Wang X, Wang W, Du J, Wei J, Zhang Y, Wang J, Hou Y. Altered long non-coding RNA expression profile in rabbit atria with atrial fibrillation: TCONS_00075467 modulates atrial electrical remodeling by sponging miR-328 to regulate CACNA1C. J Mol Cell Cardiol. 2017;108:73–85.
35. Zhu P, Yang M, Ren H, Shen G, Chen J, Zhang J, Liu J, Sun C. Long noncoding RNA MALAT1 downregulates cardiac transient outward potassium

current by regulating miR-200c/HMGB1 pathway. J Cell Biochem. 2018;119(12):10239–49.
36. Girmatsion Z, Biliczki P, Bonauer A, Wimmer-Greinecker G, Scherer M, Moritz A, Bukowska A, Goette A, Nattel S, Hohnloser SH, Ehrlich JR. Changes in microRNA-1 expression and IK1 up-regulation in human atrial fibrillation. Heart Rhythm. 2009;6(12):1802–9.
37. D'Souza A, Pearman CM, Wang Y, Nakao S, Logantha S, Cox C, Bennett H, Zhang Y, Johnsen AB, Linscheid N, Poulsen PC, Elliott J, Coulson J, McPhee J, Robertson A, da Costa Martins PA, Kitmitto A, Wisloff U, Cartwright EJ, Monfredi O, Lundby A, Dobrzynski H, Oceandy D, Morris GM, Boyett MR. Targeting miR-423-5p reverses exercise training-induced HCN4 channel Remodeling and sinus bradycardia. Circ Res. 2017;121(9):1058–68.

Non-coding RNAs and Atrial Fibrillation

19

Diego Franco, Amelia Aranega, and Jorge N. Dominguez

Abstract

Atrial fibrillation is the most frequent type of cardiac arrhythmia in humans, with an estimate incidence of 1–2% in the general population, rising up to 8–10% in the elderly. Cardiovascular risk factors such as diabetes, obesity, hypertension and hyperthyroidism can increase the occurrence of AF. The onset of AF triggers additional AF episodes, leading to structural and electrical remodeling of the diseased heart. Understanding the molecular bases of atrial fibrillation have greatly advance over the last decade demonstrating a pivotal role of distinct ion channels in AF pathophysiology. A new scenario has opened on the understanding of the molecular mechanisms underlying AF, with the discovery of non-coding RNAs and their wide implication in multiple disease states, including cardiac arrhythmogenic pathologies. microRNAs are small non-coding RNAs of 22–24 nucleotides that are capable of regulating gene expression by interacting with the mRNA transcript 3′UTRs and promoting mRNA degradation and/or protein translation blockage. Long non-coding RNAs are a more diverse group of non-coding RNAs, providing transcriptional and post-transcriptional roles and subclassified according to their functional properties. In this chapter we summarized current state-of-the-art knowledge on the functional of microRNAs and long non-coding RNAs as well as their cross-talk regulatory mechanisms in atrial fibrillation.

Keywords

microRNAs · lncRNAs · Atrial fibrillation · Biomakers

1 Background

Atrial fibrillation is the most frequent type of cardiac arrhythmia in humans, with an estimate incidence of 1–2% in the general population [1]. In the elderly, AF can rise up to 8–10%. Cardiovascular risk factors such as diabetes, obesity, hypertension and hyperthyroidism can increase the occurrence of AF [2–4]. Importantly, AF can be also secondary to surgical interventions, inflammatory processes and obstructive sleep apnea [5]. The onset of AF triggers additional AF episodes, leading to electrical and structural remodeling of the diseased heart, a condition quoted as "AF begets AF". Electrical remodeling leads to progressive changes in the

D. Franco (✉) · A. Aranega · J. N. Dominguez
Cardiovascular Development Group, Department of Experimental Biology, University of Jaen, Jaen, Spain
e-mail: dfranco@ujaen.es

J. Xiao (ed.), *Non-coding RNAs in Cardiovascular Diseases*, Advances in Experimental Medicine and Biology 1229, https://doi.org/10.1007/978-981-15-1671-9_19

cardiac electrical properties, coursing with early after depolarizations (EADs), delayed after depolarizations (DADs) and/or changes in the action potential duration (APD) configuration culminating thus in rotor formation [6]. Structural remodeling normally courses with atrial fibrosis, inflammation and/or dilatation [7].

Epidemiological studies have undoubtedly demonstrated that cardiovascular risk factors, such as those previously mentioned, enhance AF occurrence. Importantly there are also unquestionable evidences that AF courses in absence of previous risk factors, i.e. a condition dubbed lone AF [8]. Seminal studied by Brugada et al. [9] demonstrate a familiar genetic component in lone AF. Subsequent screening of candidate genes in familiar AF kindreds identified a large number of point mutations in distinct genes encoding for proteins involved in cardiac electrophysiology. Yet, despite this advancement, genetic identification of causative genes in AF only explains 10–15% of all AF patients [10]. In recent years, genome-wide association analyses (GWAS) lightened the discovery of new genes associated to AF. Pioneer worked by Gubdjartsson et al. [11] firstly identify common risk variants highly associated to the onset of lone AF in distinct ethnic cohorts. More recently additional GWAS studies and meta-GWAS have further identified new candidate genes for AF pathophysiology, with over 70 genes potentially involved [12].

Understanding the molecular bases of atrial fibrillation have greatly advance over the last decade. Beside the involvement of genes encoding of distinct ion channels involved in the configuration of the cardiac action potential, the discovery of potential candidate genes by GWAS, and subsequently the functional analyses have unraveled novel pathways [13]. Among them, the most explored to date is driven by Pitx2, leading to Wnt, microRNAs and ion channel remodeling [14–16]. Importantly, a new scenario has opened on the understanding of the molecular mechanisms underlying AF, with the discovery of non-coding RNAs and their wide implication in multiple disease states, including therein cardiac structural and arrhythmogenic pathologies [17].

Non-coding RNAs can be grossly subclassified into two major groups; small non coding RNAs (shorten that 200 nucleotides in length) and long non coding RNAs (longer that 200 nucleotides in length). Small non-coding RNAs contain distinct subclasses such as piwi-RNAs, snoRNAs, siRNAs, and the most numerous and well-studied group of microRNAs [18, 19]. microRNAs are small non-coding RNAs of 22–24 nucleotide that are capable of regulating gene expression by interacting with the mRNA transcript 3′UTRs are promoting mRNA degradation and/or protein translation blockage [20]. Long non-coding RNAs are equally an heterogenous group of non-coding RNAs that are basically subclassified according to their functional properties yet such a classification is complex and imprecise given our limited understanding of their transcriptional and post-transcriptional function [21]. Furthermore, complex interplays between long non coding RNAs and microRNAs are also operative, opening a completely novel landscape of gene regulation.

2 microRNAs as Biomarkers of AF

Non coding RNAs are becoming acknowledged as novel biomarkers in distinct cardiovascular pathologies, including AF (see for recent reviews [22, 23]). Wang et al. [24] recently demonstrated that two distinct microRNAs are significantly decreased in post-ablation AF patients compared to non-ablated AF patients. Importantly, using an experimental model of AF, in pigs, they further corroborated that AF ablation significantly diminished miR-155 and miR-24 expression. Biochemical and molecular analysis demonstrated that these two microRNAs can influence nitric oxide (NO) and endothelial nitric oxide synthase (eNOS) are altered, supporting the role of NO/eNOS pathway in AF. Feldman et al. [25] recently demonstrated that circulating miR-23 and miR-26 were significantly decreased while Harling et al. identified that plasma circulating miR-483 was significantly increased in postoperative patients developing AF as compared to those that did not develop AF, suggesting a functional role for these microRNAs in the onset of post-operative AF. More recently Liu et al. reported that AF catheter ablation restores miR-409-3p and miR-432 plasma levels, further supporting a pivotal role for microRNAs in AF pathophysiology. Soeki et al. [26] nicely demonstrated that expression of miR-328 and miR-1 were increased in AF patients as compared to control, displaying enhanced expression in the left atrium and pulmonary vein plasma as compared to systemic plasma expression. These evidence support a plausible role for local miR-328 production in relation to atrial substrate remodeling. Similar findings were also reported by Zhou et al. [27]. Overall these data demonstrate that microRNAs might serve as biomarkers to identify and probably to predict the onset and/or course of AF pathophysiology.

3 SNV in microRNAs Associated to AF

Genomic variations on the promoter sequences driving microRNA expression or within the precursors/seed sequences of microRNAs have been reported to be associated to increase rate of AF occurrence. In particular, three distinct microRNAs have been already described, miR-125a, miR-196a2 and miR-146 [28–30]. A miR-125a polymorphism is associated with recurrence of AF after ablation, an association that mechanistically links miR-125a and IL6/IL6R axis, since IL6R is a direct target of miR-125a [28]. A pre-miR-196a2 SNV is associated to increase occurrence of AF in Chinese population, a condition that is also linked with increased atrial dimensions [29]. A polymorphism in miR-146 is a prognostic biomarker for adverse cardiovascular events in AF patients following anticoagulant administration, probably involving inflammatory mechanisms, since IL6/1L6R axis is reversely correlated [30]. In addition, Hoffman et al. [31] reported coding and non-coding variants in SHOX2 gene in patients with atrial fibrillation. Non-coding variants generated a novel functional binding site for miR-92-5p. Importantly, miR-92-5p expression levels in circulating plasma were increased in those patients carrying the SNV, supporting a causative link between SHOX2 non coding SNVs, miR-92-5p expression and AF. In sum, these evidence suggest that impaired regulation of microRNAs expression can have a profound effect on AF occurrence, yet additional experimental evidence is required to fully support these findings.

4 Functional Roles of microRNAs in AF

Multiple microRNAs have been involved in electrical and structural remodeling directly linked to the course of atrial fibrillation. We provide herein evidences on the functional role of microRNAs in cell-cell coupling, electrical regulation, structural impairment as well as in additional signaling pathways related to AF pathology in the following subheadings.

4.1 Functional Roles of microRNAs in Cell-Cell Coupling

Cell-cell coupling exerted by connexin is critical for the correct electrical propagation. Two distinct microRNAs, miR-208a and miR-206, have been reported to target Cx40 and Cx43, respectively [32, 33]. Cx43 has been validated as target of miR-206 by biochemical luciferase assays. Mice over-expressing miR-206 displayed decreased atrial and ventricular Cx43 expression and thus abnormal PR interval and heart rate, leading thereafter to a shortening the life span of these mice [34]. These data postulate a plausible role for miR-208 in AF, although additional evidences are required. Li et al. [35] reported that miR-208 is increased in right atrial biopsies of AF patients, while Cx40 expression was diminished. Experimental studies demonstrate an indirect modulation of Cx40 (Gja5) by miR-208.

Curiously, Takahashi et al. [36] reported that high-fat diet increases vulnerability to atrial arrhythmia by down-regulation of Cx40 via miR-27b.

4.2 Functional Roles of microRNAs in AF Electrical Remodeling

Within the configuration of the cardiac action potential, including sodium and potassium channels. Zhao et al. [37] demonstrate that miR-192 is up-regulated in AF atrial biopsies, while SCN5A is decreased. Luciferase assays demonstrate a direct interaction and regulation of SCN5A by miR-192, leading to modulation of I_{Na} current, supporting a plausible role of these mechanism underlying AF pathophysiology.

Girmatsion et al. [38] demonstrate a complementary expression between miR-1 and Kir2.1 in left atrial AF patients biopsies, data that are concordant with increased IK1 current in LA AF patients as compared to SR patients, while connexin expression was unaffected. Furthermore, *ex vivo* stimulation also lead to similar results, supporting both a key role of miR-1/Kir2.1 in AF pathophysiology and a determinant role suggesting a primary role of atrial rate in miR-1 down-regulation and I(K1) up-regulation. Additional evidence on the role of atrial taquipacing were obtained by Jia et al. [39] using rabbit as experimental model. These authors demonstrate a clear gene expression remodeling up-regulating miR-1 and down-regulating KCNE1 and KCNB2, leading to decrease atrial effecting refractory period while increasing IK currents. In addition, KCNE1 and KCNB2 were corroborated as direct targets of miR-1. Luo et al. [40] reported impaired miR-26 expression in AF patients. Biochemical assays demonstrated that miR-26 regulates KCNJ12 expression. In vitro and in vivo manipulation of miR-26 demonstrate that if impaired, atrial fibrillation develops.

Importantly, most the microRNAs related to AF to date influence calcium homeostasis, a key event regulating onset of AF, including therein miR-21 and miR-29a modulation of CACNA1C [41–42], miR-499 regulation of CACNB2 [43] and miR-106-miR-25 regulation of RyR2 [47]. Zhao et al. [42] demonstrate that CACNA1C is a direct target of miR-21. Barana et al. [41] demonstrate miR-21 expression is up-regulated in AF vs SR atrial myocytes and that miR-21 directly regulates CACNA1C and CACNB2 provoking Ica current changes similar to those recorded in AF patients. Ling et al. [48] and Ling et al. [46] demonstrate that miR-499 directly targets CACNB2 and SK3 channels while miR-499 is significantly increased while CACNB2 and SK3 are decreased in AF patients atrial biopsies. These data similarly support a role of miR-499 in AF pathophysiology. Cañon et al. [49] reported that miR-208b was increased in human and ovine AF biopsies. Over-expression of miR-208 leads to alteration in CACNA1C and CACNB2 and SERCA both at expression and functional levels, supporting a role for miR-208 in AF.

In addition, regulation of HCN by miR-1/miR-133 [47] also plays a role on AF onset with age. Li et al. [47] demonstrate that miR-1 and miR-133 were decreased in age AF right atrial biopsies while HCN2 and HCN4 were up-regulated, supporting a role for these microRNAs in the onset of age-related AF.

Experimental animal models have also provided additional evidences on the functional roles of microRNAs in AF. Chiang et al. [48] demonstrated that deletion of the microRNA-106b-25 cluster in mice promotes atrial fibrillation by enhancing ryanodine receptor type-2 expression and calcium release. Wang et al. [49] and Chinchilla et al. [14] also demonstrated that Pitx2 deficiency disrupt microRNA expression that are linked to atrial arrhythmogenesis, a signaling pathway that also involves regulation of Wnt and Wnt-driven microRNAs expression [15], which is highly susceptible to alteration of cardiovascular risk factors such as hyperthyroidism, hypertension and redox homeostasis imbalance [16]. In dogs, expression of miR-30 and miR-133 is impaired in chronic atrial fibrillation [50] and down-regulation of miR-133 and miR-590 contributes to nicotine-induced atrial remodeling [51].

4.3 Functional Roles of microRNAs in AF Structural Remodeling

Structural remodeling in AF invariably courses with intramyocardial fibrosis. Multiple pathways have been involved in triggering fibrosis and similarly, several reports highlight the functional roles of microRNAs governing this process. Ang-II driven fibrosis is controlled by miR-27 [52], while miR-30c [53] modulated Tgfb-driven fibrosis.

miR-27 can diminished angiotensin II-induced fibrosis, by modulating collagen I/III, plasminogen activator inhibitor type 1 and alpha smooth muscle actin expression by targeting Alk5, a tgf-beta1 receptor as well as inhibiting Smad2/3 phosphorylation without altering Smad1 activity [52]. Furthermore, In isolated perfused hearts, miR-27b restoration markedly attenuated AngII-induced increase in interatrial conduction time, AF incidence and AF duration.

Xu et al. [53] demonstrate that miR-30c directly regulates Tgfbr2 as well as fibroblast proliferation, differentiation, migration and collagen production of cardiac fibroblasts. Therefore, modulating miR-30c expression can provide beneficial effects reversing AF induced atrial fibrosis.

miR-132 influences CTGF activation [54] and miR-30 regulates Snail [58]. Importantly, the most well-described microRNA favouring fibrosis in AF is miR-21, including herein the regulation of CADM1/STAT2 [59], WWP1 [57] as well as other unidentified pathways [58–59]. In addition to fibrosis, structural remodeling in AF also courses with activation of apoptosis. Two distinct microRNAs have been reported to activate apoptosis in AD, miR-122 [60] and miR-1/miR-133 [61].

Quiao et al. [54] demonstrated that miR-132 expression was decreased and CTGF increased in the human and canine models with AF. The expression of miR-132 and CTGF protein levels were upregulated in Ang II stimulated cardiac fibroblasts of adult rats. Furthermore, when miR-132 was introduced into cardiac fibroblasts, the expression of miR-132 increased significantly whereas the expression of CTGF decreased, supporting miR-132 may target CTGF in regulating fibrosis in Ang II-treated cardiac fibroblasts.

Yuan et al. [55] reported an inverse correlation between miR-30a and Snail1 and periostin expression in AngII-induced fibrosis in cardiac fibroblasts. However, the putative mechanisms behind these findings remains unexplored. Cao et al. [56] demonstrated that miR-21 overexpression promotes cardiac fibrosis via STAT3 signaling pathway by decrease CADM1 expression in cell culture models of cardiac fibrosis, supporting that miR-21 might be an important signaling molecule for cardiac fibrotic remodeling and AF.

Tao et al. [57] demonstrated that TGF-β1, collagen I and collagen III levels are significantly elevated in AF patients, miR-21 expression is increased, while the WWP-1 expression was decreased. miR-21 transfected cardiac fibroblasts decreased WWP-1 expression, while opposite effects were observed after miR-21 inhibitor administration. Therefore these data indicated that miR-21 inhibits cardiac fibroblasts proliferation by inactivating the TGF-β1/Smad2 signaling pathway via up-regulation of WWP-1. Yang et al. [62] demonstrated that miR-23b and miR-27b were up-regulated in AF left atrial samples as well as in angiotensin II treated fibroblasts. Overexpression of these microRNAs enhance collagen expression, a process that is TGFBR3 dependent. These data support a functional role for miR-23b and miR-27b in AF fibrosis.

4.4 Functional Roles of microRNAs in Additional AF Related Pathways

Besides electrical and structural remodeling associated to AF, other signaling pathways have been reported to play a role in AF and several microRNAs have been associated to modulate such signaling pathways. Ankyrin B is regulated by miR-34 [63], PTEN/PI3K, STAT3 and Smad7 by miR-21 [64–66] dystrophin by miR-31 [70] and SIRT1 by miR-199 [68]. Overall, these data suggest an increasing important role of microRNAs modulating AF pathophysiology.

5 Transcriptomic Analyses of microRNAs in AF Conditions

Multiple studies have been performed searching for the transcriptomic fingerprints of atrial fibrillation. Some of these studies were exclusively done using a candidate approach on the expression of a limited number of microRNAs, already demonstrating differential expression in human AF. In this context, Da Silva et al. [69] identified increased plasma expression of miR-133b, miR-328 and miR-499 in patients with acute new onset of AF as compared to controls and well-controlled patients. miR-21 on the contrary was decreased in well-controlled patients as compared to controls and new-onset AF patients.

More recently, microRNA microarray analyses provided additional evidences on the differential expression in distinct tissue involved in AF pathogenesis. For example, Zhang et al. [70] analyzed the microRNA fingerprint of the cardiac autonomic nervous plexus and identified 16 differentially expressed microRNAs in atrial taquipaced dogs as compared to controls. These authors further demonstrating that miR-206 controls SOD1 expression, balancing therefore redox homeostasis in atrial taquipaced dogs. In an experimental model of induced AF, Torrado et al. [71] reported the early microRNA signature of AF.

Importantly, great efforts have been devoted to understand the differential contribution of the left and right atrial chambers in AF pathology. Slagsvold et al. [72–73] microRNA array of selected microRNAs between RA and LA, in AF and SR after coronary bypass surgery or valve replacement. They demonstrate rather similar differences between RA and LA atrial analyses in both AF and SR patients, whereas more differences were observed when comparing RA AF vs RA SR and LA AF vs LA SR. In other words, right and left atrial chambers display mostly similar microRNA expression patterns in AF and SR, respectively while AF distinctly affect both RA and LA. Doñate-Puertas et al. [74] analyzed the differential distribution of 662 microRNAs in the left atrium of AF patients with valvular heart disease by microarrays. These authors reported that 42 microRNAs were differentially expressed in AF as compared to controls. A similar report was performed by Liu et al. [75] in AF patients with mitral stenosis. From 1962 microRNAs, only 22 microRNAs were differentially expressed, using microarrays. Xiao et al. [76] similarly investigated differential microRNA expression in AF patients with mitral stenosis but data were obtained from the right atrium instead of the left atrium. Using microarrays against 773 human microRNAs, these authors identified 28 differentially expressed microRNAs. Importantly, side-to-side comparison of the differentially expressed microRNAs in LA AF vs SR resulted in no shared microRNAs between the three distinct studies. Only four microRNAs (miR-18, miR-25, miR-20 and miR-451) were shared by the studies of Slagsvold et al. [72–73] and Doñate-Puertas et al. [74] (Fig. 19.1a). The overall lack of coincidence can be explained on the one hand by a large variability of the human patients cohorts collected on each study, the tissue samples selected or the distinct microRNA microarray platforms used but also it could be attributed to large biological variability that it is current beyond our understanding. Importantly, efforts should be done to solve the puzzle. Secondly, a minimal common microRNA signature is found when comparing LA and RA AF samples (7% of all differentially expressed microRNA in AF samples) (Fig. 19.1b), merging all three studies together, supporting that distinct post-transcriptional regulatory mechanisms are distinct driving AF expression in the LA as compared to the RA.

In addition, a large number of experiments have been performed using whole genome transcriptomics. Cooley et al. [77], Liu et al. [78] and Yan et al. [79] identified the microRNA signature of left and right atrial chambers in the context of AF with valvular heart disease. The authors reported a wide array of microRNA differential gene expression supporting the notion that both AF and valvular heart disease distinct affect the microRNA pattern of both left and right atrial chambers. Importantly, both left and right atrial chambers are distinctly affected by disease progression and by the development of AF. Liu et al.

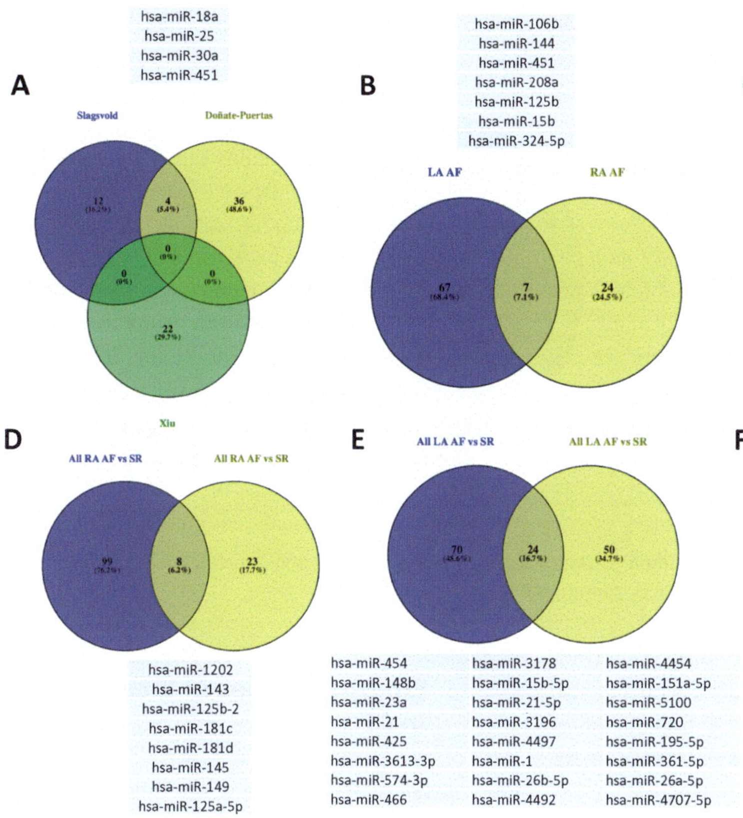

Fig. 19.1 Transcriptomic analyses of microRNAs in AF conditions

[78] reported significant decreased expression of miR-146, miR-150 and miR-199 in blood of patients with paroxysmal and permanent AF, while miR-21 was increased but only in those with permanent AF using massive parallel sequencing.

Surprisingly, a common hallmark of AF is poorly achieved in both RA and LA signatures using massive RNA sequencing technologies; i.e. 2 microRNAs are shared in the RA; miR-133 and miR-331 (Fig. 19.1c); none in LA (Fig. 19.1d). Side-to-side comparison of microarray analyses and RNAseq strategies unraveled a relatively low commonality in the RA AF samples (6.2%; 8 microRNAs) (Fig. 19.1e) but a more robust and significant shared microRNAs in the LA AF (17%; 22 microRNAs) (Fig. 19.1f). Thus, these analyses are promising in providing a core microRNA signature of LA AF remodeling, opening new ways to explore the functional consequences and roles of differentially expressed microRNAs in the context of AF.

However, the large incongruency between studies might be highly related to the large variability on the tissue sample analyzed (systemic plasma, cardiac plasma, atrial biopsies, remnants of cardiac surgery), patients inclusion criteria and methodological approaches used. For example, several studies analyzed differences in AF in the context of valve diseases [74, 76, 78] while only a single study has been reported in absence of valve diseases [80]. In this context Wang et al. [80] analyzed the microRNA expression signature of the LA in AF patients without valve disease by low density microarrays, leading to the identification of 10 differentially expressed microRNAs. Surprisingly, none of the microRNAs in the non valvular AF signature is shared with those previously reported in valvular AF (Fig. 19.2a). Therefore, given the large variability

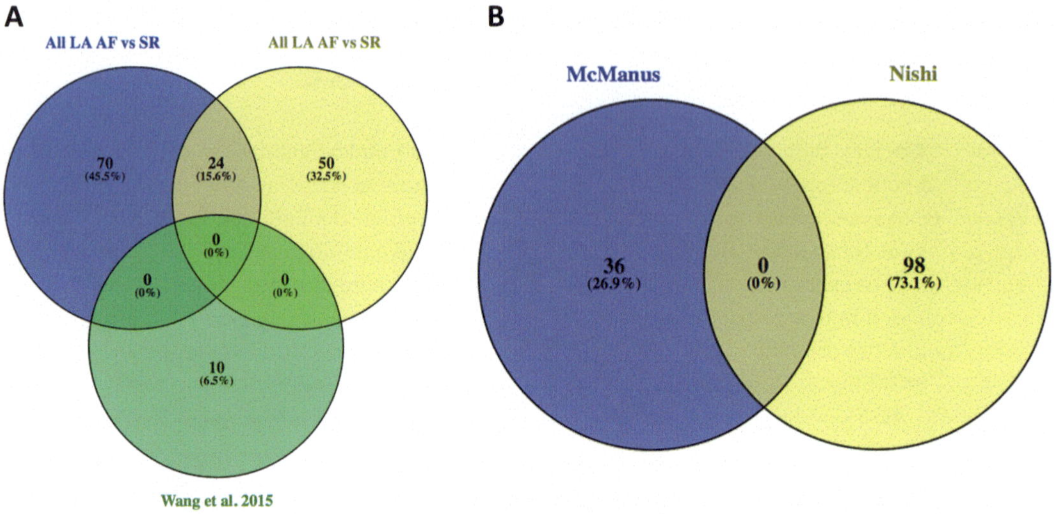

Fig. 19.2 Large variability on the tissue sample analyzed, patients inclusion criteria and methodological approaches used induced large incongruency of microRNAs transcriptomic

of the subjects analyzed, confounding comorbidities such as valvular heart diseases, seems to also greatly influence the microRNA fingerprint of AF, and thus it is hard to find an common AF transcriptomic hallmark.

Transcriptomic analyses were also done in AF post-surgery [81–82]. McManus et al. [84] analyzed 86 microRNAs by qPCR in circulating plasma and atrial tissue samples in patients before and after catheter surgery. They reported 21 differentially expressed microRNAs in AF plasma and 33 up-regulated after surgery. Among these, miR-21 and miR-150 increased threefold, supporting a plausible role for these microRNAs on the regulation of the gene regulatory networks governing AF. Nishi et al. [82] using a similar approach reported 98 differentially expressed microRNA in right atrial samples of AF vs controls. Two microRNAs, miR-21 and miR-208 were elevated after surgery. Interestingly, miRNA-21 expression was highest in patients with chronic AF or an unsuccessful maze procedure, and gradually decreased in order from those with a successful maze procedure to SR patients. Similarly as in previous comparative studies, no microRNA commonality is observed in the results provided by McManus et al. [81] and Nishi et al. [82] (Fig. 19.2b).

6 Emerging Roles of lncRNAs in AF

Our current understanding of the functional roles of long non coding RNAs is on its infancy. Yet solid evidences for the plausible role of discrete lncRNAs in AF have already been provided. For example, Gore-Panter et al. [83] identified PANCR, a lncRNA adjacent to PITX2 in humans. PANCR subcellular localization is mainly cytoplasmic and its expression is independent in sinus rhythm disturbances. Importantly, PANCR silencing significantly modifies PITX2 expression, mimicking thereafter the effects of PITX2 knockdown. However, its current role in AF remains elusive. Shen et al. [84] using a candidate approach analyses reported that KCNQ1OT1 is up-regulated in an AF mouse model as well as in AngII-treated mice. Furthermore these authors demonstrate the functional role of KCNQ1OT1 modulating several electrophysiological parameters such as the effective refractory period and the interatrial conduction. In addition, silencing KCNQ1OT1 leads to diminish the incidence of AF and AF episodes during AngII-treatment. Mechanistically, KCNQ1OT1 regulates CACNA1C by sponging miR-384, supporting thus a pivotal role of this lncRNA in AF pathophysiology. Zhao et al. [88] investigated the modulative effects of lncRNA TCONS_00202959 on autonomic neural function and myocardial functions in atrial fibrillation rat model. They show that over-expression of this lncRNA in an experimental rat AF model enhances the atrial effective refractory period and diminishes the AF induction rate. More recently, Cao et al. [86] demonstrate increased expression of lncRNA PVT1 in human AF atrial biopsies as compared to controls and they also demonstrate a role for PVT1 directing atrial fibroblast proliferation and collagen deposition by sponging miR-128-3p that in turn facilitated Sp1 expression and thus Tgfb/Smads signaling.

In addition to our knowledge of discrete lncRNA in AF, several studies have been carried out to provide a more global picture of the lncRNA profile in AF. Ruan et al. [87] analyzed by microarray the LA profile of lncRNAs in AF patients with rheumatic valve disease. They identified 219 differentially expressed lncRNAs. Similarly, Mei et al. [88] analyzed the RA profile of lncRNAs in AF patients and identified 182 differentially expressed lncRNA. Wu et al., [89] lncRNA transcriptomic analyses by microarrays using atrial tissue samples (both right and left). 16 lncRNA and 5 mRNA were found to be differentially expressed in AF patients. Chen et al. [90] performed a microarray analyses using pulmonary vein myocardium and the surrounding myocardium and compared to LA appendage. The authors reported 94 differentially expressed lncRNAs, among which AK055347 was one of lncRNAs most significantly altered. Experimental manipulation of this lncRNAs demonstrate a role in mitochondria energy production. Comparison of all the data provides by these authors demonstrate no single match between them (data not shown), raising up the poor robustness of these findings that might be due to technical or biological variables. In addition, how these lncRNAs can influence AF phenotype remains mostly unsolved.

In addition to the lncRNAs hallmark in the AF diseased myocardium, additional studies have been carried out in leucocytes. Su et al. [91] reported the differentially expressed lncRNAs profiles in leucocytes of paroxysmal AF as compared to controls. A total of 2095 lncRNAs were differentially expressed. Two of these lncRNAs (ENST00000559960 and uc004aef.3) were further validated and identified as biomarkers of AF.

Additional evidences on the differential lncRNA expression profile in AF have been reported in two distinct experimental models. Li et al. [92] analyzed the expression profile of lncRNAs by RNAseq in RA samples of experimental rabbit AF model. These authors identified 1220 differentially expressed lncRNAs. They further explore the functional role of one of these differentially expressed lncRNA, i.e. TCONS_00075467, showing that silencing leads to a decrease in L-type calcium current and thus the action potential duration. They further demonstrate that TCONS_00075467 can sponge the microRNA miR-328 and thus regulate the downstream protein CACNA1C, supporting thus a pivotal role in AF pathophysiology. Wang et al. [93] analyzed the lncRNA profile in fat pads from experimental canine model of AF. These authors reported 576 differentially expressed lncRNA (166 down-regulated and 410 up-regulated). In vivo silencing of two of these differentially expressed lncRNAs, TCONS_00032546 and TCONS_00026102, significantly shorten or prolong the atrial effective refractory period thereby increasing or preventing AF inducibility by promoting or inhibiting the neurogenesis, respectively. The lack of evolutionary lncRNA conservation hampers comparison with data obtained in human tissues and thus provides an additional obstacle to dissect the AF lncRNA transcriptomic hallmark.

7 Perspectives

In this study we provide convincing evidence on the functional role of microRNAs and lncRNAs in atrial fibrillation. A wealth of knowledge is currently available of the role of microRNAs in atrial fibrillation, including therein major contributions impacting on both electrical and structural remodeling. In addition several other microRNA-regulated pathways have been reported although additional experimental evidences are required to fully understand their contribution to AF. Importantly, large discrepancies are observed when transcriptomic analyses are compared. Therefore, efforts should be made to understand the nature of such discrepancy and to search for a common pathways that will serve us to undoubtfully unravel the transcriptomic hallmarks of AF pathophysiology.

Importantly, novel layers of complexity lay ahead of us requiring to decipher gene-gene interactions [94], microRNA-mRNA interactions [95–96] and microRNA-lncRNAs [100] in AF pathophysiology.

Understanding the functional impact of lncRNAs in AF is also major challenge. At present our understanding of lncRNAs is on its infancy. LncRNAs provide a wide array of cellular functions, impacting on both transcriptional and post-transcriptional regulation. They are evolutionarily poorly conserved and our current picture of the transcriptomics profile in AF reflects more controversy and doubts than certainties. Importantly integrative pathways also involved lncRNAs, including microRNAs [97] and mRNAs [98–99] regulation. In addition, disecting whether these non-coding RNAs exert their function in circulating plasma [100–101] or exosome-contained [102] will be of great important to solve current discrepancies. In the next coming years we will witness increasing evidences of the functional impact of lncRNAs in AF pathology as well as od additional non-coding RNAs, i.e. circRNAs, that just entered this arena [103–104].

References

1. Hakim FA, Shen WK. Atrial fibrillation in the elderly: a review. Fut Cardiol. 2014;10:745–58.
2. Abed HS, Wittert GA. Obesity and atrial fibrillation. Obes Rev. 2013;14:929–38.
3. Vargas-Uricoechea H, Sierra-Torres CH. Thyroid hormones and the heart. Horm Mol Biol Clin Investig. 2014;18:15–26.
4. Goudis CA, Korantzopoulos P, Ntalas IV, Kallergis EM, Liu T, Ketikoglou DG. Diabetes mellitus and atrial fibrillation: pathophysiological mechanisms and potential upstream therapies. Int J Cardiol. 2015;184:617–22.
5. Qaddoura A, Kabali C, Drew D, et al. Obstructive sleep apnea as a predictor of atrial fibrillation after coronary artery bypass grafting: a systematic review and meta-analysis. Can J Cardiol. 2014;30:1516–2522.
6. Akoum N, Marrouche N. Assessment and impact of cardiac fibrosis on atrial fibrillation. Curr Cardiol Rep. 2014;16:518.
7. Berenfeld O, Jalife J. Mechanisms of atrial fibrillation: rotors, ionic determinants, and excitation frequency. Cardiol Clin. 2014;32:495–506
8. Potpara TS, Lip GY. A brief history of 'lone' atrial fibrillation: from 'a peculiar pulse irregularity' to a modern public health concern. Curr Pharm Des. 2015;21:679–96.
9. Brugada R, Tapscott T, Czernuszewicz GZ, et al. Identification of a genetic locus for familial atrial fibrillation. N Engl J Med. 1997;336:905–11.
10. Lozano-Velasco E, Garcia-Padilla C, Aránega AE, Franco D. Genetics of atrial Fibrilation: in search of novel therapeutic targets. Cardiovasc Hematol Disord Drug Targets. 2019 Feb 6.
11. Gudbjartsson DF, Arnar DO, Helgadottir A, Gretarsdottir S, Holm H, Sigurdsson A, Jonasdottir A, Baker A, Thorleifsson G, Kristjansson K, Palsson A, Blondal T, Sulem P, Backman VM, Hardarson GA, Palsdottir E, Helgason A, Sigurjonsdottir R, Sverrisson JT, Kostulas K, Ng MC, Baum L, So WY, Wong KS, Chan JC, Furie KL, Greenberg SM, Sale M, Kelly P, CA MR, Smith EE, Rosand J, Hillert J, Ma RC, Ellinor PT, Thorgeirsson G, Gulcher JR, Kong A, Thorsteinsdottir U, Stefansson K. Variants conferring risk of atrial fibrillation on chromosome 4q25. Nature. 2007 Jul 19;448(7151):353–7.
12. Roselli C, Chaffin MD, Weng LC, Aeschbacher S, Ahlberg G, Albert CM, Almgren P, Alonso A, Anderson CD, Aragam KG, Arking DE, Barnard J, Bartz TM, Benjamin EJ, Bihlmeyer NA, Bis JC, Bloom HL, Boerwinkle E, Bottinger EB, Brody JA, Calkins H, Campbell A, Cappola TP, Carlquist J, Chasman DI, Chen LY, Chen YI, Choi EK, Choi SH, Christophersen IE, Chung MK, Cole JW, Conen D, Cook J, Crijns HJ, Cutler MJ, Damrauer SM, Daniels BR, Darbar D, Delgado G, Denny JC, Dichgans M, Dörr M, Dudink EA, Dudley SC, Esa N, Esko T, Eskola M, Fatkin D, Felix SB, Ford I, Franco OH, Geelhoed B, Grewal RP, Gudnason V, Guo X, Gupta N, Gustafsson S, Gutmann R, Hamsten A, Harris TB, Hayward C, Heckbert SR, Hernesniemi J, Hocking LJ, Hofman A, ARVR H, Huang J, Huang PL, Huffman J, Ingelsson E, Ipek EG, Ito K, Jimenez-Conde J, Johnson R, Jukema JW, Kääb S, Kähönen M, Kamatani Y, Kane JP, Kastrati A, Kathiresan S, Katschnig-Winter P, Kavousi M, Kessler T, Kietselaer BL, Kirchhof P, Kleber ME, Knight S, Krieger JE, Kubo M, Launer LJ, Laurikka J, Lehtimäki T, Leineweber K, Lemaitre RN, Li M, Lim HE, Lin HJ, Lin H, Lind L, Lindgren CM, Lokki ML, London B, RJF L, Low SK, Lu Y, Lyytikäinen LP, Macfarlane PW, Magnusson PK, Mahajan A,

Malik R, Mansur AJ, Marcus GM, Margolin L, Margulies KB, März W, DD MM, Melander O, Mohanty S, Montgomery JA, Morley MP, Morris AP, Müller-Nurasyid M, Natale A, Nazarian S, Neumann B, Newton-Cheh C, Niemeijer MN, Nikus K, Nilsson P, Noordam R, Oellers H, Olesen MS, Orho-Melander M, Padmanabhan S, Pak HN, Paré G, Pedersen NL, Pera J, Pereira A, Porteous D, Psaty BM, Pulit SL, Pullinger CR, Rader DJ, Refsgaard L, Ribasés M, Ridker PM, Rienstra M, Risch L, Roden DM, Rosand J, Rosenberg MA, Rost N, Rotter JI, Saba S, Sandhu RK, Schnabel RB, Schramm K, Schunkert H, Schurman C, Scott SA, Seppälä I, Shaffer C, Shah S, Shalaby AA, Shim J, Shoemaker MB, Siland JE, Sinisalo J, Sinner MF, Slowik A, Smith AV, Smith BH, Smith JG, Smith JD, Smith NL, Soliman EZ, Sotoodehnia N, Stricker BH, Sun A, Sun H, Svendsen JH, Tanaka T, Tanriverdi K, Taylor KD, Teder-Laving M, Teumer A, Thériault S, Trompet S, Tucker NR, Tveit A, Uitterlinden AG, Van Der Harst P, Van Gelder IC, Van Wagoner DR, Verweij N, Vlachopoulou E, Völker U, Wang B, Weeke PE, Weijs B, Weiss R, Weiss S, Wells QS, Wiggins KL, Wong JA, Woo D, Worrall BB, Yang PS, Yao J, Yoneda ZT, Zeller T, Zeng L, Lubitz SA, Lunetta KL, Ellinor PT. Multi-ethnic genome-wide association study for atrial fibrillation. Nat Genet. 2018 Jun 11;50(9):1225–33.

13. Wang J, Klysik E, Sood S, Johnson RL, Wehrens XH, Martin JF. Pitx2 prevents susceptibility to atrial arrhythmias by inhibiting left-sided pacemaker specification. Proc Natl Acad Sci U S A. 2010 May 25;107(21):9753–8.
14. Chinchilla A, Daimi H, Lozano-Velasco E, Dominguez JN, Caballero R, Delpón E, Tamargo J, Cinca J, Hove-Madsen L, Aranega AE, Franco D. PITX2 insufficiency leads to atrial electrical and structural remodeling linked to arrhythmogenesis. Circ Cardiovasc Genet. 2011 Jun;4(3):269–79.
15. Lozano-Velasco E, Hernández-Torres F, Daimi H, Serra SA, Herraiz A, Hove-Madsen L, Aránega A, Franco D. Pitx2 impairs calcium handling in a dosedependent manner by modulating Wnt signalling. Cardiovasc Res. 2016 Jan 1;109(1):55–66.
16. Lozano-Velasco E, Wangensteen R, Quesada A, Garcia-Padilla C, Osorio JA, Ruiz-Torres MD, Aranega A, Franco D. Hyperthyroidism, but not hypertension, impairs PITX2 expression leading to Wnt-microRNA-ion channel remodeling. PLoS One. 2017 Dec 1;12(12):e0188473.
17. Dueñas A, Expósito A, Aranega A, Franco D. The role of non-coding RNA in congenital heart diseases. J Cardiovasc Dev Dis. 2019 Apr 1;6(2). pii:E15.
18. Lozano-Velasco E, Garcia-Padilla C, Aránega AE, Franco D. Genetics Of Atrial Fibrilation: In Search Of Novel Therapeutic Targets. Cardiovasc Hematol DisordDrug Targets. 2019 Feb 6.
19. Rynkeviciene R, Simiene J, Strainiene E, Stankevicius V, Usinskiene J, Miseikyte Kaubriene E, Meskinyte I, Cicenas J, Suziedelis K. Non-coding RNAs in glioma. Cancers (Basel). 2018 Dec 22;11(1).. pii):E17.
20. Yamamoto T, Saitoh N. Non-coding RNAs and chromatin domains. Curr Opin Cell Biol. 2019 Jan 22;58:26–33.
21. Expósito-Villén A, E Aránega A, Franco D. Functional Role of Non-Coding RNAs during Epithelial-To-Mesenchymal Transition. Noncoding RNA. 2018 May 28;4(2).. pii:E14.
22. Fico A, Fiorenzano A, Pascale E, Patriarca EJ, Minchiotti G. Long non-coding RNA in stem cell pluripotency and lineage commitment: functions and evolutionary conservation. Cell Mol Life Sci. 2019 Apr;76(8):1459–71.
23. Saeedi Borujeni MJ, Esfandiary E, Baradaran A, Valiani A, Ghanadian M, Codoñer-Franch P, Basirat R, Alonso-Iglesias E, Mirzaei H, Yazdani A. Molecular aspects of pancreatic β-cell dysfunction: oxidative stress, microRNA, and long noncoding RNA. J Cell Physiol. 2019 Jun;234(6):8411–25.
24. Orenes-Piñero E, Quintana-Giner M, Romero-Aniorte AI, Valdés M, Marín F. Novel biomarkers in cardiology: MicroRNAs in atrial fibrillation. Arch Cardiol Mex. 2015 Jul-Sep;85(3):225–9.
25. Tsiachris D, Giannopoulos G, Kossyvakis C, Deftereos S, Tsioufis C, Siasos G, Oikonomou E, Gatzoulis K, Tousoulis D, Stefanadis C. Biomarkers determining prognosis of atrial fibrillation ablation. Curr Med Chem. 2018 Mar 20;
26. Wang M, Sun L, Ding W, Cai S, Zhao Q. Ablation alleviates atrial fibrillation by regulating the signaling pathways of endothelial nitric oxide synthase/nitric oxide via miR-155-5p and miR-24-3p. J Cell Biochem. 2019 Mar;120(3):4451–62.
27. Feldman A, Moreira DAR, Gun C, Wang HL, Hirata MH, de Freitas GJ, Leite GGS, Farsky P. Analysis of circulating miR-1, miR-23a, and miR-26a in atrial fibrillation patients undergoing coronary bypass artery grafting surgery. Ann Hum Genet. 2017 May;81(3):99–105.
28. Harling L, Lambert J, Ashrafian H, Darzi A, Gooderham NJ, Athanasiou T. Elevated serum microRNA 483-5p levels may predict patients at risk of postoperative atrial fibrillation. Eur J Cardiothorac Surg. 2017 Jan;51(1):73–8.
29. Liu T, Zhong S, Rao F, Xue Y, Qi Z, Wu S. Catheter ablation restores decreased plasmamiR-409-3p and miR-432 in atrial fibrillation patients. Europace. 2016 Jan;18(1):92–9.
30. Soeki T, Matsuura T, Bando S, Tobiume T, Uematsu E, Ise T, Kusunose K, Yamaguchi K, Yagi S, Fukuda D, Yamada H, Wakatsuki T, Shimabukuro M, Sata M. Relationship between local production of microRNA-328 and atrial substrate remodeling in atrial fibrillation. J Cardiol. 2016 Dec;68(6):472–7.
31. Zhou Q, Maleck C, von Ungern-Sternberg SNI, Neupane B, Heinzmann D, Marquardt J, Duckheim M, Scheckenbach C, Stimpfle F, Gawaz M, Schreieck J, Seizer P, Gramlich M. Circulating MicroRNA-21

correlates with left atrial Low-voltage areas and is associated with procedure outcome in patients undergoing atrial fibrillation ablation. Circ Arrhythm Electrophysiol. 2018 Jun;11(6):e006242.
32. Shen XB, Zhang SH, Li HY, Chi XD, Jiang L, Huang QL, Xu SH. Rs12976445 Polymorphism is associated with post-ablation recurrence of atrial fibrillation by modulating the expression of MicroRNA-125a and interleukin-6R. Med Sci Monit. 2018 Sep 11;24:6349–58.
33. Su YM, Li J, Guo YF, Cai F, Cai XX, Pan HY, Deng XT, Pan M. A functional single-nucleotide polymorphism in pre-microRNA-196a2 is associated with atrial fibrillation in Han Chinese. Clin Lab. 2015;61(9):1179–85.
34. Jin Y, Zhou TY, Cao JN, Feng QT, Fu YJ, Xu X, Yang CJ. MicroRNA-206 downregulates Connexin43 in cardiomyocytes to induce cardiac arrhythmias in a transgenic mouse model. Heart Lung Circ. 2018 Oct 4;S1443–9506(18). pii:): 31917–6.
35. Li S, Jiang Z, Wen L, Feng G, Zhong G. MicroRNA-208a-3p contributes to connexin40 remolding in human chronic atrial fibrillation. Exp Ther Med. 2017 Dec;14(6):5355–62.
36. Takahashi K, Sasano T, Sugiyama K, Kurokawa J, Tamura N, Soejima Y, Sawabe M, Isobe M, Furukawa T. High-fat diet increases vulnerability to atrial arrhythmia by conduction disturbance via miR-27b. J Mol Cell Cardiol. 2016 Jan;90:38–46.
37. Zhao Y, Huang Y, Li W, Wang Z, Zhan S, Zhou M, Yao Y, Zeng Z, Hou Y, Chen Q, Tu X, Wang QK, Huang Z. Post-transcriptional regulation of cardiac sodium channel gene SCN5A expression and function by miR-192-5p. Biochim Biophys Acta. 2015 Oct;1852(10 Pt A):2024–34.
38. Girmatsion Z, Biliczki P, Bonauer A, Wimmer-Greinecker G, Scherer M, Moritz A, Bukowska A, Goette A, Nattel S, Hohnloser SH, Ehrlich JR. Changes in microRNA-1 expression and IK1 up-regulation in human atrial fibrillation. Heart Rhythm. 2009 Dec;6(12):1802–9.
39. Jia X, Zheng S, Xie X, Zhang Y, Wang W, Wang Z, Zhang Y, Wang J, Gao M, Hou Y. MicroRNA-1 accelerates the shortening of atrial effective refractory period by regulating KCNE1 and KCNB2 expression: an atrial tachypacing rabbit model. PLoS One. 2013 Dec 30;8(12):e85639.
40. Luo X, Pan Z, Shan H, Xiao J, Sun X, Wang N, Lin H, Xiao L, Maguy A, Qi XY, Li Y, Gao X, Dong D, Zhang Y, Bai Y, Ai J, Sun L, Lu H, Luo XY, Wang Z, Lu Y, Yang B, Nattel S. MicroRNA-26 governs profibrillatory inward-rectifier potassium current changes in atrial fibrillation. J Clin Invest. 2013 May;123(5):1939–51.
41. Barana A, Matamoros M, Dolz-Gaitón P, Pérez-Hernández M, Amorós I, Núñez M, Sacristán S, Pedraz Á, Pinto Á, Fernández-Avilés F, Tamargo J, Delpón E, Caballero R. Chronic atrial fibrillation increases microRNA-21 in human atrial myocytes decreasing L-type calcium current. Circ Arrhythm Electrophysiol. 2014 Oct;7(5):861–8.
42. Zhao Y, Yuan Y, Qiu C. Underexpression of CACNA1C caused by overexpression of microRNA-29a underlies the pathogenesis of atrial fibrillation. Med Sci Monit. 2016 Jun 24;22:2175–81.
43. Ling TY, Wang XL, Chai Q, Lu T, Stulak JM, Joyce LD, Daly RC, Greason KL, Wu LQ, Shen WK, Cha YM, Lee HC. Regulation of cardiac CACNB2 by microRNA-499: potential role in atrial fibrillation. BBA Clin. 2017 Feb 9;7:78–84.
44. Chiang DY, Zhang M, Voigt N, Alsina KM, Jakob H, Martin JF, Dobrev D, Wehrens XH, Li N. Identification of microRNA-mRNA dysregulations in paroxysmal atrial fibrillation. Int J Cardiol. 2015 Apr 1;184:190–7.
45. Ling TY, Wang XL, Chai Q, Lau TW, Koestler CM, Park SJ, Daly RC, Greason KL, Jen J, Wu LQ, Shen WF, Shen WK, Cha YM, Lee HC. Regulation of the SK3 channel by microRNA-499DOUBLE-HYPHENpotential role in atrial fibrillation. Heart Rhythm. 2013 Jul;10(7):1001–9.
46. Cañón S, Caballero R, Herraiz-Martínez A, Pérez-Hernández M, López B, Atienza F, Jalife J, Hove-Madsen L, Delpón E, Bernad A. miR-208b upregulation interferes with calcium handling in HL-1 atrial myocytes: implications in human chronic atrial fibrillation. J Mol Cell Cardiol. 2016 Oct;99:162–73.
47. Li YD, Hong YF, Yusufuaji Y, Tang BP, Zhou XH, Xu GJ, Li JX, Sun L, Zhang JH, Xin Q, Xiong J, Ji YT, Zhang Y. Altered expression of hyperpolarizationactivated cyclic nucleotide-gated channels and microRNA-1 and -133 in patients with age-associated atrial fibrillation. Mol Med Rep. 2015 Sep;12(3):3243–8.
48. Chiang DY, Kongchan N, Beavers DL, Alsina KM, Voigt N, Neilson JR, Jakob H, Martin JF, Dobrev D, Wehrens XH, Li N. Loss of microRNA-106b-25 cluster promotes atrial fibrillation by enhancing ryanodine receptor type-2 expression and calcium release. Circ Arrhythm Electrophysiol. 2014 Dec;7(6):1214–22.
49. Wang J, Bai Y, Li N, Ye W, Zhang M, Greene SB, Tao Y, Chen Y, Wehrens XH, Martin JF. Pitx2-microRNA pathway that delimits sinoatrial node development and inhibits predisposition to atrial fibrillation. Proc Natl Acad Sci U S A. 2014 Jun 24;111(25):9181–6.
50. Li H, Li S, Yu B, Liu S. Expression of miR-133 and miR-30 in chronic atrial fibrillation in canines. Mol Med Rep. 2012 Jun;5(6):1457–60.
51. Shan H, Zhang Y, Lu Y, Zhang Y, Pan Z, Cai B, Wang N, Li X, Feng T, Hong Y, Yang B. Downregulation of miR-133 and miR-590 contributes to nicotineinduced atrial remodelling in canines. Cardiovasc Res. 2009 Aug 1;83(3):465–72.
52. Wang Y, Cai H, Li H, Gao Z, Song K. Atrial overexpression of microRNA-27b attenuates angiotensin II-induced atrial fibrosis and fibrillation by targeting ALK5. Hum Cell. 2018 Jul;31(3):251–60.

53. Xu J, Wu H, Chen S, Qi B, Zhou G, Cai L, Zhao L, Wei Y, Liu S. MicroRNA-30c suppresses the profibrogenic effects of cardiac fibroblasts induced by TGF-β1 and prevents atrial fibrosis by targeting TGFβRII. J Cell Mol Med. 2018 Jun;22(6):3045–57.
54. Qiao G, Xia D, Cheng Z, Zhang G. miR-132 in atrial fibrillation directly targets connective tissue growth factor. Mol Med Rep. 2017 Oct;16(4):4143–50.
55. Yuan CT, Li XX, Cheng QJ, Wang YH, Wang JH, Liu CL. MiR-30a regulates the atrial fibrillation-induced myocardial fibrosis by targeting snail 1. Int J Clin Exp Pathol. 2015 Dec 1;8(12):15527–36.
56. Cao W, Shi P, Ge JJ. miR-21 enhances cardiac fibrotic remodeling and fibroblast proliferation via CADM1/STAT3 pathway. BMC Cardiovasc Disord. 2017 Mar 23;17(1):88.
57. Tao H, Zhang M, Yang JJ, Shi KH. MicroRNA-21 via dysregulation of WW domain-containing protein 1 regulate atrial fibrosis in atrial fibrillation. Heart Lung Circ. 2018 Jan;27(1):104–13.
58. Cardin S, Guasch E, Luo X, Naud P, Le Quang K, Shi Y, Tardif JC, Comtois P, Nattel S. Role for MicroRNA-21 in atrial profibrillatory fibrotic remodeling associated with experimental postinfarction heart failure. Circ Arrhythm Electrophysiol. 2012 Oct;5(5):1027–35.
59. Adam O, Löhfelm B, Thum T, Gupta SK, Puhl SL, Schäfers HJ, Böhm M, Laufs U. Role of miR-21 in the pathogenesis of atrial fibrosis. Basic Res Cardiol. 2012 Sep;107(5):278.
60. Zhang X, Jing W. Upregulation of miR-122 is associated with cardiomyocyte apoptosis in atrial fibrillation. Mol Med Rep. 2018 Aug;18(2):1745–51.
61. Tsoporis JN, Fazio A, Rizos IK, Izhar S, Proteau G, Salpeas V, Rigopoulos A, Sakadakis E, Toumpoulis IK, Parker TG. Increased right atrial appendage apoptosis is associated with differential regulation of candidate MicroRNAs 1 and 133A in patients who developed atrial fibrillation after cardiac surgery. J Mol Cell Cardiol. 2018 Aug;121:25–32.
62. Yang Z, Xiao Z, Guo H, Fang X, Liang J, Zhu J, Yang J, Li H, Pan R, Yuan S, Dong W, Zheng XL, Wu S, Shan Z. Novel role of the clustered miR-23b-3p and miR-27b-3p in enhanced expression of fibrosis-associated genes by targeting TGFBR3 in atrial fibroblasts. J Cell Mol Med. 2019 Feb;7
63. Zhu Y, Feng Z, Cheng W, Xiao Y. MicroRNA-34a mediates atrial fibrillation through regulation of Ankyrin-B expression. Mol Med Rep. 2018 Jun;17(6):8457–65.
64. Zhang K, Zhao L, Ma Z, Wang W, Li X, Zhang Y, Yuan M, Liang X, Li G. Doxycycline attenuates atrial remodeling by interfering with MicroRNA-21 and downstream phosphatase and Tensin homolog (PTEN)/phosphoinositide 3-kinase (PI3K) signaling pathway. Med Sci Monit. 2018 Aug 11;24:5580–7.
65. Huang Z, Chen XJ, Qian C, Dong Q, Ding D, Wu QF, Li J, Wang HF, Li WH, Xie Q, Cheng X, Zhao N, Du YM, Liao YH. Signal transducer and activator of transcription 3/MicroRNA-21 feedback loop contributes to atrial fibrillation by promoting atrial fibrosis in a rat sterile pericarditis model. Circ Arrhythm Electrophysiol. 2016 Jul;9(7). pii:e003396.
66. He X, Zhang K, Gao X, Li L, Tan H, Chen J, Zhou Y. Rapid atrial pacing induces myocardial fibrosis by down-regulating Smad7 via microRNA-21 in rabbit. Heart Vessel. 2016 Oct;31(10):1696–708.
67. Reilly SN, Liu X, Carnicer R, Recalde A, Muszkiewicz A, Jayaram R, Carena MC, Wijesurendra R, Stefanini M, Surdo NC, Lomas O, Ratnatunga C, Sayeed R, Krasopoulos G, Rajakumar T, Bueno-Orovio A, Verheule S, Fulga TA, Rodriguez B, Schotten U, Casadei B. Up-regulation of miR-31 in human atrial fibrillation begets the arrhythmia by depleting dystrophin and neuronal nitric oxide synthase. Sci Transl Med. 2016 May 25;8(340):340ra74.
68. Yamac AH, Kucukbuzcu S, Ozansoy M, Gok O, Oz K, Erturk M, Yilmaz E, Ersoy B, Zeybek R, Goktekin O, Kilic U. Altered expression of micro-RNA 199a and increased levels of cardiac SIRT1 protein are associated with the occurrence of atrial fibrillation after coronary artery bypass graft surgery. Cardiovasc Pathol. 2016 May-Jun;25(3):232–6.
69. da Silva AMG, de Araújo JNG, de Oliveira KM, Novaes AEM, Lopes MB, de Sousa JCV, Filho AAA, Luchessi AD, de Rezende AA, Hirata MH, Silbiger VN. Circulating miRNAs in acute new-onset atrial fibrillation and their target mRNA network. J Cardiovasc Electrophysiol. 2018 Aug;29(8):1159–66.
70. Zhang Y, Zheng S, Geng Y, Xue J, Wang Z, Xie X, Wang J, Zhang S, Hou Y. MicroRNA profiling of atrial fibrillation in canines: miR-206 modulates intrinsic cardiac autonomic nerve remodeling by regulating SOD1. PLoS One. 2015 Mar 27;10(3):e0122674.
71. Torrado M, Franco D, Lozano-Velasco E, Hernández-Torres F, Calviño R, Aldama G, Centeno A, Castro-Beiras A, Mikhailov A. A MicroRNA-transcription factor blueprint for early atrial Arrhythmogenic remodeling. Biomed Res Int. 2015;2015:263151.
72. Slagsvold KH, Johnsen AB, Rognmo O, Høydal M, Wisløff U, Wahba A. Comparison of left versus right atrial myocardium in patients with sinus rhythm or atrial fibrillation - an assessment of mitochondrial function and microRNA expression. Physiol Rep. 2014 Aug 28;2(8). pii:e12124.
73. Slagsvold KH, Johnsen AB, Rognmo O, Høydal MA, Wisløff U, Wahba A. Mitochondrial respiration and microRNA expression in right and left atrium of patients with atrial fibrillation. Physiol Genomics. 2014 Jul 15;46(14):505–11.
74. Doñate Puertas R, Jalabert A, Meugnier E, Euthine V, Chevalier P, Rome S. Analysis of the microRNA signature in left atrium from patients with valvular heart disease reveals their implications in atrial fibrillation. PLoS One. 2018 May 3;13(5):e0196666.
75. Liu H, Chen GX, Liang MY, Qin H, Rong J, Yao JP, Wu ZK. Atrial fibrillation alters the microRNA

expression profiles of the left atria of patients with mitral stenosis. BMC Cardiovasc Disord. 2014 Jan 25;14:10.

76. Xiao J, Liang D, Zhang Y, Liu Y, Zhang H, Liu Y, Li L, Liang X, Sun Y, Chen YH. MicroRNA expression signature in atrial fibrillation with mitral stenosis. Physiol Genomics. 2011 Jun 15;43(11):655–64.
77. Cooley N, Cowley MJ, Lin RC, Marasco S, Wong C, Kaye DM, Dart AM, Woodcock EA. Influence of atrial fibrillation on microRNA expression profiles in left and right atria from patients with valvular heart disease. Physiol Genomics. 2012 Feb 13;44(3):211–9.
78. Liu H, Qin H, Chen GX, Liang MY, Rong J, Yao JP, Wu ZK. Comparative expression profiles of microRNA in left and right atrial appendages from patients with rheumatic mitral valve disease exhibiting sinus rhythm or atrial fibrillation. J Transl Med. 2014 Apr 6;12:90.
79. Yan Y, Shi R, Yu X, Sun C, Zang W, Tian H. Identification of atrial fibrillation-associated microRNAs in left and right atria of rheumatic mitral valve disease patients. Genes Genet Syst. 2018 Dec 24;
80. Wang J, Song S, Xie C, Han J, Li Y, Shi J, Xin M, Wang J, Luo T, Meng X, Yang B. MicroRNA profiling in the left atrium in patients with non-valvular paroxysmal atrial fibrillation. BMC Cardiovasc Disord. 2015 Aug 29;15:97.
81. McManus DD, Tanriverdi K, Lin H, Esa N, Kinno M, Mandapati D, Tam S, Okike ON, Ellinor PT, Keaney JF Jr, Donahue JK, Benjamin EJ, Freedman JE. Plasma microRNAs are associated with atrial fibrillation and change after catheter ablation (the miRhythm study). Heart Rhythm. 2015 Jan;12(1):3–10.
82. Nishi H, Sakaguchi T, Miyagawa S, Yoshikawa Y, Fukushima S, Saito S, Ueno T, Kuratani T, Sawa Y. Impact of microRNA expression in human atrial tissue in patients with atrial fibrillation undergoing cardiac surgery. PLoS One. 2013 Sep 12;8(9):e73397.
83. Gore-Panter SR, Hsu J, Barnard J, Moravec CS, Van Wagoner DR, Chung MK, Smith JD. PANCR, the PITX2 adjacent noncoding RNA, is expressed in human left atria and regulates PITX2c expression. Circ Arrhythm Electrophysiol. 2016 Jan;9(1):e003197.
84. Shen C, Kong B, Liu Y, Xiong L, Shuai W, Wang G, Quan D, Huang H. YY1-induced upregulation of lncRNA KCNQ1OT1 regulates angiotensin II-induced atrial fibrillation by modulating miR-384b/CACNA1C axis. Biochem Biophys Res Commun. 2018 Oct 20;505(1):134–40.
85. Zhao JB, Zhu N, Lei YH, Zhang CJ, Li YH. Modulative effects of lncRNA TCONS_00202959 on autonomic neural function and myocardial functions in atrial fibrillation rat model. Eur Rev Med Pharmacol Sci. 2018 Dec;22(24):8891–7.
86. Cao F, Li Z, Ding WM, Yan L, Zhao QY. LncRNA PVT1 regulates atrial fibrosis via miR-128-3p-SP1-TGF-β1-Smad axis in atrial fibrillation. Mol Med. 2019 Mar 20;25(1):7.
87. Ruan Z, Sun X, Sheng H, Zhu L. Long non-coding RNA expression profile in atrial fibrillation. Int J Clin Exp Pathol. 2015 Jul 1;8(7):8402–10.
88. Mei B, Liu H, Yang S, Liang MY, Yue Y, Huang SQ, Hou J, Chen GX, Wu ZK. Long non-coding RNA expression profile in permanent atrial fibrillation patients with rheumatic heart disease. Eur Rev Med Pharmacol Sci. 2018 Oct;22(20):6940–7.
89. Wu J, Han D, Shi R, Chen M, Sun J, Tian H, Yan Y. Identification of atrial fibrillation-associated lncRNAs in atria from patients with rheumatic mitral valve disease. Microsc Res Tech. 2019 Apr 11;
90. Chen G, Guo H, Song Y, Chang H, Wang S, Zhang M, Liu C. Long non-coding RNA AK055347 is upregulated in patients with atrial fibrillation and regulates mitochondrial energy production in myocardiocytes. Mol Med Rep. 2016 Dec;14(6):5311–7.
91. Su Y, Li L, Zhao S, Yue Y, Yang S. The long non-coding RNA expression profiles of paroxysmal atrial fibrillation identified by microarray analysis. Gene. 2018 Feb 5;642:125–34.
92. Li Z, Wang X, Wang W, Du J, Wei J, Zhang Y, Wang J, Hou Y. Altered long non-coding RNA expression profile in rabbit atria with atrial fibrillation: TCONS_00075467 modulates atrial electrical remodeling by sponging miR-328 to regulate CACNA1C. J Mol Cell Cardiol. 2017 Jul;108:73–85.
93. Wang W, Wang X, Zhang Y, Li Z, Xie X, Wang J, Gao M, Zhang S, Hou Y. Transcriptome analysis of canine cardiac fat pads: involvement of two novel long non-coding RNAs in atrial fibrillation neural remodeling. J Cell Biochem. 2015 May;116(5):809–21.
94. Huang Y, Wang C, Yao Y, Zuo X, Chen S, Xu C, Zhang H, Lu Q, Chang L, Wang F, Wang P, Zhang R, Hu Z, Song Q, Yang X, Li C, Li S, Zhao Y, Yang Q, Yin D, Wang X, Si W, Li X, Xiong X, Wang D, Huang Y, Luo C, Li J, Wang J, Chen J, Wang L, Wang L, Han M, Ye J, Chen F, Liu J, Liu Y, Wu G, Yang B, Cheng X, Liao Y, Wu Y, Ke T, Chen Q, Tu X, Elston R, Rao S, Yang Y, Xia Y, Wang QK. Molecular basis of gene-gene interaction: cyclic cross-regulation of gene expression and post-GWAS gene-gene interaction involved in atrial fibrillation. PLoS Genet. 2015 Aug 12;11(8):e1005393.
95. Wang T, Wang B. Identification of microRNA-mRNA interactions in atrial fibrillation using microarray expression profiles and bioinformatics analysis. Mol Med Rep. 2016 Jun;13(6):4535–40.
96. Wang J, Wang Y, Han J, Li Y, Xie C, Xie L, Shi J, Zhang J, Yang B, Chen D, Meng X. Integrated analysis of microRNA and mRNA expression profiles in the left atrium of patients with nonvalvular paroxysmal atrial fibrillation: role of miR-

146b-5p in atrial fibrosis. Heart Rhythm. 2015 May;12(5):1018–26.

97. Qian C, Li H, Chang D, Wei B, Wang Y. Identification of functional lncRNAs in atrial fibrillation by integrative analysis of the lncRNA-mRNA network based on competing endogenous RNAs hypothesis. J Cell Physiol. 2018 Nov;27
98. Yu XJ, Zou LH, Jin JH, Xiao F, Li L, Liu N, Yang JF, Zou T. Long noncoding RNAs and novel inflammatory genes determined by RNA sequencing in human lymphocytes are up-regulated in permanent atrial fibrillation. Am J Transl Res. 2017 May 15;9(5):2314–26.
99. Xu Y, Huang R, Gu J, Jiang W. Identification of long non-coding RNAs as novel biomarker and potential therapeutic target for atrial fibrillation in old adults. Oncotarget. 2016 Mar 8;7(10):10803–11.
100. Lu Y, Hou S, Huang D, Luo X, Zhang J, Chen J, Xu W. Expression profile analysis of circulating microRNAs and their effects on ion channels in Chinese atrial fibrillation patients. Int J Clin Exp Med. 2015 Jan 15;8(1):845–53.
101. Natsume Y, Oaku K, Takahashi K, Nakamura W, Oono A, Hamada S, Yamazoe M, Ihara K, Sasaki T, Goya M, Hirao K, Furukawa T, Sasano T. Combined analysis of human and experimental murine samples identified novel circulating MicroRNAs as biomarkers for atrial fibrillation. Circ J. 2018 Mar 23;82(4):965–73.
102. Mun D, Kim H, Kang JY, Park H, Park H, Lee SH, Yun N, Joung B. Expression of miRNAs in circulating exosomes derived from patients with persistent atrial fibrillation. FASEB J. 2019 Feb 12:fj201801758R.
103. Hu M, Wei X, Li M, Tao L, Wei L, Zhang M, Cheng H, Yuan Y. Circular RNA expression profiles of persistent atrial fibrillation in patients with rheumatic heart disease. Anatol J Cardiol. 2019 Jan;21(1):2–10.
104. Zhang Y, Ke X, Liu J, Ma X, Liu Y, Liang D, Wang L, Guo C, Luo Y. Characterization of circRNA-associated ceRNA networks in patients with nonvalvular persistent atrial fibrillation. Mol Med Rep. 2019 Jan;19(1):638–50.

Y RNAs: Biogenesis, Function and Implications for the Cardiovascular System

20

Nedyalka Valkov and Saumya Das

Abstract

In recent years, progress in the field of high-throughput sequencing technology and its application to a wide variety of biological specimens has greatly advanced the discovery and cataloging of a diverse set of non-coding RNAs (ncRNAs) that have been found to have unexpected biological functions. Y RNAs are an emerging class of highly conserved, small ncRNAs. There is a growing number of reports in the literature demonstrating that Y RNAs and their fragments are not just random degradation products but are themselves bioactive molecules. This review will outline what is currently known about Y RNA including biogenesis, structure and functional roles. In addition, we will provide an overview of studies reporting the presence and functions attributed to Y RNAs in the cardiovascular system.

Keywords

Non-coding RNA · Y RNA · Cardiovascular diseases

N. Valkov · S. Das (✉)
Cardiovascular Research Center of Massachusetts General Hospital and Harvard Medical School, Boston, MA, USA
e-mail: sdas@mgh.harvard.edu

1 Introduction and Historical Overview

Only about 1.5% of the human genome is made up of protein-coding genes, but at least 80% of the genome is dynamically transcribed, creating a transcriptional landscape mainly dominated by non-coding RNAs (ncRNAs) [1, 2]. Nowadays, regulatory ncRNAs, such as the well-studied microRNAs (miRNAs) or long non-coding RNAs (lncRNAs) are recognized as essential functional molecules, and have significantly impacted our understanding of development, homeostasis and disease in various fields, including cardiovascular biology [3, 4], cancer [5, 6] and metabolic disorders [7, 8]. There are numerous examples in the literature of ncRNAs demonstrated to control key genes involved in both normal development and disease [9, 10]. There are also many instances highlighting how ncRNA dysregulation is tightly linked to the pathogenesis of many human disorders, including cardiovascular diseases (CVDs) [11–13]. From this body of research, the possibility of using ncRNAs as potential therapeutic targets and diagnostic tools has generated considerable interest among academic scientists and pharma/biotechnology commercial entities alike.

While miRNA and lncRNAs have garnered the most attention among the different types of ncRNAs, recent investigations have illuminated the increasingly diverse functions of other types

J. Xiao (ed.), *Non-coding RNAs in Cardiovascular Diseases*, Advances in Experimental Medicine and Biology 1229, https://doi.org/10.1007/978-981-15-1671-9_20

of ncRNAs [14–17]. Among the ncRNAs, Y RNAs are among the least studied species, but are recently gaining attention. Y RNAs were discovered in the early 1980s, during the characterization of serum from patients with the autoimmune disease systemic lupus erythematosis (SLE) [18]. Lerner and colleagues set out to uncover the molecular nature of the targets of the antibodies produced during the autoimmune response. Initially the group immunoprecipitated nuclear cell extracts from mouse derived tumor cells using serum from SLE patients containing antibodies against the proteins Ro and La, common autoantigens and targets of the immune system in rheumatic diseases like SLE. They discovered a class of small nuclear ncRNA, U RNA, associated with ribonucleoproteins (RNPs), as autoantigens [19]. In a following study, they used whole cell extracts and reacted with serum containing antibodies to Ro and La [18]. In the second time of experiments, they identified small cytoplasmic RNAs associated with RNPs, which they termed Y RNAs, to differentiate them from the nuclear U RNAs [18]. After these initial observations, Y RNAs have been reported to participate in other ribonucleoprotein complexes, leading to the proposition that Y-RNAs may play a role in scaffolding and assembly of RNA-protein complexes, but that their diverse functions are dependent in part, on the composition of the interacting proteins present in the complexes [20]. Y RNAs are highly conserved throughout evolution, and have been found in all vertebrates [21, 22], and related orthologs have also been reported in some bacteria [23] and nematodes [24, 25], but so far not in plants, fungi or insects. Y RNAs are expressed in all human cells; however levels of different Y RNAs vary among cell types [21]. Their expression also differs among human tissue types, with high levels reported in the heart and brain and lower amounts in the liver [26]. Furthermore, differential Y RNA expression has also been found in disease, including coronary artery disease [27] and cancer [28], pointing towards potential involvement of Y RNAs in the pathogenesis of these disorders. Finally, although the field of Y RNA has developed slowly since their discovery, functional roles of Y RNAs are beginning to be unveiled in various research fields, providing evidence that these ncRNAs may themselves be bioactive, and not simply structural RNAs involved only in scaffolding and assembly. This review will focus on the current state of knowledge about the biogenesis, structure and functional roles of Y RNAs. In addition, we will provide an updated summary of examples of Y RNAs, known or suggested to be involved in cardiovascular functions.

2 Biogenesis, Structure and Localization of Y RNAs

Y RNAs are encoded by individual genes and tend to reside in close proximity to each other, usually clustered on the same chromosome [29, 30]. There are four Y RNA genes denoted, Y1, Y3, Y4 and Y5 (Y2 is a truncated form of Y1) [31]. The number of individual Y RNAs differ between species. For example, in humans, all four Y RNAs are expressed, and range in size from 84 to 113 nts [32]. Rodents, on the other hand have only two Y RNAs, which are orthologs of human hY1 and hY3, but their genomes have a redundant Y5 RNA gene that is no longer expressed [33]. Both human and mouse Y RNAs have been shown to have few if any modified nucleotides [31]. Along with the annotated genes, the human genome has numerous Y RNA sequences documented as pseudogenes that are transcribed, in contrast to mice which have few [33, 34]. Y RNAs are transcribed in the nucleus by RNA polymerase III (Fig. 20.1) [32]. Transcription stops within a T-rich stretch, producing a 3′ oligo-uridinylated (Oligo-U) sequence, which serves as a binding site for La protein. Binding of La to the 3′ Oligo-U tail of Y-RNA protects YRNA from 3′ to 5′ exonucleolytic degradation and promotes its nuclear retention [35, 36]. In addition to La protein, the newly synthesized transcript also associates with Ro60 [21, 37]. The resulting Ro-RNP complex is then exported to the cytoplasm, which is mediated by Ran GTPase and exportin-5 [38]. Some Ro-RNPs, however, like the Y5 RNP remain in the nucleus

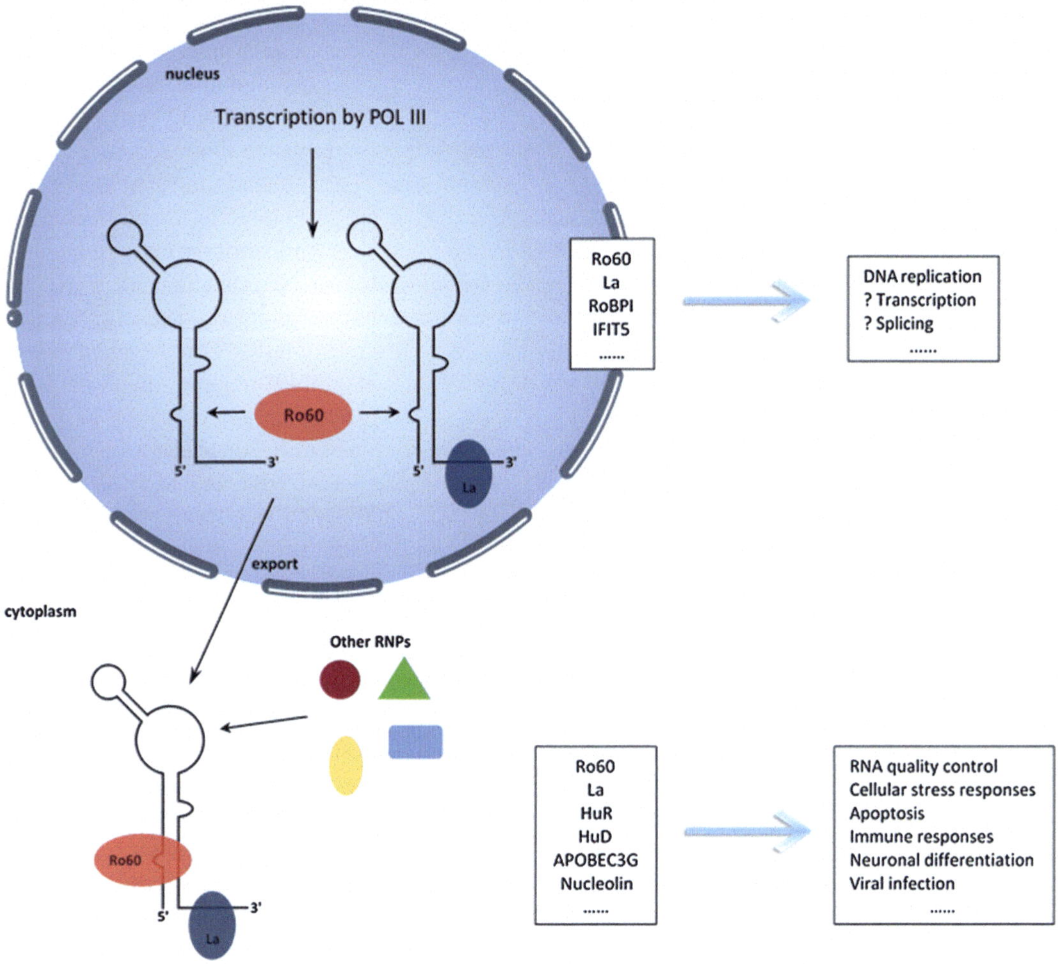

Fig. 20.1 Y RNAs cellular functions based on the association with RNA binding proteins (RNPs)

[39], while others, such as Y3 RNA, can be exported by an alternative pathway through binding of Y3 RNP with zipcode binding protein (ZBP1), allowing export by exportin-1 [40]. It is currently unknow whether Y RNA is bound in a complex with La during the nuclear export, or it could be that La re-associates with Y-RNA after translocation (Fig. 20.1).

Structural experiments have revealed that Y RNAs fold into distinct hairpin-containing structures, formed by base-pairing the 3′ and 5′ ends of the mature form of Y RNA (Fig. 20.2) [42, 43]. A defining feature of vertebrate Y RNAs is that these RNAs have at least two main stems each, separated by a large pyrimidine-rich single stranded loop [32], but individual Y-RNAs differ slightly in their primary and secondary structures [43]. The Y RNA stems are usually not ideal double strands. Often within the stem, there is also a bulged helix region. One of these, the main stem at the 5′/3′ end, is a highly conserved cytosine bulge, which is the high affinity binding site for Ro60 [44]. It has been shown that mutation or cleavage of this cite inhibits Ro60 binding and disrupts the entire Y RNA folding [35, 44, 45]. In addition, it has been demonstrated that the lower stem structure of Y RNA is important for efficient nuclear export, as cleavage of the lower stem of hY1 RNA in Xenopus laevis oocyte blocks export of the Y RNA into the cytoplasm [38].

Ro60 is both nuclear and cytoplasmic [37, 46] and is found in most animal cells and in some

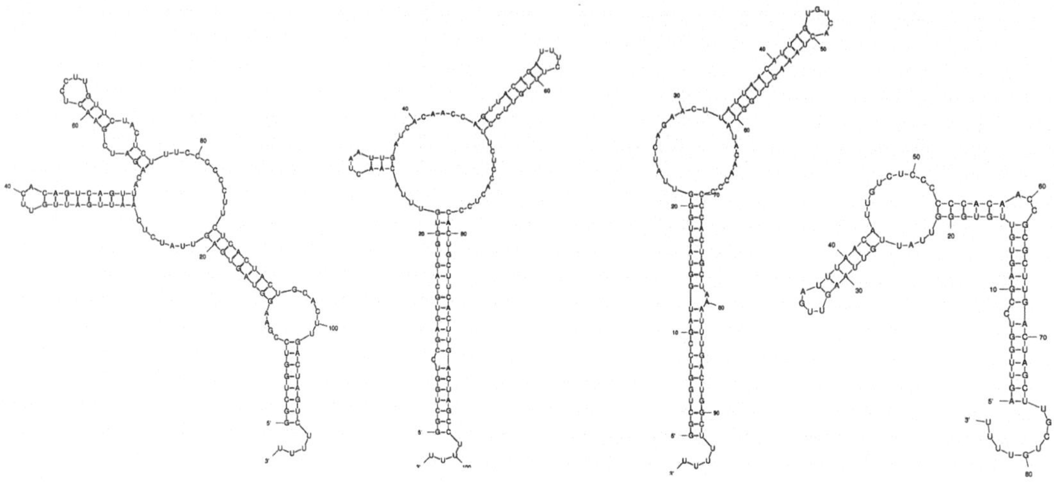

hY1 (113nt) hY3 (102nt) hY4 (96nt) hY5 (84nt)

Fig. 20.2 Full-length human Y RNA (hY) secondary structure. Structures are drawn using Mfold software [41]

bacteria [45]. Immunoprecipitation studies from human and mouse cells have shown that most Y RNAs exist as Ro60 RNP complexes [32, 37]. Ro60 binding to Y RNA was found to be important for successful Y RNA nuclear export [35] and to stabilize Y RNA in the cytoplasm, as siRNAs mediated knockdown of Ro60 in human keratinocytes was shown to significantly reduce Y RNA levels [47]. In contrast to the highly conserved lower stem region, the loops of Y RNAs differ greatly among individual Y RNAs and are quite flexible in nature [42]. Importantly, the loop domain has been reported to bind various proteins such as polypyrimidine tract-binding protein (PTB/hnRNP I) [48], nucleolin [49], and ZBP1 (Fig. 20.1) [50]. The effects of Y RNA interactions with these proteins are largely unknown, but it has been proposed that they could impact Y RNA localization and function [51]. Evidence for this was provided in experiments demonstrating that depletion of mouse IGF2BP1 and its chicken ortholog ZBP1, both of which directly associate with Y3, leads to nuclear accumulation of Ro60 and Y3, suggesting participation of these proteins in the nuclear export of Ro60/Y RNA complex [40, 52]. On the other hand, Y RNA itself can affect the subcellular distribution of Y RNA binding proteins. This was supported by the finding that depletion of Y RNA in mouse cells results in nuclear accumulation of Ro60, while binding of Y RNA to a Ro60 nuclear localization signal sequence promotes retaining of the RoRNPs in the cytosol [20, 45].

There are discrepancies in the literature in terms of the relative Y RNA distribution in the cytoplasm and nucleus, which may be attributed to the different experimental procedures used in the studies and/or the physiological state of the cells [53–55]. Initial cell fractionation studies in mammalian cultures and X laevis oocytes showed that Y RNAs were primarily cytoplasmic [37, 56, 57]. Later it was demonstrated that human and mouse Y5 localizes mainly to the nucleus, while Y1, Y3 and Y4 were found to be mostly cytoplasmic [39]. By using, ultrastructural and *in situ* hybridization experiments in human cells, others have demonstrated that Y RNAs can accumulate in both the nucleus and the cytosol at distinct compartments [58, 59]. Furthermore, in an *in vitro* system, where G1 phase template nuclei were incubated with fluorescently-labeled hY RNAs, it was found that all four hY RNAs bind with chromatin. Moreover, hY5 was recruited mostly to the nucleoli, while hY1, hY3 and hY4 were found to bind predominantly early replicating euchromatin [55]. It was also shown that the loop domain directs the targeting of of hY RNAs to euchromatin, since hY RNAs with mutated loop domains were shown to bind unselectively to chromatin, suggesting that this part of the hY RNA structure is important for promoting selective Y RNA chromatin association [55]. Despite inconsistent reports with regards to Y RNA distribution, growing evidence now demonstrate that Y RNAs are present in both the cytoplasm and nucleus of eukaryotic cells.

It was reported that the subcellular localization of Y RNA within the cell can be cell cycle dependent and can change during environmental stress [55, 60, 61]. Indeed, both Y RNAs and Ro60 were found to accumulate in the nucleus upon UV irradiation or oxidative stress in several organisms [20, 40, 60, 61]. This observation suggests a possible stress dependent role of Ro60/Y RNA, but on the other hand the accumulation of the complex in the nucleus can also result from suppression of the nuclear export, triggered by stress induced impairment of the RanGTP gradient, as this was shown to be the case for other proteins [62].

Y RNAs have also been detected in various retroviruses including murine leukemia virus (MLV) and human immunodeficiency virus (HIV) [63, 64]. These viruses are known to incorporate other ncRNAs as well including tRNA and miRNAs [65, 66]. The mechanisms of viral encapsulation are not very well understood, but it has been suggested that this process happens when the newly synthesized host Y RNA are still in the nucleus and seems to be independent of Ro60 binding [64]. Whether Y RNAs modulate viral function is still unknown, however several proteins involved in virus infection such as YBX1, hnRNP K and nucleolin were reported to bind to Y RNAs [67]. Consistent with this, it has been suggested that Y RNAs may promote an antiviral immune response by stimulating TLR7 [68] in the newly infected cells, or may act as scaffolds for virus packaging [63, 69].

3 Biological Functions of Y RNAs: Ongoing Work

Although Y RNAs were initially discovered more than three decades ago, a relatively small number of studies have been published regarding their biological roles, with most of the literature describing their structure and protein interactions. Reported functions of Y RNAs include involvement in DNA replication [51], and regulation of RNA stability and cellular stress responses [70, 71]. Y RNAs were identified as being essential factors for initiation of chromosomal DNA replication in cell-free reactions, in which isolated G1-phase nuclei were incubated with fractioned cellular extracts from actively proliferating human cells [72]. Using this system, Christov et al. found that adding the fraction containing purified Y RNA subtypes, increased the proportion of replicating nuclei in a dose-dependent manner [72]. Depletion of hY1-RNA by RNA interference, inhibited cell proliferation and reduced significantly the percentages of human cells in S-phase, during which DNA replication occurs [72]. Further studies by the same group discovered that Y RNAs function redundantly with regards to their role in DNA replication, as any of the four hY RNAs, in the absence of the others, is sufficient to stimulate DNA replication [72]. Another interesting finding is that inhibition of replication, resulting from siRNA-mediated degradation of a hY RNA, can be rescued by adding any vertebrate Y RNA, but not non-vertebrate Y RNAs [73]. The functional redundancy observed among the hY RNAs was attributed to the presence of an evolutionary conserved upper stem region of vertebrate Y RNAs, which was shown to be necessary and sufficient for Y RNA function in DNA replication [73, 74]. In contrast, the loop domains and the lower stem of Y RNAs seem unessential with regards to Y RNA role in DNA replication, as DNA replication remained unaffected when they were mutated [73].

As mentioned earlier, Y RNA binds to euchromatin throughout the cell cycle. Evidence was provided that this association increases during S-phase and declines in G1 phase or mitosis [75].

Furthermore, the dynamics of Y RNA association with chromatin was shown to correlate with that of the origin replication complex (ORC), implying that Y RNAs and ORC likely participate in a common functional pathway [75]. Constituently, all four hY RNAs were shown to interact with members of the ORC, as well as with proteins participating in the initiation of DNA replication, but not with proteins involved in DNA replication elongation, suggesting that Y RNAs act specifically in the initiation stage of replication [55, 76]. Consistent with a function in DNA replication and cell proliferation, Y RNA levels were found to correlate with the proliferative condition of the cells [75] and to increase in solid human tumors compared to healthy controls [77]. In another study, however, it was reported that mouse Ro60 knockout cells, which had about 30-fold lower Y-RNA levels, did not demonstrate decreased growth rates, indicating that chromosomal replication can still occur in the absence of Ro60 [61, 78]. And therefore, while there are increasing examples in the literature supporting a role of Y RNA in DNA replication, the exact molecular mechanisms by which Y RNA regulates DNA replication are still unknown.

Growing amount of experimental data supports the role of YRNAs in RNA stability and quality control via the interaction with Ro60. It has been shown that Ro60 binds and process [79, 80] defective non-coding RNAs such as misfolded 5S rRNA, pre-tRNAs and U2 snRNA in various organisms, including C. elegans, X. laevis, and mouse [61, 79, 81, 82]. It was found that under normal conditions Y RNAs compete with misfolded RNAs for association with Ro60 [44]. Structural and biochemical studies have demonstrated that Y RNAs bind to the outer surface of Ro60, while misfolded RNAs pass through the Ro60 cavity and also bind to the Ro60 outer surface at portions overlapping with the Y RNA-binding region [70, 79]. Because, Y RNAs bind Ro60 with higher affinity and sequence complementarity compared to misfolded RNAs, the 'steric occlusion' model was proposed suggesting that bound Y RNAs sterically hinders the binding of misfolded RNAs to Ro60. [70, 79]. And thus, it appears that Y RNAs serve as guards for Ro60 function in regulating RNA quality, permitting access only when needed [80, 83]. Consistently, under conditions of stress, such as exposure to UV-irradiation, Ro60/Y RNA complex can function as cellular stress sensors. This was supported by the finding that Ro60 can dissociate from Y RNAs and rescue misfolded RNAs, thereby helping cellular recovery [45]. The mechanism that regulates dissociation of Y RNAs from Ro, however, is currently unknown. Furthermore, it has been showed that Y RNAs can not only regulate Ro60 access to RNA substrates, but also can contribute to recognition of misfolded ncRNAs and recruit other proteins involved in RNA metabolism [83, 84]. In the bacterium D. radiodurans, Y RNA function as a scaffold, tethering the exonuclease PNPase to the bacterial ortholog of Ro (rosixty related, Rsr), thus forming an RNA degradation complex which mediates RNA decay [47, 83]. In contrast to prokaryotes, in mammals PNPases reside inside mitochondria and since Ro60 RNPs are predominantly cytosolic, it is possible that PNPases RNA degradation machine in mammalian cells does not form. It was suggested, however, that Y RNA can scaffold Ro60 to other proteins playing a role in RNA metabolism, including helicases, exoribonucleases or RNA chaperones [47]. With regards to eukaryotes, however, association of exoribonucleases with RoRNPs and their Y RNAs to this date have not been reported. In fact, one study, using tandem affinity purifications of mouse Ro60, reported that it was unable to detect association with any ribonuclease [40].

To this date, by mostly pull down assays, more than 20 proteins with roles in the regulation of various cellular processes, have been reported to interact with Y RNAs [85]. For example, Argonaute (Ago) and MOV10 have key functions in miRNA-mediated gene silencing, others like HuR influence cytokine production, and still others regulate mRNA transcripts splicing or processing, virus infection and innate immunity. The effects from these interactions are mostly unknown, however, it has been proposed that they could impose specific cellular functions through binding with Y RNAs (Fig. 20.1). In addition, not all of the identified proteins were shown to associate with all four hY RNAs, implying that depending on their bound proteins, different Y-RNAs could have different functions. [28, 80]. Support for this notion was provided in several studies. For example, HuR, a protein specifically expressed in neuronal cells, was demonstrated to influence cytokine production by a mechanism involving association of HuR with Y3-RNA and AU-rich elements in mRNA transcripts [86, 87]. Similarly, CPSF, a protein with a role in mRNA splicing, was shown to regulate human histone-H3 mRNA synthesis and processing in cooperation with a fragment derived from Y3 RNA [88]. Accordingly, within the group of proteins reported to directly interact with Y RNAs, there are some, such as calcineurin and nulceolin, with documented roles in the heart [89–91]. It is interesting, whether Y RNA interaction with these proteins is of functional significance, e.g., influencing specific processes in the heart.

Interestingly, most of the reported roles of Y RNAs involve nuclear functions. But at steady state Y RNAs are predominantly cytoplasmic. Therefore, it is conceivable that Y RNAs could play functions in modulating not only nuclear but cytoplasmic mRNAs as well. In this line of thought, one can speculate that in addition to Ro60, other RBPs could also be sequestered by Y RNAs in a similar way. Thus, they may serve an analogous function to long ncRNAs, for instance, which have been reported to regulate gene expression by acting as scaffolds or sponges [92, 93]. In support to this notion, recently it was found that Y3 RNA can function as a molecular sponge for the HuD enhancer [94]. HuD plays a role in regulating neuronal cell fate by promoting gene expression through interacting with many mRNAs involved in motor neuron neurogenesis [95]. It was found that binding of Y3 RNA to HuD, altered HuD localization, limiting HuD access to the polysomal compartment, which subsequently reduced expression of the involved mRNAs (PMID: [94]). Future investigations on the Y RNA compartment specific function would be interesting and useful, as it could shed more light on the Y RNA roles in regulating cytoplasmic mRNA functions. In addition to understanding the cellular role of Y RNA, future work is also needed to inform on the physiological significance of Y RNAs during normal and pathological conditions, for example by using genetic models.

Y RNAs do not solely exist in their full length. A growing number of RNA sequencing studies have identified small RNA fragments of about 25–35 nt, comprising parts of Y RNAs [96, 97]. Fragmentation, performed by RNAse L [98] was shown to increase in apoptotic cells and upon activation of the innate immune system [99, 100]. Interestingly, it was found that these Y RNA fragments were still associated with Ro60 and La, suggesting that the binding of the proteins could have a protective role, preventing Y RNA degradation by exonucleases [99]. Despite the fact that Y RNA fragmentation increases significantly during apoptosis, Y RNA products have also been detected in non-apoptotic, proliferating cells, at amounts comparable to that of known miRNAs [100]. Since Y RNA fragments are produced from conserved ends of the hairpin containing Y RNAs, and their structure resembles that of the pre-miRNAs, some of these Y RNA fragments were originally annotated as a new kind of miRNA [101, 102]. Experimental evidence of Y RNA-encoded regulatory microRNAs, however, has not been reported to date [99]. Studies have shown that the biogenesis of Y RNA fragments is independent of the classical miRNA biogenesis pathway [100], evidenced by the findings that Y RNA fragments do not interact with Ago proteins [100, 103] and their processing is independent of Dicer [104]. Moreover, luciferase reporter assay studies have shown that reporter mRNA constructs could not be suppressed by Y RNAs, unlike miRNAs, further providing evidence that the identified fragments are not produced by the canonical miRNA pathway and do not act as miRNAs [101]. Apart from cells, Y RNA fragments have also been reported in various biofluids, either as cell-free RNPs or within extracellular vesicles and were shown to comprise a significant fraction of the RNA component in human serum and plasma [105–107]. Furthermore, differences in circulating Y RNA products were detected in disease [27, 106, 108]. For instance, increased levels of 3′ Y-RNA fragments were found in the plasma of patients with breast cancer [106], while full length and 5′ fragments of hY4 were elevated in chronic lymphocytic leukemia (CLL) patients, compared with healthy controls [108]. Elevated amounts of extracellular Y-RNA products have also been detected in patients with atherosclerosis and coronary artery disease [27]. These findings together with the observation that similar to miRNAs, Y RNA fragments are stable in human plasma [27], suggest that they may be further investigated as biomarkers for disease. Whether these Y RNA fragments are biologically significant is still unclear, but for some of them functional relevance has recently been ascribed, e.g., in the context of heart disease and cancer [108–111].

4 Y RNAs in Cardiovascular Biology and Disease

Given that Y RNAs have only recently started to gain more attention, knowledge about their roles in the heart is still limited, and the full impact of this field on the cardiovascular system is yet to be determined. Here we highlight examples of Y RNAs, known or suggested to be involved in cardiovascular functions. The few reports that exist only hint at the Y RNA roles that are yet to be revealed and which potentially may lead to the identification of novel therapeutic targets.

Myocardial infarction (MI), and subsequent ischemic heart failure remains a significant contributor to the global burden of cardiovascular disease. Patients who survive MI often will develop heart failure (HF) and will consequently be at increased risk for premature death [112]. Cardiosphere-derived cells (CDCs) are stem cells derived from cardiac tissue itself that have shown promising clinical results in reducing infarct size and improving cardiovascular function [113, 114]. They had been initially hypothesized to improve tissue repair and boost cardiac function by triggering native cardiomyocyte proliferation, recruiting endogenous progenitor cells and exerting potent anti-inflammatory, antifibrotic and angiogenic effects [115–117]. The regenerative benefits of CDCs in vivo are shown to be mediated mostly via paracrine effects, particularly through secretion of exosomes (EVs) [118–120]. These endogenous vesicles mediate intercellular communication, transferring various cargo of RNAs, proteins and lipids [120]. Y RNAs were shown to be particularly abundant in EVs [120]. In a recent study, it was shown that after tRNAs, Y RNAs and their fragments make up the largest portion of small RNAs in CDC-EVs, accounting for about 20% of the total small exosomal RNAs [109]. One particular 5′ fragment of Y4-RNA was found to be specifically enriched, being the most abundant individual small RNA present in CDC-EVs, compared to normal human dermal fibroblast EVs [109]. It was demonstrated that Y4-fragment can be transferred to bone-marrow derived macrophages via EVs and this was shown to promote cardioprotection by altering gene expression. In an in vitro setting, Y4-fragment was shown to act indirectly on cardiomyocytes by modulating the cytokine profile secreted by macrophages. In particular, overexpression of Y4-fragment in macrophages, when cocultured with oxidatively stressed cardiomyocytes, was shown to suppress cardiomyocyte death by inducing strong and prolonged upregulation of the anti-inflammatory cytokine IL10. Furthermore, similar cardioprotective response was observed in vivo when it was demonstrated that administration of this Y4-product triggered IL10 release and reduced infarct size in a rat model of ischemia/reperfusion injury (I/R). Finally, evidence was provided that the abundance of Y4- fragments in CDC-exosomes correlated with the CDCs functional benefit of mitigating damage after myocardial infarction [109].

Later, in a follow up study from the same group, their initial findings were further expanded by demonstrating that the same highly abundant Y4-fragment promotes beneficial effects in a mouse model of cardiac hypertrophy induced by Ang II infusion [110]. Intravenous administration of Y4-fragment was shown to mitigate the progression of LV remodeling by decreasing cardiac hypertrophy, fibrosis and inflammation in the murine hypertensive model. Some of the benefits on the heart were attributed to the increased levels of IL-10 protein detected in the plasma after systemic injection of Y4-fragment. Y4-fragment was shown to replenish normal levels of IL-10 in heart after Ang II infusion. It was proposed that the expression of Y4-fragment in heart after administration promotes effects at the site of injury likely via activation of cardiac-resident macrophages. Y4-fragment was shown to suppress inflammatory response by reducing the levels of the proinflammatory cytokines IL1b and IL6 in the heart and decreasing expression of CD68 and F4/80 markers of infiltrating inflammatory macrophages. Adding to initial findings, it was demonstrated that the release of IL-10 by macrophages induced by Y4-fragment, counteracts Ang II effect in cultured cardiomyocytes and cardiac fibroblasts. Decreased atrial natriuretic peptide (ANP) expression in cultured cardiomyocytes or IL6 in cardiac fibroblasts upon Ang II treatment were only detected in the presence of macrophage-conditioned media containing increased Y4-fragment, demonstrating again evidence of the direct Y4-fragment effect on macrophage activation and underscoring the importance of cellular cross-talk during myocardial damage. Additionally, the favorable actions ofY4-fragment on the heart were detected in the absence of elevated blood pressure, suggesting thatY4-fragment prevents Ang II local actions on the heart without affecting its hemodynamic effects. Importantly, both the Y4-fragment and CDC-EVs were demonstrated to act in the same direction, producing similar beneficial effect on the heart, suggesting that CDC cardioprotective properties are at least in part mediated by this single fragment, further implying that the fragment may be useful therapeutically either by itself or at enhanced levels in EVs [110].

Y RNAs have also been implicated in cardiac neonatal lupus (NL) [121]. Cardiac NL is an autoimmune disease in which tissue injury in the fetus is believed to be related to the transplacental passage of maternal autoantibodies targeting Ro/SSA (Sjögren syndrome type A antigen) and/or La/SSB (Sjögren syndrome type B antigen) ribonuclear proteins [122–124]. The most common cardiac manifestation of cardiac NL is complete congenital heart block (CHB) that may be accompanied by valvular abnormalities, endocardial fibroelastosis, and/or dilated cardiomyopathy [125, 126]. Increased physiological apoptosis has been proposed as a link between anti-Ro60 antibodies and injury, providing a mechanism by which these typically inaccessible Ro and La antigens can be translocated to the surface of the heart fetal cells and become available to maternal antibodies to initiate injury [127–129]. Evidence was provided that Y3 RNA is required for Ro60 membrane translocation and subsequent formation of immune complexes capable of inducing a toll-like receptor (TLR) dependent proinflammatory cascade [121]. In this study, two experimental approaches were used to address the dependence of Y RNA for Ro60 trafficking to the cell membrane: siRNA-mediated knockdown of mouse Y3 RNA and a single point mutation of Ro60 that blocks RNA binding. It was found that depletion of Y3 RNA in murine fibroblasts undergoing apoptosis prevented cell surface translocation of Ro60, and similarly the mutated Ro60 (unbound Y RNA) construct but not the wild type form was unable to get exposed on the cell surface. Based on these findings, it was suggested that Y3 RNA masks a nuclear localization signal on Ro60, allowing for translocation and surface accessibility of cytosolic Ro60/mY3 RNA complexes. Moreover, upon opsonization with anti-Ro60 antibodies, these apoptotic fibroblasts promoted TLR7 dependent TNFα secretion from cocultured macrophages. Interestingly, apoptosis is known to promote caspase-dependent cleavage of Y RNAs, which somewhat conflicts the findings in this study [99]. However, as mentioned earlier, the small fragments produced during apoptotic driven degradation arise from the most highly conserved part of the Y RNA and remain associated with Ro60 [99]. It is therefore possible that these Y RNA products would still be capable of blocking the Ro60 nuclear localization signal, allowing and even facilitating surface accessibility of cytosolic Ro60/mY3 RNA complexes and may be even sufficient to induce proinflammatory response [130].

Complementing the findings of this study, again in the context of autoimmune associated

CHB, another paper demonstrated that the complex of human Ro60-associated Y3 RNA with anti-Ro60 IgG is required for activation of both TLR7 and FcγR dependent proinflammatory responses [131]. Macrophages transfected with both synthetic hY3 RNA that binds Ro60 and an immune complex produced by incubation of hY3/Ro60 with IgG from a CHB mother (anti-Ro60 present in serum) was shown to induce strong TNF-α release. Moreover, collagen secretion and fibrosis markers were markedly increased in cultured fetal cardiac fibroblasts exposed to supernatants of macrophages transfected with hY3 RNA. In contrast to healthy heart, immunohistological evaluation of autopsy tissue from a fetus diagnosed with CHB revealed TLR7 expression in the conduction system with TLR7 positive cells located near the atrioventricular groove. Based on the findings, Ro60-hY3 was proposed as a link between inflammation and fetal cardiac fibrosis in CHB, providing a mechanism by which hY3/Ro60 binds to anti-Ro antibodies and form immune complexes capable of inducing immune response which promotes fibrosis [131].

In addition to modulating inflammatory responses during cardiac injury, Y RNAs have also been shown to induce apoptosis in atherosclerosis [132]. In atherosclerosis, cholesterol deposition into the arterial wall triggers increased accumulation of macrophages and promotes apoptosis in these cells [133]. The induction of macrophage apoptosis speeds up the progression of atherosclerosis by promoting the development of a necrotic core, which on the other hand contributes to plaque disruption and acute thrombosis [134, 135]. Significant upregulation of fragmented Y RNA has been detected in the medium of cultured macrophages treated with lipids, as well as in the blood of mouse models for atherosclerosis and in the serum of patients with coronary artery disease (CAD) [27]. In addition, biostatistical analysis associated fragmented Y-RNA with atherosclerosis burden by demonstrating a strong positive correlation between the levels of one specific 5′ fragment of Y1-RNA (RNY1-5p) into the serum and CAD risk [27]. Importantly, RNY1-5p was shown to associate better with CAD status in comparison to some CAD-specific miRNAs (e.g., miRNA-17, miRNA-133, miRNA-155), suggesting potential diagnostic application of RNY1-5p measurement as a biomarker for CAD risk assessment [27]. In another study, it was demonstrated that macrophage activation upon treatment with atherogenic lipids triggers the processing of Y RNAs into small Y RNA products in these cells [132]. *In vitro* gain- and loss-of-function studies showed that Y RNA fragments, but not full-length Y RNAs from which they were derived, activated both caspase 3 and NF-κB pathways, promoting cell death and inflammation in the macrophages [132]. In addition, it was found that not only intracellular but also extracellular Y RNA fragments induce apoptosis and inflammation in macrophages [132]. Specifically, it was shown that extracellular affinity purified Y RNA fragment/Ro60 complex from apoptotic HEK293T cells could trigger cell death in macrophages. Interestingly, synthetic Y RNA fragment alone was not able to induce macrophage activation, implying that the fragments must be bound in a complex with Ro60 in order to get incorporated in the cell and subsequently produce a biological response [132]. Based on these findings, Y RNA fragment/Ro60 complex released by macrophages could contribute to the progression of CAD by participating in a negative feed-back loop in which increasing number of macrophages die by apoptosis in the lipid abundant arterial wall and by this possibly reinforce the pathogenesis of atherosclerosis [132].

5 Conclusion

In summary, Y RNAs have been shown to participate in a range of cellular processes including DNA replication, RNA quality control and cellular stress responses. More recently, accumulating evidence suggest functional involvement of Y RNAs in disease such as cancer and immune related pathologies. Roles of Y RNAs in cardiovascular biology are also starting to emerge. In this context, Y RNAs have been reported to mediate both beneficial and adverse effects on the cardiovascular system. However, investigations on Y RNAs are still at a very early stage, and there are many questions that remain to be answered. Improved functional and mechanistic understanding of Y RNAs will provide valuable insights into normal human physiology and disease pathogenesis.

Acknowledgements SD is funded by RO1 HL122547 and AHA SFRN grant.

Competing Financial Interests The authors declare no competing financial interests.

References

1. Birney E. Evolutionary genomics: come fly with us. Nature. 2007;450(7167):184–5.
2. Carninci P, Kasukawa T, Katayama S, Gough J, Frith MC, Maeda N, Oyama R, Ravasi T, Lenhard B, Wells C, Kodzius R, Shimokawa K, Bajic VB, Brenner SE, Batalov S, Forrest AR, Zavolan M, Davis MJ, Wilming LG, Aidinis V, Allen JE, Ambesi-Impiombato A, Apweiler R, Aturaliya RN, Bailey TL, Bansal M, Baxter L, Beisel KW, Bersano T, Bono H, Chalk AM, Chiu KP, Choudhary V, Christoffels A, Clutterbuck DR, Crowe ML, Dalla E, Dalrymple BP, de Bono B, Della Gatta G, di Bernardo D, Down T, Engstrom P, Fagiolini M, Faulkner G, Fletcher CF, Fukushima T, Furuno M, Futaki S, Gariboldi M, Georgii-Hemming P, Gingeras TR, Gojobori T, Green RE, Gustincich S, Harbers M, Hayashi Y, Hensch TK, Hirokawa N, Hill D, Huminiecki L, Iacono M, Ikeo K, Iwama A, Ishikawa T, Jakt M, Kanapin A, Katoh M, Kawasawa Y, Kelso J, Kitamura H, Kitano H, Kollias G, Krishnan SP, Kruger A, Kummerfeld SK, Kurochkin IV, Lareau LF, Lazarevic D, Lipovich L, Liu J, Liuni S, McWilliam S, Madan Babu M, Madera M, Marchionni L, Matsuda H, Matsuzawa S, Miki H, Mignone F, Miyake S, Morris K, Mottagui-Tabar S, Mulder N, Nakano N, Nakauchi H, Ng P, Nilsson R, Nishiguchi S, Nishikawa S, Nori F, Ohara O, Okazaki Y, Orlando V, Pang KC, Pavan WJ, Pavesi G, Pesole G, Petrovsky N, Piazza S, Reed J, Reid JF, Ring BZ, Ringwald M, Rost B, Ruan Y, Salzberg SL, Sandelin A, Schneider C, Schonbach C, Sekiguchi K, Semple CA, Seno S, Sessa L, Sheng Y, Shibata Y, Shimada H, Shimada K, Silva D, Sinclair B, Sperling S, Stupka E, Sugiura K, Sultana R, Takenaka Y, Taki K, Tammoja K, Tan SL, Tang S, Taylor MS, Tegner J, Teichmann SA, Ueda HR, van Nimwegen E, Verardo R, Wei CL, Yagi K, Yamanishi H, Zabarovsky E, Zhu S, Zimmer A, Hide W, Bult C, Grimmond SM, Teasdale RD, Liu ET, Brusic V, Quackenbush J, Wahlestedt C, Mattick JS, Hume DA, Kai C, Sasaki D, Tomaru Y, Fukuda S, Kanamori-Katayama M, Suzuki M, Aoki J, Arakawa T, Iida J, Imamura K, Itoh M, Kato T, Kawaji H, Kawagashira N, Kawashima T, Kojima M, Kondo S, Konno H, Nakano K, Ninomiya N, Nishio T, Okada M, Plessy C, Shibata K, Shiraki T, Suzuki S, Tagami M, Waki K, Watahiki A, Okamura-Oho Y, Suzuki H, Kawai J, Hayashizaki Y, Consortium F, Group RGER, Genome Science G. The transcriptional landscape of the mammalian genome. Science. 2005;309(5740):1559–63.
3. Thum T. MicroRNA therapeutics in cardiovascular medicine. EMBO Mol Med. 2012;4(1):3–14.
4. Greco S, Salgado Somoza A, Devaux Y, Martelli F. Long noncoding RNAs and cardiac disease. Antioxid Redox Signal. 2018;29(9):880–901.
5. Huarte M. The emerging role of lncRNAs in cancer. Nat Med. 2015;21(11):1253–61.
6. Hayes J, Peruzzi PP, Lawler S. MicroRNAs in cancer: biomarkers, functions and therapy. Trends Mol Med. 2014;20(8):460–9.
7. Fan B, Luk AOY, Chan JCN, Ma RCW. MicroRNA and diabetic complications: a clinical perspective. Antioxid Redox Signal. 2018;29(11):1041–63.
8. Giroud M, Scheideler M. Long non-coding RNAs in metabolic organs and energy homeostasis. Int J Mol Sci. 2017;18(12).
9. Sayed D, Abdellatif M. MicroRNAs in development and disease. Physiol Rev. 2011;91(3):827–87.
10. Ng SY, Lin L, Soh BS, Stanton LW. Long noncoding RNAs in development and disease of the central nervous system. Trends Genet. 2013;29(8):461–8.
11. Duan L, Xiong X, Liu Y, Wang J. miRNA-1: functional roles and dysregulation in heart disease. Mol Omics Mol Biosyst. 2014;10(11):2775–82.
12. Iorio MV, Croce CM. MicroRNA dysregulation in cancer: diagnostics, monitoring and therapeutics. A comprehensive review. EMBO Mol Med. 2012;4(3):143–59.
13. Iorio MV, Croce CM. Causes and consequences of microRNA dysregulation. J Cancer. 2012;18(3):215–22.
14. Abbott JA, Francklyn CS, Robey-Bond SM. Transfer RNA and human disease. Front Genet. 2014;5:158.
15. Wang Q, Lee I, Ren J, Ajay SS, Lee YS, Bao X. Identification and functional characterization of tRNA-derived RNA fragments (tRFs) in respiratory syncytial virus infection. Mol Ther. 2013;21(2):368–79.
16. Ozata DM, Gainetdinov I, Zoch A, O'Carroll D, Zamore PD. PIWI-interacting RNAs: small RNAs with big functions. Nat Rev Genet. 2019;20(2):89–108.
17. Assumpcao CB, Calcagno DQ, Araujo TM, Santos SE, Santos AK, Riggins GJ, Burbano RR, Assumpcao PP. The role of piRNA and its poten-

tial clinical implications in cancer. Epigenomics. 2015;7(6):975–84.
18. Lerner MR, Boyle JA, Hardin JA, Steitz JA. Two novel classes of small ribonucleoproteins detected by antibodies associated with lupus erythematosus. Science. 1981;211(4480):400–2.
19. Lerner MR, Steitz JA. Antibodies to small nuclear RNAs complexed with proteins are produced by patients with systemic lupus erythematosus. Proc Natl Acad Sci U S A. 1979;76(11):5495–9.
20. Sim S, Weinberg DE, Fuchs G, Choi K, Chung J, Wolin SL. The subcellular distribution of an RNA quality control protein, the Ro autoantigen, is regulated by noncoding Y RNA binding. Mol Biol Cell. 2009;20(5):1555–64.
21. Pruijn GJ, Wingens PA, Peters SL, Thijssen JP, van Venrooij WJ. Ro RNP associated Y RNAs are highly conserved among mammals. BBA-Mol Basis Dis. 1993;1216(3):395–401.
22. Mosig A, Guofeng M, Stadler BM, Stadler PF. Evolution of the vertebrate Y RNA cluster. Theory Biosci. 2007;126(1):9–14.
23. Sim S, Wolin SL. Bacterial Y RNAs: gates, tethers, and tRNA Mimics. Microbiol Spectr. 2018;6(4).
24. Van Horn DJ, Eisenberg D, O'Brien CA, Wolin SL. Caenorhabditis elegans embryos contain only one major species of Ro RNP. RNA Biol. 1995;1(3):293–303.
25. Boria I, Gruber AR, Tanzer A, Bernhart SH, Lorenz R, Mueller MM, Hofacker IL, Stadler PF. Nematode sbRNAs: homologs of vertebrate Y RNAs. J Mol Evol. 2010;70(4):346–58.
26. Wolin SL, Steitz JA. The Ro small cytoplasmic ribonucleoproteins: identification of the antigenic protein and its binding site on the Ro RNAs. Proc Natl Acad Sci U S A. 1984;81(7):1996–2000.
27. Repetto E, Lichtenstein L, Hizir Z, Tekaya N, Benahmed M, Ruidavets JB, Zaragosi LE, Perret B, Bouchareychas L, Genoux A, Lotte R, Ruimy R, Ferrieres J, Barbry P, Martinez LO, Trabucchi M. RNY-derived small RNAs as a signature of coronary artery disease. BMC Med. 2015;13:259.
28. Langley AR, Chambers H, Christov CP, Krude T. Ribonucleoprotein particles containing non-coding Y RNAs, Ro60, La and nucleolin are not required for Y RNA function in DNA replication. PLoS One. 2010;5(10):e13673.
29. Maraia RJ, Sasaki-Tozawa N, Driscoll CT, Green ED, Darlington GJ. The human Y4 small cytoplasmic RNA gene is controlled by upstream elements and resides on chromosome 7 with all other hY scRNA genes. Nucleic Acids Res. 1994;22(15):3045–52.
30. Maraia R, Sakulich AL, Brinkmann E, Green ED. Gene encoding human Ro-associated autoantigen Y5 RNA. Nucleic Acids Res. 1996;24(18):3552–9.
31. Hendrick JP, Wolin SL, Rinke J, Lerner MR, Steitz JA. Ro small cytoplasmic ribonucleoproteins are a subclass of La ribonucleoproteins: further characterization of the Ro and La small ribonucleoproteins from uninfected mammalian cells. Mol Biol Cell. 1981;1(12):1138–49.
32. Wolin SL, Steitz JA. Genes for two small cytoplasmic Ro RNAs are adjacent and appear to be single-copy in the human genome. Cell. 1983;32(3):735–44.
33. Perreault J, Noel JF, Briere F, Cousineau B, Lucier JF, Perreault JP, Boire G. Retropseudogenes derived from the human Ro/SS-A autoantigen-associated hY RNAs. Nucleic Acids Res. 2005;33(6):2032–41.
34. Perreault J, Perreault JP, Boire G. Ro-associated Y RNAs in metazoans: evolution and diversification. Mol Biol Evol. 2007;24(8):1678–89.
35. Simons FH, Rutjes SA, van Venrooij WJ, Pruijn GJ. The interactions with Ro60 and La differentially affect nuclear export of hY1 RNA. RNA Biol. 1996;2(3):264–73.
36. Wolin SL, Cedervall T. The La protein. Annu Rev Biochem. 2002;71:375–403.
37. Peek R, Pruijn GJ, van der Kemp AJ, van Venrooij WJ. Subcellular distribution of Ro ribonucleoprotein complexes and their constituents. J Cell Sci. 1993;106(Pt 3):929–35.
38. Rutjes SA, Lund E, van der Heijden A, Grimm C, van Venrooij WJ, Pruijn GJ. Identification of a novel cis-acting RNA element involved in nuclear export of hY RNAs. RNA Biol. 2001;7(5):741–52.
39. Gendron M, Roberge D, Boire G. Heterogeneity of human Ro ribonucleoproteins (RNPS): nuclear retention of Ro RNPS containing the human hY5 RNA in human and mouse cells. Clin Exp Immunol. 2001;125(1):162–8.
40. Sim S, Yao J, Weinberg DE, Niessen S, Yates JR 3rd, Wolin SL. The zipcode-binding protein ZBP1 influences the subcellular location of the Ro 60-kDa autoantigen and the noncoding Y3 RNA. RNA Biol. 2012;18(1):100–10.
41. Zuker M. Mfold web server for nucleic acid folding and hybridization prediction. Nucleic Acids Res. 2003;31(13):3406–15.
42. Teunissen SW, Kruithof MJ, Farris AD, Harley JB, Venrooij WJ, Pruijn GJ. Conserved features of Y RNAs: a comparison of experimentally derived secondary structures. Nucleic Acids Res. 2000;28(2):610–9.
43. van Gelder CW, Thijssen JP, Klaassen EC, Sturchler C, Krol A, van Venrooij WJ, Pruijn GJ. Common structural features of the Ro RNP associated hY1 and hY5 RNAs. Nucleic Acids Res. 1994;22(13):2498–506.
44. Green CD, Long KS, Shi H, Wolin SL. Binding of the 60-kDa Ro autoantigen to Y RNAs: evidence for recognition in the major groove of a conserved helix. RNA Biol. 1998;4(7):750–65.
45. Sim S, Wolin SL. Emerging roles for the Ro 60-kDa autoantigen in noncoding RNA metabolism. Wiley Interdiscip Rev Rna. 2011;2(5):686–99.
46. Xia PZ, Fritz KA, Geoghegan WD, Jordon RE. The particulate (speckled-like thread) nuclear staining pattern: species and cellular distribution of Ro/SSA antigen. J Clin Lab Immunol. 1987;22(3):101–5.

47. Wolin SL, Belair C, Boccitto M, Chen X, Sim S, Taylor DW, Wang HW. Non-coding Y RNAs as tethers and gates: insights from bacteria. RNA Biol. 2013;10(10):1602–8.
48. Fabini G, Raijmakers R, Hayer S, Fouraux MA, Pruijn GJ, Steiner G. The heterogeneous nuclear ribonucleoproteins I and K interact with a subset of the ro ribonucleoprotein-associated Y RNAs in vitro and in vivo. J Biol Chem. 2001;276(23):20711–8.
49. Fouraux MA, Bouvet P, Verkaart S, van Venrooij WJ, Pruijn GJ. Nucleolin associates with a subset of the human Ro ribonucleoprotein complexes. J Mol Biol. 2002;320(3):475–88.
50. Kohn M, Lederer M, Wachter K, Huttelmaier S. Near-infrared (NIR) dye-labeled RNAs identify binding of ZBP1 to the noncoding Y3-RNA. RNA Biol. 2010;16(7):1420–8.
51. Kowalski MP, Baylis HA, Krude T. Non-coding stem-bulge RNAs are required for cell proliferation and embryonic development in C. elegans. J Cell Sci. 2015;128(11):2118–29.
52. Wolin SL, Sim S, Chen X. Nuclear noncoding RNA surveillance: is the end in sight? Trends Genet. 2012;28(7):306–13.
53. Hall AE, Dalmay T. Discovery of novel small RNAs in the quest to unravel genome complexity. Biochem Soc Trans. 2013;41(4):866–70.
54. Pruijn GJ, Simons FH, van Venrooij WJ. Intracellular localization and nucleocytoplasmic transport of Ro RNP components. Eur J Cell Biol. 1997;74(2):123–32.
55. Zhang AT, Langley AR, Christov CP, Kheir E, Shafee T, Gardiner TJ, Krude T. Dynamic interaction of Y RNAs with chromatin and initiation proteins during human DNA replication. J Cell Sci. 2011;124(Pt 12):2058–69.
56. O'Brien CA, Margelot K, Wolin SL. Xenopus Ro ribonucleoproteins: members of an evolutionarily conserved class of cytoplasmic ribonucleoproteins. Proc Natl Acad Sci U S A. 1993;90(15):7250–4.
57. Simons FH, Pruijn GJ, van Venrooij WJ. Analysis of the intracellular localization and assembly of Ro ribonucleoprotein particles by microinjection into Xenopus laevis oocytes. J Cell Biol. 1994;125(5):981–8.
58. Farris AD, Puvion-Dutilleul F, Puvion E, Harley JB, Lee LA. The ultrastructural localization of 60-kDa Ro protein and human cytoplasmic RNAs: association with novel electron-dense bodies. Proc Natl Acad Sci U S A. 1997;94(7):3040–5.
59. Matera AG, Frey MR, Margelot K, Wolin SL. A perinucleolar compartment contains several RNA polymerase III transcripts as well as the polypyrimidine tract-binding protein, hnRNP I. J Cell Biol. 1995;129(5):1181–93.
60. Chen X, Quinn AM, Wolin SL. Ro ribonucleoproteins contribute to the resistance of Deinococcus radiodurans to ultraviolet irradiation. Genes Dev. 2000;14(7):777–82.
61. Chen X, Smith JD, Shi H, Yang DD, Flavell RA, Wolin SL. The Ro autoantigen binds misfolded U2 small nuclear RNAs and assists mammalian cell survival after UV irradiation. Curr Biol. 2003;13(24):2206–11.
62. Kohn M, Pazaitis N, Huttelmaier S. Why YRNAs? About versatile RNAs and their functions. Biomol Ther. 2013;3(1):143–56.
63. Garcia EL, Onafuwa-Nuga A, Sim S, King SR, Wolin SL, Telesnitsky A. Packaging of host mY RNAs by murine leukemia virus may occur early in Y RNA biogenesis. J Virol. 2009;83(23):12526–34.
64. Wang T, Tian C, Zhang W, Luo K, Sarkis PT, Yu L, Liu B, Yu Y, Yu XF. 7SL RNA mediates virion packaging of the antiviral cytidine deaminase APOBEC3G. J Virol. 2007;81(23):13112–24.
65. Huang Y, Mak J, Cao Q, Li Z, Wainberg MA, Kleiman L. Incorporation of excess wild-type and mutant tRNA(3Lys) into human immunodeficiency virus type 1. J Virol. 1994;68(12):7676–83.
66. Balasubramaniam M, Pandhare J, Dash C. Are microRNAs important players in HIV-1 infection? An update. Viruses. 2018;10(3).
67. Stake M, Singh D, Singh G, Marcela Hernandez J, Kaddis Maldonado R, Parent LJ, Boris-Lawrie K. HIV-1 and two avian retroviral 5′ untranslated regions bind orthologous human and chicken RNA binding proteins. Virology. 2015;486:307–20.
68. Telesnitsky A, Wolin SL. The host RNAs in retroviral particles. Viruses. 2016;8(8).
69. Eckwahl MJ, Sim S, Smith D, Telesnitsky A, Wolin SL. A retrovirus packages nascent host noncoding RNAs from a novel surveillance pathway. Genes Dev. 2015;29(6):646–57.
70. Stein AJ, Fuchs G, Fu C, Wolin SL, Reinisch KM. Structural insights into RNA quality control: the Ro autoantigen binds misfolded RNAs via its central cavity. Cell. 2005;121(4):529–39.
71. Chen X, Sim S, Wurtmann EJ, Feke A, Wolin SL. Bacterial noncoding Y RNAs are widespread and mimic tRNAs. RNA Biol. 2014;20(11):1715–24.
72. Christov CP, Gardiner TJ, Szuts D, Krude T. Functional requirement of noncoding Y RNAs for human chromosomal DNA replication. Mol Biol Cell. 2006;26(18):6993–7004.
73. Gardiner TJ, Christov CP, Langley AR, Krude T. A conserved motif of vertebrate Y RNAs essential for chromosomal DNA replication. RNA Biol. 2009;15(7):1375–85.
74. Wang I, Kowalski MP, Langley AR, Rodriguez R, Balasubramanian S, Hsu ST, Krude T. Nucleotide contributions to the structural integrity and DNA replication initiation activity of noncoding y RNA. Biochemistry. 2014;53(37):5848–63.
75. Kheir E, Krude T. Non-coding Y RNAs associate with early replicating euchromatin in concordance with the origin recognition complex. J Cell Sci. 2017;130(7):1239–50.
76. Krude T, Christov CP, Hyrien O, Marheineke K. Y RNA functions at the initiation step of mamma-

lian chromosomal DNA replication. J Cell Sci. 2009;122(Pt 16):2836–45.
77. Christov CP, Trivier E, Krude T. Noncoding human Y RNAs are overexpressed in tumours and required for cell proliferation. Br J Cancer. 2008;98(5):981–8.
78. Xue D, Shi H, Smith JD, Chen X, Noe DA, Cedervall T, Yang DD, Eynon E, Brash DE, Kashgarian M, Flavell RA, Wolin SL. A lupus-like syndrome develops in mice lacking the Ro 60-kDa protein, a major lupus autoantigen. Proc Natl Acad Sci U S A. 2003;100(13):7503–8.
79. Fuchs G, Stein AJ, Fu C, Reinisch KM, Wolin SL. Structural and biochemical basis for misfolded RNA recognition by the Ro autoantigen. Nat Struct Mol Biol. 2006;13(11):1002–9.
80. Hogg JR, Collins K. Human Y5 RNA specializes a Ro ribonucleoprotein for 5S ribosomal RNA quality control. Genes Dev. 2007;21(23):3067–72.
81. Labbe JC, Hekimi S, Rokeach LA. Assessing the function of the Ro ribonucleoprotein complex using Caenorhabditis elegans as a biological tool. Biochem Cell Biol. 1999;77(4):349–54.
82. O'Brien CA, Wolin SL. A possible role for the 60-kD Ro autoantigen in a discard pathway for defective 5S rRNA precursors. Genes Dev. 1994;8(23):2891–903.
83. Chen X, Taylor DW, Fowler CC, Galan JE, Wang HW, Wolin SL. An RNA degradation machine sculpted by Ro autoantigen and noncoding RNA. Cell. 2013;153(1):166–77.
84. Chen X, Wurtmann EJ, Van Batavia J, Zybailov B, Washburn MP, Wolin SL. An ortholog of the Ro autoantigen functions in 23S rRNA maturation in D. radiodurans. Genes Dev. 2007;21(11):1328–39.
85. Driedonks TAP, Nolte-'t Hoen ENM. Circulating Y-RNAs in extracellular vesicles and ribonucleoprotein complexes; implications for the immune system. Front Immunol. 2018;9:3164.
86. Katsanou V, Papadaki O, Milatos S, Blackshear PJ, Anderson P, Kollias G, Kontoyiannis DL. HuR as a negative posttranscriptional modulator in inflammation. Mol Cell. 2005;19(6):777–89.
87. Herdy B, Karonitsch T, Vladimer GI, Tan CS, Stukalov A, Trefzer C, Bigenzahn JW, Theil T, Holinka J, Kiener HP, Colinge J, Bennett KL, Superti-Furga G. The RNA-binding protein HuR/ELAVL1 regulates IFN-beta mRNA abundance and the type I IFN response. Eur J Immunol. 2015;45(5):1500–11.
88. Kohn M, Ihling C, Sinz A, Krohn K, Huttelmaier S. The Y3** ncRNA promotes the 3′ end processing of histone mRNAs. Genes Dev. 2015;29(19):1998–2003.
89. Wilkins BJ, Molkentin JD. Calcineurin and cardiac hypertrophy: where have we been? Where are we going? J Physiol. 2002;541(Pt 1):1–8.
90. Parra V, Rothermel BA. Calcineurin signaling in the heart: the importance of time and place. J Mol Cell Cardiol. 2017;103:121–36.
91. Jiang B, Zhang B, Liang P, Chen G, Zhou B, Lv C, Tu Z, Xiao X. Nucleolin protects the heart from ischaemia-reperfusion injury by up-regulating heat shock protein 32. Cardiovasc Res. 2013;99(1):92–101.
92. Gaiti F, Hatleberg WL, Tanurdzic M, Degnan BM. Sponge Long non-coding RNAs are expressed in specific cell types and conserved networks. Noncoding RNA. 2018;4(1).
93. Wang KC, Chang HY. Molecular mechanisms of long noncoding RNAs. Mol Cell. 2011;43(6):904–14.
94. Tebaldi T, Zuccotti P, Peroni D, Kohn M, Gasperini L, Potrich V, Bonazza V, Dudnakova T, Rossi A, Sanguinetti G, Conti L, Macchi P, D'Agostino V, Viero G, Tollervey D, Huttelmaier S, Quattrone A. HuD Is a neural translation enhancer acting on mTORC1-responsive genes and counteracted by the Y3 small non-coding RNA. Mol Cell. 2018;71(2):256–270 e210.
95. Bolognani F, Contente-Cuomo T, Perrone-Bizzozero NI. Novel recognition motifs and biological functions of the RNA-binding protein HuD revealed by genome-wide identification of its targets. Nucleic Acids Res. 2010;38(1):117–30.
96. Rother S, Meister G. Small RNAs derived from longer non-coding RNAs. Biochimie. 2011;93(11):1905–15.
97. Tuck AC, Tollervey D. RNA in pieces. Trends Genet. 2011;27(10):422–32.
98. Donovan J, Rath S, Kolet-Mandrikov D, Korennykh A. Rapid RNase L-driven arrest of protein synthesis in the dsRNA response without degradation of translation machinery. RNA. 2017;23(11):1660–71.
99. Rutjes SA, van der Heijden A, Utz PJ, van Venrooij WJ, Pruijn GJ. Rapid nucleolytic degradation of the small cytoplasmic Y RNAs during apoptosis. J Biol Chem. 1999;274(35):24799–807.
100. Nicolas FE, Hall AE, Csorba T, Turnbull C, Dalmay T. Biogenesis of Y RNA-derived small RNAs is independent of the microRNA pathway. FEBS Lett. 2012;586(8):1226–30.
101. Meiri E, Levy A, Benjamin H, Ben-David M, Cohen L, Dov A, Dromi N, Elyakim E, Yerushalmi N, Zion O, Lithwick-Yanai G, Sitbon E. Discovery of microRNAs and other small RNAs in solid tumors. Nucleic Acids Res. 2010;38(18):6234–46.
102. Verhagen AP, Pruijn GJ. Are the Ro RNP-associated Y RNAs concealing microRNAs? Y RNA-derived miRNAs may be involved in autoimmunity. BioEssays. 2011;33(9):674–82.
103. Chen CJ, Heard E. Small RNAs derived from structural non-coding RNAs. Methods. 2013;63(1):76–84.
104. Langenberger D, Cakir MV, Hoffmann S, Stadler PF. Dicer-processed small RNAs: rules and exceptions. J Exp Zool Part B-Mol Dev Evol. 2013;320(1):35–46.
105. Dhahbi JM, Spindler SR, Atamna H, Boffelli D, Mote P, Martin DI. 5′-YRNA fragments derived by processing of transcripts from specific YRNA genes and pseudogenes are abundant in human serum and plasma. Physiol Genomics. 2013;45(21):990–8.

106. Dhahbi JM. Circulating small noncoding RNAs as biomarkers of aging. Ageing Res Rev. 2014;17:86–98.
107. Vojtech L, Woo S, Hughes S, Levy C, Ballweber L, Sauteraud RP, Strobl J, Westerberg K, Gottardo R, Tewari M, Hladik F. Exosomes in human semen carry a distinctive repertoire of small non-coding RNAs with potential regulatory functions. Nucleic Acids Res. 2014;42(11):7290–304.
108. Haderk F, Schulz R, Iskar M, Cid LL, Worst T, Willmund KV, Schulz A, Warnken U, Seiler J, Benner A, Nessling M, Zenz T, Gobel M, Durig J, Diederichs S, Paggetti J, Moussay E, Stilgenbauer S, Zapatka M, Lichter P, Seiffert M. Tumor-derived exosomes modulate PD-L1 expression in monocytes. Sci Immunol. 2017;2(13).
109. Cambier L, de Couto G, Ibrahim A, Echavez AK, Valle J, Liu W, Kreke M, Smith RR, Marban L, Marban E. Y RNA fragment in extracellular vesicles confers cardioprotection via modulation of IL-10 expression and secretion. EMBO Mol Med. 2017;9(3):337–52.
110. Cambier L, Giani JF, Liu W, Ijichi T, Echavez AK, Valle J, Marban E. Angiotensin II-induced end-organ damage in mice is attenuated by human exosomes and by an Exosomal Y RNA fragment. Hypertension. 2018;72(2):370–80.
111. Chakrabortty SK, Prakash A, Nechooshtan G, Hearn S, Gingeras TR. Extracellular vesicle-mediated transfer of processed and functional RNY5 RNA. RNA. 2015;21(11):1966–79.
112. Jhund PS, McMurray JJ. Heart failure after acute myocardial infarction: a lost battle in the war on heart failure? Circulation. 2008;118(20): 2019–21.
113. Marban E, Cingolani E. Direct reprogramming: bypassing stem cells for therapeutics. J Am Med Assoc. 2015;314(1):19–20.
114. Marban E. Breakthroughs in cell therapy for heart disease: focus on cardiosphere-derived cells. Mayo Clin Proc. 2014;89(6):850–8.
115. Barile L, Milano G, Vassalli G. Beneficial effects of exosomes secreted by cardiac-derived progenitor cells and other cell types in myocardial ischemia. Stem Cell Investig. 2017;4:93.
116. Tseliou E, Fouad J, Reich H, Slipczuk L, de Couto G, Aminzadeh M, Middleton R, Valle J, Weixin L, Marban E. Fibroblasts rendered Antifibrotic, Antiapoptotic, and Angiogenic by priming with Cardiosphere-derived extracellular membrane vesicles. J Am Coll Cardiol. 2015;66(6):599–611.
117. de Couto G, Liu W, Tseliou E, Sun B, Makkar N, Kanazawa H, Arditi M, Marban E. Macrophages mediate cardioprotective cellular postconditioning in acute myocardial infarction. J Clin Investig. 2015;125(8):3147–62.
118. Ibrahim A, Marban E. Exosomes: fundamental biology and roles in cardiovascular physiology. Annu Rev Physiol. 2016;78:67–83.
119. Vandergriff AC, de Andrade JB, Tang J, Hensley MT, Piedrahita JA, Caranasos TG, Cheng K. Intravenous cardiac stem cell-derived exosomes ameliorate cardiac dysfunction in doxorubicin induced dilated cardiomyopathy. Stem Cells Int. 2015;2015:960926.
120. Valadi H, Ekstrom K, Bossios A, Sjostrand M, Lee JJ, Lotvall JO. Exosome-mediated transfer of mRNAs and microRNAs is a novel mechanism of genetic exchange between cells. Nat Cell Biol. 2007;9(6):654–9.
121. Reed JH, Sim S, Wolin SL, Clancy RM, Buyon JP. Ro60 requires Y3 RNA for cell surface exposure and inflammation associated with cardiac manifestations of neonatal lupus. J Immunol. 2013;191(1):110–6.
122. Brucato A, Cimaz R, Caporali R, Ramoni V, Buyon J. Pregnancy outcomes in patients with autoimmune diseases and anti-Ro/SSA antibodies. Clin Rev Allergy Immunol. 2011;40(1):27–41.
123. Brucato A, Frassi M, Franceschini F, Cimaz R, Faden D, Pisoni MP, Muscara M, Vignati G, Stramba-Badiale M, Catelli L, Lojacono A, Cavazzana I, Ghirardello A, Vescovi F, Gambari PF, Doria A, Meroni PL, Tincani A. Risk of congenital complete heart block in newborns of mothers with anti-Ro/SSA antibodies detected by counterimmunoelectrophoresis: a prospective study of 100 women. Arthritis Rheum. 2001;44(8):1832–5.
124. Buyon JP, Winchester R. Congenital complete heart block. A human model of passively acquired autoimmune injury. Arthritis Rheum. 1990;33(5):609–14.
125. Izmirly PM, Saxena A, Sahl SK, Shah U, Friedman DM, Kim MY, Buyon JP. Assessment of fluorinated steroids to avert progression and mortality in anti-SSA/Ro-associated cardiac injury limited to the fetal conduction system. Ann Rheum Dis. 2016;75(6):1161–5.
126. Izmirly PM, Saxena A, Kim MY, Wang D, Sahl SK, Llanos C, Friedman D, Buyon JP. Maternal and fetal factors associated with mortality and morbidity in a multi-racial/ethnic registry of anti-SSA/Ro-associated cardiac neonatal lupus. Circulation. 2011;124(18):1927–35.
127. Casciola-Rosen LA, Anhalt G, Rosen A. Autoantigens targeted in systemic lupus erythematosus are clustered in two populations of surface structures on apoptotic keratinocytes. J Exp Med. 1994;179(4):1317–30.
128. Miranda-Carus ME, Boutjdir M, Tseng CE, DiDonato F, Chan EK, Buyon JP. Induction of antibodies reactive with SSA/Ro-SSB/La and development of congenital heart block in a murine model. J Immunol. 1998;161(11):5886–92.
129. Clancy RM, Neufing PJ, Zheng P, O'Mahony M, Nimmerjahn F, Gordon TP, Buyon JP. Impaired clearance of apoptotic cardiocytes is linked to anti-SSA/Ro and -SSB/La antibodies in the patho-

genesis of congenital heart block. J Clin Investig. 2006;116(9):2413–22.
130. Vollmer J, Tluk S, Schmitz C, Hamm S, Jurk M, Forsbach A, Akira S, Kelly KM, Reeves WH, Bauer S, Krieg AM. Immune stimulation mediated by autoantigen binding sites within small nuclear RNAs involves Toll-like receptors 7 and 8. J Exp Med. 2005;202(11):1575–85.
131. Clancy RM, Alvarez D, Komissarova E, Barrat FJ, Swartz J, Buyon JP. Ro60-associated single-stranded RNA links inflammation with fetal cardiac fibrosis via ligation of TLRs: a novel pathway to autoimmune-associated heart block. J Immunol. 2010;184(4):2148–55.
132. Hizir Z, Bottini S, Grandjean V, Trabucchi M, Repetto E. RNY (YRNA)-derived small RNAs regulate cell death and inflammation in monocytes/macrophages. Cell Death Dis. 2017;8(1):e2530.
133. Moore KJ, Tabas I. Macrophages in the pathogenesis of atherosclerosis. Cell. 2011;145(3):341–55.
134. Tabas I, Williams KJ, Boren J. Subendothelial lipoprotein retention as the initiating process in atherosclerosis: update and therapeutic implications. Circulation. 2007;116(16):1832–44.
135. Naghavi M, Libby P, Falk E, Casscells SW, Litovsky S, Rumberger J, Badimon JJ, Stefanadis C, Moreno P, Pasterkamp G, Fayad Z, Stone PH, Waxman S, Raggi P, Madjid M, Zarrabi A, Burke A, Yuan C, Fitzgerald PJ, Siscovick DS, de Korte CL, Aikawa M, Juhani Airaksinen KE, Assmann G, Becker CR, Chesebro JH, Farb A, Galis ZS, Jackson C, Jang IK, Koenig W, Lodder RA, March K, Demirovic J, Navab M, Priori SG, Rekhter MD, Bahr R, Grundy SM, Mehran R, Colombo A, Boerwinkle E, Ballantyne C, Insull W Jr, Schwartz RS, Vogel R, Serruys PW, Hansson GK, Faxon DP, Kaul S, Drexler H, Greenland P, Muller JE, Virmani R, Ridker PM, Zipes DP, Shah PK, Willerson JT. From vulnerable plaque to vulnerable patient: a call for new definitions and risk assessment strategies: part I. Circulation. 2003;108(14):1664–72.

Translational Potential of Non-coding RNAs for Cardiovascular Disease

21

Jenny Y. Y. Ooi and Bianca C. Bernardo

Abstract

Heart failure is the end result of a variety of cardiovascular disease states. Heart failure remains a challenge to treat, and the incidence continues to rise with an aging population, and increasing rates of diabetes and obesity. Non-coding RNAs, once considered as "junk DNA", have emerged as powerful transcriptional regulators and potential therapeutic targets for the treatment of heart failure. Different classes of non-coding RNAs exist, including small non-coding RNAs, referred to as microRNAs, and long non-coding RNAs. Both microRNAs and long non-coding RNAs play a role in cardiac development as well as in the pathogenesis of cardiovascular disease, prompting many studies to investigate their role as potential therapeutic targets. Most studies manipulate miRNAs and lncRNAs of interest via antisense oligonucleotides; however, several challenges remain limiting their potential clinical value. As such, viral and non-viral delivery methods are being developed to achieve targeted delivery *in vivo*.

Keywords

Non-coding RNAs · Long non-coding RNAs · microRNAs · Cardiovascular disease · Heart failure · Antisense oligonucleotides

1 Background

Heart failure (HF) is the end result of a variety of disease states, including coronary artery disease and hypertension. It is a devastating disorder characterized by chamber remodeling, hypertrophy, fibrosis and poor heart function. It is a significant global health problem which is increasing in prevalence as the population ages [1, 2]. Despite improvements in cardiovascular therapies, medical management and prevention, mortality rates remain high, with almost 50% patients with HF dying within 5 years of diagnosis [3]. As a multifactorial clinical syndrome, HF represents an epidemic threat; highlighting the need to better understand disease mechanisms. The increasing burden of HF on health systems has prompted a number of investigations to identify and develop

J. Y. Y. Ooi
Baker Heart and Diabetes Institute, Melbourne, VIC, Australia

Department of Diabetes, Central Clinical School, Monash University, Clayton, VIC, Australia

B. C. Bernardo (✉)
Baker Heart and Diabetes Institute, Melbourne, VIC, Australia

Department of Diabetes, Central Clinical School, Monash University, Clayton, VIC, Australia

Department of Paediatrics, University of Melbourne, Melbourne, VIC, Australia
e-mail: bianca.bernardo@baker.edu.au

J. Xiao (ed.), *Non-coding RNAs in Cardiovascular Diseases*, Advances in Experimental Medicine and Biology 1229, https://doi.org/10.1007/978-981-15-1671-9_21

new therapies for the prevention and treatment of HF [4].

Advances in genome-wide profiling has found that over 90% of the genome encodes a vast range of non-coding RNAs (ncRNAs) instead of protein-coding messenger RNA. NcRNAs can differ in length, from small ncRNAs of approximately 18–25 nucleotides (i.e. microRNAs [miRNAs]), to larger ncRNAs of over 200 nucleotides called long non-coding RNAs (lncRNAs). There are many different types of ncRNAs and they are generally classified into groups based on their length and mechanism of gene regulation (see review [5]). These types include small interfering (siRNAs), miRNAs, piwi-associated RNAs, circular RNAs, small nucleolar RNAs, small nuclear RNAs and lncRNAs [6]. Of these, miRNAs have been extensively studied in the heart, where they have a role in cardiac biology and can influence cardiac remodeling in cardiovascular disease (see reviews [7–11]). Evidence from preclinical studies points to potential applications of miRNAs for diagnostic and therapeutic purposes (see reviews [9, 10, 12–15]). In contrast, less is known about lncRNAs, but they have a demonstrated role in cardiac development and prognostic potential in the clinic [16, 17].

Earlier chapters in this series have discussed in detail the biology of ncRNAs, as well as the research progress of ncRNAs and heart failure. This particular chapter will focus on miRNAs and lncRNAs and aims to provide readers with an updated summary on those miRNAs and lncRNAs with translational potential for cardiovascular disease, with an emphasis on translational hurdles and new technologies that are being developed to deliver ncRNAs to the heart.

2 Therapeutic Applications of ncRNAs

2.1 Targeting miRNAs in the Heart

Among all the ncRNAs, miRNAs have the capacity to target several genes simultaneously within a similar signaling network or pathway; therefore, they may serve as preferable therapeutic targets compared with other ncRNAs. Two main strategies are used to manipulate the expression of miRNAs: chemically modified inhibitors and miRNA mimics. These strategies aim to normalize miRNA expression in the tissue by either silencing over-expressed miRNAs (using inhibitors) or restoring miRNAs (using miRNA mimics) that have a deficit in expression under pathological conditions (for review see [9]). As miRNAs have been shown to control pathophysiological changes of the heart, including cardiomyocyte cell death, autophagy, contractility, fibrosis and hypertrophy, researchers have investigated the therapeutic potential of miRNAs intensively for the treatment of cardiovascular disease. These studies have been reviewed elsewhere, and have mainly focused on inhibiting miRNAs [9, 10, 13, 18, 19]. Here we present an example of a miRNA that may have a dual therapeutic effect, and the need to consider miRNAs in respect to sex and severity of disease.

miR-208a is a potential therapeutic candidate demonstrating the synergistic effect of miRNAs. Not only did pharmacologic inhibition of miR-208a prevent pathological cardiac remodeling, improve cardiac function and survival in a rat hypertensive model [20] (Fig. 21.1), it was also found to control whole-body metabolism, by protecting mice against high fat diet-induced obesity, despite being a cardiac specific miRNA [21]. These protective actions of miR-208a are due to upregulation of its target gene, thyroid hormone-associated protein 1 (THRAP1, also known as MED13) in cardiac tissue. Thus, pharmacological inhibition of miR-208a potentially has a dual effect not only to improve cardiac function in patients following a cardiac insult, but also in those patients with co-morbidities such a diabetes or a metabolic syndrome to improve whole-body metabolism.

Recently, it has become apparent that the pharmacological effect of miRNA inhibitors is dependent on type and severity of disease, and sex, which may determine therapeutic outcome [22–25]. In our own studies using inhibitors against the miR-34 family and miR-34a in heart

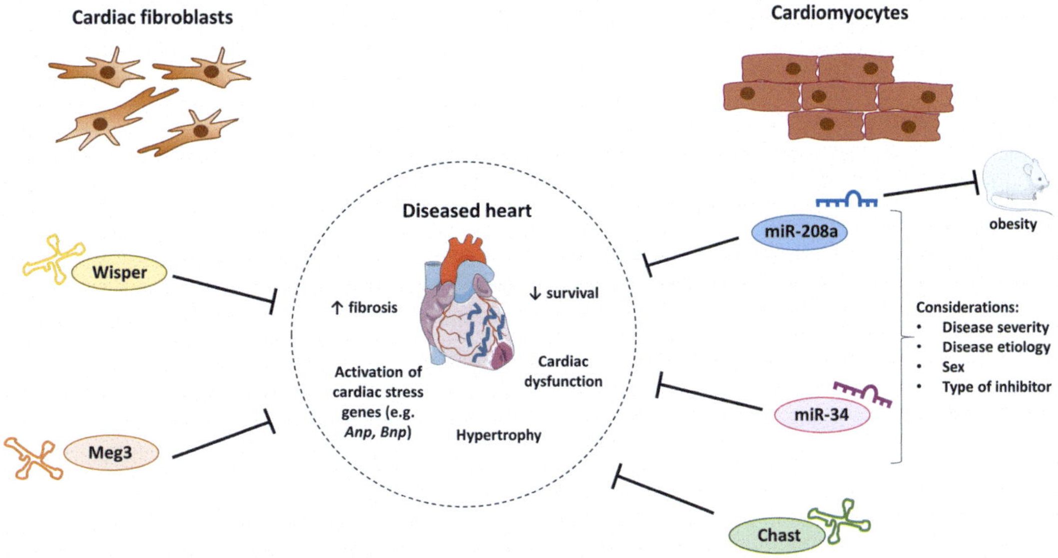

Fig. 21.1 Non-coding RNA therapies for the failing heart. A schematic showing examples of microRNAs and long non-coding RNAs that are dysregulated in the failing heart and have been successfully targeted in preclinical models of cardiac disease. For microRNA therapeutics, disease severity, disease etiology, sex and type of inhibitor can influence therapeutic outcome. miR-208a has a dual-therapeutic affect having also been shown to protect against high fat diet induced obesity in mice

failure mouse models, we found that inhibiting the miR-34 family was therapeutically more effective at protecting the heart against myocardial infarction than inhibiting miR-34a alone [23] (Fig. 21.1). Further, inhibiting miR-34a alone was able to attenuate cardiac pathology in a moderate mouse model of hypertrophic cardiomyopathy, but was ineffective in a more severe model [22] suggesting that therapies that inhibit miR-34a alone may have limited potential in settings of established cardiac pathology. Our follow up studies on miR-34a further confirmed that treatment with miR-34a inhibitors showed little benefit in a setting of severe dilated cardiomyopathy associated with atrial fibrillation, when compared to a setting of moderate dilated cardiomyopathy [24]. In the same study, we showed that males and females respond differently to a miRNA-34a based drug, and identified sex- & treatment-dependent regulation of miRNAs in the diseased heart [24]. Several other studies have reported sexual dimorphism in the miRNA transcriptome. Whole genome wide studies have reported differentially-expressed miRNAs between males and females across four human tissues including brain, colorectal mucosa, peripheral blood, and cord blood [26], as well as in human and murine normal and diseased heart [27], indicating that gender specific treatment strategies may need to be considered. More recently, sex-specific regulation of miRNAs targeting proteins involved in mitochondrial metabolism in the heart were identified [28].

Further, Eding and colleagues [25] demonstrated that the pharmacological effect of antimiR-208a was (i) stronger under disease conditions (compared to basal) in both small and large animal models of cardiac stress, (ii) target regulation can be dependent on the type of stress, and (iii) that both the type and severity of disease determine the therapeutic outcome [25].

Collectively, these studies indicate that disease etiology and sex influences the therapeutic outcome of miRNA-based drug therapies. These factors will be important to consider when assessing the therapeutic dose and predicting therapeutic outcome in the clinic.

2.2 Targeting lncRNAs in the Heart

LncRNAs have been identified to play a role in cardiovascular health and disease and have recently been extensively reviewed [5, 6, 29–33]. Here, we will focus on those lncRNAs that show promise for therapeutic application in cardiovascular disease (Fig. 21.1). One of the most widely used antisense oligonucleotides (ASOs) to inhibit lncRNAs are GapmeRs. GapmeRs are highly potent, single-stranded ASOs that function by RNase H-dependent degradation of complementary RNA targets [34]. GapmeRs are designed to have 2–5 locked nucleic acid (LNA) moieties at each terminus which flank a central "gap" of 5–10 single stranded DNA nucleotides [35]. The LNA:DNA nucleotide combination increases binding affinity, half-life and improved stability of the GapmeR, as well as facilitating unassisted cellular uptake [35]. Only recently have GapmeRs been used to inhibit lncRNAs in preclinical models of heart failure [36, 37]. Three lncRNAs with translation potential into clinical scenarios (due to identification of a human homolog) are cardiac hypertrophy-associated transcript *(Chast)* [37], Wisp2 super-enhancer-associated RNA *(Wisper)* [36] and maternally expressed gene 3 *(Meg3)* [38] (Fig. 21.1).

The lncRNA *Chast* was identified from whole-genome lncRNA profiling, and upregulated in hypertrophic mouse hearts [37]. Of translational relevance for humans, a human homolog of *CHAST* was identified and found to be conserved in sequence and structure. Further highlighting the potential translational relevance, *CHAST* expression was upregulated in the hearts from patients with aortic stenosis (which causes hypertrophy of the heart) compared to healthy hearts [37]. The therapeutic potential of *Chast* inhibition using GapmeRs was tested in a preclinical mouse model of established cardiac disease (induced by transverse aortic constriction, TAC). *Chast* inhibition in TAC mice resulted in attenuation of cardiac hypertrophy, smaller cardiomyocyte size and improved cardiac function compared to TAC animals treated with the control-GapmeR [37] (Fig. 21.1). Importantly, there were no signs of toxicological side effects from GapmeR treatment [37].

Wisper is a heart enriched lncRNA that is highly expressed in cardiac fibroblasts and upregulated in the fibrotic myocardial tissue following myocardial infarction [36]. As *Wisper* was found to correlate with cardiac fibrosis in both a mouse model of myocardial infarction, and in heart tissue from patients with aortic stenosis [36], it represents a potential anti-fibrotic therapy. To determine whether *Wisper* could be a potential therapy to combat cardiac fibrosis, *Wisper* was inhibited in a mouse model of myocardial infarction two and nine days after injury using GapmeRs. At both seven and 28 days post-myocardial infarction, *Wisper*-depleted myocardial infarction mice had (i) improved cardiac function, (ii) decreased expression of the fibrotic gene program, (iii) reduction of infarct size, and (iv) attenuation of cardiac fibrosis compared to control treated myocardial infarction mice [36] (Fig. 21.1). These findings in a preclinical mouse model, coupled with the observation that human *WISPER* expression correlates with fibrosis in patients with aortic stenosis, identifies *Wisper* as a potential therapeutic target to treat cardiac fibrosis and prevent pathological remodeling in the diseased heart [36].

Another lncRNA with potential to be an anti-fibrotic therapy is *Meg3*. *Meg3* was identified from global profiling of lncRNAs in cardiac fibroblasts from hearts of mice that had undergone 13 weeks of pressure overload (induced by TAC) [38]. *Meg3* is a fibroblast-enriched lncRNA which was downregulated following TAC. GapmeR-mediated silencing of *Meg3* one week after TAC (i) prevented the development of cardiac fibrosis, (ii) attenuated cardiomyocyte hypertrophy, (iii) decreased the expression of the cardiac stress genes atrial natriuretic peptide and B-type natriuretic peptide, (iv) inhibited matrix metalloproteinase 2; and (v) improved diastolic function of the heart [38] (Fig. 21.1). *Meg3* is highly conserved across species, and a human homolog of MEG3 has been identified [39, 40], demonstrating the translational potential of *Meg3* as a target for the prevention of extracellular matrix remodeling in the heart.

Together, these studies support translation into the clinic, although careful consideration into GapmeR design and delivery will need to be considered (discussed further in Sect. 3.2).

2.3 Circulating Non-coding RNAs as Potential Biomarkers

The detection and stability of circulating miRNAs (ci-miRNAs) in plasma, and with emerging techniques that can detect ci-miRNAs in a quantitative manner (e.g. quantitative PCR, droplet digital PCR, RNA sequencing) suggests that ci-miRNAs can be used as clinical biomarkers for cardiovascular disease. Indeed, several groups have characterized the levels of miRNAs in the circulation of patients with cardiovascular disease ([41–44]; also see reviews [45, 46]). Studies suggest that in some conditions measurement of a panel of ci-miRNAs may be an alternative way to conventional markers for early detection in acute myocardial infarction [47, 48]. Whilst ci-miRs may be useful for diagnostics and monitoring approaches, further studies are still required before ci-miRNAs can be eventually used as biomarkers for cardiovascular pathologies.

Although not as extensively studied compared to ci-miRNAs, there have been several studies reporting lncRNAs in circulation as useful predictors of disease prognosis ([32, 49, 50]). The lncRNA long intergenic noncoding RNA predicting cardiac remodeling (LIPCAR) is an example of a potential biomarker as increased plasma levels were associated with left ventricular remodeling post myocardial infarction, and increased risk of cardiovascular death in heart failure patients [16]. In addition, numerous other lncRNAs have been identified as potential biomarkers. The lncRNA GAS5 was found to be downregulated in the plasma of patients with coronary artery disease, which might be a promising biomarker for the diagnosis of coronary artery disease [51]. Myocardial infarction-associated transcript (MIAT) and smooth muscle and endothelial cell-enriched migration/differentiation-associated long noncoding RNA (SENCR) were associated with left ventricular remodeling in patients with diabetic cardiomyopathy [52]. Vausort and colleagues [50] identified a number of lncRNAs to be dysregulated in peripheral blood cells of patients with acute myocardial infarction which may help predict outcome. Other potential lncRNAs as biomarkers for acute myocardial infarction include Zinc finger antisense 1 (ZFAS1), Cdr1 antisense (CDR1AS), urothelial carcinoma-associated 1 (UCA1), HOX antisense intergenic RNA (HOTAIR) [53–55], and for heart failure are non-coding repressor of NFAT (NRON) and myosin heavy-chain-associated RNA transcripts (MHRT) [56]. Collectively, these findings encourage future studies to determine the value of lncRNAs as novel cardiac biomarkers.

2.4 miRNAs in Clinical Trials

Despite convincing preclinical studies demonstrating therapeutic effect of miRNA inhibitors there are currently no miRNA targeted clinical trials for heart disease. However, there are positive progresses of RNA-based treatments (siRNAs and miRNAs) in other fields of disease [57]. Translational efficacy and safety of miRNA-based therapeutics to patients (an inhibitor against miR-122, miravisen) has been shown in phase IIa clinical trials for the treatment of hepatitis C virus, where results indicate that the treatment was well tolerated [58]. In July 2018, miRAgen Therapeutics Inc. announced they would initiate a Phase 2 clinical trial to evaluate MRG-201 (a synthetic mimic of miRNA-29) in patients with a predisposition for keloid formation (keloids are raised overgrowths of scar tissue). This follows successful testing of MRG-201 in Phase 1 clinical trials which demonstrated MRG-201 could reduce fibrogenesis in patients after skin trauma (http://www.miragen.com/pipeline/). miR-29 targets proteins involved in fibrosis including collagens, fibrillins and elastin, thus representing a potential therapeutic target for tissue fibrosis in other pathological conditions. Despite the well-documented role of miR-29 in cardiac remodelling and fibrosis [59, 60], there have been confounding studies that may influence the development of miR-29 as a therapy for the treatment of heart failure [59–61].

MiRagen, in collaboration with Servier, are also developing a synthetic miRNA inhibitor of miRNA-92a (MRG-110) to promote the revascularization process for treatment of ischemic heart failure. Other clinical trials using novel oligonucleotides to inhibit miR-17 (RGLS4326) for the treatment of autosomal dominant polycystic kidney disease are being studied in Phase 1 trials.

No clinical trials targeting lncRNAs for cardiovascular disease have been reported so far.

3 Translational Hurdles of ncRNAs

3.1 miRNAs

Most of preclinical and clinical studies use antisense oligonucleotides (ASOs) to inhibit the miRNA of interest. They have been chemically modified to improve stability, binding affinity and nuclease resistance, most commonly with 2′ sugar modifications such as 2′-*O*-methyl (2′-OMe), 2′-O-Methyoxyethyl (2′-Moe), 2′-fluoro (2′-F) or LNA, incorporation of phosphodiester and phosphorothioate linkages or conjugation to cholesterol (see reviews [5, 8, 9]). Often referred to as "antagomiRs" [cholesterol conjugated] or "antimiRs" [LNA based], these inhibitors are non-tissue specific and impact on several organs (such as liver and kidney) upon systemic administration. Given the ubiquitous expression of some miRNAs, and the different functions of miRNAs in various tissues and/or oncogenic efficacies, this may be problematic. For example, inhibition of miR-34 in the heart is protective [22, 23], but miR-34 is also recognized as a master regulator of tumor suppression and miR-34 replacement therapy is being investigated as a cancer treatment [62]. Under these conditions, a targeted-tissue specific method may be preferable. Furthermore, miRNA inhibitors have the potential to affect RNA species beyond their intended targets [63, 64], which may make clinical intervention complex.

Over the years, there have been significant progresses in next generation sequencing and miRNA systems biology. Recent studies have demonstrated that not only do miRNAs regulate their target mRNAs, but miRNAs in the heart can also regulate the expression of other secondary miRNAs in the heart [63, 65]. Thus, a better understanding of miRNA-miRNA crosstalk and complex signaling networks in a normal and diseased state will be important for the successful design of miRNA-based therapies for cardiovascular disease.

Further complicating the use of ASOs are inconsistent results when investigators have used antagomiRs or antimiRs targeting the same miRNA in preclinical mouse models of cardiac disease [59, 60, 66, 67]. Whilst one group reported that inhibition of miR-21 (using antagomiRs) prevented cardiac hypertrophy and fibrosis in a mouse model of pressure overload [67], another group was unable to replicate these findings using a LNA-antimiR-21 approach [66]. Similarly, mice subjected to pressure overload were less susceptible to cardiac fibrosis and hypertrophy following inhibition of miR-29 using LNA-antimiRs [59], whereas earlier reports suggested inhibition of miR-29b with antagomiRs promoted the fibrotic response [60]. The disparity in these studies may be partially explained by different oligonucleotide chemistries, specific targeting of an individual miRNA vs. a miRNA family, experimental protocols utilized, or different effects of miRNAs in different cells types (e.g. cardiomyocytes vs fibroblasts). These inconsistencies have yet to be resolved, demonstrating that further studies are required before these miRNAs can enter clinical trials as a therapeutic for cardiac fibrosis and hypertrophy.

3.2 lncRNAs

Several challenges need to be resolved before a lncRNA based therapy enters the clinic for cardiovascular disease (see reviews [29, 30, 68, 69]). The most challenging issue is target specificity. A single lncRNA has pleiotropic actions, where some act through more than one mechanism, can regulate multiple signaling pathways and have a number of functions within an organism. For example, the lncRNA gene, antisense non-coding RNA in the INK4 locus (ANRIL) is associated with an increased risk of atherosclerotic cardiovascular disease [70], but also has a role in cancer cell proliferation [71], thus making it a difficult therapeutic target.

LncRNAs are not well conserved across species which may limit the use of animal models for preclinical studies. This is illustrated by lncRNAs, such as Braveheart *(Bvht;* regulates cardiac cell fate*)*, *Mirt1* and *Mirt2* (thought to have a protective role on cardiac function and left ventricular remodeling post myocardial infarction), in which a human homolog has not been identified [72, 73]. Further, for those potentially important lncRNAs that have no rodent homolog, experimental analysis is restricted to human cells and tissues, making translation from bench to bedside more difficult. The low homology between species makes characterization and clinical testing of human lncRNAs more difficult. However, it is thought that the secondary structure of lncRNAs is conserved rather than the primary sequence, and that structure may be more important to function than sequence [29]. Thus, lncRNAs may have structural homologs in other species, which may allow the use of animal models for preclinical testing. However, the relationship between lncRNA structure and function is not well understood and needs to be studied further.

Another hurdle facing the development of lncRNAs as therapeutic targets is cellular location. LncRNAs have widely varying subcellular distributions. Some lncRNAs reside in the cytoplasm, nucleus, mitochondria and other extracellular locations, and can even shuttle to various subcellular locations [74]. The same lncRNA can reside in multiple cellular compartments and have a functional effect in each, which may make therapeutic intervention complex. Antisense and RNAi-based gene-knockdown methods vary in efficacy between different cellular compartments [74], thus the subcellular distribution of lncRNAs need to be determined in order to employ the best potential therapeutic approach [75].

ASOs (such as GapmeRs) are commonly used to inhibit lncRNAs, however, potency, toxicity, route of delivery, dose, duration of treatment, off-target effects, stability and specificity need to be considered when developing and testing ASOs as pharmacological agents. With the use of bioinformatics tools and gene sequence databases, the sequence of GapmeRs, specifically of the DNA gap and flanking LNAs, need to be carefully designed before they can be used *in vivo*. A carefully designed GapmeR should have favourable therapeutic properties including high target affinity, specificity, stability and favourable pharmacokinetic and tissue-penetrating properties.

Overexpression of lncRNA is also possible with the use of viral vectors, nanoparticles and RNA mimics, although these approaches also have their limitations. Challenges facing viral delivery of lncRNAs include (i) efficiency of lncRNA upregulation, (ii) low packaging limit of adeno-associated virus (AAV) vectors and these cannot be used for packaging lncRNA >3–4 kb; and (iii) ability to overexpress the lncRNA in the subcellular localization in which it resides [32]. Despite these challenges, two studies have used viral-mediated overexpression of lncRNAs in a mouse model of myocardial infarction demonstrating feasibility of this approach [76, 77]. The elevated risk of toxicity needs to be considered when using nanoparticles, and RNA mimics are prone to degradation and can have difficulties entering the cell [78].

4 Emerging Approaches to Deliver ncRNAs to the Heart

There are intense efforts to identify agents that are capable of targeted delivery of oligonucleotides to tissues and cells (see reviews [5, 9, 79, 80]). One common method to achieve targeted delivery is using viral approaches. AAV is the preferred method, and allows for greater flexibility as there are a number of AAV serotypes, promoters and reporter genes to choose from to enhance tissue specificity [81]. AAVs have been shown to be effective in delivering protein coding genes in preclinical models [82], and no side-effects were reported from clinical trials in patients with heart failure [83], demonstrating translational potential. AAVs are commonly employed to deliver miRNA "sponges" or "tough decoys" to inhibit miRNAs in the tissue of interest [84–88], although developing a cardiac-specific technology may be more difficult [89].

Other non-viral methods have recently been demonstrated to have the potential to deliver miRNA therapeutics to the heart. Ultrasound microbubbles coupled with a specific single-chain antibody has allowed targeted delivery of miRNA-126 mimics in abdominal aortic aneurysm [90], although antibodies specifically targeting cardiomyocytes need to be developed. Light-induced antimiR activation (a technique which facilitates local delivery) against miR-92a to improve angiogenesis has been demonstrated in human cells [91]. Coronary angiogenesis is reduced in hearts as they undergo pathological remodeling and this contributes towards the transition to heart failure [92]. This particular method of local delivery could potentially be applied at open-heart surgery in the clinic. An unlockable core-shell nanocomplex (Hep@PGEA) was used to deliver miR-499 to the hearts of mice following myocardial infarction [93]. This approach suppressed cardiomyocyte apoptosis and promoted cardiac repair, without showing any obvious toxic effects in other tissues [93]. Hydrogels are cross-linked polymers which can carry and release therapeutics after injection in tissues, are safe in large animal models [94], and successfully used to deliver miR-302 mimics to the heart to promote cardiomyocyte proliferation and regeneration following myocardial infarction [95]. These hydrogels could be delivered to the heart by catheter in a clinical setting. Negatively-charged calcium phosphate nanoparticles (CaP-NPs) for the delivery of miRNAs to cardiac cells *in vitro* and *in vivo* have been developed and used successfully [96], with a follow-up study showing an inhalation approach was effective for the delivery of therapeutics via CaP-NPs to the diseased heart [97]. Finally, CRISPR/cas9 technology is a powerful ncRNAs editing tool and has been shown to be an efficient and stable technology for inhibiting miRNA *in vitro* and *in vivo* [98].

5 Conclusion

NcRNAs have emerged as critical regulators of gene expression and function. Studies conducted over the last two decades clearly demonstrate that miRNAs and lncRNAs play an pivotal role in cardiovascular health and disease. Functional studies targeting these classes of ncRNAs demonstrate their therapeutic potential in treating pathology associated with cardiovascular disease such as hypertrophy, fibrosis and cardiac dysfunction. As a result of these favorable outcomes in preclinical models, approaches to deliver ncRNAs to the heart are being continually developed. However, further studies are necessary to clarify the role and regulation of ncRNAs in the heart to develop effective treatments for cardiovascular disease.

Acknowledgments The authors would like to thank Julie R. McMullen at Baker Heart & Diabetes Institute for proofreading the manuscript. The authors acknowledge funding support from the Sir Edward Dunlop Medical Research Foundation (to J.Y.Y.O and B.C.B). B.C.B is supported by an Alice Baker and Eleanor Shaw Fellowship (The Baker Foundation, Melbourne, Australia).

Competing Financial Interests The authors declare no competing financial interests.

References

1. Braunwald E. The war against heart failure: the Lancet lecture. Lancet. 2015;385(9970):812–24.
2. Mozaffarian D, Benjamin EJ, Go AS, Arnett DK, Blaha MJ, Cushman M, de Ferranti S, Després J-P, Fullerton HJ, Howard VJ, Huffman MD, Judd SE, Kissela BM, Lackland DT, Lichtman JH, Lisabeth LD, Liu S, Mackey RH, Matchar DB, McGuire DK, Mohler ER, Moy CS, Muntner P, Mussolino ME, Nasir K, Neumar RW, Nichol G, Palaniappan L, Pandey DK, Reeves MJ, Rodriguez CJ, Sorlie PD, Stein J, Towfighi A, Turan TN, Virani SS, Willey JZ, Woo D, Yeh RW, Turner MB. Heart disease and stroke statistics—2015 update: a report from the American Heart Association. Circulation. 2015;131:e29–e322.

3. Liu L, Eisen HJ. Epidemiology of heart failure and scope of the problem. Cardiol Clin. 2014;32(1):1–8.
4. Bernardo BC, Blaxall BC. From bench to bedside: new approaches to therapeutic discovery for heart failure. Heart Lung Circ. 2016;25(5):525–34.
5. Das A, Samidurai A, Salloum FN. Deciphering non-coding RNAs in cardiovascular health and disease. Front Cardiovasc Med. 2018;5:73.
6. Wadley GD, Lamon S, Alexander SE, McMullen JR, Bernardo BC. Non-coding RNAs regulating cardiac muscle mass. J Appl Physiol (Bethesda, Md: 1985). 2018.
7. Barwari T, Joshi A, Mayr M. MicroRNAs in cardiovascular disease. J Am Coll Cardiol. 2016;68(23):2577–84.
8. Bernardo BC, Charchar FJ, Lin RCY, McMullen JR. A MicroRNA guide for clinicians and basic scientists: background and experimental techniques. Heart Lung Circ. 2012;21(3):131–42.
9. Bernardo BC, Ooi JYY, Lin RCY, McMullen JR. miRNA therapeutics: a new class of drugs with potential therapeutic applications in the heart.Future. Med Chem. 2015;7(13):1771–92.
10. Hata A. Functions of MicroRNAs in cardiovascular biology and disease. Annu Rev Physiol. 2013;75(1):69–93.
11. Xiao J, Chen Y-H. MicroRNAs: novel regulators of the heart. J Thorac Dis. 2010;2(1):43–7.
12. Gidlöf O, Erlinge D. MicroRNAs in the failing heart – novel therapeutic targets? Scand Cardiovasc J. 2014;48(6):328–34.
13. Ooi JYY, Bernardo BC, McMullen JR. The therapeutic potential of microRNAs regulated in settings of physiological cardiac hypertrophy. Future Med Chem. 2014;6(2):205–22.
14. Wronska A, Kurkowska-Jastrzebska I, Santulli G. Application of microRNAs in diagnosis and treatment of cardiovascular disease. Acta Physiol. 2015;213(1):60–83.
15. Zhou SS, Jin JP, Wang JQ, Zhang ZG, Freedman JH, Zheng Y, Cai L. miRNAS in cardiovascular diseases: potential biomarkers, therapeutic targets and challenges. Acta Pharmacol Sin. 2018;39(7):1073–84.
16. Kumarswamy R, Bauters C, Volkmann I, Maury F, Fetisch J, Holzmann A, Lemesle G, de Groote P, Pinet F, Thum T. Circulating long noncoding RNA, LIPCAR, predicts survival in patients with heart failure. Circ Res. 2014;114(10):1569–75.
17. Kumarswamy R, Thum T. Non-coding RNAs in cardiac remodeling and heart failure. Circ Res. 2013;113(6):676–89.
18. Small EM, Olson EN. Pervasive roles of microRNAs in cardiovascular biology. Nature. 2011; 469(7330):336–42.
19. Lv D, Liu J, Zhao C, Sun Q, Zhou Q, Xu J, Xiao J. Targeting microRNAs in cardiac hypertrophy and heart failure. Mini Rev Med Chem. 2015
20. Montgomery RL, Hullinger TG, Semus HM, Dickinson BA, Seto AG, Lynch JM, Stack C, Latimer PA, Olson EN, van Rooij E. Therapeutic inhibition of miR-208a improves cardiac function and survival during heart failure/clinical perspective. Circulation. 2011;124(14):1537–47.
21. Grueter CE, van Rooij E, Johnson BA, DeLeon SM, Sutherland LB, Qi X, Gautron L, Elmquist JK, Bassel-Duby R, Olson EN. A cardiac microRNA governs systemic energy homeostasis by regulation of MED13. Cell. 2012;149(3):671–83.
22. Bernardo BC, Gao XM, Tham YK, Kiriazis H, Winbanks CE, Ooi JY, Boey EJ, Obad S, Kauppinen S, Gregorevic P, Du XJ, Lin RC, McMullen JR. Silencing of miR-34a attenuates cardiac dysfunction in a setting of moderate, but not severe, hypertrophic cardiomyopathy. PLoS One. 2014;9(2):e90337.
23. Bernardo BC, Gao XM, Winbanks CE, Boey EJ, Tham YK, Kiriazis H, Gregorevic P, Obad S, Kauppinen S, Du XJ, Lin RC, McMullen JR. Therapeutic inhibition of the miR-34 family attenuates pathological cardiac remodeling and improves heart function. Proc Natl Acad Sci U S A. 2012;109(43):17615–20.
24. Bernardo BC, Ooi JYY, Matsumoto A, Tham YK, Singla S, Kiriazis H, Patterson NL, Sadoshima J, Obad S, Lin RCY, McMullen JR. Sex differences in response to miRNA-34a therapy in mouse models of cardiac disease: identification of sex-, disease- and treatment-regulated miRNAs. J Physiol. 2016;594(20):5959–74.
25. Eding JE, Demkes CJ, Lynch JM, Seto AG, Montgomery RL, Semus HM, Jackson AL, Isabelle M, Chimenti S, van Rooij E. The efficacy of cardiac anti-miR-208a therapy is stress dependent. Mol Ther. 2017;25(3):694–704.
26. Cui C, Yang W, Shi J, Zhou Y, Yang J, Cui Q, Zhou Y. Identification and analysis of human sex-biased MicroRNAs. Genomics Proteomics Bioinformatics. 2018;16(3):200–11.
27. Tsuji M, Kawasaki T, Matsuda T, Arai T, Gojo S, Takeuchi JK. Sexual dimorphisms of mRNA and miRNA in human/murine heart disease. PLoS One. 2017;12(7):e0177988.
28. Sanchez-Ruderisch H, Queiros AM, Fliegner D, Eschen C, Kararigas G, Regitz-Zagrosek V. Sex-specific regulation of cardiac microRNAs targeting mitochondrial proteins in pressure overload. Biol Sex Differ. 2019;10(1):8.
29. Gomes CPC, Spencer H, Ford KL, Michel LYM, Baker AH, Emanueli C, Balligand JL, Devaux Y, Cardiolinc network. The function and therapeutic potential of Long non-coding RNAs in cardiovascular development and disease. Mol Ther Nucleic Acids. 2017;8:494–507.
30. Greco S, Salgado Somoza A, Devaux Y, Martelli F. Long noncoding RNAs and cardiac disease. Antioxid Redox Signal. 2018;29(9):880–901.
31. Hermans-Beijnsberger S, van Bilsen M, Schroen B. Long non-coding RNAs in the failing heart and vasculature. Non-coding RNA Res. 2018;3(3):118–30.
32. Hobuss L, Bar C, Thum T. Long non-coding RNAs: at the heart of cardiac dysfunction? Front Physiol. 2019;10:30.

33. Shen S, Jiang H, Bei Y, Xiao J, Li X. Long non-coding RNAs in cardiac remodeling. Cell Physiol Biochem. 2017;41(5):1830–7.
34. Castanotto D, Lin M, Kowolik C, Wang L, Ren XQ, Soifer HS, Koch T, Hansen BR, Oerum H, Armstrong B, Wang Z, Bauer P, Rossi J, Stein CA. A cytoplasmic pathway for gapmer antisense oligonucleotide-mediated gene silencing in mammalian cells. Nucleic Acids Res. 2015;43(19):9350–61.
35. Frieden M, Christensen SM, Mikkelsen ND, Rosenbohm C, Thrue CA, Westergaard M, Hansen HF, Orum H, Koch T. Expanding the design horizon of antisense oligonucleotides with alpha-L-LNA. Nucleic Acids Res. 2003;31(21):6365–72.
36. Micheletti R, Plaisance I, Abraham BJ, Sarre A, Ting CC, Alexanian M, Maric D, Maison D, Nemir M, Young RA, Schroen B, Gonzalez A, Ounzain S, Pedrazzini T. The long noncoding RNA Wisper controls cardiac fibrosis and remodeling. Sci Transl Med. 2017;9(395)
37. Viereck J, Kumarswamy R, Foinquinos A, Xiao K, Avramopoulos P, Kunz M, Dittrich M, Maetzig T, Zimmer K, Remke J, Just A, Fendrich J, Scherf K, Bolesani E, Schambach A, Weidemann F, Zweigerdt R, de Windt LJ, Engelhardt S, Dandekar T, Batkai S, Thum T. Long noncoding RNA Chast promotes cardiac remodeling. Sci Transl Med. 2016;8(326):326ra322.
38. Piccoli MT, Gupta SK, Viereck J, Foinquinos A, Samolovac S, Kramer FL, Garg A, Remke J, Zimmer K, Batkai S, Thum T. Inhibition of the cardiac fibroblast-enriched lncRNA Meg3 prevents cardiac fibrosis and diastolic dysfunction. Circ Res. 2017;121(5):575–83.
39. Miyoshi N, Wagatsuma H, Wakana S, Shiroishi T, Nomura M, Aisaka K, Kohda T, Surani MA, Kaneko-Ishino T, Ishino F. Identification of an imprinted gene, Meg3/Gtl2 and its human homologue MEG3, first mapped on mouse distal chromosome 12 and human chromosome 14q. Genes Cells. 2000;5(3):211–20.
40. Zhang X, Rice K, Wang Y, Chen W, Zhong Y, Nakayama Y, Zhou Y, Klibanski A. Maternally expressed gene 3 (MEG3) noncoding ribonucleic acid: isoform structure, expression, and functions. Endocrinology. 2010;151(3):939–47.
41. Tijsen AJ, Creemers EE, Moerland PD, de Windt LJ, van der Wal AC, Kok WE, Pinto YM. MiR423-5p as a circulating biomarker for heart failure. Circ Res. 2010;106(6):1035–9.
42. Goren Y, Kushnir M, Zafrir B, Tabak S, Lewis BS, Amir O. Serum levels of microRNAs in patients with heart failure. Eur J Heart Fail. 2012;14(2):147–54.
43. Ovchinnikova ES, Schmitter D, Vegter EL, Ter Maaten JM, Valente MA, Liu LC, van der Harst P, Pinto YM, de Boer RA, Meyer S, Teerlink JR, O'Connor CM, Metra M, Davison BA, Bloomfield DM, Cotter G, Cleland JG, Mebazaa A, Laribi S, Givertz MM, Ponikowski P, van der Meer P, van Veldhuisen DJ, Voors AA, Berezikov E. Signature of circulating microRNAs in patients with acute heart failure. Eur J Heart Fail. 2016;18(4):414–23.
44. Vegter EL, Schmitter D, Hagemeijer Y, Ovchinnikova ES, van der Harst P, Teerlink JR, O'Connor CM, Metra M, Davison BA, Bloomfield D, Cotter G, Cleland JG, Givertz MM, Ponikowski P, van Veldhuisen DJ, van der Meer P, Berezikov E, Voors AA, Khan MA. Use of biomarkers to establish potential role and function of circulating microRNAs in acute heart failure. Int J Cardiol. 2016;224:231–9.
45. Creemers EE, Tijsen AJ, Pinto YM. Circulating microRNAs: novel biomarkers and extracellular communicators in cardiovascular disease?Circulation. Research. 2012;110(3):483–95.
46. Xu J, Zhao J, Evan G, Xiao C, Cheng Y, Xiao J. Circulating microRNAs: novel biomarkers for cardiovascular diseases. J Mol Med (Berl). 2012;90(8):865–75.
47. Wang G-K, Zhu J-Q, Zhang J-T, Li Q, Li Y, He J, Qin Y-W, Jing Q. Circulating microRNA: a novel potential biomarker for early diagnosis of acute myocardial infarction in humans. Eur Heart J. 2010;31(6):659–66.
48. Wang R, Li N, Zhang Y, Ran Y, Pu J. Circulating MicroRNAs are promising novel biomarkers of acute myocardial infarction. Intern Med. 2011;50(17):1789–95.
49. Viereck J, Thum T. Circulating noncoding RNAs as biomarkers of cardiovascular disease and injury. Circ Res. 2017;120(2):381–99.
50. Vausort M, Wagner DR, Devaux Y. Long noncoding RNAs in patients with acute myocardial infarction. Circ Res. 2014;115(7):668–77.
51. Yin Q, Wu A, Liu M. Plasma Long non-coding RNA (lncRNA) GAS5 is a new biomarker for coronary artery disease. Med Sci Monit. 2017;23:6042–8.
52. de Gonzalo-Calvo D, Kenneweg F, Bang C, Toro R, van der Meer RW, Rijzewijk LJ, Smit JW, Lamb HJ, Llorente-Cortes V, Thum T. Circulating long-non coding RNAs as biomarkers of left ventricular diastolic function and remodelling in patients with well-controlled type 2 diabetes. Sci Rep. 2016;6:37354.
53. Gao L, Liu Y, Guo S, Yao R, Wu L, Xiao L, Wang Z, Liu Y, Zhang Y. Circulating long noncoding RNA HOTAIR is an essential mediator of acute myocardial infarction. Cell Physiol Biochem. 2017;44(4):1497–508.
54. Zhang Y, Sun L, Xuan L, Pan Z, Li K, Liu S, Huang Y, Zhao X, Huang L, Wang Z, Hou Y, Li J, Tian Y, Yu J, Han H, Liu Y, Gao F, Zhang Y, Wang S, Du Z, Lu Y, Yang B. Reciprocal changes of circulating Long non-coding RNAs ZFAS1 and CDR1AS predict acute myocardial infarction. Sci Rep. 2016;6:22384.
55. Yan Y, Zhang B, Liu N, Qi C, Xiao Y, Tian X, Li T, Liu B. Circulating long noncoding RNA UCA1 as a novel biomarker of acute myocardial infarction. Biomed Res Int. 2016;2016:8079372.
56. Xuan L, Sun L, Zhang Y, Huang Y, Hou Y, Li Q, Guo Y, Feng B, Cui L, Wang X, Wang Z, Tian Y, Yu B, Wang S, Xu C, Zhang M, Du Z, Lu Y, Yang BF. Circulating long non-coding RNAs NRON and MHRT as novel predictive biomarkers of heart failure. J Cell Mol Med. 2017;21(9):1803–14.

57. Chakraborty C, Sharma AR, Sharma G, Doss CGP, Lee S-S. Therapeutic miRNA and siRNA: moving from bench to clinic as next generation medicine. Mol Ther Nucleic Acids. 2017;8:132–43.
58. Janssen HL, Reesink HW, Lawitz EJ, Zeuzem S, Rodriguez-Torres M, Patel K, van der Meer AJ, Patick AK, Chen A, Zhou Y, Persson R, King BD, Kauppinen S, Levin AA, Hodges MR. Treatment of HCV infection by targeting microRNA. N Engl J Med. 2013;368(18):1685–94.
59. Sassi Y, Avramopoulos P, Ramanujam D, Gruter L, Werfel S, Giosele S, Brunner AD, Esfandyari D, Papadopoulou AS, De Strooper B, Hubner N, Kumarswamy R, Thum T, Yin X, Mayr M, Laggerbauer B, Engelhardt S. Cardiac myocyte miR-29 promotes pathological remodeling of the heart by activating Wnt signaling. Nat Commun. 2017;8(1):1614.
60. van Rooij E, Sutherland LB, Thatcher JE, DiMaio JM, Naseem RH, Marshall WS, Hill JA, Olson EN. Dysregulation of microRNAs after myocardial infarction reveals a role of miR-29 in cardiac fibrosis. Proc Natl Acad Sci U S A. 2008;105(35):13027–32.
61. McMullen JR, Bernardo BC. Inhibition of miR-29 protects against cardiac hypertrophy and fibrosis: new insight for the role of miR-29 in the heart. Non-coding RNA Investig. 2018;2:3.
62. Slabakova E, Culig Z, Remsik J, Soucek K. Alternative mechanisms of miR-34a regulation in cancer. Cell Death Dis. 2017;8(10):e3100.
63. Ooi JYY, Bernardo BC, Singla S, Patterson NL, Lin RCY, McMullen JR. Identification of miR-34 regulatory networks in settings of disease and antimiR-therapy: implications for treating cardiac pathology and other diseases. RNA Biol. 2017;14(5):500–13.
64. Stenvang J, Petri A, Lindow M, Obad S, Kauppinen S. Inhibition of microRNA function by antimiR oligonucleotides. Silence. 2012;3(1):1.
65. Matkovich SJ, Hu Y, Dorn GW. Regulation of cardiac microRNAs by cardiac microRNAs. Circ Res. 2013;113(1):62–71.
66. Patrick DM, Montgomery RL, Qi X, Obad S, Kauppinen S, Hill JA, van Rooij E, Olson EN. Stress-dependent cardiac remodeling occurs in the absence of microRNA-21 in mice. J Clin Invest. 2010;120(11):3912–6.
67. Thum T, Gross C, Fiedler J, Fischer T, Kissler S, Bussen M, Galuppo P, Just S, Rottbauer W, Frantz S, Castoldi M, Soutschek J, Koteliansky V, Rosenwald A, Basson MA, Licht JD, Pena JT, Rouhanifard SH, Muckenthaler MU, Tuschl T, Martin GR, Bauersachs J, Engelhardt S. MicroRNA-21 contributes to myocardial disease by stimulating MAP kinase signalling in fibroblasts. Nature. 2008;456(7224):980–4.
68. McMullen JR, Drew BG. Long non-coding RNAs (lncRNAs) in skeletal and cardiac muscle: potential therapeutic and diagnostic targets? Clin Sci. 2016;130(24):2245–56.
69. Lucas T, Dimmeler S. RNA therapeutics for treatment of cardiovascular diseases: promises and challenges. Circ Res. 2016;119(7):794–7.
70. Holdt LM, Beutner F, Scholz M, Gielen S, Gabel G, Bergert H, Schuler G, Thiery J, Teupser D. ANRIL expression is associated with atherosclerosis risk at chromosome 9p21. Arterioscler Thromb Vasc Biol. 2010;30(3):620–7.
71. Zhao B, Lu YL, Yang Y, Hu LB, Bai Y, Li RQ, Zhang GY, Li J, Bi CW, Yang LB, Hu C, Lei YH, Wang QL, Liu ZM. Overexpression of lncRNA ANRIL promoted the proliferation and migration of prostate cancer cells via regulating let-7a/TGF-beta1/Smad signaling pathway. Cancer Biomark. 2018;21(3):613–20.
72. Klattenhoff CA, Scheuermann JC, Surface LE, Bradley RK, Fields PA, Steinhauser ML, Ding H, Butty VL, Torrey L, Haas S, Abo R, Tabebordbar M, Lee RT, Burge CB, Boyer LA. Braveheart, a long noncoding RNA required for cardiovascular lineage commitment. Cell. 2013;152(3):570–83.
73. Zangrando J, Zhang L, Vausort M, Maskali F, Marie PY, Wagner DR, Devaux Y. Identification of candidate long non-coding RNAs in response to myocardial infarction. BMC Genomics. 2014;15:460.
74. Lennox KA, Behlke MA. Cellular localization of long non-coding RNAs affects silencing by RNAi more than by antisense oligonucleotides. Nucleic Acids Res. 2016;44(2):863–77.
75. Batista PJ, Chang HY. Long noncoding RNAs: cellular address codes in development and disease. Cell. 2013;152(6):1298–307.
76. Wang K, Long B, Zhou LY, Liu F, Zhou QY, Liu CY, Fan YY, Li PF. CARL lncRNA inhibits anoxia-induced mitochondrial fission and apoptosis in cardiomyocytes by impairing miR-539-dependent PHB2 downregulation. Nat Commun. 2014;5:3596.
77. Wang K, Sun T, Li N, Wang Y, Wang JX, Zhou LY, Long B, Liu CY, Liu F, Li PF. MDRL lncRNA regulates the processing of miR-484 primary transcript by targeting miR-361. PLoS Genet. 2014;10(7):e1004467.
78. Kaczmarek JC, Kowalski PS, Anderson DG. Advances in the delivery of RNA therapeutics: from concept to clinical reality. Genome Med. 2017;9(1):60.
79. Biglino G, Caputo M, Rajakaruna C, Angelini G, van Rooij E, Emanueli C. Modulating microRNAs in cardiac surgery patients: novel therapeutic opportunities? Pharmacol Ther. 2017;170:192–204.
80. Kwekkeboom RF, Lei Z, Doevendans PA, Musters RJ, Sluijter JP. Targeted delivery of miRNA therapeutics for cardiovascular diseases: opportunities and challenges. Clin Sci. 2014;127(6):351–65.
81. Bass-Stringer S, Bernardo BC, May CN, Thomas CJ, Weeks KL, McMullen JR. Adeno-associated virus gene therapy: translational Progress and future prospects in the treatment of heart failure. Heart Lung Circ. 2018;27(11):1285–300.
82. Byrne MJ, Power JM, Preovolos A, Mariani JA, Hajjar RJ, Kaye DM. Recirculating cardiac delivery of AAV2/1SERCA2a improves myocardial function

in an experimental model of heart failure in large animals. Gene Ther. 2008;15(23):1550–7.
83. Zsebo K, Yaroshinsky A, Rudy JJ, Wagner K, Greenberg B, Jessup M, Hajjar RJ. Long-term effects of AAV1/SERCA2a gene transfer in patients with severe heart failure: analysis of recurrent cardiovascular events and mortality. Circ Res. 2014;114(1):101–8.
84. Jeong D, Yoo J, Lee P, Kepreotis SV, Lee A, Wahlquist C, Brown BD, Kho C, Mercola M, Hajjar RJ. miR-25 tough decoy enhances cardiac function in heart failure. Mol Ther. 2018;26(3):718–29.
85. Krol J, Busskamp V, Markiewicz I, Stadler MB, Ribi S, Richter J, Duebel J, Bicker S, Fehling HJ, Schubeler D, Oertner TG, Schratt G, Bibel M, Roska B, Filipowicz W. Characterizing light-regulated retinal microRNAs reveals rapid turnover as a common property of neuronal microRNAs. Cell. 2010;141(4):618–31.
86. Winbanks CE, Beyer C, Hagg A, Qian H, Sepulveda PV, Gregorevic P. miR-206 represses hypertrophy of myogenic cells but not muscle Fibers via inhibition of HDAC4. PLoS ONE. 2013;8(9):e73589.
87. Xie J, Ameres SL, Friedline R, Hung JH, Zhang Y, Xie Q, Zhong L, Su Q, He R, Li M, Li H, Mu X, Zhang H, Broderick JA, Kim JK, Weng Z, Flotte TR, Zamore PD, Gao G. Long-term, efficient inhibition of microRNA function in mice using rAAV vectors. Nat Methods. 2012;9(4):403–9.
88. Wang F, Fang Q, Chen C, Zhou L, Li H, Yin Z, Wang Y, Zhao CX, Xiao X, Wang DW. Recombinant Adeno-associated virus-mediated delivery of MicroRNA-21-3p lowers hypertension. Mol Ther Nucleic Acids. 2018;11:354–66.
89. Bernardo BC, Gregorevic P, Ritchie RH, McMullen JR. Generation of microRNA-34 sponges and tough decoys for the heart: developments and challenges. Front Pharmacol Transl Pharmacol. 2018;9:1090.
90. Wang X, Searle AK, Hohmann JD, Liu AL, Abraham M-K, Palasubramaniam J, Lim B, Yao Y, Wallert M, Yu E, Chen Y-C, Peter K. Dual-targeted theranostic delivery of miRs arrests abdominal aortic aneurysm development. Mol Ther. 2018;26(4):1056–65.
91. Schafer F, Wagner J, Knau A, Dimmeler S, Heckel A. Regulating angiogenesis with light-inducible AntimiRs. Angew Chem Int Ed Engl. 2013;52(51):13558–61.
92. Shiojima I, Sato K, Izumiya Y, Schiekofer S, Ito M, Liao R, Colucci WS, Walsh K. Disruption of coordinated cardiac hypertrophy and angiogenesis contributes to the transition to heart failure. J Clin Investig. 2005;115(8):2108–18.
93. Nie JJ, Qiao B, Duan S, Xu C, Chen B, Hao W, Yu B, Li Y, Du J, Xu FJ. Unlockable nanocomplexes with self-accelerating nucleic acid release for effective staged gene therapy of cardiovascular diseases. Adv Mater. 2018;30(31):e1801570.
94. Seif-Naraghi SB, Singelyn JM, Salvatore MA, Osborn KG, Wang JJ, Sampat U, Kwan OL, Strachan GM, Wong J, Schup-Magoffin PJ, Braden RL, Bartels K, DeQuach JA, Preul M, Kinsey AM, DeMaria AN, Dib N, Christman KL. Safety and efficacy of an injectable extracellular matrix hydrogel for treating myocardial infarction. J Transl Med. 2013;5(173):173ra125.
95. Wang LL, Liu Y, Chung JJ, Wang T, Gaffey AC, Lu M, Cavanaugh CA, Zhou S, Kanade R, Atluri P, Morrisey EE, Burdick JA. Sustained miRNA delivery from an injectable hydrogel promotes cardiomyocyte proliferation and functional regeneration after ischaemic injury. Nat Biomed Eng. 2017;1(12):983–92.
96. Di Mauro V, Iafisco M, Salvarani N, Vacchiano M, Carullo P, Ramirez-Rodriguez GB, Patricio T, Tampieri A, Miragoli M, Catalucci D. Bioinspired negatively charged calcium phosphate nanocarriers for cardiac delivery of MicroRNAs. Nanomedicine (Lond). 2016;11(8):891–906.
97. Miragoli M, Ceriotti P, Iafisco M, Vacchiano M, Salvarani N, Alogna A, Carullo P, Ramirez-Rodríguez GB, Patrício T, Esposti LD, Rossi F, Ravanetti F, Pinelli S, Alinovi R, Erreni M, Rossi S, Condorelli G, Post H, Tampieri A, Catalucci D. Inhalation of peptide-loaded nanoparticles improves heart failure. Sci Transl Med. 2018;10(424)
98. Chang H, Yi B, Ma R, Zhang X, Zhao H, Xi Y. CRISPR/cas9, a novel genomic tool to knock down microRNA in vitro and in vivo. Sci Rep. 2016;6:22312.

Part V

Potential Biomarkers and Therapeutic Implications

Circulating Non-coding RNAs and Cardiovascular Diseases

22

Chenglin Zhao, Yicheng Lv, Yi Duan, Guoping Li, and Zhongrong Zhang

Abstract

The discovery of noncoding RNAs (ncRNAs) including short microRNAs, long ncRNAs and circular RNAs has broaden our knowledge about mammalian genomes and transcriptomes. A growing number of evidence on aberrantly regulated ncRNAs in cardiovascular diseases has indicated that ncRNAs are critical contributors to cardiovascular pathophysiology. Moreover, multiple recent studies have reported that ncRNAs can be detected in the bloodstream that differs between health subjects and diseased patients and some of them are remarkably stable. Although our knowledge about the origin and function of the circulating ncRNAs is still limited, these molecules have been regarded as promising noninvasive biomarker for risk stratification, diagnosis and prognosis of various cardiovascular diseases. In this chapter, we have described biological characteristics of circulating ncRNAs and discussed current trends and future prospects for the usage of circulating ncRNAs as biomarkers for common cardiovascular diseases.

Keywords

Non-coding RNAs · Biomarker · Cardiovascular diseases · Heart diseases

1 Background

Only less than 3% of the human genome encodes messenger RNAs (mRNAs) that are encoded and participate in protein biosynthesis [1]. On the other hand, there are much more non-coding RNAs (ncRNAs) in the genome, most of which have undetermined functions. NcRNAs can be divided into basic ncRNAs and regulatory ncRNAs. Regulatory ncRNA can be further divided into microRNA (miRNA), long non-coding RNA (lncRNA), circular RNA (circRNA), piwi-interacting RNA (piRNA) and small interfering RNA (siRNA) [2]. Not surprisingly, regulatory ncRNAs have been found to be critical players in pathogenesis of human diseases, including cardiovascular diseases (CVDs). Numerous studies have demonstrated that miRNAs play a key role in driving gene expression changes in multiple cardiovascular pathological processes including cardiac hypertrophy, fibrosis, ischemia injury and heart failure [3, 4]. Whereas the role of lncRNAs and circRNAs are less

C. Zhao · Y. Lv · Y. Duan · Z. Zhang (✉)
Cardiac Regeneration and Ageing Lab, Institute of Cardiovascular Sciences, School of Life Science, Shanghai University, Shanghai, China

G. Li
Cardiology Division, Massachusetts General Hospital, Harvard Medical School, Boston, MA, USA

J. Xiao (ed.), *Non-coding RNAs in Cardiovascular Diseases*, Advances in Experimental Medicine and Biology 1229, https://doi.org/10.1007/978-981-15-1671-9_22

understood compared to miRNAs, to date only a few candidates have been investigated in detail in cardiovascular system. Circulating ncRNAs have been have recently emerged as promising non-invasive biomarkers because their tissue- and time-specific expression pattern in CVDs and their ability to circulate in the bloodstream in a relative stable extracellular form [5]. Here, we present a brief introduction on miRNAs, lncRNAs and circRNAs, summarize the recent discovery of these ncRNAs in related to biomarker potential for common type of CVDs and, finally, discuss the current limitations and future prospects in developing ncRNAs as CVD biomarkers.

1.1 MicroRNAs

MiRNAs are abundant family of small ncRNAs in human genomes, containing more than 2000 different loci for miRNA generation [6], it is estimated that over 30% of the cellular transcriptome is orchestrated by miRNAs [7]. MiRNA is a short 18-22 nt ncRNA produced by transcription of specific genomic locus and specialized RNA endonuclease treatment [8, 9]. MiRNA transcription is conducted by RNA Pol II and is controlled by RNA Pol II-associated transcription factors and epigenetic regulators [10–13]. The primary miRNA (pri-miRNA) then go through several steps to become mature miRNA, with the help of nuclear RNase III Drosha [14–16]. Mature miRNAs can negatively regulate expression of target genes by binding to the 3'-UTR region of mRNAs and recruiting specific silencing proteins that form RNA-induced silencing complexes (RISC) [7]. In healthy condition, miRNAs act as modulators to steady protein levels that maintain physiological homeostasis. The regulatory activity of miRNAs depends on the abundance of their targets, so the same miRNA may have different regulatory function in different cell types [17]. While during pathological process, ectopic or aberrant expression of a particular miRNA in its original tissue can result in deregulation of its target transcripts and imbalanced physical functions. MiRNAs have been found present in variety of extracellular human body fluids including plasma, serum, saliva and urine [18–21]. Blood circulating miRNAs are most studied and found that the majority of circulating miRNAs in human blood are related with a protein named Argonaute 2 (Ago2) [22]. Ago2 is the effector component of the miRNA-induced silencing complex (RISC), it can directly bind miRNAs and drive mRNA suppression [23, 24]. Therefore it has been speculated that the majority of circulating miRNAs may be products released from dead cells that remain in extracellular space because of the high stability of Ago2-miRNA complex [5], which makes them potential indicators for various pathological conditions.

1.2 Long Non-coding RNAs

Long non-coding RNAs, also known as long ncRNAs or lncRNAs, are non-coding RNA transcripts that are longer than 200 nt, similar to protein-coding genes but lacking evident ORFs [25–27]. LncRNAs represent the majority of the ncRNAs, to date more than 58,000 lncRNAs has been classified [28]. However, only a few of them has been characterized with structure, function and impact in physical or pathological process. LncRNAs are produced with RNA polymerase II, which can be antisense, interleaved or overlapping with protein-coding genes, those sequences of lncRNA that do not overlap protein-coding genes term long intervening/intergenic noncoding RNAs (lincRNAs) [29]. LncRNAs are suggested very relevant players in the regulation of cellular functions because evidence shows they can interact with genomic DNA and RNA as a flexible molecular scaffold to recruit chromatin-modifying enzymes and transcription factors and to guide their transportation to the correct functional localization [30]. In addition, lncRNAs can act as guide molecules for DNA methyltransferase and histone modifier such as polycomb repressive complex PRC2 and histone H3 lysine 9 (H3K9) methyltransferases, which lead to repressive heterochromatin and the resultant transcriptional repression [31–33]. LncRNAs have also been reported to control the activity of other ncRNAs, particularly miRNAs, as decoys or sponges that can absorb miRNAs from their mRNA targets (and thus act as competing endogenous RNAs or ceRNAs) [34]. Loss of function experiments have provided evidence for the functional importance of lncRNAs in regulation of gene expression patterns that control cellular pluripotency, differentiation and survival [35]. Because of the enormous potential of lncRNAs to regulate gene expression, there is a growing interest in the potential roles of these RNAs in disease pathogenesis. In fact, numerous studies have shown a correlation between lncRNA dysregulation, with changes in gene expression and pathogenesis. Moreover, some studies have also suggested potential role of lncRNA in gene regulation outside the cell and between different cells. Recent researches have demonstrated that it is possible to detect the presence of lncRNAs in human body fluids, indicating the possible connection between circulating lncRNA concentration and disease initiation and development, makes lncRNAs potential novel diagnostic and prognostic tools [36]. However, on the other hand, most lncRNAs rapidly evolve at sequence and expression levels, it has been suggested that tissue-specific and possible three-dimensional structures of lncRNA are only conserved among closely related species.

1.3 Circular RNAs (CircRNAs)

CircRNAs are a new class of endogenous non-coding RNAs and a field with much research activity, although the existence of circulating transcripts have been discovered for more than 20 years [37]. They are characterized by a covalently closed loop structure formed by back-splicing event that inversely connect exon boundaries [38]. These circular molecules have long been regarded as the artifacts of aberrant splicing or prerogative of several types of virus [39–41]. However, recent studies by using specific computational algorithm to identify circular molecules have demonstrated that in many cells the production of circRNA is not as rare as previously believed [42–44]. A growing number of evidence indicates that circRNAs are abundant, conserved, and stably accumulated in cells, and the expression pattern of circRNAs is highly dependent on cell type and species [45, 46]. Besides, circular RNAs are highly resistant to exonuclease RNase R, which makes them much more stable than to linear RNAs [47, 48], that explain their relative high evaluation conservation. The regulatory functions of circRNA remain to be further explored. Scientists have suggested several putative mechanisms of gene regulation by circular RNAs. (1) miRNA sponge: competitive endogenous RNA hypothesis is currently the most intensively studied and well accepted mechanism on regulatory activity of circRNAs on gene expression. CircRNA molecules contain lots of miRNA response elements (MREs) that allow them to competitively bind to miRNAs, causing suppression of the functional miRNA molecules and subsequent elevation of target miRNAs [47, 49]. (2) Interaction with RNA binding proteins (RBPs): strong direct interaction between circRNAs and their target RBPs enable gene regulation by competing with linear splicing [41]. (3) Regulation of parental gene transcription: some intronic circRNAs enhance the transcription of their hosting gene, probably by modulating RNA polymerase II in cis [50]. (4) Protein translation: some recent studies have demonstrated the potential of circRNA for direct protein translation, such as circ-ZNF609, circMbl3 and circ-SHPRH [51–53]. Furthermore, computational analysis of human transcriptomes sequencing has revealed the universal existence of circRNAs with coding potential [54, 55]. Due to their emerging role as regulators of gene expression, circRNAs are considered as important players in disease development. In addition, the stability of these circular molecule allow them to be easily identified and quantified in body fluid, which makes them high promising diagnostic biomarkers [46].

2 Circulating Non-coding RNA as Biomarkers for Cardiovascular Diseases

2.1 Myocardial Infarction

Myocardial infarction (MI) is the leading cause of death worldwide and is characterized by ischemia-induced localized heart tissue damage that induces cardiac remodeling and may progress to chronic heart failure. Appropriate therapies are required to reduce the mortality and thus a rapid diagnosis with high sensitivity and specificity is critical. MI is characterized by cell death and hypoxic stress, resulting in the release of various cardiac-specific proteins into the circulation. Classic MI biomarkers include serum concentrations of cardiac troponin (cardiac troponin T and I) and creatine kinase MB (CK-MB) [56]. Other than traditional protein markers, myocardium also releases ncRNAs into the bloodstream once injured. Numerous studies have described that single or a group of miRNAs in circulation can act as potential biomarker for cardiac injury including MI [57, 58]. MiR-1, which is abundantly expressed in cardiac and skeletal muscle and crucial in muscle differentiation and cardiac development, is firstly suggested as a circulating miRNA biomarker for acute MI [59–61]. Another high muscle-expressed miRNA miR-133, which is a crucial regulator of muscle development and pathophysiological alterations, has also been suggested to be a diagnostic biomarker for acute MI without prognostic potential on future left ventricular remodeling after MI [61, 62]. Cardiac-specific miRNAs miR-499 and miR-208a/b expressed by cardiac myosin genes have been suggested as biomarkers for myocardial damage and infarct severity [63]. In addition, results from patient and animal models showed a positive correlation between muscle and myocardial circulating miRNAs and acute MI with T-segment elevation (STEMI). The circulating levels of miRNAs including miR-1, miR-499-5p, miR-133a and miR-133b and followed the same pattern as rising of cardiac troponin T level and left ventricular ejection fraction (LVEF) in STEMI patients. Therefore, these miRNAs were regarded to be related to the extent of myocardial damage and necrosis after infarction [60]. It is worth mention that circulating non-muscle miRNA levels in patients with STEMI, such as liver miR-122-5p or pancreas-specific miR-375, showed an opposite pattern of muscle and cardiac-specific miRNAs, which was down-regulated in STEMI group of patients. These results were not consistent with the results observed in animal models of cardiogenic shock, in which plasma levels of liver-specific miR-122 showed a massive increase after external cardiac intervention and could indicate the time of infarction [64]. Additionally, a recent study has shown that plasma miR-122 levels measured less than 8 h after infarction demonstrated the same pattern of increase as that in animal models and miR-122-5p/133b ratio can act as a prognostic biomarker for successful stratification of STEMI patients [65]. Level of miR-133b in MI was measured in infarct-related artery (IRA) occlusion, without ST-segment elevation. Patients with closed IRA were found with higher levels of miR-133a, miR-133b then patients with patented IRA, but there was no difference in troponin T levels. These resulted suggested that elevated circulating miRNAs reveal the degree of IRA in MI and may indicate patients requiring urgent coronary revascularization [66].

Circulating miRNAs have also been used to predict individual risk for future fatal acute MI in healthy individuals [67]. The HUNT study examined 112 healthy subjects and identified 10 plasma miRNAs that were differentially expressed between lethal cases and controls. The best miRNA expression model for prediction of future fatal MI consists of miR-106a, miR-424, let-7 g, miR-144 and miR-660 levels, which provided a correct risk assessment of 77.6% (74.1% and 81.8% for men and woman respectively). Other circulating miRNAs such as miR-34a, miR-192 and miR-194 have also been shown to be good predictors of risk assessment for heart failure after MI [68]. These miRNAs are expressed in a p53-dependent manner, linking them to other miRNAs that have been described as driving factors for CVDs [69]. Collectively, multiple studies have confirmed the ideas that circulating miRNA may serve as sensitive and specific biomarkers for MI, the combination of miRNA with cardiac troponin might be accurate diagnostic and prognostic tool for patients.

Recently, some circulating lncRNAs and circRNAs have also been explored as potential biomarkers of acute MI. CDR1 antisense (CDR1AS) and cyclic zinc finger antisense 1 (ZFAS1) showed significant differential expression between acute MI patients and healthy subjects; and similar changes in circulating CDR1AS and ZFAS1 were also consistently observed in the mouse models. Thereby researchers suggested changes in circulating CDR1AS and ZFAS1 could independently predict acute MI [70]. Another lncRNA urothelial carcinoma associated 1 (UCA1) was studied as well, which was found to be expressed in bladder and lung cancer and suggested as a predictive biomarker. UCA1 is specifically expressed in the heart of healthy adult individuals; while plasma UCA1 levels are reduced in the early state of patients with acute MI and increased on day 3 post-MI. The level of UCA1 circulating was also found negatively correlated with the expression of miR-177 [71].

2.2 Coronary Artery Disease

Coronary Artery Disease (CAD) is caused by the formation of atherosclerotic plaques, resulting in structural remodeling of the arterial wall, activation of endothelial cells and inflammatory cells may eventually lead to myocardial ischemia [72]. Activation of endothelial cells is critical for atherosclerosis; it is a potential source to seek new biomarkers for early diagnosis and identification of instable plaque, which eventually allow risk stratification of patients. It has been suggested that miRNAs associated with cellular components formed by atherogenesis are deregulated in CAD [73]. However, the cyclic signature data of CAD miRNAs are not consistent. Endothelial cells (miR-17, miR-92a and miR-126), inflammation (miR-155) and smooth muscle cell-associated (miR-145) miRNA were found to decrease in the circulation of CAD patients, while plasma myocardium and muscle miRNA (miR- 133a, miR-208a and miR-499) were increased. It was believed that miRNA may be cleared from the bloodstream by ingestion of atherosclerotic lesions or vasculature, and that enhanced release and elevation of miRNA may reflect myocardial damage [74]. In contrast, the miRNA signature of miR-126 and miR-17/92a cluster was up-regulated together with miR-451, miR-106b/25 cluster and miR-21/590-5p family in vulnerable CAD and was suggested as a novel biomarker [75]. Consistent with previous results, miR-1, miR-133a/b, miR-122, miR-126 and miR-199a have been reported elevated in the circulation of stable and unstable angina patients and miR-92a and miR-486 were associated with high-density lipoprotein components identified as potential circulating biomarkers for coronary plaque [76–78]. In addition, the severity of CAD for patients with hyperlipidemia was found associated with increased plasma levels of lipid metabolism-related miR-122 and miR-370 [79]. MiRNA signatures for risk assessment in patients with symptomatic obstructive CAD and chest pain were explored. MiR-134, miR-2861 and miR-3135b were associated with coronary artery calcification and were altered in patients with obstructive CAD [80]. A prognostic analysis evaluated circulating vascular and endothelial miRNAs in patients with CAD and found expression level of miR-126 and miR-199a contained in microvesicles but not freely circulating miRNA could predict the occurrence of cardiovascular events in patients with stable CAD [81]. Collectively, blood miRNAs have the potential to improve CAD diagnosis and prognosis, whereas, replication and validation of these findings in large independent cohorts are still required.

Recently, lncRNAs have get attention as CAD biomarkers. Microarray-based screening of plasma in CAD patients identified a transcript called CoroMarker as a marker for stability, sensitivity, and specificity of the CAD [82, 83]. This lncRNA is present in extracellular vesicles and circulating monocytes in peripheral blood. The same group reported another lncRNA LncPPARδ, which was elevated in circulating peripheral blood mononuclear cells, as another CAD biomarker in combination with other risk factors [84]. The combined use of circRNAs and miRNAs as biomarker for carotid plaque rupture was also investigated and found the ratio of serum circR-284/has-miR-221 was significantly increased in acutely symptomatic patients with carotid disease. This combination demonstrated favorable characteristics to be a prognostic biomarker of plaque rapture and stroke [85].

2.3 Cardiomyopathy

Cardiomyopathies are a group of heart diseases characterized by morphological and functional abnormalities in the myocardium. When they originate from myocardial dysfunction or changes in the body, they can be classified as primary or intrinsic cardiomyopathy; and when their pathogenic factors are external factors for the heart, they can be classified as secondary or extrinsic cardiomyopathy [72]. Intrinsic cardiomyopathy can be obtained with a genetic basis or in response to stress on the myocardium. Inherited cardiomyopathies are the most common form of the disease, hence genetic testing is the most common diagnosis. Also, patients with cardiomyopathy often receive a series of biochemical tests to detect biomarkers that can assist diagnose [86]. Several therapies for cancer and other diseases can cause serious side effects that affect cardiovascular health. Cardiotoxicity and damage impede heart function and cause high blood pressure, apoptosis, arrhythmia, fibrosis, and finally heart failure. Therefore, minimizing or preventing these side effects by early monitoring of drug-induced cardiotoxicity and damage would be very significant for treatment strategies [87]. A few studies have evaluated ncRNA plasma levels in drug-induced cardiomyopathies. An in vivo study evaluating isoproterenol-induced cardiactoxic model in rats reported an increase in serum miR-208 level in a time-dependent manner and was associated with traditional myocardial injury cardiac troponin I [88]. Other animal studies support the response of miR-208 to isoproterenol, metaproterenol, allylamine and mitoxantrone [89–91]. On the other hand, miR-208 did not respond to a single administration of doxorubicin, and doxorubicin treatment induced other muscle and heart-specific miRNAs. In the chemotherapy treatment of doxorubicin, circulating miR-208a was not detected in the bloodstream of breast cancer patients [92]. These differences may be due to species-specificity, time- or dose-dependent effects, or indicate that different drugs may cause different circulating miRNA patterns. Therefore, other miRNAs should be considered to be biomarkers of drug-induced cardiotoxicity. Zhao et al. determined whether detectable levels of specific miRNAs are released into the circulation for bevacizumab-induced cardiotoxicity. They identified two cancer-associated miRNAs (miR-579 and miR-1254) that were specifically elevated in the circulation of bevacizumab-induced cardiotoxic patients and distinguish this patient group from AMI patients. MiR-1254 also showed strong correlation to the clinical diagnosis of bevacizumab-induced cardiotoxicity [93].

3 Prospects and Challenges

We have accumulated a great deal about the association of circulating miRNAs with various types of human heart diseases and injuries. Other circulating ncRNAs species as lncRNAs and circRNAs are also promising biomarkers of CVDs, however their physiological or pathological roles in the context of CVDs remain largely unknown. The study of circulating lncRNAs asa cardiac biomarkers is not as advanced as miRNA, partially because of the general assumption that lncRNAs are unstable in body fluids and the findings that lncRNAs are not conserved among species as miRNAs. However, recent data indicate that most lncRNAs are stable in neuroblastoma cell lines, although this study does not address the problem of extracellular stability [94]. Additionally, due to the emerging role of circRNA as regulators of gene expression, circRNA is likely to be an important player in the initiation and progress of diseases including CVDs. Research on the circular and stable RNA molecules has just begun and is a completely new field of research that will help to better understand the pathogenesis of CVDs. Regulatory networks occur in complex organisms and the surprising stability of these molecules suggests that circRNAs have great potential to be developed as CVD biomarkers.

Nevertheless, currently the use of ncRNA is still limited by (1) insufficient knowledge about the origin and function of ncRNAs especially for lncRNA and circRNAs; (2) diversity of RNA extraction and ncRNA detection methods without a standard protocol; (3) lack of consistency and standardization in different studies on same type of CVDs; (4) a relatively small patient cohort to date [95]. Still, some circulating ncRNAs appear to have stronger diagnostic and prognostic value than conventional biomarkers, not only because of their tissue and disease-specific expression patterns, but also because of the high physicochemical properties and their high stability in circulation system [96–98]. Whether circulating ncRNAs represent attractive diagnostic and prognostic biomarkers required future studies of large cohorts with standardized protocol for processing body fluid and RNA procreation and consistent analysis method.

Acknowledgements This work was supported by the grants from National Natural Science Foundation of China.

Competing Financial Interests The authors declare no competing financial interests.

References

1. Lander ES, Linton LM, Birren B, Nusbaum C, Zody MC, Baldwin J, Devon K, Dewar K, Doyle M, FitzHugh W, Funke R, Gage D, Harris K, Heaford A, Howland J, Kann L, Lehoczky J, LeVine R, McEwan P, McKernan K, Meldrim J, Mesirov JP, Miranda C, Morris W, Naylor J, Raymond C, Rosetti M, Santos R, Sheridan A, Sougnez C, Stange-Thomann Y, Stojanovic N, Subramanian A, Wyman D, Rogers J, Sulston J, Ainscough R, Beck S, Bentley D, Burton J, Clee C, Carter N, Coulson A, Deadman R, Deloukas P, Dunham A, Dunham I, Durbin R, French L, Grafham D, Gregory S, Hubbard T, Humphray S, Hunt A, Jones M, Lloyd C, McMurray A, Matthews L, Mercer S, Milne S, Mullikin JC, Mungall A, Plumb R, Ross M, Shownkeen R, Sims S, Waterston RH, Wilson RK, Hillier LW, McPherson JD, Marra MA, Mardis ER, Fulton LA, Chinwalla AT, Pepin KH, Gish WR, Chissoe SL, Wendl MC, Delehaunty KD, Miner TL, Delehaunty A, Kramer JB, Cook LL, Fulton RS, Johnson DL, Minx PJ, Clifton SW, Hawkins T, Branscomb E, Predki P, Richardson P, Wenning S, Slezak T, Doggett N, Cheng JF, Olsen A, Lucas S, Elkin C, Uberbacher E, Frazier M, Gibbs RA, Muzny DM, Scherer SE, Bouck JB, Sodergren EJ, Worley KC, Rives CM, Gorrell JH, Metzker ML, Naylor SL, Kucherlapati RS, Nelson DL, Weinstock GM, Sakaki Y, Fujiyama A, Hattori M, Yada T, Toyoda A, Itoh T, Kawagoe C, Watanabe H, Totoki Y, Taylor T, Weissenbach J, Heilig R, Saurin W, Artiguenave F, Brottier P, Bruls T, Pelletier E, Robert C, Wincker P, Smith DR, Doucette-Stamm L, Rubenfield M, Weinstock K, Lee HM, Dubois J, Rosenthal A, Platzer M, Nyakatura G, Taudien S, Rump A, Yang H, Yu J, Wang J, Huang G, Gu J, Hood L, Rowen L, Madan A, Qin S, Davis RW, Federspiel NA, Abola AP, Proctor MJ, Myers RM, Schmutz J, Dickson M, Grimwood J, Cox DR, Olson MV, Kaul R, Raymond C, Shimizu N, Kawasaki K, Minoshima S, Evans GA, Athanasiou M, Schultz R, Roe BA, Chen F, Pan H, Ramser J, Lehrach H, Reinhardt R, McCombie WR, de la Bastide M, Dedhia N, Blocker H, Hornischer K, Nordsiek G, Agarwala R, Aravind L, Bailey JA, Bateman A, Batzoglou S, Birney E, Bork P, Brown DG, Burge CB, Cerutti L, Chen HC, Church D, Clamp M, Copley RR, Doerks T, Eddy SR, Eichler EE, Furey TS, Galagan J, Gilbert JG, Harmon C, Hayashizaki Y, Haussler D, Hermjakob H, Hokamp K, Jang W, Johnson LS, Jones TA, Kasif S, Kaspryzk A, Kennedy S, Kent WJ, Kitts P, Koonin EV, Korf I, Kulp D, Lancet D, Lowe TM, McLysaght A, Mikkelsen T, Moran JV, Mulder N, Pollara VJ, Ponting CP, Schuler G, Schultz J, Slater G, Smit AF, Stupka E, Szustakowki J, Thierry-Mieg D, Thierry-Mieg J, Wagner L, Wallis J, Wheeler R, Williams A, Wolf YI, Wolfe KH, Yang SP, Yeh RF, Collins F, Guyer MS, Peterson J, Felsenfeld A, Wetterstrand KA, Patrinos A, Morgan MJ, de Jong P, Catanese JJ, Osoegawa K, Shizuya H, Choi S, Chen YJ, Szustakowki J, International Human Genome Sequencing C. Initial sequencing and analysis of the human genome. Nature. 2001;409(6822):860–921.
2. Thum T. Facts and updates about cardiovascular non-coding RNAs in heart failure. ESC Heart Failure. 2015;2(3):108–11.
3. Papait R, Kunderfranco P, Stirparo GG, Latronico MV, Condorelli G. Long noncoding RNA: a new player of heart failure? J Cardiovasc Transl Res. 2013;6(6):876–83.
4. Thum T, Condorelli G. Long noncoding RNAs and microRNAs in cardiovascular pathophysiology. Circ Res. 2015;116(4):751–62.
5. Turchinovich A, Weiz L, Langheinz A, Burwinkel B. Characterization of extracellular circulating microRNA. Nucleic Acids Res. 2011;39(16):7223–33.
6. Kozomara A, Griffiths-Jones S. miRBase: annotating high confidence microRNAs using deep sequencing

data. Nucleic Acids Res. 2014;42(Database issue):D68–73.
7. Bartel DP. MicroRNAs: target recognition and regulatory functions. Cell. 2009;136(2):215–33.
8. Zhuo Y, Gao G, Shi JA, Zhou X, Wang X. miRNAs: biogenesis, origin and evolution, functions on virus-host interaction. Cell Physiol Biochem. 2013;32(3):499–510.
9. Lee Y, Jeon K, Lee JT, Kim S, Kim VN. MicroRNA maturation: stepwise processing and subcellular localization. Eur Mol Biol Organ J. 2002;21(17):4663–70.
10. Krol J, Loedige I, Filipowicz W. The widespread regulation of microRNA biogenesis, function and decay. Nat Rev Genet. 2010;11(9):597–610.
11. Lee Y, Kim M, Han J, Yeom KH, Lee S, Baek SH, Kim VN. MicroRNA genes are transcribed by RNA polymerase II. Eur Mol Biol Organ J. 2004;23(20):4051–60.
12. Kim VN, Han J, Siomi MC. Biogenesis of small RNAs in animals. Nat Rev Mol Cell Biol. 2009;10(2):126–39.
13. Davis-Dusenbery BN, Hata A. Mechanisms of control of microRNA biogenesis. Biochem Med. 2010;148(4):381–92.
14. Lee Y, Ahn C, Han J, Choi H, Kim J, Yim J, Lee J, Provost P, Radmark O, Kim S, Kim VN. The nuclear RNase III Drosha initiates microRNA processing. Nature. 2003;425(6956):415–9.
15. Denli AM, Tops BB, Plasterk RH, Ketting RF, Hannon GJ. Processing of primary microRNAs by the Microprocessor complex. Nature. 2004;432(7014):231–5.
16. Han J, Lee Y, Yeom KH, Nam JW, Heo I, Rhee JK, Sohn SY, Cho Y, Zhang BT, Kim VN. Molecular basis for the recognition of primary microRNAs by the Drosha-DGCR8 complex. Cell. 2006;125(5):887–901.
17. Lu J, Clark AG. Impact of microRNA regulation on variation in human gene expression. Genome Res. 2012;22(7):1243–54.
18. Mitchell PS, Parkin RK, Kroh EM, Fritz BR, Wyman SK, Pogosova-Agadjanyan EL, Peterson A, Noteboom J, O'Briant KC, Allen A, Lin DW, Urban N, Drescher CW, Knudsen BS, Stirewalt DL, Gentleman R, Vessella RL, Nelson PS, Martin DB, Tewari M. Circulating microRNAs as stable blood-based markers for cancer detection. Proc Natl Acad Sci U S A. 2008;105(30):10513–8.
19. Zubakov D, Boersma AW, Choi Y, van Kuijk PF, Wiemer EA, Kayser M. MicroRNA markers for forensic body fluid identification obtained from microarray screening and quantitative RT-PCR confirmation. Int J Leg Med. 2010;124(3):217–26.
20. Gupta SK, Bang C, Thum T. Circulating microRNAs as biomarkers and potential paracrine mediators of cardiovascular disease. Circ Cardiovasc Genet. 2010;3(5):484–8.
21. Wang L, Lv Y, Li G, Xiao J. MicroRNAs in heart and circulation during physical exercise. J Sport Health Sci. 2018;7(4):433–41.
22. Arroyo JD, Chevillet JR, Kroh EM, Ruf IK, Pritchard CC, Gibson DF, Mitchell PS, Bennett CF, Pogosova-Agadjanyan EL, Stirewalt DL, Tait JF, Tewari M. Argonaute2 complexes carry a population of circulating microRNAs independent of vesicles in human plasma. Proc Natl Acad Sci U S A. 2011;108(12):5003–8.
23. Song JJ, Liu J, Tolia NH, Schneiderman J, Smith SK, Martienssen RA, Hannon GJ, Joshua-Tor L. The crystal structure of the Argonaute2 PAZ domain reveals an RNA binding motif in RNAi effector complexes. Nat Struct Biol. 2003;10(12):1026–32.
24. Ma JB, Ye K, Patel DJ. Structural basis for overhang-specific small interfering RNA recognition by the PAZ domain. Nature. 2004;429(6989):318–22.
25. Dey BK, Mueller AC, Dutta A. Long non-coding RNAs as emerging regulators of differentiation, development, and disease. Transcription. 2014;5(4):e944014.
26. Rinn JL, Chang HY. Genome regulation by long noncoding RNAs. Annu Rev Biochem. 2012;81:145–66.
27. Anderson DM, Anderson KM, Chang CL, Makarewich CA, Nelson BR, McAnally JR, Kasaragod P, Shelton JM, Liou J, Bassel-Duby R, Olson EN. A micropeptide encoded by a putative long noncoding RNA regulates muscle performance. Cell. 2015;160(4):595–606.
28. Iyer MK, Niknafs YS, Malik R, Singhal U, Sahu A, Hosono Y, Barrette TR, Prensner JR, Evans JR, Zhao S, Poliakov A, Cao X, Dhanasekaran SM, Wu YM, Robinson DR, Beer DG, Feng FY, Iyer HK, Chinnaiyan AM. The landscape of long noncoding RNAs in the human transcriptome. Nat Genet. 2015;47(3):199–208.
29. Ransohoff JD, Wei Y, Khavari PA. The functions and unique features of long intergenic non-coding RNA. Nat Rev Mol Cell Biol. 2018;19(3):143–57.
30. Gupta RA, Shah N, Wang KC, Kim J, Horlings HM, Wong DJ, Tsai MC, Hung T, Argani P, Rinn JL, Wang Y, Brzoska P, Kong B, Li R, West RB, van de Vijver MJ, Sukumar S, Chang HY. Long non-coding RNA HOTAIR reprograms chromatin state to promote cancer metastasis. Nature. 2010;464(7291):1071–6.
31. Zhao J, Sun BK, Erwin JA, Song JJ, Lee JT. Polycomb proteins targeted by a short repeat RNA to the mouse X chromosome. Science. 2008;322(5902):750–6.
32. Nagano T, Mitchell JA, Sanz LA, Pauler FM, Ferguson-Smith AC, Feil R, Fraser P. The Air noncoding RNA epigenetically silences transcription by targeting G9a to chromatin. Science. 2008;322(5908):1717–20.
33. Pandey RR, Mondal T, Mohammad F, Enroth S, Redrup L, Komorowski J, Nagano T, Mancini-Dinardo D, Kanduri C. Kcnq1ot1 antisense noncoding RNA mediates lineage-specific transcriptional silencing through chromatin-level regulation. Mol Cell. 2008;32(2):232–46.
34. Wang Y, Hou J, He D, Sun M, Zhang P, Yu Y, Chen Y. The emerging function and mechanism of ceRNAs in Cancer. Trends Genet. 2016;32(4):211–24.
35. Chen ZH, Wang WT, Huang W, Fang K, Sun YM, Liu SR, Luo XQ, Chen YQ. The lnc RNA HOTAIRM1 regulates the degradation of PML-RARA oncoprotein

and myeloid cell differentiation by enhancing the autophagy pathway. Cell Death Differ. 2017;24(2):212–24.
36. Huang X, Yuan T, Tschannen M, Sun Z, Jacob H, Du M, Liang M, Dittmar RL, Liu Y, Liang M, Kohli M, Thibodeau SN, Boardman L, Wang L. Characterization of human plasma-derived exosomal RNAs by deep sequencing. BMC Genomics. 2013;14:319.
37. Nigro JM, Cho KR, Fearon ER, Kern SE, Ruppert JM, Oliner JD, Kinzler KW, Vogelstein B. Scrambled exons. Cell. 1991;64(3):607–13.
38. Lasda E, Parker R. Circular RNAs: diversity of form and function. RNA. 2014;20(12):1829–42.
39. Kos A, Dijkema R, Arnberg AC, van der Meide PH, Schellekens H. The hepatitis delta (delta) virus possesses a circular RNA. Nature. 1986;323(6088):558–60.
40. Sanger HL, Klotz G, Riesner D, Gross HJ, Kleinschmidt AK. Viroids are single-stranded covalently closed circular RNA molecules existing as highly base-paired rod-like structures. Proc Natl Acad Sci U S A. 1976;73(11):3852–6.
41. Ashwal-Fluss R, Meyer M, Pamudurti NR, Ivanov A, Bartok O, Hanan M, Evantal N, Memczak S, Rajewsky N, Kadener S. circ RNA biogenesis competes with pre-mRNA splicing. Mol Cell. 2014;56(1):55–66.
42. Salzman J, Gawad C, Wang PL, Lacayo N, Brown PO. Circular RNAs are the predominant transcript isoform from hundreds of human genes in diverse cell types. PLoS One. 2012;7(2):e30733.
43. Wu Q, Wang Y, Cao M, Pantaleo V, Burgyan J, Li WX, Ding SW. Homology-independent discovery of replicating pathogenic circular RNAs by deep sequencing and a new computational algorithm. Proc Natl Acad Sci U S A. 2012;109(10):3938–43.
44. Jeck WR, Sorrentino JA, Wang K, Slevin MK, Burd CE, Liu J, Marzluff WF, Sharpless NE. Circular RNAs are abundant, conserved, and associated with ALU repeats. RNA. 2013;19(2):141–57.
45. Danan M, Schwartz S, Edelheit S, Sorek R. Transcriptome-wide discovery of circular RNAs in Archaea. Nucleic Acids Res. 2012;40(7):3131–42.
46. Burd CE, Jeck WR, Liu Y, Sanoff HK, Wang Z, Sharpless NE. Expression of linear and novel circular forms of an INK4/ARF-associated non-coding RNA correlates with atherosclerosis risk. PLos Genet. 2010;6(12):e1001233.
47. Memczak S, Jens M, Elefsinioti A, Torti F, Krueger J, Rybak A, Maier L, Mackowiak SD, Gregersen LH, Munschauer M, Loewer A, Ziebold U, Landthaler M, Kocks C, le Noble F, Rajewsky N. Circular RNAs are a large class of animal RNAs with regulatory potency. Nature. 2013;495(7441):333–8.
48. Enuka Y, Lauriola M, Feldman ME, Sas-Chen A, Ulitsky I, Yarden Y. Circular RNAs are long-lived and display only minimal early alterations in response to a growth factor. Nucleic Acids Res. 2016;44(3):1370–83.
49. Tay Y, Rinn J, Pandolfi PP. The multilayered complexity of ceRNA crosstalk and competition. Nature. 2014;505(7483):344–52.
50. Zhang Y, Zhang XO, Chen T, Xiang JF, Yin QF, Xing YH, Zhu S, Yang L, Chen LL. Circular intronic long noncoding RNAs. Mol Cell. 2013;51(6):792–806.
51. Legnini I, Di Timoteo G, Rossi F, Morlando M, Briganti F, Sthandier O, Fatica A, Santini T, Andronache A, Wade M, Laneve P, Rajewsky N, Bozzoni I. Circ-ZNF609 Is a Circular RNA that Can Be Translated and Functions in Myogenesis. Mol Cell. 2017;66(1):22–37.. e29
52. Pamudurti NR, Bartok O, Jens M, Ashwal-Fluss R, Stottmeister C, Ruhe L, Hanan M, Wyler E, Perez-Hernandez D, Ramberger E, Shenzis S, Samson M, Dittmar G, Landthaler M, Chekulaeva M, Rajewsky N, Kadener S. Translation of CircRNAs. Mol Cell. 2017;66(1):9–21.. e27
53. Begum S, Yiu A, Stebbing J, Castellano L. Novel tumour suppressive protein encoded by circular RNA, circ-SHPRH, in glioblastomas. Oncogene. 2018;37(30):4055.
54. Abe N, Matsumoto K, Nishihara M, Nakano Y, Shibata A, Maruyama H, Shuto S, Matsuda A, Yoshida M, Ito Y, Abe H. Rolling circle translation of circular RNA in living human cells. Sci Rep. 2015;5:16435.
55. Yang Y, Fan X, Mao M, Song X, Wu P, Zhang Y, Jin Y, Yang Y, Chen LL, Wang Y, Wong CC, Xiao X, Wang Z. Extensive translation of circular RNAs driven by N(6)-methyladenosine. Cell Res. 2017;27(5):626–41.
56. Hachey BJ, Kontos MC, Newby LK, Christenson RH, Peacock WF, Brewer KC, McCord J. Trends in use of biomarker protocols for the evaluation of possible myocardial infarction. J Am Heart Assoc. 2017;6(9)
57. Goldberg L, Tirosh-Wagner T, Vardi A, Abbas H, Pillar N, Shomron N, Nevo-Caspi Y, Paret G. Circulating microRNAs: a potential biomarker for cardiac damage, inflammatory response, and left ventricular function recovery in pediatric viral myocarditis. J Cardiovasc Transl Res. 2018;11(4):319–28.
58. Deddens JC, Vrijsen KR, Colijn JM, Oerlemans MI, Metz CH, van der Vlist EJ, Nolte-'t Hoen EN, den Ouden K, Jansen Of Lorkeers SJ, van der Spoel TI, Koudstaal S, Arkesteijn GJ, Wauben MH, van Laake LW, Doevendans PA, Chamuleau SA, Sluijter JP. Circulating extracellular vesicles contain miRNAs and are released as early biomarkers for cardiac injury. J Cardiovasc Transl Res. 2016;9(4):291–301.
59. Ai J, Zhang R, Li Y, Pu J, Lu Y, Jiao J, Li K, Yu B, Li Z, Wang R, Wang L, Li Q, Wang N, Shan H, Li Z, Yang B. Circulating microRNA-1 as a potential novel biomarker for acute myocardial infarction. Biochem Biophys Res Commun. 2010;391(1):73–7.
60. D'Alessandra Y, Devanna P, Limana F, Straino S, Di Carlo A, Brambilla PG, Rubino M, Carena MC, Spazzafumo L, De Simone M, Micheli B, Biglioli P, Achilli F, Martelli F, Maggiolini S, Marenzi G, Pompilio G, Capogrossi MC. Circulating microRNAs are new and sensitive biomarkers of myocardial infarction. Eur Heart J. 2010;31(22):2765–73.

61. Kuwabara Y, Ono K, Horie T, Nishi H, Nagao K, Kinoshita M, Watanabe S, Baba O, Kojima Y, Shizuta S, Imai M, Tamura T, Kita T, Kimura T. Increased microRNA-1 and microRNA-133a levels in serum of patients with cardiovascular disease indicate myocardial damage. Circ Cardiovasc Genet. 2011;4(4):446–54.
62. Bauters C, Kumarswamy R, Holzmann A, Bretthauer J, Anker SD, Pinet F, Thum T. Circulating miR-133a and miR-423-5p fail as biomarkers for left ventricular remodeling after myocardial infarction. Int J Cardiol. 2013;168(3):1837–40.
63. Wang GK, Zhu JQ, Zhang JT, Li Q, Li Y, He J, Qin YW, Jing Q. Circulating microRNA: a novel potential biomarker for early diagnosis of acute myocardial infarction in humans. Eur Heart J. 2010;31(6):659–66.
64. Andersson P, Gidlof O, Braun OO, Gotberg M, van der Pals J, Olde B, Erlinge D. Plasma levels of liver-specific miR-122 is massively increased in a porcine cardiogenic shock model and attenuated by hypothermia. Shock. 2012;37(2):234–8.
65. Cortez-Dias N, Costa MC, Carrilho-Ferreira P, Silva D, Jorge C, Calisto C, Pessoa T, Robalo Martins S, de Sousa JC, da Silva PC, Fiuza M, Diogo AN, Pinto FJ, Enguita FJ. Circulating miR-122-5p/miR-133b ratio is a specific early prognostic biomarker in acute myocardial infarction. Circ J. 2016;80(10):2183–91.
66. Gacon J, Kablak-Ziembicka A, Stepien E, Enguita FJ, Karch I, Derlaga B, Zmudka K, Przewlocki T. Decision-making microRNAs (miR-124, -133a/b, −34a and −134) in patients with occluded target vessel in acute coronary syndrome. Kardiologia Polska. 2016;74(3):280–8.
67. Bye A, Rosjo H, Nauman J, Silva GJ, Follestad T, Omland T, Wisloff U. Circulating microRNAs predict future fatal myocardial infarction in healthy individuals – The HUNT study. J Mol Cell Cardiol. 2016;97:162–8.
68. Matsumoto S, Sakata Y, Suna S, Nakatani D, Usami M, Hara M, Kitamura T, Hamasaki T, Nanto S, Kawahara Y, Komuro I. Circulating p53-responsive microRNAs are predictive indicators of heart failure after acute myocardial infarction. Circ Res. 2013;113(3):322–6.
69. Evans S, Mann DL. Circulating p53-responsive microRNAs as predictive biomarkers in heart failure after acute myocardial infarction: the long and arduous road from scientific discovery to clinical utility. Circ Res. 2013;113(3):242–4.
70. Zhang Y, Sun L, Xuan L, Pan Z, Li K, Liu S, Huang Y, Zhao X, Huang L, Wang Z, Hou Y, Li J, Tian Y, Yu J, Han H, Liu Y, Gao F, Zhang Y, Wang S, Du Z, Lu Y, Yang B. Reciprocal changes of circulating long non-coding RNAs ZFAS1 and CDR1AS predict acute myocardial infarction. Sci Rep. 2016;6:22384.
71. Mentz RJ, O'Connor CM. Pathophysiology and clinical evaluation of acute heart failure. Nat Rev Cardiol. 2016;13(1):28–35.
72. Maron BJ, Towbin JA, Thiene G, Antzelevitch C, Corrado D, Arnett D, Moss AJ, Seidman CE, Young JB, American Heart A, Council on Clinical Cardiology HF, Transplantation C, Quality of C, Outcomes R, Functional G, Translational Biology Interdisciplinary Working G, Council on E, Prevention. Contemporary definitions and classification of the cardiomyopathies: an American heart association scientific statement from the council on clinical cardiology, heart failure and transplantation committee; quality of care and outcomes research and functional genomics and translational biology interdisciplinary working groups; and council on epidemiology and prevention. Circulation. 2006;113(14):1807–16.
73. Lu M, Yuan S, Li S, Li L, Liu M, Wan S. The exosome-derived biomarker in atherosclerosis and its clinical application. J Cardiovasc Transl Res. 2019;12(1):68–74.
74. Fichtlscherer S, De Rosa S, Fox H, Schwietz T, Fischer A, Liebetrau C, Weber M, Hamm CW, Roxe T, Muller-Ardogan M, Bonauer A, Zeiher AM, Dimmeler S. Circulating microRNAs in patients with coronary artery disease. Circ Res. 2010;107(5):677–84.
75. Ren J, Zhang J, Xu N, Han G, Geng Q, Song J, Li S, Zhao J, Chen H. Signature of circulating microRNAs as potential biomarkers in vulnerable coronary artery disease. PLoS One. 2013;8(12):e80738.
76. D'Alessandra Y, Carena MC, Spazzafumo L, Martinelli F, Bassetti B, Devanna P, Rubino M, Marenzi G, Colombo GI, Achilli F, Maggiolini S, Capogrossi MC, Pompilio G. Diagnostic potential of plasmatic MicroRNA signatures in stable and unstable angina. PLoS One. 2013;8(11):e80345.
77. Niculescu LS, Simionescu N, Sanda GM, Carnuta MG, Stancu CS, Popescu AC, Popescu MR, Vlad A, Dimulescu DR, Simionescu M, Sima AV. MiR-486 and miR-92a identified in circulating HDL discriminate between stable and vulnerable coronary artery disease patients. PLoS One. 2015;10(10):e0140958.
78. Al-Muhtaresh HA, Salem AH, Al-Kafaji G. Upregulation of circulating cardiomyocyte-enriched miR-1 and miR-133 associate with the risk of coronary artery disease in Type 2 diabetes patients and serve as potential biomarkers. J Cardiovasc Transl Res. 2019;12(4):347–57.
79. Gao W, He HW, Wang ZM, Zhao H, Lian XQ, Wang YS, Zhu J, Yan JJ, Zhang DG, Yang ZJ, Wang LS. Plasma levels of lipometabolism-related miR-122 and miR-370 are increased in patients with hyperlipidemia and associated with coronary artery disease. Lipids Health Dis. 2012;11:55.
80. Liu W, Ling S, Sun W, Liu T, Li Y, Zhong G, Zhao D, Zhang P, Song J, Jin X, Xu Z, Song H, Li Q, Liu S, Chai M, Dai Q, He Y, Fan Z, Zhou YJ, Li Y. Circulating microRNAs correlated with the level of coronary artery calcification in symptomatic patients. Sci Rep. 2015;5:16099.
81. Jansen F, Yang X, Proebsting S, Hoelscher M, Przybilla D, Baumann K, Schmitz T, Dolf A, Endl E, Franklin BS, Sinning JM, Vasa-Nicotera M, Nickenig G, Werner N. MicroRNA expression in circulating microvesicles predicts cardiovascular events in

patients with coronary artery disease. J Am Heart Assoc. 2014;3(6):e001249.
82. Cai Y, Yang Y, Chen X, Wu G, Zhang X, Liu Y, Yu J, Wang X, Fu J, Li C, Jose PA, Zeng C, Zhou L. Circulating 'lncRNA OTTHUMT00000387022' from monocytes as a novel biomarker for coronary artery disease. Cardiovasc Res. 2016;112(3):714–24.
83. Yang Y, Cai Y, Wu G, Chen X, Liu Y, Wang X, Yu J, Li C, Chen X, Jose PA, Zhou L, Zeng C. Plasma long non-coding RNA, CoroMarker, a novel biomarker for diagnosis of coronary artery disease. Clin Neurosci Res. 2015;129(8):675–85.
84. Cai Y, Yang Y, Chen X, He D, Zhang X, Wen X, Hu J, Fu C, Qiu D, Jose PA, Zeng C, Zhou L. Circulating "LncPPARdelta" from monocytes as a novel biomarker for coronary artery diseases. Medicine. 2016;95(6):e2360.
85. Tijsen AJ, Creemers EE, Moerland PD, de Windt LJ, van der Wal AC, Kok WE, Pinto YM. MiR423-5p as a circulating biomarker for heart failure. Circ Res. 2010;106(6):1035–9.
86. Coats CJ, Heywood WE, Mills K, Elliott PM. Current applications of biomarkers in cardiomyopathies. Expert Rev Cardiovasc Ther. 2015;13(7):825–37.
87. Sandhu H, Maddock H. Molecular basis of cancer-therapy-induced cardiotoxicity: introducing microRNA biomarkers for early assessment of subclinical myocardial injury. Clin Neurosci Res (Lond). 2014;126(6):377–400.
88. Ji X, Takahashi R, Hiura Y, Hirokawa G, Fukushima Y, Iwai N. Plasma miR-208 as a biomarker of myocardial injury. Clin Chem. 2009;55(11):1944–9.
89. Nishimura Y, Kondo C, Morikawa Y, Tonomura Y, Torii M, Yamate J, Uehara T. Plasma miR-208 as a useful biomarker for drug-induced cardiotoxicity in rats. J Appl Toxicol. 2015;35(2):173–80.
90. Calvano J, Achanzar W, Murphy B, DiPiero J, Hixson C, Parrula C, Burr H, Mangipudy R, Tirmenstein M. Evaluation of microRNAs-208 and 133a/b as differential biomarkers of acute cardiac and skeletal muscle toxicity in rats. Toxicol Appl Pharmacol. 2016;312:53–60.
91. Glineur SF, De Ron P, Hanon E, Valentin JP, Dremier S, Nogueira da Costa A. Paving the route to plasma miR-208a-3p as an acute cardiac injury biomarker: preclinical rat data supports its use in drug safety assessment. Toxicol Sci. 2016;149(1):89–97.
92. Oliveira-Carvalho V, Ferreira LR, Bocchi EA. Circulating mir-208a fails as a biomarker of doxorubicin-induced cardiotoxicity in breast cancer patients. J Appl Toxicol. 2015;35(9):1071–2.
93. Zhao Z, He J, Zhang J, Liu M, Yang S, Li N, Li X. Dysregulated miR1254 and miR579 for cardiotoxicity in patients treated with bevacizumab in colorectal cancer. Tumor Biol. 2014;35(6):5227–35.
94. Clark MB, Johnston RL, Inostroza-Ponta M, Fox AH, Fortini E, Moscato P, Dinger ME, Mattick JS. Genome-wide analysis of long noncoding RNA stability. Genome Res. 2012;22(5):885–98.
95. Moldovan L, Batte KE, Trgovcich J, Wisler J, Marsh CB, Piper M. Methodological challenges in utilizing miRNAs as circulating biomarkers. J Cell Mol Med. 2014;18(3):371–90.
96. Quinn JJ, Chang HY. Unique features of long non-coding RNA biogenesis and function. Nat Rev Genet. 2016;17(1):47–62.
97. Chen X, Ba Y, Ma L, Cai X, Yin Y, Wang K, Guo J, Zhang Y, Chen J, Guo X, Li Q, Li X, Wang W, Zhang Y, Wang J, Jiang X, Xiang Y, Xu C, Zheng P, Zhang J, Li R, Zhang H, Shang X, Gong T, Ning G, Wang J, Zen K, Zhang J, Zhang CY. Characterization of microRNAs in serum: a novel class of biomarkers for diagnosis of cancer and other diseases. Cell Res. 2008;18(10):997–1006.
98. Arita T, Ichikawa D, Konishi H, Komatsu S, Shiozaki A, Shoda K, Kawaguchi T, Hirajima S, Nagata H, Kubota T, Fujiwara H, Okamoto K, Otsuji E. Circulating long non-coding RNAs in plasma of patients with gastric cancer. Anticancer Res. 2013;33(8):3185–93.

23 Small Interfering RNAs and RNA Therapeutics in Cardiovascular Diseases

Parveen Bansal and Malika Arora

Abstract

Ribonucleic acid (RNA) is being exploited and understood in its many aspects of function and structure for development of valuable tools in the therapeutics of various diseases such as cardiovascular etc. The expanded knowledge regarding function of RNA in the genomics and inside the cell has dramatically changed the therapeutic strategies in the past few years. RNA has become a spotlight of attention for developing novel therapeutic schemes and hence variety of therapeutic strategies is being coming into the picture that includes RNA interference, use of aptamers, role of microRNA (miRNA) that can alter the complex gene expression patterns. It is due to the fact that RNA offers various advantages in disease management as it can be edited and modified in its various forms such as secondary and tertiary structures. Although scientists are in process of manufacturing RNA-targeting therapies using variety of endogenous gene silencing regulators, Small interfering RNAs (Si RNAs), aptamers and microRNA for cardiovascular diseases yet the development of a novel, risk free therapeutic strategy is a major challenge and need of the hour in cardiovascular medicine. In this regard these agents are required to overcome pleothra of barriers such as stability of drug targets, immunogenicity, adequate binding, targeted delivery etc. to become effective drugs. Recent years have witnessed the progress of RNA therapeutic strategies in cardiovascular diseases that are likely to significantly expand the cardiovascular therapeutic repertoire within the next decade. The present manuscript has been compiled to summarize various approaches of siRNA based therapies in cardiovascular diseases along with the advantages, outcomes and limitations if any in this regard. In addition, the future prospects of RNA therapeutic modalities in cardiovascular diseases are summarized.

Keywords

Cardiovascular disease (CVD) · Small interfering RNAs (Si RNAs) · Aptamer · microRNA

P. Bansal (✉)
University Centre of Excellence in Research, Baba Farid University of Health Sciences, Faridkot, India

M. Arora
Multidisciplinary Research Unit, Guru Gobind Singh Medical College, Faridkot, India

J. Xiao (ed.), *Non-coding RNAs in Cardiovascular Diseases*, Advances in Experimental Medicine and Biology 1229, https://doi.org/10.1007/978-981-15-1671-9_23

1 Introduction

Cardiovascular disease (CVD) is becoming a leading cause of morbidity, mortality as well as disability across the globe despite of the advancements in therapeutics and risk management strategies [1].The disease has been reported to be chronic in nature and the symptoms of the disease deteriorate as time period increases. Besides noteworthy therapeutic achievements in CVD, there are multiple undesirable risk factors associated with therapeutic modalities such as drug toxicity, complexity, resistance and many more. Hence the development of a novel, risk free therapeutic strategy is a major challenge and need of the hour in cardiovascular medicine. As per the availability of current literature, several lines of evidences are available supporting the function of RNA specifically the application of small interfering RNAs in silencing the disease causing genes in cardiovascular diseases [2]. It has been considered that RNA plays dynamic and versatile role in regulating the gene expression by acting as an intermediate molecule between DNA and proteins [3, 4].

RNA can offer various advantage in disease management as it can be edited and modified in its various forms such as secondary and tertiary structures. Moreover it may undergo tight, dynamic and various post transcriptional regulatory modifications by using plenty of RNA binding proteins [5, 6]. Hence RNA interference (RNAi) can propose major advantage over pharmacological therapy as they can target specific pathogenic genes that are associated with CVD with low toxicity and high potency. In addition to it, it is pertinent to mention that various biotechnology companies are already in process of manufacturing RNA-targeting therapies using various drug- able targets. For the same purpose, variety of endogenous gene silencing regulators, Small interfering RNAs (Si RNAs), aptamers and microRNA are being exploited to investigate the potential therapeutic agents [7].

It has been observed that novel technologies involved multiple types of small RNA that include miRNA, siRNA, snRNA, piRNA and snoRNA etc. Recent studies are evidencing the extremely broad spectrum of RNA species. Amongst these classes, the expression of mRNA target is inhibited by using siRNA whereas the miRNA are either used for inhibiting other miRNA or to mimic as some other miRNA which will be antagonizing the function of endogenous miRNA due to mimic behaviour [8]. This hypothesis explains how subclasses/varieties of RNA talk to each other and respond differently that leads to altered functional genetic information playing a vital role in various pathological conditions such as CVD etc. To date, therapies involving RNA agents are being exploited to treat various diseases such as cancer [9], infectious [10] and neurodegenerative diseases [11] as well.

The therapeutic potential of RNA based agents are being explored in multiple clinical trials in context to cardiovascular diseases. This manuscript focuses to summarize three such approaches that include siRNA, miRNA and aptamers as well along with the clinical trials conducted in this regard. Further the future directions of RNA therapeutics alongwith their outcomes and limitations in regard to cardiovascular diseases are critically summarized.

2 RNA and Its World: Traditional Concept vs. Current Concept

2.1 Traditional Concept of RNA World

As per the description of various classical studies, it has been observed that a large amount of RNA is transcribed into the cell. The structure and function of variety of RNA transcribed in the cell is becoming better understood with respect to their role in molecular biology as well as their therapeutic potential. Most of the RNA transcribed in the cell do not encode for proteins rather only a part of it (such as tRNA and rRNA) is involved in the process of translation and its regulation. As per the traditional knowledge, RNAs were considered to be transmitters of genetic information i.e. from DNA to RNA and then to the ribosome for proteins synthesis, and

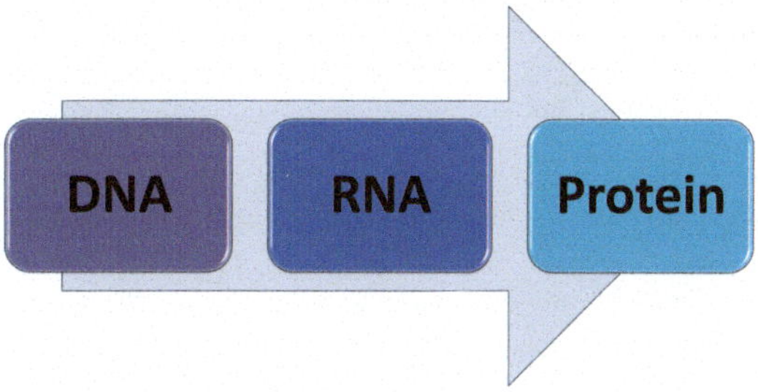

Fig. 23.1 Representation of traditional classical central dogma of molecular biology

hence considered to be the regulators of protein synthesis/Gene expression [12]. The traditional concept of RNA and its role in gene expression was dictated in central dogma which is represented as follows in Fig. 23.1.

2.2 Current Concept of RNA World

Since last decade the multiple studies have expended the role of RNA within the cell and as other catalytic RNAs [13, 14]. As per current status, it is obvious that RNA is not only the intermediary molecule to encode proteins from genes rather some of its types may act as functional end products to control the gene expression in a different but strategic manner. Moreover, recent studies are evidencing the use of new classes of small RNAs such as miRNA as well as siRNA which are generated as a product of some novel biosynthetic pathways and are helpful to mediate regulatory functions [15]. Earlier it was considered that RNA are of two types that include coding RNA (that codes for proteins) and Non coding RNA (which do not encode for proteins). The various types of RNA include rRNA, tRNA, mRNA, snRNA, siRNA and snoRNA etc. The availability of different types of RNA along with their percentage is shown in Fig. 23.2.

Although a variety of RNAs are known to the scientist still the current understanding of RNA molecules and its function is only the tip of the iceberg. The RNA research is gaining momentum on a fast pace due to the rapid development of the molecular biotechnology as well as the various classes of RNA have attracted considerable attention of the scientists to unfold their role in gene regulation and in developing novel drug discovery and development targets. Amongst the above mentioned classes, microRNAs (miRNAs) as well as small interfering RNAs (siRNAs) are being highly exploited for their therapeutic potential and has been depicted by number of scientists against various deadly diseases such as cancer and others [16, 17]. Moreover these small molecules have a potential to become non-druggable target to cure plethora of diseases without undergoing drug induced side effects [18].

3 Small Interfering RNAs

SiRNAs are small non-coding RNA; a novel class of RNA based therapeutic agent with an important role in gene expression. siRNAs have a well-defined structure usually varying in its length from 20 to 24-bp with phosphorylation on 5′ end and hydroxylation on 3′ end [19]. In addition to it, siRNAs exists with overhanging nucleotides on both the sides. In the cell itself, the Dicer enzyme is responsible for the production of siRNAs from either long dsRNAs or small hairpin RNAs. Although these molecules are only of length 20–25 base pairs yet they work to inhibit the gene expression. These are the key molecules to direct post transcriptional gene silencing process called RNA interference (RNAi) rather their existence was first defined by the participation of siRNA in RNAi. It has been demonstrated that the siRNA are derived from the longer transcripts and the processing involves an enzyme named as DICER [20]. The general properties of the siRNA are shown in Table 23.1.

4 Mechanism of Action of siRNA

siRNAs are double stranded RNAs that direct post transcriptional gene silencing process called RNAi. These dsRNAs can be introduced into the cell with the help of transfection method. With the help of complementary siRNA sequence any

Fig. 23.2 Representation of various types of RNA and its availability in eukaryotic cell

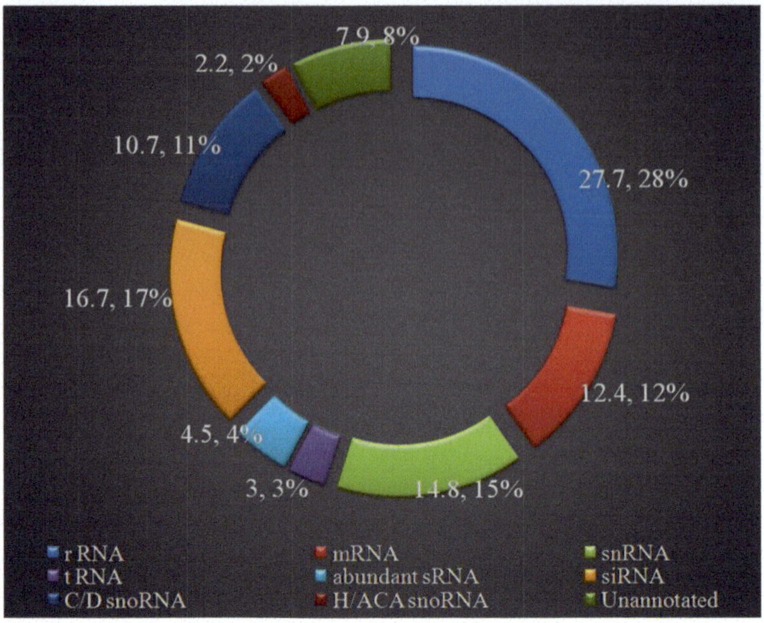

of the gene can be knocked down and hence this RNA class is becoming an important tool for validating the gene functions as well as drug targeting. RNAi is a normal process that took place in almost all the eukaryotic cells. In this highly conserved process, dsRNA molecules i.e. siRNAs silence the post transcriptional effect of any gene of interest [7, 21]. Now a day, synthetic siRNAs are being synthesized by various biotechnology companies that are used to silence the effect of some pre-decided target genes. The knockdown of the target genes is entirely based upon the complementarily between a siRNA and the target gene [22]. Although, synthetic siRNAs are designed to silence targeted gene, but sometime unintended genes may also get knock down, due to imperfect complementarily to non-targeted mRNAs [22].

Table 23.1 Representation of general properties of siRNA

S. no.	Features	Property of siRNA
1.	Before processing DICER	Double-stranded RNA having nucleotides from30–100
2.	Structure	RNA duplex having 21–23 nucleotide with 2 nucleotides overhanging on 3′termial
3.	Complementary	Fully complementary to mRNA
4.	mRNA target	Single
5.	Gene regulation mechanism	mRNA having Endonucleolytic cleavage
6.	Clinical applications	Therapeutic agent

The steps involved in the RNA interference are as follows:

1. **Synthesis of siRNA**: The synthesis of siRNA is the main stage of RNAi. To achieve the synthesis of siRNA, long dsRNAs are transfected inside the cell followed by cleavage of the ds DNA by an endo-ribonuclease enzyme. The enzyme used for the cleavage of the dsRNA is known as Dicer. This enzyme helps to cut a long piece of dsRNA into smaller pieces of 21–25 bp dsRNAs having 2 nucleotides on the 3′ terminus alongwith phosphate groups on 5′ terminus. The smaller dsRNA produced in this process are known either as silencing RNA or short interfering RNA [23].
2. **Incorporation of siRNA to RISC**: In this step, siRNA duplexes are inserted into the RNA-induced silencing complex (RISC). RISC complex plays a crucial role in RNAi. It is a RNA/protein nuclease complex that ini-

tially binds to the siRNA duplexes [24]. For the incorporation of siRNA to RISC, 5′- terminal phosphorylation of the siRNA is compulsory. RISC has two domains named as PAZ and PIWI that help to recognize the 5′-terminus and 3′-terminus of the actual guiding strand followed by targeting the homologous regions in the guiding strand [25].

3. **Gene silencing**: After incorporation into RISC complex, siRNAs are identified by RNA-induced silencing complex (RISC) as well as Argonaute 2 (AGO2) followed by uncoiling of the dssiRNAs into single strands [26–28]. Single stranded siRNA are recognized by their complementary mRNA and after binding with perfect complementary strands target mRNA is finally degraded by exonucleases and hence mRNA cleavage is induced. After the mRNA cleavage, the same will not be recognized by the cell as it is recognized as abnormal mRNA which will in turn silence the gene due to no translation [29, 30]. The step to step process of RNA interference is shown in Fig. 23.3.

There are several advantages of siRNA over conventional drugs [19, 31]. Detection of target sites is pretty easier with high flexibility since both the target siRNA and mRNA are sequences-specific. The inhibitory effect of the siRNA may be realized by targeting particular region of the mRNA [32]. In the process of gene silencing only a small amount of siRNA is required to reduce the concentration of homologous mRNA drastically within a period of 24 h. Physiological impact of cells is not altered by siRNA [33]. The transcripts of interest are destroyed selectively by high level homology of siRNA to the target region of cognate transcription. In the absence of the target sequences, the siRNA remain dormant in the cells and in the presence of the target sequence, the genes are silenced stably. siRNAs displays long term biological effects [34].

5 Chronological Representation of Discoveries in the Area of RNAi

The field of RNAi is not new to us. As far as the discovery of RNAi is concerned, geneticists Craig Mello and Andrew Fire discovered that upon injecting double-stranded RNA (dsRNA) into small worms some of the corresponding genes get switched off and hence the concept of the RNAi came into picture [35]. Finally research-

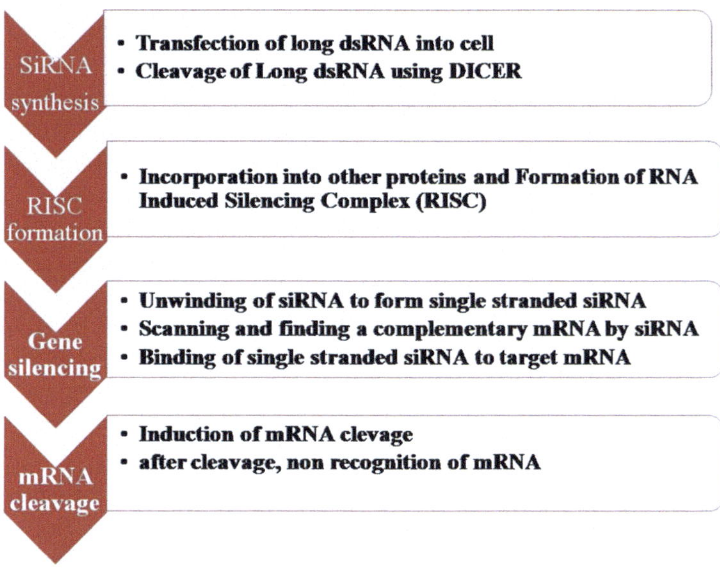

Fig. 23.3 Representation of step to step process of RNA interference

Table 23.2 Representation of chronological discoveries in the area of RNAi

Year	Discoveries in the area of RNAi	References
1998	When double stranded RNA (dsRNA), called small interfering RNA (siRNA), is injected into worms, it switches off the corresponding gene, which leads to the identification of RNA interference (RNAi) as a whole new cellular pathway.	[36]
2002	RNAi is a pathway common to mammals.	[37]
	One of the biggest RNAi companies *i.e.* Alnylam was established.	
2004	First clinical trial of an RNAi was conducted in patients having age-related macular degeneration.	[38, 39]
2005	Novartis agreed to purchase almost 20% of Alnylam's stock	[40]
2006	Mello and Fire won the Nobel Prize for Medicine and Physiology for their work	[41, 42]
	Merck purchases biotechnology company Sirna for US$1.1bn	
2007	Roche purchases just under 5% of Alnylam's stock and RNAi company, Dicerna, was founded	[43]
2008	A phase III trial of RNAi in wet age-related macular degeneration is terminated because of a lack of efficacy	[44]
2012	Alnylam discovers that a sugar molecule called N-acetylgalactosamine is key to getting RNAi into liver cells	[45]
2016	Alnylam reports an "imbalance of deaths" in a phase III study for a drug called revusiran, designed to treat hereditary transthyretin amyloidosis, and development is subsequently discontinued.	[46]
	Dicerna scraps the first two of its drugs to make it to clinical trials because preliminary results do not meet the company's expectations, USFDA refused to grant approval for further clinical trials of any of Arrowhead's RNAi drugs because of unexplained deaths in chimpanzees.	
2017	Alnylam's drug patisiran is found to be effective and safe in a phase III trial for treating hereditary transthyretin amyloidosis (pictured) with neuropathy	[47]
2018	Several of the key companies expect to start numerous clinical trials of new RNAi therapeutics.	[48]
	First ever gene-silencing drug won FDA approval	

ers were awarded with Noble Prize for Medicine and Physiology in 2006. Some of the chronological discoveries in the area of RNAi are shown in Table 23.2.

6 RNA Interference in Cardiovascular Diseases

The technique is used to down regulate the desired gene expression using easily formulated small interfering RNA fragments. The method is quickly evolving against various diseases since its discovery and is becoming a routine application in many of the laboratories. There are number of studies that explain the success of RNA interference in treatment of human diseases.

RNAi induced by siRNA has emerged as a crucial technique for screening new therapeutic targets and searching molecular mechanisms of cardiovascular diseases [49]. siRNAs can be used to inhibit the overproduction of proteins that are associated with cardiovascular disease. Proprotein convertase subtilisin/kexin type 9 (PCSK9) has been reported to increase the levels of cholesterol in plasma; inhibition of the enzyme decreases the chances of hypercholesterolemia [50]. Studies have been carried out on the monkeys and it has been concluded that the special siRNA delivery by lipidoid nanoparticles against PCSK9 can decrease the cholesterol effectively [51]. siRNA have been found to silence the CCR2 i.e. chemokine receptor that results in enhanced recovery from myocardial infarction as it reduces the penetration of inflammatory cells into the infracted area [52].

Apart from inflammation, cardiomyocyte apoptosis is also observed during myocardial in fraction. Cardiomyocyte apoptosis results in reduced cardiac contractility as observed in mouse models with myocardial infarction (MI). Post myocardial infarction, apoptosis is mediated by tyrosine phosphatase Src homology region 2 domain-containing phosphatase 1 (SHP-1) [53].

It has been reported that RNAi against SHP-1 rescues cardiomyocytes from apoptosis among mouse MI model [54]. Addition, a hurdle in RNA therapeutics has been observed in mouse MI model but it resulted in non-specific gene silencing because of the off-target binding of siRNAs [55]. To reduce off-target binding of siRNA is also very important in RNA therapy. Tough decoy (TuD) RNA has been introduced which is meant to silence the sense strand of the siRNA duplex [56]. Recently, RNAi-based gene silencing methods are being established in humans and varieties of clinical trials are ongoing which may act as a promising therapy for the fatal diseases such as cardiovascular, neurological diseases etc.

It has been observed that upcoming cardiovascular RNA drugs are used to address multiple organ systems. It is not always mandatory to address heart or vasculature directly rather the disease can be managed by targeting liver RNA drugs. Liver targeted RNA drugs are gaining success and are developed in the field of cardiovascular diseases. Another system such as immune system involving monocytes or macrophages can be targeted for delivering RNA drug to its tissue target [57]. Various studies involving the role of RNAi specifically in cardiovascular diseases are shown in Table 23.3.

7 SiRNA Based Drugs: FDA Approval

Though the idea of the gene silencing has been revealed two decades ago, yet, the researchers are desperate and making critical steps for seeking approval for newly manufactured/to be manufactured new siRNA based medicines from US Food and Drug Administration (FDA). It has been observed that there is entry of FDA approved drugs into the market and amongst those drugs the drugs for various diseases are enlisted. The FDA approval for few of the siRNA has led the field of gene silencing to the new heights due to the fact that RNAi has the flexibility to design as many as novel targets against many different genes/diseases with high specificity. Few such drugs are enlisted in Table 23.4.

8 Future Perspective

The flexibility of RNAs makes them crucial therapeutics modality for number of human diseases. Exploring new classes of RNA that possess therapeutic potential will help in its successful translation to the clinic. Understanding the mode of action of various RNAs including long-noncoding RNAs (lncRNAs), miRNA, siRNA, etc. in CVD will help in improved therapeutics among patients. lncRNAs are distinct form of short noncoding RNAs that binds the targets through complimentary base pairing. lncRNAsfold into specific tertiary structures and interact with its proteins targets and the function of lncRNAs in MI have revealed [85]. The role of lncRNAs is only partially known and recently unfolded in cardiac development and the progression of MI [86]. Hence studies relating to regulation of long-noncoding RNAs for reversal of the diseased state and triggering the endogenous regenerative process can be a promising therapeutic tool for CVD patients [87, 88]. Many diseases result from multigene dysregulation; so administration of more than one therapeutic target will be beneficial for good outcome. Combination of RNA therapeutics with protein or small molecule drugs may also become promising therapy [89]. Delivery of RNAs will improve cell-based therapies. Cell based therapies will be promising approach for rejuvenation of ischemic myocardium since adult cardiomyocytes have restricted regenerative capacity [90]. However, this therapeutic approach has some obstacles like less cell retention and poor cell survival in infracted regions. These therapeutic challenges can be improved by incorporating few RNA agents. Delivery of mRNA encoding angiogenic factors along with RNAi that is responsible for decreased inflammation and fibrosis in the host tissue may improve survival [91]. For implementation of this approach few new strategies needs to be designed for effective cell and RNAs delivery. To achieve this goal, a new strategy should be designed for effective deliver of cells and RNAs to infracted area. Role of RNA therapeutics in treating MI has been successfully demonstrated in small animals however preclinical studies on large animals and

Table 23.3 Representation of studies involving RNAi as therapeutic agents in cardiovascular diseases

Clinical trials identification number	Recruiting status	Conditions of diseases	No. phases	Treatment	No of enrolments	Study completion date	References
NCT03060577 (ORION-3)	Not recruiting, active	Atherosclerotic cardiovascular disease	2	Inclisiran (ALN-PCSSC)	490	2022	[58]
		Symptomatic atherosclerosis		Evolocumab (REPATHA)			
		Familial hypercholesterolemia					
		Type2 diabetes					
NCT03792607	Recruiting	Type 2 diabetes mellitus			50	March 5, 2019	[59]
		Cardiovascular disease					
NCT03705234	Recruiting	Atherosclerotic cardiovascular disease	3	Inclisiran	15,000	March 25, 2019	[60]
				Placebo			
NCT03399370	Active, not recruiting	ASCVD	3	Inclisiran sodium	1561	April 17, 2019	[61]
		Elevated cholesterol		Placebo			
NCT03400800	Active, not recruiting	ASCVD	3	Inclisiran sodium	1617	April 17, 2019	[62]
		Elevated cholesterol		Placebo			
NCT03515772	Recruiting	HIV infections		Co-administration of darunavir with a cardiovascular	60	October 31, 2019	[63]
		Drug interactions					
		Cardiovascular diseases					
NCT03672994	Recruiting	Asthma			650	April 30, 2019	[64]
		COPD					
		Heart failure					
		Community-acquired PneumoniaHealthy					
		Breathlessness					
NCT02527343 (BROADEN study)	Active, not recruiting	Familial partial Lipodystrophy	2 and 3	Volanesorsen (ISIS 304801, IONIS-APOCIIIRx)	60	September, 2021	[65]
				Placebo			
NCT03371355	Recruiting	NAFLD	2	ISIS 703802 (AKCEA-ANGPTL3-LRx, IONIS-ANGPTL3-LRx)	144	September 26, 2018	[66]
		Diabetes mellitus,					
		Type 2Hypertriglyceridemia					
		Fatty liver, nonalcoholic		Placebo (sterile Normal saline (0.9% NaCl))			

NCT03455777	Withdrawn (study withdrawn due to lack of available patients meeting entry criteria)	Homozygous familial Hypercholesterolemia	2	AKCEA-ANGPTL3-LRX (ISIS 703802)	0	December 3, 2018	[67]
NCT02900027	Completed	Elevated triglycerides (TG)	1	Placebo comparator APOC-III-L-Rx	56	May 22, 2018	[68]
NCT02963311 (ORION-2)	Completed	Lipid metabolism disorders dyslipidemias hypercholesterolemia Hyperlipidemias Hyperlipoproteinemia type II	2	ALN-PCSSC (PCSK9) Standard of care/low density lipoprotein-cholesterol (LDL-C)	4	December 21, 2018	[69]
NCT03159416 (ORION-7)	Completed	Renal insufficiency Kidney diseases Urologic diseases	1	Inclisiran (ALN-PCSSC)	31	November 9, 2018	[70]
NCT03360747	Completed	Lipoprotein lipase Deficiency Hyperlipoproteinemia type 1 Familial Chylomicronemia syndrome	2	AKCEA-ANGPTL3-LRX (ISIS 703802)	3	April 25, 2019	[71]
NCT03070782	Completed	Elevated lipoprotein(a) Cardiovascular disease	2	Placebo (sterile Normal saline (0.9% NaCl) ISIS 681257	286	December 13, 2018	[72]
NCT02824003	Completed	Type 2 diabetes	2	ISIS-GCGRRx Placebo	15	May 8, 2018	[73]
NCT02583919	Completed	Type 2 diabetes	2	ISIS-GCGRRx (Isis 449884) Placebo	79	June 25, 2018	[74]

Table 23.4 List of FDA approved siRNA drugs used for treatment of various diseases

Drugs	Disease treatment
ONPATTRO (Patisiran)	Used for the treatment of polyneuropathy in people with hereditary transthyretin-mediated amyloidosis (fatal rare disease) [75].
Givosiran (ALN-AS1)	It is available in a dosage form for subcutaneous administration for treating acute hepatic porphyria (AHP) and other porphyrias like acute intermittent, variegate and hereditary coproporphyria. It is also employed in ALAD-deficiency porphyria (ADP) [76].
Fitusiran (ALN-AT3)	Subcutaneous dosage form targeting antithrombin used for treatment of hemophilia and rare bleeding disorders (RBDs) [77].
Inclisiran (ALN-PCSsc)	Subcutaneous dosage form targeting proprotein convertase subtilisin kexin type 9 (PCSK9) used for the treatment of hypercholesterolemia [78].
Lumasiran (ALN-GO1)	Subcutaneous dosage form targeting glycolate oxidase (GO) used for the treatment of Primary Hyperoxaluria Type 1 (PH1) [79].
Vutrisiran (ALN-TTRsc02)	Subcutaneous dosage form targeting transthyretin (TTR) used for the treatment of transthyretin-mediated (ATTR) amyloidosis [80].
Cemdisiran (ALN-CC5)	Subcutaneous dosage form targeting the C5 component of the complement pathway and being used for various complement-mediated diseases [81].
ALN-AAT02	Subcutaneous dosage form targeting alpha-1 antitrypsin (AAT) used for the treatment of AAT deficiency-associated liver disease [82, 83].
ALN-HBV02 (VIR-2218)	Subcutaneous dosage form targeting the hepatitis B virus (HBV) genome used for the treatment of chronic HBV infection [82, 83].
ALN-AGT	Subcutaneous dosage form targeting angiotensinogen (AGT) used for the treatment of hypertension [82, 84].

patients will further explore/establish their efficacy in future. To maximize benefits and to avoid adverse effects, there is a need to draw stringent standard operative procedures for delivery strategies, development and improvement of RNA-based MI therapeutics.

References

1. Benjamin EJ, Blaha MJ, Chiuve SE, Cushman M, Das SR, Deo R, de Ferranti SD, Floyd J, Fornage M, Gillespie C, Isasi CR, Jimenez MC, Jordan LC, Judd SE, Lackland D, Lichtman JH, Lisabeth L, Liu S, Longenecker CT, Mackey RH, Matsushita K, Mozaffarian D, Mussolino ME, Nasir K, Neumar RW, Palaniappan L, Pandey DK, Thiagarajan RR, Reeves MJ, Ritchey M, Rodriguez CJ, Roth GA, Rosamond WD, Sasson C, Towfighi A, Tsao CW, Turner MB, Virani SS, Voeks JH, Willey JZ, Wilkins JT, Wu JH, Alger HM, Wong SS, Muntner P, American Heart Association Statistics Committee and Stroke Statistics Subcommittee. Heart disease and stroke statistics-2017 update: a report from the American Heart Association. Circulation. 2017;135(10):e146–603.
2. Tang Y, Ge YZ, Yin JQ. Exploring in vitro roles of siRNA in cardiovascular disease. Acta Pharmacol Sin. 2007;28(1):1–9.
3. Kapranov P, Willingham AT, Gingeras TR. Genome-wide transcription and the implications for genomic organization. Nat Rev Genet. 2007;8(6):413–23.
4. Mercer TR, Dinger ME, Mattick JS. Long non-coding RNAs: insights into functions. Nat Rev Genet. 2009;10(3):155–9.
5. Stellos K. The rise of epitranscriptomic era: implications for cardiovascular disease. Cardiovasc Res. 2017;113(5):e2–3.
6. Stellos K, Gatsiou A, Stamatelopoulos K, Perisic Matic L, John D, Lunella FF, Jae N, Rossbach O, Amrhein C, Sigala F, Boon RA, Furtig B, Manavski Y, You X, Uchida S, Keller T, Boeckel JN, Franco-Cereceda A, Maegdefessel L, Chen W, Schwalbe H, Bindereif A, Eriksson P, Hedin U, Zeiher AM, Dimmeler S. Adenosine-to-inosine RNA editing controls cathepsin S expression in atherosclerosis by enabling HuR-mediated post-transcriptional regulation. Nat Med. 2016;22(10):1140–50.
7. Siomi H, Siomi MC. On the road to reading the RNA-interference code. Nature. 2009;457(7228):396–404.
8. Carthew RW, Sontheimer EJ. Origins and mechanisms of miRNAs and siRNAs. Cell. 2009;136(4):642–55.
9. Moreno PM, Pego AP. Therapeutic antisense oligonucleotides against cancer: hurdling to the clinic. Front Chem. 2014;2:87.
10. Schluep T, Lickliter J, Hamilton J, Lewis DL, Lai CL, Lau JY, Locarnini SA, Gish RG, Given BD. Safety, tolerability, and pharmacokinetics of ARC-520 injection, an RNA interference-based therapeutic for the treatment of chronic hepatitis B virus infection, in healthy volunteers. Clin Pharmacol Drug Dev. 2017;6(4):350–62.
11. Scoles DR, Meera P, Schneider MD, Paul S, Dansithong W, Figueroa KP, Hung G, Rigo F, Bennett CF, Otis TS, Pulst SM. Antisense oligonucleotide therapy for spinocerebellar ataxia type 2. Nature. 2017;544(7650):362–6.

12. Roly ZY, Backhouse B, Cutting A, Tan TY, Sinclair AH, Ayers KL, Major AT, Smith CA. The cell biology and molecular genetics of Mullerian duct development. Wiley Interdiscip Rev Dev Biol. 2018;7(3):e310.
13. Warf MB, Berglund JA. Role of RNA structure in regulating pre-mRNA splicing. Trends Biochem Sci. 2010;35(3):169–78.
14. Lippman Z, Martienssen R. The role of RNA interference in heterochromatic silencing. Nature. 2004;431(7006):364–70.
15. Jacquier A. The complex eukaryotic transcriptome: unexpected pervasive transcription and novel small RNAs. Nat Rev Genet. 2009;10(12):833–44.
16. Davidson BL, McCray PB Jr. Current prospects for RNA interference-based therapies. Nat Rev Genet. 2011;12(5):329–40.
17. Burnett JC, Rossi JJ. RNA-based therapeutics: current progress and future prospects. Chem Biol. 2012;19(1):60–71.
18. Lares MR, Rossi JJ, Ouellet DL. RNAi and small interfering RNAs in human disease therapeutic applications. Trends Biotechnol. 2010;28(11):570–9.
19. Wittrup A, Lieberman J. Knocking down disease: a progress report on siRNA therapeutics. Nat Rev Genet. 2015;16(9):543–52.
20. Liu X, Jiang F, Kalidas S, Smith D, Liu Q. Dicer-2 and R2D2 coordinately bind siRNA to promote assembly of the siRISC complexes. RNA. 2006;12(8):1514–20.
21. Donze O, Picard D. RNA interference in mammalian cells using siRNAs synthesized with T7 RNA polymerase. Nucleic Acids Res. 2002;30(10):e46.
22. Jackson AL, Linsley PS. Recognizing and avoiding siRNA off-target effects for target identification and therapeutic application. Nat Rev Drug Discov. 2010;9(1):57–67.
23. Carthew RW. Synthesis of siRNA for RNAi in Drosophila. CSH Protoc. 2006;2006(3) https://doi.org/10.1101/pdb.prot4512.
24. Matranga C, Tomari Y, Shin C, Bartel DP, Zamore PD. Passenger-strand cleavage facilitates assembly of siRNA into Ago2-containing RNAi enzyme complexes. Cell. 2005;123(4):607–20.
25. Ameres SL, Martinez J, Schroeder R. Molecular basis for target RNA recognition and cleavage by human RISC. Cell. 2007;130(1):101–12.
26. Sledz CA, Holko M, de Veer MJ, Silverman RH, Williams BR. Activation of the interferon system by short-interfering RNAs. Nat Cell Biol. 2003;5(9):834–9.
27. Liu J, Carmell MA, Rivas FV, Marsden CG, Thomson JM, Song JJ, Hammond SM, Joshua-Tor L, Hannon GJ. Argonaute2 is the catalytic engine of mammalian RNAi. Science. 2004;305(5689):1437–41.
28. Meister G. Argonaute proteins: functional insights and emerging roles. Nat Rev Genet. 2013;14(7):447–59.
29. Hammond SM, Bernstein E, Beach D, Hannon GJ. An RNA-directed nuclease mediates post-transcriptional gene silencing in Drosophila cells. Nature. 2000;404(6775):293–6.
30. Cerutti H. RNA interference: traveling in the cell and gaining functions? Trends Genet. 2003;19(1):39–46.
31. Sioud M. Therapeutic siRNAs. Trends Pharmacol Sci. 2004;25(1):22–8.
32. Tan FL, Yin JQ. RNAi, a new therapeutic strategy against viral infection. Cell Res. 2004;14(6):460–6.
33. McManus MT, Sharp PA. Gene silencing in mammals by small interfering RNAs. Nat Rev Genet. 2002;3(10):737–47.
34. Agrawal N, Dasaradhi PV, Mohmmed A, Malhotra P, Bhatnagar RK, Mukherjee SK. RNA interference: biology, mechanism, and applications. Microbiol Mol Biol Rev. 2003;67(4):657–85.
35. Parrish S, Fleenor J, Xu S, Mello C, Fire A. Functional anatomy of a dsRNA trigger: differential requirement for the two trigger strands in RNA interference. Mol Cell. 2000;6(5):1077–87.
36. Fire A, Xu S, Montgomery MK, Kostas SA, Driver SE, Mello CC. Potent and specific genetic interference by double-stranded RNA in Caenorhabditis elegans. Nature. 1998;391(6669):806–11.
37. Mello CC, Conte D Jr. Revealing the world of RNA interference. Nature. 2004;431(7006):338–42.
38. Gehrs KM, Anderson DH, Johnson LV, Hageman GS. Age-related macular degeneration – emerging pathogenetic and therapeutic concepts. Ann Med. 2006;38(7):450–71.
39. Paddison PJ, Silva JM, Conklin DS, Schlabach M, Li M, Aruleba S, Balija V, O'Shaughnessy A, Gnoj L, Scobie K, Chang K, Westbrook T, Cleary M, Sachidanandam R, McCombie WR, Elledge SJ, Hannon GJ. A resource for large-scale RNA-interference-based screens in mammals. Nature. 2004;428(6981):427–31.
40. Wadman M. Swooping for biotech. Nature. 2005;437(7058):475.
41. Bernards R. The Nobel Prize in Physiology or Medicine for 2006 for the discovery of RNA interference. Ned Tijdschr Geneeskd. 2006;150(52):2849–53.
42. Mack GS. MicroRNA gets down to business. Nat Biotechnol. 2007;25(6):631–8.
43. Haussecker D. The business of RNAi therapeutics. Hum Gene Ther. 2008;19(5):451–62.
44. Palanki MS, Akiyama H, Campochiaro P, Cao J, Chow CP, Dellamary L, Doukas J, Fine R, Gritzen C, Hood JD, Hu S, Kachi S, Kang X, Klebansky B, Kousba A, Lohse D, Mak CC, Martin M, McPherson A, Pathak VP, Renick J, Soll R, Umeda N, Yee S, Yokoi K, Zeng B, Zhu H, Noronha G. Development of prodrug 4-chloro-3-(5-methyl-3-{[4-(2-pyrrolidin-1-ylethoxy)phenyl]amino}-1,2,4-benzotria zin-7-yl) phenyl benzoate (TG100801): a topically administered therapeutic candidate in clinical trials for the treatment of age-related macular degeneration. J Med Chem. 2008;51(6):1546–59.
45. Haussecker D. The business of RNAi therapeutics in 2012. Mol Ther Nucleic Acids. 2012;1:e8.
46. Garber K. Alnylam terminates revusiran program, stock plunges. Nat Biotechnol. 2016;34(12):1213–4.

47. Rizk M, Tuzmen S. Update on the clinical utility of an RNA interference-based treatment: focus on Patisiran. Pharmgenomics Pers Med. 2017;10:267–78.
48. Chakraborty C, Sharma AR, Sharma G, Doss CGP, Lee SS. Therapeutic miRNA and siRNA: moving from bench to clinic as next generation medicine. Mol Ther Nucleic Acids. 2017;8:132–43.
49. Bartz F, Kern L, Erz D, Zhu M, Gilbert D, Meinhof T, Wirkner U, Erfle H, Muckenthaler M, Pepperkok R, Runz H. Identification of cholesterol-regulating genes by targeted RNAi screening. Cell Metab. 2009;10(1):63–75.
50. Tibolla G, Norata GD, Artali R, Meneghetti F, Catapano AL. Proprotein convertase subtilisin/kexin type 9 (PCSK9): from structure-function relation to therapeutic inhibition. Nutr Metab Cardiovas Dis. 2011;21(11):835–43.
51. Frank-Kamenetsky M, Grefhorst A, Anderson NN, Racie TS, Bramlage B, Akinc A, Butler D, Charisse K, Dorkin R, Fan Y, Gamba-Vitalo C, Hadwiger P, Jayaraman M, John M, Jayaprakash KN, Maier M, Nechev L, Rajeev KG, Read T, Rohl I, Soutschek J, Tan P, Wong J, Wang G, Zimmermann T, de Fougerolles A, Vornlocher HP, Langer R, Anderson DG, Manoharan M, Koteliansky V, Horton JD, Fitzgerald K. Therapeutic RNAi targeting PCSK9 acutely lowers plasma cholesterol in rodents and LDL cholesterol in nonhuman primates. Proc Natl Acad Sci U S A. 2008;105(33):11915–20.
52. Majmudar MD, Keliher EJ, Heidt T, Leuschner F, Truelove J, Sena BF, Gorbatov R, Iwamoto Y, Dutta P, Wojtkiewicz G, Courties G, Sebas M, Borodovsky A, Fitzgerald K, Nolte MW, Dickneite G, Chen JW, Anderson DG, Swirski FK, Weissleder R, Nahrendorf M. Monocyte-directed RNAi targeting CCR2 improves infarct healing in atherosclerosis-prone mice. Circulation. 2013;127(20):2038–46.
53. Sugano M, Tsuchida K, Hata T, Makino N. RNA interference targeting SHP-1 attenuates myocardial infarction in rats. FASEB J. 2005;19(14):2054–6.
54. Kim D, Hong J, Moon HH, Nam HY, Mok H, Jeong JH, Kim SW, Choi D, Kim SH. Anti-apoptotic cardioprotective effects of SHP-1 gene silencing against ischemia-reperfusion injury: use of deoxycholic acid-modified low molecular weight polyethyleneimine as a cardiac siRNA-carrier. J Control Release. 2013;168(2):125–34.
55. Burchard J, Jackson AL, Malkov V, Needham RH, Tan Y, Bartz SR, Dai H, Sachs AB, Linsley PS. MicroRNA-like off-target transcript regulation by siRNAs is species specific. RNA. 2009;15(2):308–15.
56. Mockenhaupt S, Grosse S, Rupp D, Bartenschlager R, Grimm D. Alleviation of off-target effects from vector-encoded shRNAs via codelivered RNA decoys. Proc Natl Acad Sci U S A. 2015;30:E4007–16.
57. Xu F, Jin L, Jin Y, Nie Z, Zheng H. Long noncoding RNAs in autoimmune diseases. J Biomed Mater Res A. 2019;107(2):468–75.
58. Hur K, Kim SH, Kim JM. Potential implications of long noncoding RNAs in autoimmune diseases. Immune Netw. 2019;19(1):e4.
59. Qie Y, Sheng Y, Xu H, Jin Y, Ma F, Li L, Li X, An D. Identification of a new powdery mildew resistance gene pmDHT at or closely linked to the Pm5 locus in the Chinese wheat Landrace Dahongtou. Plant Dis. 2019;103:2645–51.
60. Rapanelli M, Tan T, Wang W, Wang X, Wang ZJ, Zhong P, Frick L, Qin L, Ma K, Qu J, Yan Z. Behavioral, circuitry, and molecular aberrations by region-specific deficiency of the high-risk autism gene Cul3. Mol Psychiatry. 2019; https://doi.org/10.1038/s41380-019-0498-x.
61. Nissen PH, Rejmark L. Expanding the spectrum of genetic variants in the calcium sensing receptor (CASR) gene in hypercalcemic individuals. Clin Endocrinol (Oxf). 2019;91(5):683–90.
62. Moreno AM, Palmer N, Aleman F, Chen G, Pla A, Jiang N, Chew WL, Law M, Mali P. Author correction: immune-orthogonal orthologues of AAV capsids and of Cas9 circumvent the immune response to the administration of gene therapy. Nat Biomed Eng. 2019;3(10):842.
63. Meng Q, Sun S, Luo Z, Shi B, Shan A, Cheng B. Maternal dietary resveratrol alleviates weaning-associated diarrhea and intestinal inflammation in pig offspring by changing intestinal gene expression and microbiota. Food Funct. 2019;10(9):5626–43.
64. Manor E, Gonen R, Sarussi B, Keidar-Friedman D, Kumar J, Tang HT, Tassone F. The role of AGG interruptions in the FMR1 gene stability: A survey in ethnic groups with low and high rate of consanguinity. Mol Genet Genomic Med. 2019;7(10):e00946.
65. Liu Z, Chen X. A novel missense mutation in human Receptor Roundabout-1 (ROBO1) gene associated with pituitary stalk interruption syndrome. J Clin Res Pediatr Endocrinol. 2019; https://doi.org/10.4274/jcrpe.galenos.2019.2018.0309.
66. Liu C, Kanazawa T, Tian Y, Mohamed Saini S, Mancuso S, Mostaid MS, Takahashi A, Zhang D, Zhang F, Yu H, Doo Shin H, Sub Cheong H, Ikeda M, Kubo M, Iwata N, Woo SI, Yue W, Kamatani Y, Shi Y, Li Z, Everall I, Pantelis C, Bousman C. The schizophrenia genetics knowledgebase: a comprehensive update of findings from candidate gene studies. Transl Psychiatry. 2019;9(1):205.
67. Li XZ, Yan Y, Zhang JF, Sun JF, Sun B, Yan CG, Choi SH, Johnson BJ, Kim JK, Smith SB. Oleic acid in the absence of a PPARgamma agonist increases adipogenic gene expression in bovine muscle satellite cells. J Anim Sci. 2019;97(10):4114–23.
68. Asghar O, Alam U, Hayat SA, Aghamohammadzadeh R, Heagerty AM, Malik RA. Obesity, diabetes and atrial fibrillation; epidemiology, mechanisms and interventions. Curr Cardiol Rev. 2012;8(4):253–64.
69. Assis R. Out of the testis, into the ovary: biased outcomes of gene duplication and deletion in Drosophila. Evolution. 2019;73(9):1850–62.

70. Attaran S, Saleh HZ, Shaw M, Ward A, Pullan M, Fabri BM. Does the outcome improve after radiofrequency ablation for atrial fibrillation in patients undergoing cardiac surgery? A propensity-matched comparison. Eur J Cardiothorac Surg. 2012;41(4):806–10.. discussion 810-801
71. Ahmad K, Spens AE. Separate Polycomb Response Elements control chromatin state and activation of the vestigial gene. PLoS Genet. 2019;15(8):e1007877.
72. Ahuja V, Powers-Lee SG. Human carbamoyl-phosphate synthetase: insight into N-acetylglutamate interaction and the functional effects of a common single nucleotide polymorphism. J Inherit Metab Dis. 2008;31(4):481–91.
73. Ai L, Liu J, Jiang Y, Guo W, Wei P, Bai L. Specific PCR method for detection of species origin in biochemical drugs via primers for the ATPase 8 gene by electrophoresis. Mikrochim Acta. 2019;186(9):634.
74. Akhbari M, Khalili M, Shahrabi-Farahani M, Biglari A, Bandarian F. Expression level of circulating cell free miR-155 gene in serum of patients with diabetic nephropathy. Clin Lab. 2019;65(8) https://doi.org/10.7754/Clin.Lab.2019.190209.
75. Yang J. Patisiran for the treatment of hereditary transthyretin-mediated amyloidosis. Expert Rev Clin Pharmacol. 2019;12(2):95–9.
76. Sardh E, Harper P, Balwani M, Stein P, Rees D, Bissell DM, Desnick R, Parker C, Phillips J, Bonkovsky HL, Vassiliou D, Penz C, Chan-Daniels A, He Q, Querbes W, Fitzgerald K, Kim JB, Garg P, Vaishnaw A, Simon AR, Anderson KE. Phase 1 trial of an RNA interference therapy for acute intermittent porphyria. N Engl J Med. 2019;380(6):549–58.
77. Pasikowska M, Walsby E, Apollonio B, Cuthill K, Phillips E, Coulter E, Longhi MS, Ma Y, Yallop D, Barber LD, Patten P, Fegan C, Ramsay AG, Pepper C, Devereux S, Buggins AG. Phenotype and immune function of lymph node and peripheral blood CLL cells are linked to transendothelial migration. Blood. 2016;128(4):563–73.
78. Ray KK, Landmesser U, Leiter LA, Kallend D, Dufour R, Karakas M, Hall T, Troquay RP, Turner T, Visseren FL, Wijngaard P, Wright RS, Kastelein JJ. Inclisiran in patients at high cardiovascular risk with elevated LDL cholesterol. N Engl J Med. 2017;376(15):1430–40.
79. Kitagawa H, Ohbuchi K, Munekage M, Fujisawa K, Kawanishi Y, Namikawa T, Kushida H, Matsumoto T, Shimobori C, Nishi A, Sadakane C, Watanabe J, Yamamoto M, Hanazaki K. Phenotyping analysis of the Japanese Kampo medicine maoto in healthy human subjects using wide-targeted plasma metabolomics. J Pharm Biomed Anal. 2019;164:119–27.
80. Vita G, Vita GL, Stancanelli C, Gentile L, Russo M, Mazzeo A. Genetic neuromuscular disorders: living the era of a therapeutic revolution. Part 1: Peripheral neuropathies. Neurol Sci. 2019;40(4):661–9.
81. Tarantini G, Masiero G, Fovino LN, Mojoli M, Varricchio A, Loi B, Gistri R, Misuraca L, Gabrielli G, Cortese B, Pisano F, Moretti L, Tumminello G, Olivari Z, Mazzarotto P, Colombo A, Calabro P, Nicolino A, Tellaroli P, Corrado D, Durante A, Steffenino G, RAIi a. "Full-plastic jacket" with everolimus-eluting Absorb bioresorbable vascular scaffolds: Clinical outcomes in the multicenter prospective RAI registry (ClinicalTrials.gov Identifier: NCT02298413). Int J Cardiol. 2018;266:67–74.
82. Weng Y, Xiao H, Zhang J, Liang XJ, Huang Y. RNAi therapeutic and its innovative biotechnological evolution. Biotechnol Adv. 2019;37(5):801–25.
83. Turner L. ClinicalTrials.gov, stem cells and 'pay-to-participate' clinical studies. Regen Med. 2017;12(6):705–19.
84. Yang A, Baxi S, Korenstein D. ClinicalTrials.gov for facilitating rapid understanding of potential harms of new drugs: the case of checkpoint inhibitors. J Oncol Pract. 2018;14(2):72–6.
85. Mercer TR, Mattick JS. Structure and function of long noncoding RNAs in epigenetic regulation. Nat Struct Mol Biol. 2013;20(3):300–7.
86. Devaux Y, Zangrando J, Schroen B, Creemers EE, Pedrazzini T, Chang CP, Dorn GW 2nd, Thum T, Heymans S, Cardiolinc Network. Long noncoding RNAs in cardiac development and ageing. Nat Rev Cardiol. 2015;12(7):415–25.
87. Vausort M, Wagner DR, Devaux Y. Long noncoding RNAs in patients with acute myocardial infarction. Circ Res. 2014;115(7):668–77.
88. Ounzain S, Pedrazzini T. Long non-coding RNAs in heart failure: a promising future with much to learn. Ann Transl Med. 2016;4(15):298.
89. Jones SK, Merkel OM. Tackling breast cancer chemoresistance with nano-formulated siRNA. Gene Ther. 2016;23(12):821–8.
90. Baumann V, Winkler J. miRNA-based therapies: strategies and delivery platforms for oligonucleotide and non-oligonucleotide agents. Future Med Chem. 2014;6(17):1967–84.
91. Zangi L, Lui KO, von Gise A, Ma Q, Ebina W, Ptaszek LM, Spater D, Xu H, Tabebordbar M, Gorbatov R, Sena B, Nahrendorf M, Briscoe DM, Li RA, Wagers AJ, Rossi DJ, Pu WT, Chien KR. Modified mRNA directs the fate of heart progenitor cells and induces vascular regeneration after myocardial infarction. Nat Biotechnol. 2013;31(10):898–907.

Part VI

Future Prospects

Prospective Advances in Non-coding RNAs Investigation

24

Muhammad Ishtiaq Jan, Tahir Ali, Ayesha Ishtiaq, Iram Mushtaq, and Iram Murtaza

Abstract

Non-coding RNAs (ncRNAs) play significant roles in numerous physiological cellular processes and molecular alterations during pathological conditions including heart diseases, cancer, immunological disorders and neurological diseases. This chapter is focusing on the basis of ncRNA relation with their functions and prospective advances in non-coding RNAs particularly miRNAs investigation in the cardiovascular disease management.

The field of ncRNAs therapeutics is a very fascinating and challenging too. Scientists have opportunity to develop more advanced therapeutics as well as diagnostic approaches for cardiovascular conditions. Advanced studies are critically needed to deepen the understanding of the molecular biology, mechanism and modulation of ncRNAs and chemical formulations for managing CVDs.

Keywords

CVD management · ncRNA · miRNA · Therapeutics · Diagnostics

M. I. Jan · T. Ali · A. Ishtiaq · I. Mushtaq
I. Murtaza (✉)
Department of Biochemistry, Signal Transduction Laboratory, Faculty of Biological Sciences, Quaid-i-Azam University, Islamabad, Pakistan
e-mail: irambch@qau.edu.pk

1 Prospective Advances in Non-coding RNAs Investigation

It is believed that basic goal of biology is to understand the relationship between the DNA sequence and the instructions encoded in DNA, which are used to create and maintain an organism. Data obtained from whole genome sequencing projects proposed that, remarkably similar numbers of protein-coding genes are present in the genome of different species [1–3]. It shows that, the complexity in numerous aspect of organisms arise from non-coding region of the genome. These non-coding regions include various regulatory and functional units including non-coding RNAs. The discovery of non-coding RNAs revolutionized the landscape of molecular genetics [4–7]. Numerous experimental and bioinformatics strategies have been taken to study, identify and address the novel ncRNAs in the different model organisms from *Escherichia coli* to human [8, 9]. Documented results from these investigation revealed that the anticipated numbers of the ncRNAs were much lesser [4, 10]. Advanced technology such as next generation sequencing (SOLiD or Genome analyzer) have a significant contribution in the high-throughput detection of ncRNAs [11]. Recently, not only non-invasive diagnosis tools used to monitor ncRNA concentration in the body fluids but also silencing and inhibitions or replacement

J. Xiao (ed.), *Non-coding RNAs in Cardiovascular Diseases*, Advances in Experimental Medicine and Biology 1229, https://doi.org/10.1007/978-981-15-1671-9_24

and re-activation are also included in the translational opportunities [12].

The screening of the ncRNA in the model organism is based on the bio-computational prediction of ncRNA and sequencing after isolation from cells, tissues or entire organism by direct biochemical analysis. In the Experimental RNomics basically four methods are commonly used to identify ncRNAs. These methods are: RNA sequencing which is the most traditional method, the parallel cloning of many ncRNAs by generating cDNA library, the microarray analysis and genomics SELEX (selected evolution of ligands by exponential enrichment). Further, different computational approaches including Pfold, RNAfold, RNAz, EvoFold, QRNA, CMFinder and FOLDALIGN) RNAalifold are mostly used to identify ncRNAs [11–19].

Recently, in the last decade the interest on ncRNA has been remarkably increased [12]. Numerous studies focusing on the deregulation of ncRNAs and their relationship with diseases including cardiovascular diseases has been reported recently, thus increasing their importance as therapeutic potential tools for diseases. Moreover, inhibition or over expression of long or small ncRNA has a strong therapeutic strategy for the various types of cardiac pathologies such as CVDs [4, 12, 20–26]. As reported by Rayner et al. [27] upon inhibition of miR-33a/b, VLDL triglycerides were reduced and HDL level was increased, supporting the role of these small ncRNA in dyslipidemia and related diseases including atherosclerosis. Thus, the antimiRs/BlockmiRs of these miRNAs are a potential therapeutic tool for various dyslipidemia related disorders. Similarly, the over expression with mimic or adeno-virus mediated miRNA, such as miR-378, has a key anti-apoptotic as well as anti-hypertrophic potential in cardiac cells [28], proposing a potential treatment of heart abnormalities including ischemic heart diseases. Further, from clinical point of view, numerous studies are focusing on the ncRNA (small circulatory RNA) as a biomarker of various diseases including cancer and CVDs. For instance, circulatory hsa-miR-21-5p, hsa-miR-218-5 and hsa-miR-211 have prominent roles in the diabetes mellitus induced atherosclerosis and have been documented as confirmed biomarkers for the atherosclerosis progression. Studies also reported the role of some miRNA * in CVDs too. miRNA* originates from the same hairpin structure (pre and pri miRNA) of the main miRNA and it is supposed to be complementary to the main miRNA. MiR-208a has been considered promising MI (STEMI) biomarkers, because of its potent characteristics including: high specificity, high sensitivity and superior kinetics over gold standard cTn, because it can be detected within 2 h (earlier then cTn) and allow early diagnosis of AMI. Within 24 h miR-208a decline to baseline in proposed minor cardiac events after major infarction [29–34].

The "Transcriptomic medicine", means therapeutic targeting of RNA, basically comprised of two strategies, single-stranded antisense oligonucleotides (ASO) and double-stranded RNA-mediated interference (RNAi). ASO are synthetic agents of 20 base pair (bp) in length that target pre-mRNA, mRNA and noncoding RNA. The action mechanism of ASO depends upon the ASO hybridization site and chemical properties of ASO. ASO mainly stimulates RNAase H activity to inhibit protein production via mRNA degradation and prevent splicing factor binding to induce alternative splicing [35–40]. Unlike ASO, RNAi are double stranded RNA molecules of 19 to 25 bp in length, used as a synthetic mediator of RNAi to silence the target gene. Beside the target gene silencing, RNAi (siRNA) could also induce knock down of unintended gene either via miRNA gene regulation machinery or through imperfect complimentary binding to mRNA [39, 41–46]. Similar to RNAi, miRNA also regulates gene expression at post transcriptional level and could also induce numerous mRNA silencing unlike one target siRNA silencing. ASOs (antagomirs) bind to miRISC preventing them to bind with mRNA. Miravirsen is the only miRNA therapeutic agent involve in the miR-122 inhibition, has been assessed in the clinical trials (NCT01200420) for the patients with chronic hepatitis C [47–53]. Aptamer is another class of DNA or RNA based synthetic therapeutics as well as diagnosis agents that bind to their specific target via SELEX. Up to date numerous aptamers have been generated for targeting various molecules including protein, whole cells, viruses, bacteria as well as small metal ions. Aptamers have similar functional capabilities as chemical antibodies. Other properties of the aptamers include small size, high selectivity and affinity, while most important is their flexible structure and can be engendered *in vitro*. In addition as attractive therapeutic strategy, aptamers can be used as an antagonist to inhibit target efficiently. For instance, Macugen is the first aptamer (FDA approved) used in age-related macular degradation (AMD) by targeting vascular endothelial growth factor (VEGF), but unfortunately was not effective than VEGF-specific monoclonal antibody [54–57].

Mipomersen (20 bp) is an ASO which target apolipoprotein B (ApoB) mRNA and subsequently induced inhibition of protein synthesis by activating RNase H activation. Apolipoprotein B is the key component of atherogenic lipoprotein and determinant of risk factor for cardio vascular diseases. PCSK9 (proprotein convertase subtilisin/kexin-9) is another target of antisense technology getting attention in the field of cardiac diseases. PCSK9 enhanced circulatory LDL-C levels via reducing LDL receptor expression, transported into hepatocytes. The synthesis of PCSK9 can be inhibited via long-acting RNAi therapeutic agent known as 'Inclisiran'. Inclisiran is now in the clinical trial phase 2 showing virtuous results [58, 59]. Apolipoprotein C3 (AOCP-III) elevates in hypertriglyceridemia and in insulin resistance condition and considered as risk factor for CVDs. Therefore AOCP-III is the key target of antisense technology and volansesorsen is an ASO which target AOCP-III mRNA. Volansesorsen is recently in the phase 3 clinical trial and has been assessed for familial chylomicronemia syndrome patients [60–62]. In addition, angiopoietin-like 3 (ANGPT3) and angiopoietin-like 4 are the promising risk factors for CVDs. Any mutation in the gene coding of ANGPTL3 and ANGPTL4 can induce loss of function of these genes and are linked with low levels of plasma LDL, HDL, triglycerides as well as reduced insulin resistance. IONIS-ANGPTL3-L_{Rx} (ANGPTL3-L_{RX}) is the ligand conjugated ASO of second generation that targets mRNA (ANGPTL3 and ANGPTL4). This drug is in the phase 1 clinical trial and currently studied in human individuals [63–68].

Inflammation has a prominent role in the development of CVDs and CRP is an inflammatory marker whose elevation is the risk factor for CVDs. Therefore, CRP is also considered as the key target for ASO associated medicine/drugs. Recently, ISIS-CRPRx an ASO was used against endotoxin induced CRP increased level. This drug is also in the clinical trial (phase 2) for the patients with inflammation associated atrial fibrillation (AF). However, the CRP level was reduced with ISIS-CRPRx pre-treatment, but the AF progression was not reduced. This finding showed that, ISIS-CRPRx has anti-inflammatory potential. Moreover, ISIS-CRPRx reduced high sensitivity CRP (hs-CRPRx) elevated during rheumatoid arthritis is in a phase 2 clinical trial for 36 days [69–76]. Overall, numerous clinical trial/studies comprised of small interfering RNA and ASO treatments are going on to reduced/attenuate the burden of CVDs.

Regenerative medicines have got remarkable attention since ancient times. Like, other mammalian, human being possess most modest tissues regenerative ability, but still at cellular level tissues can repair themselves due to stem cells. Hence, stem cells can be used as regenerative starting point to produce suitable cell types for therapeutic purposes. Even, in organs such as adult heart that don't possess meaningful stem cell, somatic cell types can be stimulated to evoke repair of stem cell devoid tissues through the cellular reprograming and lineage specific differentiation [77, 78]. However, more new strategies are needed to establish a link between physiology and stem cell biology. In this context genome based new concepts and strategies are arising continuously. It is well known that, 80% of our genome is transcribed into numerous non-coding RNAs which have regulatory functions (https://www.encodeproject.org/). Due to these regulatory functions, the non-coding RNAs are considered as the key frontier in the regenerative medicine and it is assumed that the deeper understanding of ncRNA which are thought to be involved in the pluripotency, differentiation and cellular plasticity can transmute present medicine towards more specific and personalized pathological diagnosis and therapies. Recently, microRNA and lncRNA either with transcription factors or completely on their own have been documented as key players for reprograming fully differentiated mature cells into pluripotent stem cells (iPSCs) or inducing trans-differentiating cells into different lineages [79–82].

Skeletal muscles have impressive and remarkable regenerative ability due to their muscle specific stem cells (satellite cells). H19 gene which contains IncRNA sequence is exceedingly expressed in the satellite cells. Experimental data from the recent research demonstrate that, targeted deletion of H19 will cause loss (50%) of satellite cells in the adult muscles. This shows that, imprinted gene encoding the H19 gene IncRNA is essential for the satellite cells quiescent state. In addition miR-499 and miR-208b role have also been reported during maturation of regenerating myofibers by targeting/repressing transcriptional repressors Purb, Hp-1b, Sp3 and Sox6. Further, the slow genes can also be silenced by Linc-MYH, a ncRNA (IncRNA), which is located in the cluster of fast MYH genes [83–87].

Heart muscles have very low regenerative abilities. It has been observed that, few hours after heart attack 25% of total heart muscles (left ventricle) are lost and ultimately exchanged by non-contracting scar. To resolve this issue, researcher around the world are applying array of approaches such as direct delivery of regenerative cells isolated from different sources (e.g. embryonic stem cells, heart biopsies/liposuction, bone marrow, induced pluripotent stem cells), implantations of functional patches to engineered tissues, inducing stimulation (*in vivo*) of resident cells via reprogramming factors delivery, or re-entry of cardiomyocytes in cell cycle via different inducers [88–92].

In the present decade, it is well known that, ncRNA represents a keystone for the treatment of various pathologies, including cardiovascular disorders [93]. However, there are limitations in the field for controlled, efficient and safe systematic delivery to specific and desired tissues while using ncRNA as a drug. It is also considered that, answer to these limitations could be obtained from nano-medicine. Nano-particles (1–100 nm) are a smart class of engineered nano-carriers for drugs to the targeted cells/tissues. Upon release of the loaded drug within the cells, damage can be reduced. In addition, as NPs provide protection to drug against enzyme degradation, a great interest has been shown by the scientific community to promote this technology towards innovative medical methodologies, to overcome the present conventional medicine limitations e.g. impaired target specificity, organ toxicity and poor drug bioavailability. However, the use of NPs in the field of cardiovascular diseases is much less then cancer. But, after successful pre-clinical and clinical outcomes from the oncological therapy, NPs are becoming innovative keys for future clinical studies in the field of CVDs [93–98]. Recently, ncRNA-loaded-NPs have been used in the field of oncology, e.g. polyethylene glycol-polyethylenimine nano-complexes can successfully deliver miR-150 to chronic myeloid leukemia cells [99].

Furthermore, the rate of tumor growth in the lungs can be reduced by targeting key oncogenes via miR-29b delivered by miR-29b-cationic lipoplexes-based carriers [100]. Di Mauro et al., first time reported that, negatively charged calcium-phosphate bio-inspired NPs can be used (both in *vivo* and in *vitro*) to efficiently deliver miRNAs into cardiomyocytes [101].

2 Prospective Roles of miRNAs in Cardiovascular Diseases

Several years of research showed that among nc-RNAs, miRNAs possess the significant potential to be employed as diagnostic tool or therapeutic agent. The detailed overview of the miRNA utilization in modulating CVDs has been addressed in the Sect. 24.1 "An overview of non-coding RNAs and cardiovascular system". Briefly they can be employed with respect to their modulation strategies as miRNA sponges or erasers, miRNA targets-sites protectors, Small molecule inhibitors, Anti-Sense oligodeoxyribonucleotides (ASOs) or as Anti-miRNA oligodeoxyribonucleotides (AMOs). The detailed prospective analysis of various miRNAs in multiple cardiovascular diseases is addressed in following section.

2.1 Prospective of miRNAs Therapeutic Role in Cardiac Development and Hypertrophy

The irreversible enlargement of cardiomyocytes (cardiac hypertrophy) is a compensatory mechanism occurs in response to various pathophysiological stimuli including pressure over load. The pressure overload can also be occurred due to valve dysfunction. The enlargement of the cardiac cells occur to normalize the stress but chronically it produces cardiac hypertrophy which can also lead to sudden death and heart failure (HF). To date, various studies proposed different pathways which can cause cardiac hypertrophy at molecular level but the exact mechanism is still under investigation. *In vitro* and *in vivo* studies showed that cardiac remolding of heart with changes in expression profile of genes occurs as a result of various stimuli. The emerging roles and increasing evidences of different miRNAs in cardiac hypertrophy reveal that miRNAs are the key modulator of cardiac development and cardiac hypertrophy.

miR-208a is transcribed with its host gene myosin heavy chain α MHC. Their expression is relatively stable and plays an important role in the expression of β MHC response to cardiac stress in the cardiac hypertrophy [142]. Mir-208a targets thyroid hormones receptor protein 1 (THRAP1) that negatively regulates β MHC. Null mice showed no hypertrophy in response to pressure overload after thoracic aortic constriction because β MHC was unable to upregulate. LNA modified antimiR-208 study showed prevention in pathological cardiac remodeling in diastolic heart disease. The beneficial effect was verified by reducing the plasma level of miR-208a. The expression analysis based on these notions confirmed the pro-hypertrophic nature of miR-208a. Thus miR-208a and its downstream effectors are the important therapeutic targets in cardiac remodeling [102]. The pathological effect was also confirmed by transgenic over expression of miR-208a followed by detouring to normal texture of ventricular walls [103].

miR-21 is a dynamically regulated miRNA which plays key role in various pathological diseases including heart diseases. Thum *et al* showed that *in vivo* knockdown experiment of antagomir prevent cardiac hypertrophy and interstitial fibrosis after thoracic bending. miR-21 regulates MAP kinase signaling pathway in cardiac disease through its target *spry1* while antagomirs of miR-21 regulates spry1 [104]. miR-21 has a contradictory role regarding its inhibitory effect in regulating cardiac remodeling which needs more exploration [105, 106]. miR-21 has a key role in circulating angiogenic cells. Increased oxidative stress and impaired migratory capacity was observed in up regulation of miR-21 via nitric oxide synthase inhibitor asymmetric di-methyl arginine (ADMA) in angiogenic cells by targeting superoxide dismutase 2 and Map kinase inhibitor *sprouty 2* both *in vivo* and *in vitro* [107]. Thus targeting miR-21 in angiogenic cell provides a good platform to use this miR-21 as a therapeutic in cardiovascular diseases. miR-21 antagonist block fibrosis and cardiac hypertrophy in mice model by inhibition of endothelial mesenchymal cell transition in TGFβ treated endothelial cells [108]. In balloon injured rat carotid artery model anti miR-21 strategy blocked restenosis [109]. miR-21 is over expressed in cardiovascular diseases like atherosclerosis. The abnormal proliferation of vascular smooth muscle cells (VSMCs) and neointimal lesion results in post angio-plasticity restenosis as the consequences of miR-21 overexpression [110]. In knock down experiment of miR-21, reduction was observed in neointimal lesion formation while over expressing miR-21 strategy enhanced VSMCs proliferation. It is therefore identified that miR-21 targets both PTEN and bcl-2 in proliferation and apoptosis of VSMCs [109].

Cellular fibroblasts maintain extracellular matrix in healthy individuals. Cardiac fibrosis which is a hallmark of cardiac hypertrophy occurs along with proliferation and activation of fibroblasts. In fibrosis the monolayer of fibroblasts produces extracellular matrix, proteinase, cytokines and growth factors which interact with myocyte cells [111]. The upregulation of miR-21 is linked with up regulation of factors which triggers cardiac fibrosis. miR- 21 targets sprout 1 which acts as a repressor of endogenous ERK/MAP pathway. In mice ventricle pressure overload was significantly improved after treatment with miR-21 antagomir. In contrast, in mice cardiac fibroblasts, the over expression of miR-21 is responsible for cardiac ischemic/reperfusion injury (IR) [112]. miR-21 also targets *PTEN* and as a result increases level of p-AkT and MMP-2 which increases fibrotic response. *In vitro* experiments revealed that miR-21 is stimulated by angiotensin II or phenylephrine which is further confirmed by *in vivo* analysis that miR-21 expression was increased by four folds during cardiac hypertrophy after aortic bending. However, modulating miR-21 via antisense showed a negative effect on cardiac hypertrophy [113]. The miR-21 knock down experiment showed decrease in proliferation and increase apoptosis in rat cultured aortic vascular smooth muscles cells (VSMCs) thus miR-21 possess both proliferative and anti-apoptotic activity due to the involvement of bcl2 [114]. Moreover, miR-21 attenuates the AKT/mTOR pathway by targeting *tensin* homolog (Pten) and phosphatase which ultimately leads to cardiac hypertrophy [115]. The passenger strand of miR-21-3p also exerts its cardiac hypertrophic effect by targeting sorbin and SH3 domain-containing protein 2 (Sorbs2), PDZ-LIM domain 5 (Pdlim5) and histone deacetylase-8 (Hdac8) [116].

Ischemia/reperfusion injury is the pathological cause of oxidative stress and apoptosis among cardiovascular diseases. miR-1 is up regulated and has a pro-apoptotic role in ischemia which also enhances arrhythmogenicity [103]. Calcium and calmodulin signaling pathways play important roles in cardiac hypertrophy which is negatively regulated by miR-1 [117]. The level of miR-1 is reduced in αMHC calcineurin mice. Calm1 and calm2 are the effectors of calmodulin which are the targets of miR-1. Mef2a is a pro hypertrophic transcription factors which is directly targeted by miR-1. Adenovirus induced miR-1 over expression blocked cardiac hypertrophic response and calcium calmodulin signaling pathway [118] . Arrhythmogenesis may also occurs due to the over expression of miR-1. When the expression level of miR-1 was reduced by antagomirs in infarcted hearts, it protected conductive potential by reducing the level of ion channel proteins, KCN2 and GJAI [119]. Neonatal cardiac hypertrophy can be prevented via over expression of miR-1. In such study miR-1 inhibited the expression of its targets including cyclin-dependent kinase 9, Ras guanosine-triphosphatase activating protein, Ras homolog enriched in brain and fibronectin [120] Protein phosphatase PP2A is targeted by miR-1 which in turns lead to CaMKII dependent hyper phosphorylation of RyR2 that plays a critical role in arrhythmia by calcium release. Muscle specific miR-1 deletion is responsible for arrhythmia and ventricular septal defects [121]. The cardiac transcription factor, (Irx5) can block potassium channel subunit Kv4.2 which is responsible for rapid potassium current. However, experiments showed that Irx5 is the valid target of miR-1 [122]. Basic helix loop helix transcription factor Hand2 has a major role in cardiogenesis. Due to down regulation of Hand2 as a effector response of miR-1 over expression, mice were unable to survive due to insufficient development of myocardial cell. Moreover, miR-I also targets serum response factor (SRF), myogenic differentiation factor (Myo D) and myocyte enhancing factor 2 (Mef2) during development of heart which bears thin wall texture of ventricle, HF and cardio-genesis arrest at embryonic stage [123]. It has also been found that various genes are targeted by miR-1 in silico including cyclin-dependent kinase 9 (Cdk9), Ras GTPase-activating protein (RasGAP, fibronectin and Ras homolog enriched in brain (Rheb) [120]. Cardiac hypertrophy can also be mitigated by down-regulation of insulin-like growth factor (Igf1), extracellular matrix (ECM) remodeling factor, twinfilin 1 (Twf1) and heart and neural crest derivatives expressed 2 (Hand2) [124]. The downstream transcription factor GATA4 is also regulated by miR-1 showing their pivotal role during cardiac hypertrophy [125]. Twinfilin 1 (Twf1) is a cytoskeletal regulatory protein which prevent the assembly of actin monomers in to filaments [126]. During stress signals it can induce hypertrophy in neonatal cardiomyocytes with the down regulation of miR-1. It confirmed that Twf1 is a putative targets of miR-1 while the up regulation of this miRNA can be used therapeutically to reduce the level of Twf1 [125]. Insulin like growth factor (IGF-1) is also a validated target of miR-1 [127] In various cardiac hypertrophic failure models there is reciprocal expression of miR-1 and IGF-1. However, previous studies showed that expression of miR-1 depends on activation of IGF-1 via PI3K/AKT pathway and attenuation of their downstream targets Foxo3a [128].

There are strong evidences which revealed that miR-133 expression is important for proper development of heart and their function. The over expression of miR-133 mitigate the cardiac hypertrophy induced through agonist while on the other hand, knock down of miR-133 with antagomeric sequence induce cardiac hypertrophy. The beneficial effect of miR-133 was also validated by sponges where the cardiac cells started proper growth. Both *in vivo* and *in vitro* study proved that miR-133 is down-regulated while calcineurin activity is enhanced during cardiac hypertrophy [129]. However, cyclosporine A inhibits the activity of calcineurin and up-regulated miR-133. It shows that miR-133 and calcineurin are reciprocal to each other during the progression of cardiac hypertrophy. Low expression of miR-133 is also associated with diabetics induced cardiomyocytes hypertrophy through SGK1 and IJGR1 [130]. *In vivo* low expression of miR-133 triggered cardiac hypertrophy by an injection of an antagomir while adenovirus mediated up regulation of miR-133 protects cardiac hypertrophy [118]. Therefore transient miR-133 mimic can also be used as a therapeutic approach to reduce cardiac hypertrophy. miR-133 targets ether-a- go-go related gene (ERG) and reduces it expression in diabetes. ERG encodes a potassium channel (IKr) which plays a major role in potassium current in myocardial cells. *In vivo* diabetes animal model studies showed that there is increase expression of miR-133 and low level of ERG protein. *In vitro* experiments showed that exogenous delivery of miR-133 reduced the level of ERG protein while miR-133 antagomir delivery halted the miR-133 and in turns increased the protein level of ERG [131] Connective tissue growth factor (CTGF) is a potential candidate of miR-133. The up-regulation of miR-133 in fibroblasts suppresses its expression level which triggers the expression of collagen synthesis in cardiac fibrosis [132]. HCN2 is an ion channel gene which is down regulated during hypertrophy being targeted by miR-133. *In vitro* inhibition of miR-133 showed increase expression of HCN2 gene [133]. In addition, *in vitro* analysis also showed that miR-133 expression can inhibit cardiac hypertrophy. On the other hand, the suppression of miR-133 by decoy sequence induced cardiac hypertrophy further confirmed their cardioprotective effect. *In vivo* study also showed increase in cardiac hypertrophy by a single antagomir infusion of miR-133. There are various targets of miR-133 which positively regulate cardiac hypertrophy including RhoA, Cdc42, and Nelf-A/WHSC2. The down regulation of respective targets with the up regulation of miR-133 can suggest their therapeutic application in cardiac hypertrophy [118]. Some transgenic mice experiments with abdominal aortic constriction (AAC) showed that insulin-like growth factor-1 (IGF-1) deficiency resists cardiac hypertrophy through mitigating down regulation of miR-133 [134]. Gain of function approaches revealed that miR-133 has the capability to reduce the expression of NFATc4 at transcription level and attenuates the cardiac hypertrophic stimuli mediated by PE in primary cardiomyocytes [126].

Circulatory miRNAs in plasma and serum contribute in various types of heart diseases and can also be used as biomarkers for diagnostic purposes. As miR-133a is expressed by cardiomyocytes [135] and it's down regulation triggers cardiac hypertrophy [136]. The targets of miR-133a includes Wolf-Hirschhorn syndrome candidate 2/Negative elongation factor A (WHSC2/NELFA), Inositol 1,4,5′-triphosphate receptor II (IP3RII), Calcineurin, Serum response factor (SRF), Ras homologue gene family member A (RhoA), Cell division control protein 42 (Cdc42), and Nuclear factor of activated T cells calcineurin-dependent 4 (Nfatc4) [137, 138]. Villar *et al* found a significantly high expression level of plasma miR-133a in 74 patients of Aortic Stenosis characterized by left ventricle elongation in post-operative patients which normalized left ventricle mass (LVM) compared with surgically pre-operative, after 1 year. miR-133a is released by myocardium in circulation and its high expression can be used as a strategy to reverse the LV hypertrophy after Aortic Valve Replacement (AVR) [138]. In this study only WHSC2/NELFA constituted a negative predictor of 1 year post-operative LVM reduction among the targets of miR-133a.

The transcription factor, Nuclear factor of activated T cells (NFAT) contains five distinct iso- forms, among these iso-forms NFATc3 is considered as a downstream key mediator of calcinerurin which play a major role in cardiac hypertrophy [139]. The knock down experiment of anti-hypertrophic factors like muscles specific ring finger protein 1 (Murf1) showed severe cardiac hypertrophy in response to pressure over load. miR-23a is a pro hypertrophic miRNA and its expression can be increased by cardiac hypertrophy signals upon treatment with Isoproterenol (Iso) or aldosterone (Aldo). Cardiac hypertrophy can be validated by its markers like atrial natriuretic peptide (ANP), brain natriuretic peptide (BNP) beta- myosin heavy chain (β-MHC) and the protein/DNA ratio analysis. The antimiR-23a (knock down) strategy revealed reduction in these markers. The promoter of miR-23a was activated but the knock down experiment of NFATc3 showed no hypertrophic signals upon treatment with Iso or Aldo which confirm that miR- 23a is a direct downstream target of NFATc3 and calcinerurin. On contrary its expression level was reduced being anti-hypertrophic factor. Murf1is the potential valid target of miR-23a proved by luciferase assay. *In vivo* experiment showed that antagomir of miR-23a reduced hypertrophic signals results in less hypertrophic phenotype of heart and their respective markers which inturn increases the expression of Murf1. miRNA transgenic mice showed that cardiac hypertrophy is positively regulated by miR-23 and increase cardiac hypertrophic markers like ANP, β MHC upon treatment with phenylephrine. On contrary, when the transgenic over expression of miR-23a was attenuated by antagomir, the heart weight was also reduced with reducing hypertrophic markers. Foxo3a is an anti- hypertrophic factor [140] and is a downstream target of miR-23 proved during luciferase assay analysis which has three distinct sites in 3' UTR of Foxo3a mRNA. Enforced over expression of mR-23a also showed a reduce level of endogenously expressed Foxo3a. The transgenic over expression of Foxa3a attenuated ROS levels through Mn-SOD target factor [141]. The over expression of miR-23a and 23b trigger hypertrophy in cardiac cultured cells [142]. miR-23a is up-regulated as a result of hypertrophic response dependent on NFAT function. *In vivo* the expression level of miR-23a was reduced by an antagomir which could not induce hypertrophy in cardiomyocytes when infected with adenovirus constructs carrying NFAT and calcineurin. miR-23a targets anti-hypertrophic MURF1 and triggers hypertrophic signals [143]. Some recent studies also demonstrated that during the progression of cardiac hypertrophy miR-23a may also regulates lysophosphatidic acid receptor 1 (Lpa1) [144].

Antagonist of miR-29 reduces apoptosis in H9C2 cells manipulated for ischemic/reperfusion injury. In cardiac injury the infarct size and apoptosis reduced after injection with miR-29 antagomir. miR-29 targets various fibrosis related effectors like collagen. miR-29 is down-regulated in cardiac fibrosis in rats which is a pathological stimulus of myocardial infarction (MI) and hypertension characterized by excessive accumulation of ECM protein. The expression level of miR-29 is reduced after MI which tends to increase the level of collagens fibrosis response. In knock down miR-29 experiment using antagomir technique *in vivo,* the collagen level was increased. miR-29 was directly applied to the myocardial infarcted tissue and it reduced the level of collagens in fibroblasts. There are also some other fibrotic genes which were also found to be the potential targets of miR-29 [145]. Boon *et al* found that LNA modified antisense has a potency of silencing miR-29 which tends to increase the level of ECM [146]. miR-29a repressed angiogenesis in mice. Mice started recovering from hind limb ischemia and MI after injection with antagomiR-29a acquiring new capillaries and smooth muscles actin positive arterioles [147]. The infarct size and apoptosis was decreased after injection with antagomiR-29a with more improvement of systolic and diastolic function. Knock down experiment of miR-29 showed a high level of collagen whereas the expression level of collagen was down in fibroblast with over expression of miR-29. It shows that collagen is a negative potential target of miR-29 [145].

Myocardial capillaries are formed by endothelial and circulating angiogenic cells. The angiogenic cells stimulate ECs for developing new vascularization. The crucial role of miRNA for vascularization was identified in Dicer transgenic mice lacking two exons in which the vessels could not developed at embryonic stage [148] . A reduced level of angiogenesis was observed in knockdown Dicer mice in response to vascular endothelial growth factors (VEGF) [149]. miR-126 plays a major role in vascular development. miR-126 deficient mice showed defects in vessels because spred 1 was highly expressed which results in reduced angiogenesis signaling through VEGF and FGF [150]. In myocardial infarcted animal model, the mice were unable to survive for 3 weeks after cardiac injury. Most of the miRNAs are transcribed from intergenic region of genes while miR-126 is located within intron of egfl7 gene. miR-126 knock down mice showed an observable defects in vascular system compare with knock down mice of egfl7 [151]. A dose of antagomir reduced the expression of miR-126 and ultimately the mice suffered from impaired vascularization after hind limb ischemia. The expression of miR-126 is up-regulated in endothelial cells. In the knock down experiment of miR-126, the mice were not able to survive because of poor angiogenesis [152] The poor vascularization in mice model reveals that miR-126 is essential for angiogenesis which shows that miR-126 mimic can be used as a therapeutic agent in ischemic conditions.

miR-34 family is highly expressed in cardiac hypertrophy and MI as a result of pressure over load. The administration of a single 8 mer LNA-antimiR 34 can better inhibits entire miR-34 family in cardiac models of TAC pressure overload. Luciferase assay showed that Vinculin, Sema4b, Pofut1, Bcl6 and VEGFs are targets of miR-34, which have cardio-protective properties. An improved systolic cardiac function which reduces fibrosis with increased akt activation, increased capillary density, lower ANP and increased expression level of respective cardio-protective genes was observed after treatment with LNA-antimiR-34 [153] The cardio-protective genes have a critical role in enhance capillary density (VEGFs), [154] as vinculin for cardiac electric function [155], pofut1 is important for Notch signaling [156], Bcl6 is important in prevention of cardiac inflammation and Sema4b inhibit IL 6 production [157].

Calcineurin elicit a serine/threonine protein phosphatase linked cardiac hypertrophy signal [158], while cyclosporine A and FK506 prevent cardiac hypertrophy by inhibiting calcineurin [159]. NFATc3 is a downstream target of calcineurin [159] which phosphorylates NFATc3 on serine residues at N termini in cytoplasm and restricted to nucleus upon dephosphorylation. Myocardin is a transcriptional co activator which expresses at high level during cardiac hypertrophic stimuli as a downstream target of NFATc3. miR-9 also target Myocardin and can reduce it expression under hypertrophic stimuli via aldosterone and isoproterenol [34]. The expression level of phosphorylated NFATc3 was reduced while myocardin was increased as a result of cardiac hypertrophic signals in mice models. Focusing on therapeutic role of miR-9 as it down regulates in cardiac hypertrophy, target validation analysis (luciferase assay) showed that miR-9 can potentially targets *myocardin*. The miR-9 mimic administration showed a reduce level of myocardin along with hypertrophic markers like β MHC and ANP in mice models [160].

miR-199a was up-regulated during cardiac hypertrophy in mice. The miR-199a expression was also high in transgenic mice of HF expressing b1-adrenergic receptor (AR) or b2-AR. The cardiac hypertrophic effect of miR-199a was also confirmed after exposure of cardiomyocytes to isoproterenol. On the other hand, miR-199a was down-regulated after insulin receptor induced activation of Akt pathway. In addition, transcription factor including hypoxia-inducible factor 1-alpha (HIF-1a), and sirtuin (Sirt1) were also up-regulated and induced cardiac hypertrophy [161]. The adenovirus mediated over expression of miR-199a showed increase in cardiomyocytes hypertrophy [162].

The activator of transcription 3 (STAT3) is one of the factors which maintain the cardiac integrity and function. The knock down experiments in animal model showed the elevated level of miR-199b. Further experiments of over expression of miR-199b revealed the disruption of sarcomere integrity. miR-199a also regulates ubiquitin conjugated enzymes (Ube2i and Ube2g1) while *in vitro* knock down experiments showed dysfunction in cardiomyocytes due to the reduction in expression of α and β MHC and loss of sarcomeres. It shows that STAT3 negatively regulates miR-199a through ubiquitin conjugating enzymes [163]. miR-199b expression is increased during mice and human heart hypertrophy, while it can also regulate calcineurin/nuclear factor of activated T cells (NFAT) pathway. The inhibition of miR-199b by antagomir in mice reduced cardiac hypertrophy and fibrosis. The dual-specificity tyrosine (Y) phosphorylation-regulated kinase 1a is also regulated by miR-199b which can also effect calcineurin-responsive gene expression during cardiac hypertrophy. The knock down experiments of miR-199b with antagomir revealed the normalization of Dyrk1a expression, reduction in NFAT activity and restoration of cardiomyocytes from hypertrophy. It demonstrates that miR-199b destabilizes the coordination of Dyrk1a and calcineurin/NFAT which ultimately leads to cardiac hypertrophy and HF [164].

The level of thioredoxin tends to increase the level of miR-98 in cardiac hypertrophy. The expression level of Ang II increased in cardiac hypertrophy, fibrosis, and in cardiomyocyte apoptosis. The expression level of Ang II was significantly reduced by mirR-98 mimic and increased by miR-98 anatgomir *in vivo*. Further studies also demonstrated that the overexpression of miR-98 reduces the cardiac hypertrophy by targeting Cyclin D2. This shows a negative co relation of Ang II with miR-98 which can also be used a therapeutic agent. Thioredoxin (Trx1) is an anti-hypertrophic protein which inhibits, Ras, apoptosis signal regulating kinase 1 (ASK1), nuclear factor kappa-light-chain enhancer of activated B cells and (NF-kB). *In vivo* experiments showed that Trx1 is a positive regulator of miR-98. Endothelin and Isoproterenol are widely used as oxidative stress based stimulus for inducing cardiac hypertrophy in animal models. However, inadequate level of reactive oxygen species (ROS) also provoke signals for cardiac hypertrophy [165–168]. Recently, in rats cardiac hypertrophic models, miR-152, miR-212 and miR-132 were up-regulated while miR-142-3p was down-regulated [169]. miR-503 expression is high in ischemic endothelial cells of hind limb in diabetic mice [170]. Treatment of diabetic mice with a decoy miR-503 completely re-perfused the ischemic region by increasing angiogenesis.

Excessive angiogenesis is harmful especially in diabetes which leads to ratinopathy and cause blindness. miR-200b is down-regulated in ratina of diabetic mice and tends to increase its targets VEGF [171]. Injection of miR-200b mimic reduce the level of diabetic- induce- VEGF and angiogenesis. It shows that in diabetes (retinopathy), miR-200b mimic can be used as a good therapeutic agent. miR-195 which is a member of miR-15 family target cell cycle regulators thus play an important role in cardiomocyte cell survival at post natal stage. The knock down experiment of miR-195 showed increase mitotic division of cardiomyocyte in neonatal mice [172]. *In vivo* and *in vitro* study showed that miR-195 is highly expressed during cardiac hypertrophy [173]. *In vitro* over expression of miR-320 triggers apoptosis in cardiomyocytes while the knock down of miR-320 with antagomir rendered apoptosis and reduced the infarct size also *in vivo* [174].

miR-33 plays a major role in atherosclerosis in up taking of cholesterol and its synthesis. It targets ABCA1 gene which is responsible for transporting and shifting of cholesterol out of cell. *In vivo* the inhibition of miR-33 results in increased expression of ABCA1 [175]. miR-33 also targets HDL which can be used as a hall mark in coronary artery disease. The inhibition of miR-33 results in increase level of HDL, low level of VLDL and TG [27]. The up-regulation of miR-92a was attributed to be anti-angiogenic in ischemic disease. In murine model studies, miR-92a was down-regulated by antagomir injection and improved capillaries were developed with increasing blood flow in ischemic condition. The expression of miR-143/145 cluster remains high in Smooth muscle cells but the expression of this cluster is decreased during re-stenosis and chronic atherosclerosis. The knock down experiment showed defect in SMCs acquiring small capacity for vasoconstriction [176].

2.2 Prospective of miRNAs Utilization in Cardiac Valvular Heart Diseases

Cardiac aortic valve stenosis due to calcification is one of the leading cause of death in adults [177]. In developed countries it is also the most common form of cardiac valvular diseases [178]. Aortic valve calcification is found in 25% of 65 year old patients [179]. Among different risk factors, calcification in bicuspid aortic valve (BAV) is also one of the risk factor of cardiac valve dysfunction which is found in 1–2% of the population [178]. Fibrosa; facing the aorta, the ventarcularis; facing the left ventricle and spongiosa; the layer between the existing two layers are the three main layers of Aortic valve. There are two types of cells in aortic valve, the interstitial cell and endothelial cell which line the valve [180]. Calcified aortic valve tissue examination in human and their *in vitro* experiments using interstitial cells (AVICs) showed that morphogenetic protein-2 (BMP-2), NOTCH1 [181] and the SMADs (Mothers against decapentaplegic) [182] provoke calcification transpiring gene pathways.

2.2.1 miRNAs in Valvular Calcification

miRNAs play various roles in the pathogenesis regulation of valvular diseases. Nigam *et al* quantified miRNAs using microarray analysis that showed the expressions of miR-16, miR- 26a, miR-27a, miR-30b, miR-130, miR-195, and miR-497 were altered. These seven miRNAs were highly expressed in aortic stenosis (AS) compared with aortic insufficiency (AI) group. The miRNAs qPCR analysis revealed that miR-26a, miR-195 and miR-30b levels were down-regulated to 65%, 59% and 62% respectively in AS compared to AI. In this study of intonation of calcification related gene analysis showed that the miR-26a has potential to reduce the expression of alkaline phosphatase (ALPL) gene by 38%, BMP2 by 36% and SMAD by 26%. The miR-26a upregulate the expression of those genes which have a role in inhibition of calcification, JAG2 by 31% and SMAD7 by 15% but the expression of two genes was increased which are considered as pro-calcific RUNX2 by 16% and SMAD5 by 21%. The miR-30b reduced the expression of genes which regulates calcification pathways, SMAD1 by 18%, SMAD3 by 12%, BMP by 39%, NOTCH1 by 19% while the levels of JAG2 and SMAD7 were increased by 14% and 40%. miR-195 increased the expression of two genes which repress calcification, JAG2 and SMAD7 by 13% and 26% while it also activated calcification related gene, BMP2 by 68%, RUNX2 by 11%, SMAD1 by 9%, SMAD3 by 4% and SMAD5 by 17% [181].

Valve Interstitial cells (VIC) keep the integrity of the valve and acquire osteoblast phenotype during its dysfunction. VIC transformation by cell differentiation and apoptosis are the main culprit of cardiac aortic valve disease (CAVD). Experiments with MC3T3-E1 cells showed that mir30b family members act as a negative regulator of osteoblastic differentiation, targeting the master osteogenic transcription factors Smad1 and Runx2. miR-30b was dramatically reduced in cultured VICs obtained from aortic calcific patients. VICs were induced to osteoblast differentiation after transfection with miR-30b inhibitor and BMP2 triggered osteoblast differentiation was characterized by ALP (Alkaline Phasphatase) assay. In such analysis high ALP level was observed. The expression level of Osteocalcin was also high which can be used as a hallmark for mature osteoblasts. miR-30b decreases the calcification of VICs in part by inhibiting the apoptosis. In vitro experiments of 293 T cell transfected with luciferase receptor showed that miR-30b directly inhibited the Runx2, Smad1, and Caspase 3 which are downstream regulators of BMP-2 signaling during osteogenesis. In addition a negative relationship was identified of miR-204 with Runx2 in osteogenesis [183].

Vascular smooth muscle cells (SMC) acquire osteoblast like phenotype that promotes calcification of vessels [184]. In these vessels the smooth muscle cells markers are decreased such as myocardin, smooth muscle myocin heavy chain, and smooth muscle alpha actin and increases the expression of bone acquiring proteins like alkaline phasphatase, osteocalcin. Runx2 is considered as a master factor for calcification of vessels. Runx2 is up-regulated as a response to pro-calcification stimuli like inflammation, stress and bone morphogenetic protein (BMP) [185]. The factors which increase the risk for calcification of vascular smooth muscles were found by Joshua *et al* that BMP decreases the expression of miR-30b and miR-30c and promotes calcification of vascular smooth muscles cells. The smooth muscles cells were treated with increasing concentrations of BMP which tend to decrease smooth muscles cells marker and increase bone morphogenic markers. In SMC the Runx2 level was increased while anti calcification miR-30b and miR-30c levels were decreased. BMP activates smad signaling pathway by phosphorylation which tends to decrease miR-30b and miR-30c expression. Runx2 was high in the cells in the presence of BMP as compared with the absence of BMP while forced expression of miR-30b and miR-30c down-regulated Runx2. BMP is a member of TGF beta which decreases the expression of miR-133 and miR-206 tends to increase the expression of Runx2 in C2C12 cells [186]. In proteoblast MC3T3-E1 cells, BMP decreased the expression of miR-208 to regulate the expression of Ets-1 and osteogenic differentiation [187]. BMP plays a very critical role in osteogenic character by high expression of Runx2 and low expression of miR-3960, results in decrease expression of home box A2 which is a repressor of Runx2 [188].

2.2.2 miRNAs in Atrial Fibrillation with Valvular Stenosis

Atrial Fibrillation (AF) is one of the most prevalent arrhythmia in developed and under developing countries. AF increases the stroke and thromboembolic complications which lead to death and disability. Chronic AF also leads to the various abnormalities associated with the dilated atria of patients with valvular heart disease (VHD). Mitral valve stenosis due to rheumatic heart disease is also considered as major cardiovascular disease in developing countries [189]. Nicola cooley *et al* found miRNAs expression profile in VHD patients with and without chronic AF. VHD patients were classified AF on the basis of clinical assessment of 1 year and the patient who did not show AF over 1 year were considered *as* sinus rhythm (SR*). Coronary artery bypass grafting-* Right atrium (CABG RA) tissue obtain from patients with normal left ventricle function were used as a control. They compare the miRNAs expression profile between VHD RAA AF (Valvular Heart Disease Right Atrial Appendage Atrial Fibrilation) and VHD LAA SR (Sinus Rhythm) through miRNA microarrays experiment and observed a considerable change in 47 different miRNA expressions, among them 15 miRNAs showed high expression in AF group while 32 showed low expression compared with SR. The greatest difference was observed in miR-146b-5p which was 6.5 fold higher while low expressions of miR-133 and 30 family were also observed in VHD RA AF than VHD RA SR basis on array experiment given in Table 24.1.

In similar study total 53 different miRNAs were showing different expressions during the

Table 24.1 Comparison miRNAs expression between VHD RAA AF and VHD LAA SR

Up-regulated miRNAs		Down-regulated miRNAs			
miR-146b-5p	miR-1308	miR-490-3p	miR-29c*	miR-99a	miR-145
miR-142-3p	miR-224	miR-378*	miR-24-1*	miR-181c	miR-367
miR-21	miR-16	miR-133a	miR-197	miR-331-3p	miR-484
miR-1202	miR-377	miR-143*	miR-30c	miR-374b	hsa-let-7c
miR-142-5p	miR-337-5p	miR-22*	miR-139-5p	miR-628-5p	miR-490-5p
miR-21*	miR-1290	miR-378	miR-125b-2*	miR-128	miR-30b
miR-483-5p	miR-198	miR-133b	miR-30e	miR-181d	miR-149
miR-22		miR-30a*	miR-99b	miR-203	miR-30a

Table 24.2 Expression profile of miRNAs in VHD-LA and healthy LA

Up-regulated miRNAs	Down-regulated miRNAs			
miR-34b*	miR-886-3p	miR-371-5p	miR-605	miR-1237
miR-10b	miR-21*	miR-134	miR-563	miR-602
miR-454	miR-17	miR-490-3p	miR-20a	hiv1-miR-H1
miR-146a	miR-939	miR-940	miR-770-5p	let-7f-1*
miR-101	miR-663	miR-33b*	miR-125a-5p	let-7b*
miR-20a*	miR-193a-5p	miR-125a-3p	miR-132	
miR-199b-5p	miR-212	miR-320a	miR-149	
miR-301a	miR-197	miR-150	miR-487b	
miR-221	miR-202	miR-1234	miR-550	
miR-148b	miR-324-3p	miR-1224-5p	miR-1274a	
miR-23a	miR-191*	miR-425*	miR-423-5p	
miR-26b	miR-1238	miR-1225-3p	miR-1228	

comparison of Valvular Heart Disease Left Atrium (VHD-LA) and healthy LA, in which 12 miRNAs were upregulated and 41miRNAs were downregulated given in Table 24.2. In addition 4 miRNAs (miR-(146b-5p, miR-21, miR-376c, miR-376a) were expressed at high level and miR-490-3p was downregulated in VHD-RA than CABG-RA. Further, differences in expression profiles of miRNAs were also been observed comparing LA with RA of VHD in which 13 miRNAs were highly expressed in LA than RA and 26 miRNAs were downregulated (Table 24.3) [190].

Hiroyuki *et al* found miRNAs expression profile in human atrial tissue in atrial fibrillation among the patients who underwent cardiac surgery in 25 valvular and 4 CABG patients after 6 months of final clinical examination. The patients were divided in three classes. Group A included those 6 patients who had atrial fibrillation and chronic AF with and without maze procedure. Group B included those 10 patients who had postoperative SR and underwent successful maze procedure and Group C included those 13 patients that underwent aortic valve replacement or CABG (coronary artery bypass grafting). In this study 94 miRNAs were differently expressed as compared with SR group of patient who did not develop postoperative AF in which 94 miRNAs were up-regulated and 4 miRNAs were down-regulated in AF based on microarray analysis given in Table 24.4. The qPCR analysis showed a high expression of miR-21 and miR-208b, while it was also observed that miR-21 expression was high in patients with chronic AF of unsuccessful and reduced in those patients of successful maze procedure. The plasma level of miR-21 was also identified which showed decrease in its expression compared with normal. There was a positive relationship of miR-21 in AF and was gradually decreased in patients with successful maze procedure [191]. Yang *et al* studied miR-21 and its downstream target *Sprouty 1(spryl)* and also found a positive relation of miR-21 with AF in the tissue obtained from left atria. There were

Table 24.3 Comparison miRNAs expression profile between LA than RA of VHD

Up-regulated miRNAs		Down-regulated miRNAs			
miR-10b	miR-499-5p	miR-575	miR-513a-5p	miR-638	miR-324-3p
miR-1	miR-34b*	miR-663	miR-939	miR-765	miR-210
miR-145*	miR-133a	miR-100	miR-630	miR-202	miR-371-5p
miR-24-1*	miR-216a	miR-125a-3p	miR-1246	miR-1275	miR-574-5p
miR-133b	miR-23b	miR-483-5p	miR-134	miR-155	miR150*
miR-22*	miR-301a	miR-1225-5p	miR-1826	miR-1224-5p	
miR-95		miR-17	miR-671-5p	miR-320a	

Table 24.4 miRNAs expression in patients with AF compared to those with SR

Expression of miRNAs						
Up						Down
let-7a	miR-152	miR-210	miR-337-5p	miR-499-5p	miR-548d-5p	miR-429
let-7d	miR-15a	miR-21	miR-34a	miR-500	miR-579	miR-31
let-7f	miR-15b	miR-215	miR-361-5p	miR-504	miR-597	miR-200b
miR-101	miR-181a	miR-216a	miR-362-5p	miR-505	miR-618	miR-885-5p
miR-103	miR-181c	miR-216b	miR-371-3p	miR-508-3p	miR-652	
miR-106b	miR-184	miR-217	miR-372	miR-509-5p	miR-660	
miR-125b	miR-185	miR-22	miR-423-5p	miR-511	miR-671-3p	
miR-127-3p	miR-187	miR-23b	miR-424	miR-517a	miR-758	
miR-129-3p	miR-190	miR-24	miR-431	miR-517c	miR-874	
miR-130a	miR-193a-3p	miR-27a	miR-449a	miR-518b	miR-886-5p	
miR-130b	miR-196b	miR-27b	miR-450a	miR-518f	miR-887	
miR-134	miR-199a-5p	miR-28-5p	miR-455-5p	miR-520e	miR-888	
miR-140-5p	miR-199b-5p	miR-320	miR-487a	miR-522	miR-93	
miR-142-3p	miR-203	miR-32	miR-487b	miR-539	miR-95	
miR-146b	miR-208b	miR-324-5p	miR-494	miR-542-5p		
miR-148b	miR-20b	miR-330-3p	miR-495	miR-545		

also increased level of atrial collagen, reduced level of *spryl* and increased level of connective tissue growth factor (CTGF), lysyl oxidase and Rac1-GTPase which can trigger AF. Due to this conspicuous role miR-21 can also be used for regulation of AF. miR-328 over expression repressed IcaL which trigger AF in patients with rheumatic heart disease [115].

The miR-21 level was also reported high in response to cardiac injury which protects fibroblast from apoptosis and results in fibrosis. Due to its critical role Ana *et al* found high expression of circulatory miR-21 in left ventricular fibrosis in patients of aortic stenosis (AS). Its major targets are TGF beta effectors which play major role in LV remodeling in response to hemodynamic stress [192]. TGF beta acts as a promoter of excessive and abnormal deposition of ECM proteins. AS affect the expression of Collagen I, Collagen III, Fibronectin, TGF-β1, Smad2, Smad3, Smad4, TAK-1, PTEN, TIMP3, PCDC4, SPRY1 and RECK [193]. It was also found that miR-21 represses some myocardial mRNAs including sprouty homolog 1 (SPRY1) [104], phosphatase and tensin homolog (PTEN), [108] and programmed cell death 4 (PDCD4) [194]. Furthermore, extra-cardiac tissues [195] such as reversion-inducing-cysteine-rich protein with kazal motifs (RECK) and the tissue inhibitor of metalloproteinase 3 (TIMP3), contributes in ECM homeostasis are considered the valid targets of miR-21 [196]. It is also found that in ECM of AS, fibrotic genes collagen I, III and fibronacten were highly expressed. Different regression analysis revealed that the expression of miR-21, smad2, TAK1, RECK and MMP were positively related to collagen I while PTCD4 is a negative predictor of collagen I [193]. The circulatory miR- 21, myocardial smad2 and TEK had also a significantly positive relation with collagen. In vitro analysis showed that repression of PTCD4 enhances the expression level of TGF beta and trans differentiation of fibroblast in myofibroblast [197].

AF and mitral stenosis both found in patients who are relatively young. There is also the greater risk for stroke and embolism. AF is also caused by mitral valve stenosis [198]. MiRNAs expression profile in nine patients having AF with mitral stenosis and four had only mitral stenosis using array analysis in which 136 miRNAs were differently expressed, 50 miRNAs were up-regulated and 86 miRNAs were down-regulated given in Table 24.5. In AF having mitral stenosis, 96 were differently expressed, 47 miRNAs were up-regulated and 49 miRNAs, were down-regulated (Table 24.6).

The pathway analysis showed that high expression of miR-212, miR-335 and miR-630 triggers TGF- signaling pathway, actin cytoskeleton and MAPK. These signaling pathways may trigger generation of AF in mitral stenosis patients. miR-212 targets: KCNK2, PAIP2, miR-335 targets: FMR1 while miR-630 targets: MYPN, LRP6, CDH2, FKBP1B and TGF were assessed. However, down regulation of miR-874, -miR-181, miR-550, miR-500, miR 149, miR-181a, miR-181c, miR-125a- 5p, miR-497 and miR-125b might also provoke MAPK signaling pathway, the TGF- signaling pathway, the regulation of the actin cytoskeleton, oxidative phosphorylation, gap junctions, and the VEGF signaling pathway in development of AF in mitral stenosis. In more detail the down-regulated miRNAs and their putative targets are given in Table 24.7.

Hai *et al* found that miRNAs expressions were altered due to AF in RA of mitral stenosis patients. They analyzed miRNAs in LAA tissue

Table 24.5 Regulation of miRNAs in AF patient compared with control

Up-regulated miRNAs		Down-regulated miRNAs			
miR-320c	miR-1915	miR-326	miR-98	miR-26b	miR-139-3p
miR-638	miR-664*	miR-143	miR-744	miR-340	miR-502-3p
miR-605	miR-483-5p	miR-484	miR-500	miR-128	miR-628-3p
miR-933	miR-134	miR-139-5p	miR-149	miR-377	miR-590-5p
miR-33b*	miR-1471	miR-9	miR-769-5p	miR-190	miR-450a
miR-550	let-7i	miR-29c*	miR-101	miR-340*	miR-452
miR-155	miR-135a*	miR-650	miR-30e*	miR-628-5p	miR-361-3p
miR-563	miR-601	miR-1305	miR-181a*	miR-99a	miR-186
miR-188-5p	miR-103	miR-362-3p	miR-19a	miR-19b	miR-486-3p
miR-505*	miR-345	miR-145	let-7e*	miR-143*	let-7a*
miR-1228	miR-1207-5p	miR-301a	miR-23b*	miR-26b*	let-7i*
miR-765	miR-1275	miR-337-3p	miR-542-5p	miR-193a-5p	
miR-1226*	miR-1224-5p	miR-338-5p	miR-10a	miR-125b-2*	
miR-342-3p	miR-923	miR-99a*	miR-17*	miR-598	
miR-370	miR-63	miR-22*	miR-9*	miR-29b	
miR-371-5p	miR-939	miR-193a-3p	miR-145*	miR-532-5p	
miR-572	miR-513b	miR-365	miR-424	miR-29c	
miR-575	miR-1202	miR-26a	miR-32	miR-7-1*	
miR-1225-5p	miR-1308	miR-215	338-3p	miR-208a	
miR-574-5p	miR-149*	miR-324-3p	miR-133b	miR-125a-5p	

(continued)

Table 24.5 (continued)

Up-regulated miRNAs		Down-regulated miRNAs			
miR-602	miR-30d	miR-455-5p	miR-133a	miR-374a	
miR-513a-5p	miR-18b*	miR-374b	miR-582-5p	miR-423-5p	
miR-1249	miR-1268	miR-33a	miR-1271	miR-181d	
miR-1181	miR-671-5p	miR-29a*,	miR-660	miR-501-5p	
miR-223	let-7b	miR-136*	miR-20a*	miR-126*	

Table 24.6 Regulation of miRNAs in MS patients compared with healthy individuals

Up-regulated miRNAs			Down-regulated miRNAs		
miR-320c	miR-602	miR-630	miR-326	miR-10a	miR-18a
miR-933	miR-513a-5p	let-7b*	miR-29a	miR-let-7a*	miR-29b
miR-33b*	miR-223	miR-574-3p	miR-650	miR-17*	miR-29c
miR-181b	miR-1915	miR-1183	miR-1305	miR-9*	miR-7-1*
miR-1539	miR-181a	miR-324-5p	miR-362-3p	miR-212	miR-208a
miR-550,	miR-664*	miR-513b	miR-1914*	miR-424	miR-374a
miR-155	miR-191*	miR-1308	miR-337-3p	miR-32	miR-335*
miR-563	miR-1471	miR-149*	miR-22*	338-3p	miR-423-5p
miR-505*	let-7i	miR-497	miR-193a-3p	miR-582-5p	miR-126*
miR-494	miR-92b	miR-425*	miR-18b	miR-660	miR-628-3p
miR-765	miR-218	miR-30d	miR-215	miR-20a*	miR-590-5p
miR-130b	miR-135a*	671-5p	miR-324-3p	miR-892b	miR-452
miR-342-3p	miR-103	let-7b	miR-455-5p	miR-340	miR-186
miR-370	miR-1238		miR-136*	miR-377	miR-486-3p
miR-371-5p	miR-1275		miR-744	miR-190	let-7i*
miR-1234	miR-1224-5p		miR-101	miR-19b	
miR-574-5p	miR-923		miR-19a	miR-335	

characterized by mitral stenosis with AF and compared with Normal SR patients. In total 22 miRNAs were dysregulated in which 10 miRNAs including miR-3613-3p, miR-3196, miR-3178, miR-466, miR-574-3p, miR-4492, miR-4707-5p, miR-15b-5p, miR-21-5p, miR-4497 were up-regulated and 12 miRNAs miR-26a-5p, miR-1, miR-195-5p, miR-26b-5p, miR-5100, miR-29a-3p, miR-24-3p, miR-361-5p, miR-151a-5p, miR-4454, miR-720, let-7 g-5p were down-regulated [199].

GO term and KEGG pathway analysis showed that potential targeted genes are associated with important biological actions that regulate transcription factor activity, protein metabolism, cell division transforming growth factor beta receptor signaling pathways. These pathways play major roles in disease progression in which miRNAs play a regulatory role at transcription level. In this study, it has been reported that mir-466, miR-574 and miR-3613 are also potentially involved in cardiovascular pathology targeting some important wnt, mTOR and Notch signaling pathways. Yang *et al* found that over expression of miR-1 play a critical role in arrhythmogenic potential by depolarizing the cytoplasmic membrane and post transcription repression of KCNJ2 (potassium inwardly-rectifying channel, subfamily J) which encode Kir2.1 (potassium ions channel subunit) and GJAI (gap junction protein alpha 1 which encodes connexin 43 [119]. miR-1 is down-regulated in some AF cases which leads to up regulation of its target gene Kir2.1 and tend to increase cardiac inward rectifier potassium current I k1 [200].

Alteration in miRNAs expression mostly implicated oncogene expression [201] and cause various types of diseases including CVD and also valvular dysfunction. Sadakatsu *et al* found

Table 24.7 Down-regulation of miRNAs in MS with AF compared with MS without AF with their putative targets

miRNAs	Targets
miR-497	CASR, FGFR1, MINK1, SCN8A, SMAD7
miR-125b	ELOVL6, ENPEP
miR-874	CACNA1E, ESR1, FMR1, ITPR2, RGS4, TFAP2B
miR-181b	CACNA2D2, GRIA2, MINK1, PIAS3
miR-550	CUGBP1, SOX5, TPM1, ATP2B3
miR-500	PDE3A, ITPR2, GRIA3
miR-149	GIT1, RAP1A
miR-181a	ATP1B1, GRIA2, MINK1, SMAD7
miR-181c	ATP1B1, GRIA2, MINK1, PIAS3, SMAD7
miR-125a-5p	BCL2, CACNB1, CACNB3, E2F2, E2F3, ENPEP, HCN4, KCNA1, KCNH4, MAPK14,MAPKAPK2, SCN2B, SCN4B, STAT3
miR-181d	ANK1, GRIA2, KCNMA1, PIAS3, SMAD7
miR-324-5p	NIPBL

Table 24.8 Regulation of miRNAs in patients with DCM

Up-regulated miRNAs			Down-regulated miRNAs		
let-7a	miR-30c	miR-150	let-7f	miR-30a-3p	miR-222
let-7b	miR-30d	miR-151*	let-7 g	miR-30a-5p	miR-335
let-7c	miR-93	miR-152	miR-1	miR-30b	miR-374
let-7d	miR-99a	miR-181a	miR-10a	miR-30e-3p	miR-422b
let-7d*	miR-99b	miR-185	miR-15a	miR-30e-5p	miR-424
let-7e	miR-100	miR-191	miR-16	miR-92	miR-483*
miR-10b	miR-103	miR-195	miR-17-5p	miR-98	miR-495
miR-15b	miR-107	miR-199a*	miR-19a	miR-101	miR-499
miR-22	miR-125a	miR-214	miR-19b	miR-106a	
miR-23a	miR-125b	miR-320	miR-20a	miR-106b	
miR-23b	miR-130a	miR-342	miR-20b	miR-126	
miR-24	miR-133a	miR-361	miR-21	miR-126*	
miR-26a	miR-133b	miR-365	miR-26b	miR-146a	
miR-27a	miR-140*	miR-423*	miR-28	miR-146b	
miR-27b	miR-143	miR-451	miR-29b	miR-191*	
miR-29a	miR-145		miR-29c	miR-208	

altered expression profile of 428 miRNAs from 67 patients including aortic stenosis, AS, ischemic cardiomyopathy, IC and dilated cardiomyopathy (DCM). In the Griffith's study of miRNAs expression [202] miR-1, miR-133 and miR-208 have great impact as regulators of heart and myocyte development and differentiation [121]. In the disease condition of DCM, 47 miRNAs were up-regulated and 40 miRNAs were down-regulated given in Table 24.8. In the disease condition with ICM, 52 miRNAs were up-regulated while 35 miRNAs were down-regulated given in Table 24.9. Human patients characterized with disease condition AS, 43 miRNAs were up-regulated while 44 miRNAs were down-regulated (Table 24.10) [203].

miR-1 expression was down-regulated in ICM but Yang *et al* reported a high expression of miR-1 in ICM while the expression of miR-133 was also not significantly reduced comparing with hypertrophic cardiomyopathy and dilated atrial myocardium reported by care *et al* [118]. This difference in miRNA expression might be due to difference in tissue samples, while miR-214 was highly up-regulated to 2 to 2.8 folds in all three respective diseases which show its contribution to cardiac hypertrophy. The miR-19 and miR-19a were mostly down-regulated in DCM and AS but not in ICM which thought to be the reason of the up regulation of such genes that can prompt a pathway lead to DCM and AS.

The up and down regulation of shear and side specific miRNAs in valvular endothelial cells (ECs) play a major role in its dysfunction in respond to shear stress which leads to alternation in gene expression profile both in vivo and in vitro [34]. In aortic disease ventricularis ECs receive

Table 24.9 miRNAs expression in patients with ICM

Up-regulated miRNAs			Down-regulated miRNAs	
let-7a	miR-27b	miR-151*	let-7f	miR-98
let-7b	miR-29a	miR-152	let-7g	miR-101
let-7c	miR-29b	miR-181a	miR-1	miR-106a
let-7d	miR-30d	miR-191	miR-17-5p	miR-126
let-7d*	miR-93	miR-195	miR-19a	miR-126*
let-7e	miR-99a	miR-199a*	miR-19b	miR-133a
miR-10a	miR-99b	miR-208	miR-20a	miR-133b
miR-10b	miR-100	miR-214	miR-20b	miR-146a
miR-15a	miR-103	miR-320	miR-26b	miR-146b
miR-15b	miR-106b	miR-342	miR-28	miR-185
miR-16	miR-107	miR-361	miR-29	miR-191*
miR-21	miR-125a	miR-365	miR-30a-3p	miR-222
miR-22	miR-125b	miR-423*	miR-30a-5p	miR-335
miR-23a	miR-130a	miR-424	miR-30b	miR-374
miR-23b	miR-140*	miR-451	miR-30c	miR-422b
miR-24	miR-143	miR-483*	miR-30e-3p	miR-495
miR-26a	miR-145		miR-30e-5p	miR-499
miR-27a	miR-150		miR-92	

Table 24.10 miRNAs expression profile in patients with AS

Up-regulated miRNAs			Down-regulated miRNAs		
let-7a	miR-93	miR-150	let-7d*,	miR-28	miR-146a
let-7b	miR-99a	miR-151*	let-7f	miR-29a	miR-146b
let-7c	miR-99b	miR-181a	let-7g	miR-29b	miR-152
let-7d	miR-100	miR-191	miR -1	miR-29c	miR-185
let-7e	miR-103	miR-195	miR-10a	miR-30a-3p	miR-191*
miR-15b	miR-106b	miR-199a*	miR-10b	miR-30a-5p	miR-208
miR-22	miR-107	miR-214	miR-15a	miR-30b	miR-222
miR-23a	miR-125a	miR-320	miR-16	miR-30e-3p	miR-335
miR-23b	miR-125b	miR-342	miR-17-5p	miR-30e-5p	miR-374
miR-24	miR-130a	miR-361	miR-19a	miR-92	miR-422b
miR-26a	miR-133a	miR-365	miR-19b	miR-98	miR-424
miR-27a	miR-133b	miR-423*	miR-20a	miR-101	miR-514
miR-27b	miR-140*	miR-483*	miR-20b	miR-106a	miR-495
miR-30c	miR-143		miR-21	miR-126	miR-499
miR-30d	miR-145		miR-26b	miR-126*	

pulsatile and uni-directional blood flow while in fibrosa ECs faces disturbed low and oscillatory blood. Recently some miRNAs like miR-23b and miR-19a were found to regulate cell growth and cyclin D1 expression be a shear response in umbilical vein ECs (HUVAECs). Microarray analysis showed the up and down expression profile of shear and side specific miRNAs in human aortic valve endothelial cells (HAVEC) by exposing non calcified fHAVECs, from fibrosa of endothelial cells and ventricularis endothelium vHAVECs. The Parallel plate flow chamber was used to expose HAVECs to steady laminar shear (LS). However, cone and plate viscometer can also be used to adopt the strategy [204] for oscillatory shear (OS). Basis on the shear strategy of HAVECs for 24 h either LS or OS were divided into four groups. In group a and b the fHAVECs were exposed to OS (FO) and LS (FL) however, in group c and d the vHAVECs were exposed to OS (VO) and LS (VL). The miRNAs expression in these groups is given in Table 24.11.

In this study the miRNAs which have inverse relation with their targets has also been identified. Two potential targets were identified for miR-139-3p, 16 potential targets for miR-187, 22 potential targets for miR-192, and 8 potential targets for miR-486-5p are given in Table 24.12 [205].

Table 24.11 Expression of miRNAs in shear strategy of HAVECs

FO versus VL		VO versus VL		FO versus FL		FL versus VL	
Up	Down	Up	Down	Up	Down	Up	Down
miR-74a	miR-486-5p	miR-21	miR-1290	miR-769-3p	miR-486-5p	miR-370	miR-485-3p
miR-187	miR-483-3p	miR-187	miR-486-5p	miR-187	miR-923		miR-485-5p
miR-217	miR-1244		miR-518e		miR-1244		
	miR-139-3p		miR-5480		miR-486-3p		
	miR- 486-3p		miR-654-3p				
	miR- 382		miR-486-3p				
	miR-923		miR-411				
	miR-543		miR-1244				
	miR-1237		miR-1300				
	miR-433		miR-647				
	miR- 485-3p		miR-192				
	miR-549		miR-923				
	miR-485-5p		miR-139-3p				

Table 24.12 miRNAs and their putative targets in shear strategy of HAVECs

miR-139-3p	fosB, Rnf41
miR-187	Cd276, Armc7, Cyyr1, Ets1, Dync1li2, Flnc, Lypd1, Ifnar1, Nfkbiz, Mbnl2, Pgm2l1, Sema3f, Snx27, Ssh2, Plod3, Trib2
miR-192	Acp1, Apln, Asb1, Atf3, C10orf10, Ccnd2, Chrnb1, Ctnnbip1, Dynlt1, Egr1, Fam129a, FosB, Hoxb5, Mcm6, Myo1d,Nav1, Ndst1, Nmt2, Nrip3, Osbpl10, Phactr2, Phlda1
miR-486-5p	Ak2, Als2cr4, Camk2n1, Ctdspl, Efna1, Mylk2, Prnd, Rnf41

2.3 miRNAs Expression in Ischemic Heart Disease (IHD)/Myocardial Infarction (MI)

Cardiovascular diseases including IHD are the leading cause of death. Inflammation is the secondary pathological effect occurs during IRI in acute myocardial infarction (AMI) of occluded coronary artery [206].

In rat AMI model the over expression of miR-214 improves hemodynamic, left ventricular function, and LV remodeling. The enhanced expression of miR-214 also showed repression in cardiomyocytes apoptosis through suppressing the Phosphatase and Tensin Homolog (PTEN) [207]. The IRI was more severe in knockdown experiment in mice with increase cardimyocytes apoptosis and increase cardiac fibrosis. miR-214 target sodium–calcium exchanger-1 which also influences calcium transport. In addition miR-214 also participates in angiogenesis which play a vital role in cardiac function [208].

In humans and animal model exercise training (ET) therapeutic strategy is used to treat different cardiovascular diseases. In human, the ET strategy produces beneficial effects on left ventricle remodeling including ejection fraction after MI [209]. In animals models, ET reduces collagen content, restored intracellular Ca^{+2} handling, and contraction of cardiomyocytes [210]. In addition, ET also modulates miRNAs which are in association with left ventricle remodeling. The sodium/calcium exchanger 1 (NCX), and sarcoplasmic reticulum calcium ATPase-2a (Serca2a), are the key regulators of cardiac function. However, miR-1 and miR-214 have the potential to target NCX and Serca2a respectively. In addition, highlighting the therapeutic values of miRNAs ET procedure can be used to normalize the expression of miR-1 and miR-214 [210]. Increase level of miR-21 expression was observed in the infarct region. The miR-21 can lead the suppression of phosphatase and tensin homolog which can also leads to the expression of fibroblast matrix metalloproteinase-2, activated fibroblast survival, and triggered fibrotic infarct remodeling. The administration of anti-miR-21 indicated beneficial results in MI rats model [211]. However, therapeutic inhibition of miR-21 showed reduction in atrial fibrosis (AF) and sustained heart function. The validation of fibroblast- specific pro survival action revealed that elevated level tends to increase fibroblast proliferation. Therapeutically, anti-miR-21 experiment showed reduction in fibroblast proliferation. This antagomeric intervention open an avenue to use anti miR-21 treatment strategy to reduce cardiac fibrosis as well as fibrosis in lungs, kidneys, and skeleton muscles [212]. The deterioration of heart function can be increased by cardiac fibrosis which may occur after MI. miR-21 has a major role in cardiac fibrosis. The miR-21 expression was increased in infarcted zone of heart in MI mice model. However, the miR-21 expression was increased in cardiac fibroblasts by TGF-β1 treatment through involving the upregulation of Col-1, α-SMA and F-actin. The treatment of anti-miR- 21 showed attenuation in cardiac fibrosis while miR-21 mimic showed an increase in fibrotic characteristics. Bioinformatics and luciferase assays showed that miR-21 directly targets Smad7 and miR-21 promotes fibroblasts activation via TGF-β/Smad7 signaling pathway [213]. *In vivo* study showed that miR-21 was significantly reduced after 6 h of AMI in infarct area however, their expression was high in boarder zone of infarction. In AMI animal model the adenovirus over expression of miR-21 reduced infarct size by 29% at 24 h with reduced cell apoptosis. In addition, decrease in dimension of left ventricles at 2 weeks after AMI was also observed. The protective effect of miR-21 was further evaluated by cardiomyocytes apoptosis induced by ischemia. miR-21 protects cardiomyocytes cell loss by targeting apoptotic target gene programmed cell death 4 (PDCD4) and activator protein 1 (AP1) pathway. It shows that therapeutically upregulation of miR-21 can be used to reduce the cardiomyocytes apoptosis and enhance cardiac function in the early phase of AMI [194]. miR-21 produces an anti-apoptotic effect by down-regulating FasL and activation of AKT through inhibition of PTEN [214]. However, inhibition of miR-21 decreases the expression level of p38 MAPK in A-498 cells. The cardioprotective effect of miR-21was enhanced when combined with miR146a. miR-146a also protects the cardiomyocytes against myocardial I/R injury by attenuating the nuclear factor κB (NF-κB) interleukin-1 receptor-associated kinase1 (IRAK1) and tumor necrosis factor (TNF) receptor-associated factor 6 (TRAF6). miR-146a together with IRAK1, TRAF6 and p-p38 constitutes a negative feed forward loop that attenuates cytokine protein synthesis in human THP-1 monocytes [215]. Previous study showed that PDCD4, PTEN, sprouty 1 (SPRY1), and SPRY2 are the valid targets of miR-21 while TRAF6 and IRAK1 are the potential targets of miR-146a. miR-21 inhibits cardiomyocytes apoptosis via PTEN/AKT–p-p38–caspase-3 and miR-146a attenuate cardiomyocytes apoptosis via TRAF6–p-p38–caspase-3 signal pathways. The combined effect of both the miRNAs (miR-21 and miR-146a) in a single mice model increases the cytoprotective therapeutic efficacy [216].

High expression level of miR-15 is associated with MI. In recent report of murine and porcine MI model, miR-15 expression was high in infarct zone [217]. However, cardiomyocytes cellular stress was decreased after endogenous silencing strategy of miR-15. In addition, the translation approach using locked-nucleic-acid–based miR therapy also showed attenuation in miR-15 expression. The role of miR-15 got more interest from researchers as it actively participating in mitochondrial function and cardiomyocyte apoptosis by targeting downstream mediators Pdk4 and Sgk1 [218].

Myocardial infarction is characterized by insufficient myocardial capillary density. This event can lead to HF and even death although the exact mechanism of angiogenesis is not well understood. Therapeutically, the overexpression of miR-24 can used to heal cardiac cells by inhibiting fibrosis via repression of fibroblast marker genes Col1a2, Col3, fibronectin, and α SMA. *In vivo* analysis of intramyocardial injection of lentiviruses showed that, miR-24 improved heart function and reduction in fibrosis was observed after

MI. Furthermore, *in vitro* experiments proved that overexpression of miR-24 reduce fibrosis. However, miR-24 also reduced differentiation and migration of cardiac fibroblasts. Further studies showed that TGF-b secretion and Smad2/3 phosphorylation in CFs were reduced during overexpression of miR-24. Cardiac fibrosis can also be activated by proteases, furin which further activates TGF-b. Bioinformatics studies revealed that furin is the valid target of miR-24 in fibrosis. It shows that miR-24 attenuates cardiac fibrosis by targeting furin–TGF-b pathway. Therapeutically, increased expression of miR-24 can be used to reduce the cardiac fibrosis after MI. The lentivirus delivery approach of miR-24 showed decrease in cardiomyocytes apoptosis by inhibiting proapoptotic pathways [219]. On the contrary, the expression level of miR-24 was increased in hypoxia and cardiac ischemia in mice ECs [220]. However, *in vitro* expression of miR-24 highlights its role as a pro-apoptotic factor in ECs by inhibiting endothelial capillary network formation on Matrigel. Luciferase assays confirmed that endothelium-enriched transcription factor GATA2 and p21-activated kinase PAK4 are the valid targets of miR-24 which have a wide role in cardiac angiogenesis. *In vitro* expression of miR-24 showed anti-angiogenic features in developing vasculature of zebrafish. However, in mouse MI model, therapeutic antagonism of miR-24 showed improvement in ischemic remodeling by cardiac EC survival. These findings showed that miR-24 has versatile characteristics on fibroblast, cardiomyocytes and endothelial cell biology within heart [220]. The cardiomyocytes loss through necrosis and apoptosis are the characteristics of AMI. The highly demanding strategy of miRNAs to salvage ischemic cardiomyocytes has a great importance to modulate gene expression towards cell survival. A wide number of different miRNAs are involved in regulation of apoptosis. miR-24 has a cardioprotective effect and plays a critical role in AMI. After MI, the ischemic border zone of the murine left ventricle showed down-regulation of miR-24. This miRNA also suppresses cardiomyocyte apoptosis by targeting BH3-only domain–containing protein Bim. Luciferase assay showed that miR-24 directly binds to Bim. However, *in vivo* overexpression of miR-24 attenuated apoptosis, reduced infarct size, and enhanced cardiac function. Therefore manipulating miR-24 level can be used as a therapy to overcome various cardiac diseases including MI [219].

miR-29 consist of three family members a, b and c. Microarray-based analysis showed that miR-29 is highly expressed in MI [145]. miR-29 is abundantly found in fibroblasts which is also playing a critical role in fibrotic ECM appearance. *In vitro* and *in vivo* experiments proved that miR-29 inhibits the expression of collagens in MI. The profibrotic properties of miR-29 with reduced collagen providing a clue for their therapeutic potential. Some other studies also confirmed that miR-29 has a direct effect on collagen expression [221]. The pharmacological effect of miR-29 was well understood by their down-regulation with reduced apoptotic rate of cardiomyocyte. The potential target of miR-29 is Mcl-1 which is an anti-apoptotic protein of Bcl-2 family. Mcl-1 acts as a regulatory subunit of p85a, phosphoinositide 3-kinase and cell division cycle [222]. The family members of miR-29 (a,b,c) positively regulates cardiomyocytes apoptosis. The inhibition of miR-29 successfully increases the level of Mcl-1 and significantly reduces the levels of apoptosis and infarct size area after I/R [223].

Endothelial miR- 92 is found within miR-17 to miR- 92 locus and has a wide role in ischemia [147]. The altered miR-92a was found in Hind limb ischemia or MI with ECs triggering angiogenic defects. The systemic administration of miR-92a antagonist showed inhibition in anti-angiogenic activities in ECs. The potential target of miR92a is Sirt1, a class III histone deacetylase and longevity gene. However, various studies shows that miR-92a is related with strong anti-angiogenic characteristics [223, 224]. On the basis of these notions, therapeutically antimiR-92a strategy can be used to increase neovascularization especially after ischemic injury.

miR-101 has two distinct isoforms including a and b. miR-101 was down-regulated in cardiac fibrosis after MI in rats. A decrease in miR-101 expression was observed in peri infarct zone. miR-101a might control the expression of collagen in cardiac fibrosis however, therapeutically the adenoviral mediated delivery of miR-101a showed beneficial effect on heart with reduce fibrotic scare [218].

Endothelial miR-126 plays a vital role for endothelial function and integrity after MI [150]. In a knock down experiment, endothelial miR-126 showed loss in neovascularization after MI due to reduce activities in angiogenic signaling and prominent chemokines vascular endothelial growth. However, the angiogenic capacity and sustained endothelial integrity were enhanced by over expression of miR-126. Importantly, endothelial miR-126 is one of the outstanding candidate among different miRNAs which can be used for neovascularization in MI [218]. The pro-angiogenic action of miR-126 showed inhibition of Sprouty-related protein-1, which acts as an intracellular inhibitor of angiogenic signaling [152] and vascular cell adhesion molecule 1 [225]. Its plasma circulatory expression level was reduced in patients with AMI. It revealed that miR-126 can also be used as a biomarker for diagnostic purposes in different cardiovascular diseases including AMI [226].

The rat's MI Model showed a high expression of miR-208a. MI was also accomplished with development of left ventricular dysfunction and fibrosis. Endoglin is an auxiliary transforming growth factor-b (TGFb) receptor that modulates TGF-b1 and TGF-b3 responses and plays critical role in vascular repair function [227]. However, it has also pro-fibrotic effects. It was proposed that miR-208a has extensive complementarity in the promoter region of endoglin. However, luciferase assay showed that miR-208a can directly modulates the expression of endoglin protein. The knock down expression of 208a abolished the stimulatory effect on the promoter region of endoglin. It shows that miR-208a enhanced the expression of endoglin during acute MI. In addition, the anti-miR-208a strategy to down regulate the expression of endoglin protein can be used as a therapeutic strategy [228]. The circulatory miR-208b was also quantified in Greek patients of AMI which support the use of this miRNA as a therapeutic marker in AMI. miR-208b is encoded by an intron of the alpha-myosin heavy chain gene (*MYH7*). During cardiac development it also regulates the production of the myosin heavy chain in cardiomyocytes [229, 230].

Plasma levels of miR-208 and miR-499 are highly increased in MI patients. There are two subunits of miR-208 including miR-208a and miR-208b. In addition increase concentrations of creatine kinase and cardiac troponin T (cTnT) were also identified. Cardiac cells release a detectable concentration of miRNAs and slightly detectable concentration of cTnT in plasma in patients with 1 h after onset of chest pain. However, patients showed highest plasma concentration of miR-208b and miR-499 and cardiac troponin T hs-cTnT within 3 h after onset of pain. However, miRNA-208a remains significantly elevated for 5 days, and even 90 days after AMI [231]. The proposed reason for this phenomena might be that miRNAs are bound to protein complex and predominantly present in cytosol while cardiac troponins mainly bound to myofibrils and a small part is found in cytosol [232]. Circulating miRNAs can be used as a rapid and powerful diagnostic markers in acute MI. Clinical data and presentation showed that initial diagnostic tools including echocardiography is nonspecific in patients with chest pain. Therefore, circulatory miRNAs can be considered good markers. The levels of miR-208b was found high up to 30 days of death in patients died with MI. Further study is required regarding diagnostic marker usage of of hs-cTnT because its concentration is also increased in apparently healthy patients with chronic stable coronary artery disease [233]. In addition to diagnostic marker the reduced expression levels of miR-208b and miR-499 with antagonist increase attention for further studies in MI.

The aberrant expression profiles of miRNAs are associated with a variety of cardiovascular diseases including cardiac hypertrophy, HF, arrhythmias and AMI [234]. The damage of cardiac tissue releases miRNAs in to circulation which also makes them suitable as biomarkers [235]. However, different cardiac cell's specific miRNAs in the blood were found modified upon initiation and remodeling of AMI. These miRNAs can also be used as a hall mark for evaluation of AMI. In addition, circulatory miR-499 was found highly expressed in patients of AMI. miR-499 is encoded by myosin and expressed in myocardium and skeletal muscle. It is specifically encoded by an intron of the Myh7b, a ventricular-specific myosin heavy chain gene [236]. It regulates the expression of the β-MHC and enhanced myocardial oxygen metabolism and tolerance [237]. In another study, miR-499 was observed in patients of AMI. The miR-499 concentration was increased within 24 h from the onset of symptoms and return back to the baseline after 7 days [238]. Plasma levels of miRNA-499 were already detectable in AMI patients after onset of 1 h of the chest pain while its levels is gradually raised within 9 h [239].

Mitochondrial fission is an important event involved in apoptosis. The knock down experiment of miR-499 showed increase in infarct size with decrease of cardiac function and increase cardiac hypertrophy in mouse model. The miR-499 inhibits cardiomyocyte apoptosis by targeting calcineurin-mediated activation of Drp1. *In vivo*, the knockdown experiment of p53 showed attenuation in the reduction of miR-499 which shows that miR-299 might also be regulated by p53 [240]. In addition, miRNA-499 also plays a key role in structural and functional differentiation of cardiac stem cells (CSCs) into cardiomyocytes [241]. Therefore, it shows that the use of miR-499 mimic therapy can be used for the recovery of cardiomyocytes after injury.

Recent advanced investigation in MI therapies has significantly reduced the rate of mortality but still is the major cause of death. MI also occurs as a result of chronic congestive HF and ventricle remodeling plaques. However a wide range of miRNAs are involved in MI including miR-93. The miR-93 plays a major role in cardiomyocyte survival via inhibiting apoptosis. miR-93 also enhances protection from ischemia by increasing angiogenesis and antioxidant effects against MI. In mice models, the knock down experiment of miR-93 showed deterioration in cardiac remodeling. It shows that therapeutically miR-93 can be used to reduce the rate of MI as a cardio-protective strategy [242].

AMI is characterized by insufficient myocardial capillary density which can leads to cardiac remodeling and HF. miRNAs play critical role in MI at transcription and translation levels. Recently, various drugs have been used which can activate the level of cardio-protective effect during transition of cardiac cells. Cardiac endothelial cell (CEC) cultured analysis revealed that miR-532 is elevated after treatment with β-arrestin-based β-adrenergic receptor antagonist (β-blocker) 'carvedilol'. This phenomenon ultimately triggers cardio-protective pathways independent of G protein-mediated second messenger signaling. The knockdown study of miR-532-5p further highlight their cardio-protective effect by increased transition to a fibroblast-like phenotype via endothelial-to-mesenchymal transition (EndMT). However, over expression of miR-532 reduced the EndMT. The inhibitory study of miR-532 in mice revealed abnormalities in function and structure of heart, reduced vascularization and reduced CEC proliferation after MI. The cardio-protective study of miR-532 was further supported by reduced expression of prss23 (a protease serine 23) which is a positive regulator of maladaptive EndMT, in CECs [243].

miR-98 is down-regulated in infarcted and ischemic myocardium of MI mice. In addition, miR-98 was also down-regulated in neonatal rat ventricular myocytes (NRVCs) after treatment with H_2O_2. The overexpression of miR-98 is cardio-protective by remarkable increase in cell viability and also inhibits H_2O_2 mediated apoptosis of NRVCs. Moreover, miR-98 overexpression also down-regulate H_2O_2-induced Bcl-2, Bax and JC-1 monomeric cells. Further, miR-98 down-regulate Fas and caspase-3 in H_2O_2-treated cardiomyocytes both at transcription and translation levels. The dual luciferase assay proved that miR-98 directly target Fas 3′-UTR which confirmed its target validation for advance studies as a candidate for therapeutic intervention in MI. The serum levels of LDH, apoptotic cells, Fas, caspase-3 activities were significantly reduced after injection of miR-98 mimic in MI mice. However, the infarct size was also reduced with improved heart function. It shows that miR-98 is an anti-apoptotic factor which reduces the activity of Fas/Caspase-3 apoptotic signal pathway [244].

miR-17-5p is interlinked with cardiac function after MI by suppressing neovascularization.

In vitro and *in vivo* analysis proved that low expression level of miR-17-5p tends to activate the ERK pathway. However, the expression of ERK was increased both at transcription and translation levels. In addition, the expression level of anti-apoptotic protein (bcl-2) was increased. However, the expression levels of bax/caspase 3/caspase 9 were decreased. The anti-miR-17-5p administration in mice showed decrease in infarct size and collagen fibers, the rate of apoptosis was also inhibited and enhancement in endothelial growth was observed. It shows that therapeutically anti-miR-17-5p can be used to restore heart function after MI by inhibiting apoptosis and repairing vascular injury [244]. The activation of promoter of miR-144/451 has been identified and regulated by a transcription factor GATA-4 [245]. miR-144 and miR-451 promote cardiomyocytes survival which is further proved by their overexpression analysis. However, the knock down experiment of miR-144 and miR-451 showed opposite effect on cardiac cells. The luciferase reporter assay revealed that both miR-144 and miR451 target ubiquitously expressed RNA-binding protein called CUG triplet repeat-binding protein 2 (CUGBP2) which further interact with COX-2, 3'untranslated region and inhibit its translation. Further, western blotting analysis showed that overexpression of miR-144 and miR-451 down-regulated CUGBP2 and up-regulated COX-2 respectively. Moreover, inhibition of COX-2 partially reduces the cardio-protective effect of miR-144 and miR-451. It shows that miR-144 and miR-451 protect cardiac cells by targeting CUGBP2-COX-2 pathway [245] during IRI.

Cardiomyocyte loss is the major event observed during various cardiac pathologies including MI. *In vitro* experiments revealed that miR-122 is up-regulated after MI. Furthermore, transcription and translation study showed that anti-miR-122 study enhances cell survival by down-regulating the pro-apoptotic protein caspase-8. On contrary, the miR-122 mimic study showed down regulation of caspase-8 both at mRNA and protein levels. It opens an avenue as a therapeutic point of view for further study of miR-122 to reduce their expression and increase cardiomyocytes viability [246].

The overexpression of miR-1 could contribute to enhance pro-apoptotic effect in myocardium by targeting sodium calcium exchanger-1 target gene in rats MI model. In cardiomyocytes and skeletal muscles, miR-1 is predominantly expressed. miR-1 is also associated with differentiation and development of cardiac tissue [247]. *In vivo* experiment showed that genetic deletion of miR-1 gene causes late embryonic lethality and HF due to arrhythmias [121]. The gap junction protein – connexin (GJA1), and potassium ion channel (KCNj2) [119] are the potential candidate proteins to regulate cardiac arrythmogenicity however miR-1 may modulate these two potential proteins. Further studies revealed that miR-1 was highly expressed both in animal and human with AMI [248]. Significantly, up-regulation of miR-1 in plasma of human AMI patients opens a therapeutic window to use anti-miR-1 to cure AMI. Some proteins like cardiac troponin I (cTnI) have been applied as a biomarker for diagnosis of AMI. However some circulatory miRNAs like miR-1 and miR-126 can also be used as a biomarkers for diagnostic purposes in different cardiovascular diseases including AMI [226]. The plasma circulatory levels of cardiac specific miRNAs (miR-1, miR-133, miR-499, miR-208) are increased due to AMI characterized by cardiac injury. However endothelial-enriched miRNAs, such as miR-126 was down-regulated [249] in patients with coronary artery disease.

miR-133 is widely found in skeletal, cardiac, and smooth muscle cells of cardiovascular system [250] miRNA-133a has a major role in regulation of cardiomyocyte proliferation. However in vivo experiment showed that genetic deletion of miRNA 133a causes lethal ventricular septal defect in embryos, dilated cardiomyopathy and HF [230]. The AMI animal model showed that the circulation levels of miR-133a increase after 1–3 h and attained a peak valve after 3-12 h, however a decrease was observed after at 12-24 h of coronary artery ligation (AMI). In addition the circulatory level of miR-133 was also significantly increased in human with AMI. The circulatory levels of miRNA-133a can also be strongly linked with cTnI with substantially high levels. The increase in level of miR-133a in early peak hours can provide a better platform to use it as early diagnostic marker [34].

Different miRNAs have been reported with a key role in cardiac ischemia including miR-16 which is up-regulated in ischemic heart. However, Beta2-adrenoreceptor (β**2**-AR) has a cardio-protective effect during ischemic injury. miR-16 was highly expressed in AMI animal model in rats induced by ligation of left coronary artery. However, oxidative injury via hydrogen peroxide in cultured neonatal rat ventricular cells (NRVCs) also showed an increased expression of miR-16. In *vivo* and *vitro* experiment also showed down regulation of cardio-protective protein β**2**-AR. In addition, the miR-16 over expression also decreases cardiomyocytes viability by increase rate of apoptosis. The miR-16 lentivirus overexpression experiments showed increase in infarct size, creatine kinase activity, lactate dehydrogenase levels, and increase cardiac dysfunction. The knock down study of miR-16 showed beneficial effect of heart. Luciferase assay further confirmed that miR-16 can target the 3'untranslated region of β**2**-AR mRNA [251]. The antimiR-16 promising therapy can be used to protect cardiac cells from ischemic cell death.

MI injury can be regulated by different miRNAs of miR-30 family. This network of miR-30 family is composed of five miRNAs (a, b, c, d, and e). The endogenous production of Hydrogen sulfide (H_2S) acts as a signaling molecule and regulates cardiovascular system. Physiologically, L-cysteine generated H_2S catalyzed by cystathionine-b-synthase, cystathionine-c-lyase (CSE), or 3-mercaptopyruvate sulfurtransferase. However, in the cardiovascular system, CSE is the predominant H_2S generating enzyme [252]. The hypoxic murine MI and ischemic NRCM models showed elevated levels of miR-30 family with significantly low expression of CSE and H_2S. The knock down of miR-30 showed increase expression of CSE and H_2S which further reduce IRI. However, luciferase assay revealed that miR-30 directly target CSE. In addition locked nucleic acid (LNA)-miR-30 family inhibitor reduced infarct size, decreased apoptosis in border zone of infarction and improved heart function. These finding showed endogenous production of H_2S via CSE in the cardiomyocytes at miRNA level and their application as a therapeutics to reduce IHD [253].

miR-22 expression is highly related to aging including mice and human. However, increase in their expression was observed with increasing age. Cardiac miR-22 acts as a strong inhibitor in the process of cardiac autophagy. *In vitro* analysis of aging, cardiomyocytes showed that miR-22 expression is increased via P53-dependent mechanism. *In vitro* study revealed that knock down of miR-22 promoted cardiac autophagy and inhibition in cardiac hypertrophy. The pharmacological inhibition of miR-22 enhanced autophagy in post MI older mice, improved cardiac function and prevention in post infarct remodeling [254]. These notions showed that moderate expression strategy of miR-22 can be used to regulate the incidents of both cardiac autophagy and cardiac hypertrophy.

The miRNA-210 gets more attention in cardiovascular research due to its association with angiogenesis in AMI. The over expression rat models showed a strong interconnection with MI. The expression of miRNA-210 was up-regulated via transfection with hepatocyte growth factor (HGF) in heart. The transcription and translation analysis revealed that up-regulation of miR-210 tends to reduce the expression of HGF. However, marked increase in HGF was observed after silencing of miR-210. In the present study micro-vessel density (MVD) of the infarcted myocardium was selected for the angiogenesis efficacy. Moreover, the anti-miR-210 also showed promotion in angiogenesis with increased MVD and improved cardiac output [255]. The reduced expression of miR-210 can be used as a therapy to reduce the risks of AMI by promoting angiogenesis.

The high level of miR-34a increases the rate of cardiomyocytes apoptosis by down-regulating anti-apoptotic enzymes including, Aldehyde dehydrogenase 2 (ALDH2). In addition, the serum level of AMI patients also showed increase expression of miR-34a with low level of ALDH2. Further, luciferase assay showed that miR-34a directly targets ALDH2 and reduces its expression both at transcription and translation levels [256]. It shows that miR-34a can be employed as a therapeutic candidate and diagnostic marker for MI.

miR-320 plays a critical role in MI. *In vivo* experiment revealed that up-regulation of miR-320 enhances cardiomyocytes loss through apoptosis during simulated I/R. However, homozygous deletion of miR-320 showed cardio-protective effect by decreased infarct size with enhanced cardiac function. The detail study of miR-320 showed that it down regulates HSP20 which is a cardio-protective protein and provide protection against IRI [257]. It shows that HSP20 is a putative target of miR-320. miR-26 inhibits the high mobility group box 1 (HMGB1) which significantly reduce IR. miR-613 expression also alters in case of IR [258].

2.4 Prospective of miRNAs Therapeutics in Cardiac Fibrosis

Cardiac fibrosis is also associated with aberrant expression of miRNAs. Several ECM mediating encoding genes for fibrillin, elastin, and collagens are associated with miR-29 family. miR-29 is down-regulated in HF. Animal model with mouse cardiac fibroblasts analysis proved that IGF-1, leukemia inhibitory factor, and pentraxin-3 (fibrosis related genes) are the valid targets of miR-29b [259]. *In vitro* inhibition experiment of miR-29 revealed an increased in cardiac fibrosis and vice versa. In addition, transfection analysis in *vivo* study showed improvement in cardiac function and attenuated cardiac fibrosis. Cardiac fibrosis signaling pathways through TGF-β/and Smad3 play a critical role in HF and is targeted by miR-29 [260]. It shows that therapeutically overexpression strategy of miR-29 can be used to overcome cardiac fibrosis.

Extracellular signal-regulated kinase (ERK) mitogen activated protein (MAP) kinase signaling pathway increases the expression of miR-21 during stimulation of cardiac fibrosis. In mouse model, the antimiR-21 study showed a reduction in fibrosis and improvement in heart function with low activity of cardiac ERK-MAP kinase. In murine cardiac fibroblasts, miR-21 increased the expression level of metalloprotease-2 (MMP-2) via the phosphatase and tensin homologue (PTEN)–AKT phosphorylation-dependent pathway [112]. In cardiac fibrosis the expression of cytokine osteopontin (OPN) is increased which also increases the level of miR-21 [261]. *In vivo* inhibitory analysis of miR-21 study revealed that PTEN and SMAD7 expressions were restored which are involved in cardiac fibrosis [262]. These results propose a promising therapeutic strategy of miR-21.

miR-24 plays a critical role in HF and other related pathways both in cardiomyocytes and fibroblasts which ultimately leads to cell death [263]. In MI model, the expression of miR-24 was down-regulated. After a short period of MI, miR-24 interacts with fibronectin, collagen, and TGF-β and triggers ECM remodeling. In mouse, MI model revealed reduction in infarct size and improvement in cardiac output after transfection of miR-24. miR-24 also regulates cardiac fibrosis via furin which ultimately secretes TGF-β [264]. In cardiac cells, miR-24 also regulates cardiomyocytes apoptosis. miR-24 significantly reduce apoptosis in transgenic animal models of MI. In addition, miR-24 also regulates excitation and contraction uncoupling of the sarcoplasmic reticulum in cardiomyocytes and T-tubules through the junctophilin-2 protein [220].

2.5 Prospective of miRNAs in Cardiac Apoptosis

Apoptosis is regulated by different miRNAs which target pro-apoptotic factors and various apoptotic pathways. Previous study showed that different miRNAs (miR-21, miR-24, miR-133, miR-210, miR-494, and miR-499) play major roles in cardiomyocytes protection against apoptosis. However, some miRNAs including miR-1, miR-29, miR-199a, and miR-320 trigger apoptosis [265]. The expression level of different miRNAs is also associated with cardiomyocytes apoptosis which further leads to cardiac valve dysfunction. In such study miR-15a and miR-29a were down regulated while miR-214 expression level was increased. Furthermore, target validation analysis proved that miR-15a targets PUMA while miR-29a targets DRP1, however miR-214 targets ARC. PUMA, DRP1 and ARC are mitochondrial membrane regulatory protein. PUMA and DRP1 expression levels were increased during apoptosis while ARC is down-regulated [166, 266]. The expression of miR-15a, miR-29a and miR-214 and its respective targets in human cardiac valve dysfunction opens up new strategy where miRNAs can be used for therapeutic intervention in future. Variety of other miRNAs have been also investigated which can regulate cardiomyocytes apoptosis like let-7 family of miRNAs, miR-34 family, miR-21 family, miR-30 family, miR-125b, and miR-138. In mice experimental model of (I/R) injury, the overexpression of miR-93 attenuates cardiomyocyte loss by targeting phosphatase and tensin homolog (PTEN) [267]. In adult cardiomyocytes (H9C2), apoptosis can be inhibited by miR-7a/b-Sp1/PARP-1 pathways [242]. However, miR-138 exhibits hypoxia-induced apoptosis via MLK3/JNK/c-jun pathway in H9C2 cardiac cells [268]. In addition, miR-142-3p and miR-613 also attenuated apoptosis by targeting high mobility group box 1 (HMGB1) [269] and PDCD10 [258]. Inhibition of miR-320 leads to up-regulate IGF1 which attenuates apoptosis by up-regulation of Bcl-2 levels and down-regulation of p-ASK, p-JNK, p-p38, Bax and Caspase-3 expression levels [270]. miR-122 is an apoptosis-related miRNA. The knockdown experiment of miR-122 showed inhibition in hypoxia/re-oxygenation induced cardiomyocytes cell apoptosis by increasing the expression of GATA-4 [271]. The expression of miR-153 was significantly high during oxidative stress. However, endogenous inhibition of miR-153 attenuated cardiomyocyte apoptosis [272]. Some miRNAs are oxidatively modified by various oxidative systems including miR-184, miR-204-3p, and miR-139-3p. Oxidation enables to establish a negative association between miRNAs and genes expression through mismatching. The oxi-miR-184 mismatches with the 3' UTRs of anti-apoptotic genes Bcl-xL and Bcl-w. The negative interaction between oxi-miR-184 and Bcl-xL and Bcl-w reduced their levels and ultimately leads to cardiomyocytes apoptosis [273]. miR-103/107 expressions are increased during MI. Inhibition analysis of miR-103/107 showed reduction in infarct size and improvement in cardiac function after IRI [273]. miR-325 is up-regulated during MI and positively regulates autophagic cell death [274]. miR-874 displays an increased in it expression profile after MI. It positively regulates MI by suppressing Foxo3a [275]. miR-873 and miR-2861 [269] are down-regulated during MI. However, these miRNAs have the ability to reduce myocardial infarct size by attenuating I/R induced programmed necrotic cell death [269]. Therefore up-regulation of miR-873 and miR-2861 has the potential to reduce infarct size and restoring cardiac activities. The expression level of miR-188-3p also reduces during MI. miR-188-3p can target ATG7 [274] which leads to reduced autophagy and MI. miR-145 promotes repair of infracted myocardium cardiomyocyte [276]. However its expression is down-regulated during MI.

2.6 miRNAs and Cardiac Progenitor Cells

Neonatal mouse cardiomyocytes have the potential to repair and regeneration after injury by MI. However, after birth the regenerative capacity of cardiac cells substantially declines within 7 days. The repair and regeneration capability become very much low in the adult cardiac cells [172]. The activation of cardiomyocytes renewal provides a new platform for the MI. Among different strategies miRNAs have the potential as new therapeutic targets for MI. miR-17~92 cluster including miR-17, miR-18a, miR-19a, miR-19b, miR-20a, and miR-92a are involved in cardiomyocytes proliferation. *In vivo* study with mice model showed that overexpression of this cluster produce beneficial results by raising the total number of cardiomyocytes which further leads to increase in wall thickness and left ventricle dimension. On the other hand, the knock down study showed reduction in cardiomyocyte proliferation and heart weight at birth time [277]. Significant proliferation in adult cardiomyocytes can be achieved by miR-548c-3p, miR-509-3p, and miR-23b-3p through translational inhibition of MEIS by regulating cell-cycle progression [278]. *In ex vivo,* miR-590 and miR-199a trigger cell cycle re-entry of adult cardiomyocytes. miR-590/miR-199a mimic showed stimulation of cardiac repair and improvement in cardiac function by regenerative processes [279].

Overexpression of miRNA-204 can trigger proliferation in neonatal and adult cardiomyocytes by targeting Jarid2. miR-204 overexpression in transgenic mice revealed excessive proliferation in cardiomyocyte throughout the embryonic and adult stages which further leads to increase in ventricular mass [280]. miR-15 family (including miR-15a, miR-15b, miR-16, miR-195, and miR-497) inhibit cardiomyocytes proliferation. The knock down experiment of miR-15b and miR-16 in mouse showed extension in the period of cardiomyocyte proliferation after birth [172]. Transgenic mice with overexpression of miR-195 showed decrease in cardiomyocytes undergoing mitosis. Furthermore, at the early postnatal period multinucleated cardiomyocytes were also remarkably increased [281]. miR-133a is an anti-proliferative marker. In zebrafish model, inhibition of miR-133 triggers cardiomyocytes proliferation [282].

The endogenous stem cells or progenitors like cardiac progenitor cells (CPCs) proliferation and differentiation can also be used an alternative strategy to compensate cardiomyocytes loss. miRNAs are also highly associated with such pathways which promote cardiomyocytes regeneration [283]. Some miRNAs including miR-302~367 clusters maintain tissue-specific progenitors in early cardiac developmental stages [284]. This cluster includes miR-302a, miR-302b, miR-302c, miR-302d and miR-367 which trigger proliferation of embryonic cardiomyocytes by targeting CPCs. The overexpression of miR-302~367 cluster in infarcted heart leads to improvement in cardiac function and exhibits attenuation in fibrosis [285]. *In vitro* study revealed that overexpression of miR-499 triggers the differentiation of human CPCs to CMs. Cardiac fibroblasts are the major constituents (50%) of the whole cells in the heart [286]. MI mice model showed that fibroblast can be reprogramed into cardiomyocytes with miRNAs in combination of some transcription factors which further produce beneficial results on heart by reducing infarct size. *In vitro* and *in vivo* analysis showed that miR-1, miR-133, miR-208 together with miR-499 also called as 'miR combo' successfully reprogrammed cardiac fibroblasts into cardiomyocytes and produce improvement in cardiac output [287].

2.7 microRNAs and Arrhythmias

Arrhythmia is mostly found in elder however, atrial fibrillation (AF) is the most common arrhythmia. Structural and electrical remodeling is the end stage manifestation due to various pathological modifications including different miRNAs. miR-1 has been demonstrated that its level reduced by ≈86% in AF. The postulated effect of miR-1 is on inward-rectifier K+ currents (IK1) [288]. miR-328 also plays a positive association with AF. miR-328 was increased by 3.5 fold in tissue of atrial sample of AF patients. The knockdown experiment of miR-328 in mouse models showed decease in AF. In addition, enhanced expression increases the risks of AF. Furthermore, miR-223 and miR-664 have been also enhanced in AF [289] suggesting their possible role as AF future therapeutic targets.

2.8 miRNAs and Hypertension

Blood pressure is regulated by renin angiotensin aldosterone system however this system is further regulated by miRNAs. The comparison study of normal and hypertensive individuals using microarray showed that miR- 181a and miR-633 are associated with down regulation of renin in kidney [290]. In animal models (rats) the expressions of miR-132 and miR-212 were increased in aorta, heart, and kidneys after infusion with angiotensin-II. The treatment of Angiotensin-II receptor type 1 blockers with internal mammary artery of patients showed down regulation of respective two miRNAs. It shows that miR-132 and miR-212 have a major role in regulating angiotensin-II mediated hypertension. Further experiments in mice model showed that knockout down of miR-143 and miR-145 significantly reduced blood pressure. However target validation analysis proved that miR-145 targets angiotensin converting enzyme (ACE) mRNA [176]. The atherosclerotic plaques showed overexpression of miR-145 in hypertensive patients undergoing carotid endarterectomy [291]. It shows the implication of miR-145 has the potential to consider blood pressure regulation and vascular damage.

2.9 miRNAs and Infective Carditis

There is no specific biomarker available for infective carditis including myocarditis and pericarditis. The diagnosis of infective carditis is mostly performed on clinical basis and some protein based biomarkers. The elevated plasma level of miR- 208b and miR-499 in viral myocarditis have been assessed to utilize as a diagnostic biomarkers for infective carditis. Furthermore, the level of expressions of these miRNAs can also be used to determine the severity of myocardial damage [292]. The miR-155 is up-regulated during acute myocarditis The experiments with viral myocarditis animal model showed an increase level of miR-155 in mouse cardiac tissue [293]. miR-221 and miR-222 are also key regulators of viral myocarditis and their response has been observed in animal models and human [294] paving way for the future research in their mechanistic regulation.

2.10 microRNAs and Atherosclerosis

Atherosclerosis is a complicated, multifaceted pathological process which is still incompletely understood. Various pathological processes including endothelial cell (EC) dysfunction, infiltration of inflammatory cells, lipid dysregulation and VSMCs differentiation are the major causes of atherosclerosis. Some miRNAs are also involved in dysfunction of endothelial cell. Atherosclerosis is characterized by the formation of plaque at arterial branching which leads to EC dysfunction due to disturbed laminar flow. miR-126-5p plays a critical role in proliferative reserve of ECs due to stress by down regulating delta-like homologue 1 (Dlk1) [295]. However, reduced expression of miR-126-5p leads to plaque formation due to reduce proliferative reserve of ECs. Infiltration of inflammatory cells occurs due to the permeability of ECs which is actively contributed by miR-155 [296]. Large numbers of miRNAs are involved in EC dysfunction given with its putative targets in Table 24.13. In response to inflammatory cell infiltration, atherosclerosis also occurs due to VSMC migration

Table 24.13 miRNAs and their targets in endothelial dysfunction

miRNAs	Targets	miRNAs	Targets
miR-1	MLCK	miR-221/222	c-Kit, eNOS, ETS-1, PAK1, p27, p57, STAT5A
miR-27a/b	SEMA6A	miR-223	IGF-1R
miR-34a	SIRT1	miR-365	BCL-2
miR-92a	KLF2, KLF4, PTEN, SOCS5	miR-492	Resistin
miR-144	IDH2	miR-513a-5p	XIAP
miR-146a	NOX4	miR-712	TIMP3
miR-155	AT1R, ETS-1, MLCK	let-7c	BCL-XL
miR-216a	BECN1	let-7g	CASP3, SMAD2, TGFBR1, THBS1
miR-217	SirT1		

from the media to the intima. miR-143/145 have been showed as critical regulators of VSMC differentiation. However, miRNAs also change its expression during inflammation which also alters the expression of its targets given in Table 24.14. VSMC differentiation and proliferation also characterized by various number of miRNAs which ultimately change the expression of its putative targets (Table 24.15) [289].

2.11 miRNAs and Heart Failure

The expression level of miRNAs is also associated with HF. These miRNAs include miR-122, miR-210, miR-423-5p, miR-499 miR-622, miR-92b, miR-30a, miR-29b, miR-21, miR-22, miR-18b∗, miR-320a, miR-200b, miR-142-3p, miR-133a, miR-129-5p, miR-1254, miR-675 and miR-499. The plasma expression of these miRNAs have been increased during HF which can also be used for diagnostic purposes [289]. The low expression level of miRNAs including miR-30b, miR-107, miR-103, miR-125b, miR126, miR-139, miR-142-3p, miR-142-5p, miR-342-3p and miR-497 can also be used for diagnostic purposes during HF.

miR-16, miR-27a, miR-101, and miR-150 are involved in the improvement of left ventricle (LV) contractility after AMI. The level of NT-proBNP can be increased during HF [297]. However, in such study NT-proBNP was an established biomarker of HF [233]. The low level of expression of miR-150 is associated with increased LV remodeling after ST segment elevation MI (STEMI) [175]. The low level of miR-150 can also be used for diagnostic and prognostic predictors of HF. The expression levels of miRNAs can be used as a prognostic indicator in the development of HF.

Table 24.14 miRNAs and their targets during inflammation

miRNAs	Targets	miRNAs	Targets
miR-9	ACAT1, PPARδ	miR-126-3p	VCAM-1
miR-10a,	MAP3K7, βTRC	miR-145	JAM-A
miR-15a	CARM1	miR-146a/b	CD40L, IRAK1, IRAK2, TLR4, TRAF6
miR-17-3p	ICAM-1	miR-155	BCL-2, ETS-1, FADD, HBP1, MAP3K10
miR-21	PPARα, TLR4	miR-181a	c-Fos
miR-29a	LPL	miR-181b	IPOA3
miR-31	E-selectin	miR-342-5p	AKT1
miR-125a-5p	ORP9		

Table 24.15 miRNAs and their targets during VSMC differentiation and proliferation

let-7 g	LOX-1	miR-133a	IGF-1R, RUNX2
let-7d	KRAS	miR-143/145	ELK1, fascin, KLF4, KLF5, PDGF-Rα, PKC-ε
miR-1	KLF4, MRTF-A, PIM-1	miR-181a	OPN
miR-21	BCL-2, PDCD4, PPARα, PTEN, TPM1	miR-195	CDC42
miR-26a	SMAD1, SMAD4	miR-208	p21
miR-29b	DNMT3b	miR-221/222	c-Kit, p27, p57
miR-125b	SP7	miR-490-3p	PAPP-A
miR-126	BCL-2, FOXO3, IRS1	miR-638	NOR1
miR-132	LRRFIP1	miR-663	JUNB, MYL9
miR-133	SP1		

References

1. Uszczynska-Ratajczak B, Lagarde J, Frankish A, Guigó R, Johnson R. Towards a complete map of the human long non-coding RNA transcriptome. Resource. 2018;8(67):276.
2. Liu G, Mattick JS, Taft RJ. A meta-analysis of the genomic and transcriptomic composition of complex life. Cell Cycle. 2013;12(13):2061–72.
3. Derrien T, Johnson R, Bussotti G, Tanzer A, Djebali S, Tilgner H, Guernec G, Martin D, Merkel A, Knowles DG. The GENCODE v7 catalog of human long noncoding RNAs: analysis of their gene structure, evolution, and expression. Genome Res. 2012;22(9):1775–89.
4. Esteller M. Non-coding RNAs in human disease. Nat Rev Genet. 2011;12(12):861.
5. Rinn JL, Euskirchen G, Bertone P, Martone R, Luscombe NM, Hartman S, Harrison PM, Nelson FK, Miller P, Gerstein M. The transcriptional activity of human chromosome 22. Genes Dev. 2003;17(4):529–40.
6. Kapranov P, Cawley SE, Drenkow J, Bekiranov S, Strausberg RL, Fodor SP, Gingeras TR. Large-scale transcriptional activity in chromosomes 21 and 22. Science. 2002;296(5569):916–9.
7. Consortium F, I RGERGP, Team I. Analysis of the mouse transcriptome based on functional annotation of 60,770 full-length cDNAs. Nature. 2002;420(6915):563.
8. Huang M-S, Zhu T, Li L, Xie P, Li X, Zhou H-H, Liu Z-Q. LncRNAs and CircRNAs from the same gene: masterpieces of RNA splicing. Cancer Lett. 2018;415:49–57.
9. Fang S, Zhang L, Guo J, Niu Y, Wu Y, Li H, Zhao L, Li X, Teng X, Sun X. NONCODEV5: a comprehensive annotation database for long non-coding RNAs. Nucleic Acids Res. 2017;46(D1):D308–14.
10. Taft RJ, Pang KC, Mercer TR, Dinger M, Mattick JS. Non-coding RNAs: regulators of disease. J Pathol. 2010;220(2):126–39.
11. Hüttenhofer A, Vogel J. Experimental approaches to identify non-coding RNAs. Nucleic Acids Res. 2006;34(2):635–46.
12. Wang J, Samuels DC, Zhao S, Xiang Y, Zhao Y-Y, Guo Y. Current research on non-coding ribonucleic acid (RNA). Genes. 2017;8(12):366.
13. Das A, Samidurai A, Salloum FN. Deciphering non-coding RNAs in cardiovascular health and disease. Front Cardiovasc Med. 2018;5:73.
14. Tang T-H, Bachellerie J-P, Rozhdestvensky T, Bortolin M-L, Huber H, Drungowski M, Elge T, Brosius J, Hüttenhofer A. Identification of 86 candidates for small non-messenger RNAs from the archaeon Archaeoglobus fulgidus. Proc Natl Acad Sci. 2002;99(11):7536–41.
15. Marker C, Zemann A, Terhörst T, Kiefmann M, Kastenmayer JP, Green P, Bachellerie J-P, Brosius J, Hüttenhofer A. Experimental RNomics: identification of 140 candidates for small non-messenger RNAs in the plant Arabidopsis thaliana. Curr Biol. 2002;12(23):2002–13.
16. Wassarman KM, Repoila F, Rosenow C, Storz G, Gottesman S. Identification of novel small RNAs using comparative genomics and microarrays. Genes Dev. 2001;15(13):1637–51.
17. Rivas E, Klein RJ, Jones TA, Eddy SR. Computational identification of noncoding RNAs in E. coli by comparative genomics. Curr Biol. 2001;11(17):1369–73.
18. Hüttenhofer A, Kiefmann M, Meier-Ewert S, O'Brien J, Lehrach H, Bachellerie JP, Brosius J. RNomics: an experimental approach that identifies 201 candidates for novel, small, non-messenger RNAs in mouse. EMBO J. 2001;20(11):2943–53.
19. Argaman L, Hershberg R, Vogel J, Bejerano G, Wagner EGH, Margalit H, Altuvia S. Novel small RNA-encoding genes in the intergenic regions of Escherichia coli. Curr Biol. 2001;11(12):941–50.
20. Zhao G. Significance of non-coding circular RNAs and micro RNAs in the pathogenesis of cardiovascular diseases. J Med Genet. 2018;55(11):713–20.
21. Xu S, Kamato D, Little PJ, Nakagawa S, Pelisek J, Jin ZG Targeting epigenetics and non-coding RNAs in atherosclerosis: from mechanisms to therapeutics. Pharmacol Ther. 2018;196:15–43.
22. Vea A, Llorente-Cortes V, de Gonzalo-Calvo D. Circular RNAs in Blood. In: Xiao J, editor. Circular Rnas: biogenesis and functions, Advances in experimental medicine and biology, vol. 1087. Cham: Springer; 2018. p. 119–30.
23. Quan G, Li J. Circular RNAs: biogenesis, expression and their potential roles in reproduction. J Ovarian Res. 2018;11(1):9.
24. Poller W, Dimmeler S, Heymans S, Zeller T, Haas J, Karakas M, Leistner D-M, Jakob P, Nakagawa S, Blankenberg S, Engelhardt S, Thum T, Weber C, Meder B, Hajjar R, Landmesser U. Non-coding RNAs in cardiovascular diseases: diagnostic and therapeutic perspectives. Eur Heart J. 2018;39(29):2704.
25. Islas JF, Moreno-Cuevas JE. A MicroRNA perspective on cardiovascular development and diseases: an update. Int J Mol Sci. 2018;19(7):2075.
26. Abbas Q, Raza SM, Biyabani AA, Jaffar MA. A review of computational methods for finding non-coding RNA genes. Genes (Basel). 2016;7(12):113.
27. Rayner KJ, Esau CC, Hussain FN, McDaniel AL, Marshall SM, van Gils JM, Ray TD, Sheedy FJ, Goedeke L, Liu X. Inhibition of miR-33a/b in non-human primates raises plasma HDL and lowers VLDL triglycerides. Nature. 2011;478(7369):404.
28. Nagalingam RS, Sundaresan NR, Gupta MP, Geenen DL, Solaro RJ, Gupta M. A cardiac-enriched microRNA, miR-378, blocks cardiac hypertrophy by targeting Ras signaling. J Biol Chem. 2013;288(16):11216–32.
29. Ai J, Zhang R, Li Y, Pu J, Lu Y, Jiao J, Li K, Yu B, Li Z, Wang R, Wang L, Li Q, Wang N, Shan H, Li Z, Yang B. Circulating microRNA-1 as a potential

novel biomarker for acute myocardial infarction. Biochem Biophys Res Commun. 2010;391(1):73–7.
30. Bialek S, Gorko D, Zajkowska A, Koltowski L, Grabowski M, Stachurska A, Kochman J, Sygitowicz G, Malecki M, Opolski G, Sitkiewicz D. Release kinetics of circulating miRNA-208a in the early phase of myocardial infarction. Kardiol Pol. 2015;73(8):613–9.
31. Cheng Y, Tan N, Yang J, Liu X, Cao X, He P, Dong X, Qin S, Zhang C. A translational study of circulating cell-free microRNA-1 in acute myocardial infarction. Clin Sci (Lond). 2010;119(2):87–95.
32. Coskunpinar E, Cakmak HA, Kalkan AK, Tiryakioglu NO, Erturk M, Ongen Z. Circulating miR-221-3p as a novel marker for early prediction of acute myocardial infarction. Gene. 2016;591(1):90–6.
33. Ji X, Takahashi R, Hiura Y, Hirokawa G, Fukushima Y, Iwai N. Plasma miR-208 as a biomarker of myocardial injury. Clin Chem. 2009;55(11):1944–9.
34. Wang GK, Zhu JQ, Zhang JT, Li Q, Li Y, He J, Qin YW, Jing Q. Circulating microRNA: a novel potential biomarker for early diagnosis of acute myocardial infarction in humans. Eur Heart J. 2010;31(6):659–66.
35. Chan JH, Lim S, Wong WS. Antisense oligonucleotides: from design to therapeutic application. Clin Exp Pharmacol Physiol. 2006;33(5–6):533–40.
36. Crooke ST. Molecular mechanisms of action of antisense drugs. Biochim Biophys Acta. 1999;1489(1):31–44.
37. Crooke ST, Wang S, Vickers TA, Shen W, Liang XH. Cellular uptake and trafficking of antisense oligonucleotides. Nat Biotechnol. 2017;35(3):230–7.
38. Dowdy SF. Overcoming cellular barriers for RNA therapeutics. Nat Biotechnol. 2017;35(3):222–9.
39. Laina A, Gatsiou A, Georgiopoulos G, Stamatelopoulos K, Stellos K. RNA therapeutics in cardiovascular precision medicine. Front Physiol. 2018;9:953.
40. Shen X, Corey DR. Chemistry, mechanism and clinical status of antisense oligonucleotides and duplex RNAs. Nucleic Acids Res. 2018;46(4):1584–600.
41. Dominski Z, Kole R. Restoration of correct splicing in thalassemic pre-mRNA by antisense oligonucleotides. Proc Natl Acad Sci U S A. 1993;90(18):8673–7.
42. Jackson AL, Linsley PS. Recognizing and avoiding siRNA off-target effects for target identification and therapeutic application. Nat Rev Drug Discov. 2010;9(1):57–67.
43. Liu J, Carmell MA, Rivas FV, Marsden CG, Thomson JM, Song JJ, Hammond SM, Joshua-Tor L, Hannon GJ. Argonaute2 is the catalytic engine of mammalian RNAi. Science (New York, NY). 2004;305(5689):1437–41.
44. Meister G. Argonaute proteins: functional insights and emerging roles. Nat Rev Genet. 2013;14(7):447–59.
45. Siomi H, Siomi MC. On the road to reading the RNA-interference code. Nature. 2009;457(7228):396–404.
46. Sledz CA, Holko M, de Veer MJ, Silverman RH, Williams BR. Activation of the interferon system by short-interfering RNAs. Nat Cell Biol. 2003;5(9):834–9.
47. Rupaimoole R, Slack FJ. MicroRNA therapeutics: towards a new era for the management of cancer and other diseases. Nat Rev Drug Discov. 2017;16(3):203–22.
48. Lam JK, Chow MY, Zhang Y, Leung SW. siRNA versus miRNA as therapeutics for gene silencing. Mol Ther Nucleic Acids. 2015;4:e252.
49. Li Z, Rana TM. Therapeutic targeting of microRNAs: current status and future challenges. Nat Rev Drug Discov. 2014;13(8):622–38.
50. Janssen HL, Reesink HW, Lawitz EJ, Zeuzem S, Rodriguez-Torres M, Patel K, van der Meer AJ, Patick AK, Chen A, Zhou Y, Persson R, King BD, Kauppinen S, Levin AA, Hodges MR. Treatment of HCV infection by targeting microRNA. N Engl J Med. 2013;368(18):1685–94.
51. Bernardo BC, Gao XM, Winbanks CE, Boey EJ, Tham YK, Kiriazis H, Gregorevic P, Obad S, Kauppinen S, Du XJ, Lin RC, McMullen JR. Therapeutic inhibition of the miR-34 family attenuates pathological cardiac remodeling and improves heart function. Proc Natl Acad Sci U S A. 2012;109(43):17615–20.
52. Rayner KJ, Sheedy FJ, Esau CC, Hussain FN, Temel RE, Parathath S, van Gils JM, Rayner AJ, Chang AN, Suarez Y, Fernandez-Hernando C, Fisher EA, Moore KJ. Antagonism of miR-33 in mice promotes reverse cholesterol transport and regression of atherosclerosis. J Clin Invest. 2011;121(7):2921–31.
53. Obad S, dos Santos CO, Petri A, Heidenblad M, Broom O, Ruse C, Fu C, Lindow M, Stenvang J, Straarup EM, Hansen HF, Koch T, Pappin D, Hannon GJ, Kauppinen S. Silencing of microRNA families by seed-targeting tiny LNAs. Nat Genet. 2011;43(4):371–8.
54. Zhou J, Rossi J. Aptamers as targeted therapeutics: current potential and challenges. Nat Rev Drug Discov. 2017;16(3):181–202.
55. Ferrara N, Adamis AP. Ten years of anti-vascular endothelial growth factor therapy. Nat Rev Drug Discov. 2016;15(6):385–403.
56. Mousa SA, Mousa SS. Current status of vascular endothelial growth factor inhibition in age-related macular degeneration. BioDrugs: clinical immunotherapeutics, biopharmaceuticals and. Gene Ther. 2010;24(3):183–94.
57. Ng EW, Shima DT, Calias P, Cunningham ET Jr, Guyer DR, Adamis AP. Pegaptanib, a targeted anti-VEGF aptamer for ocular vascular disease. Nat Rev Drug Discov. 2006;5(2):123–32.
58. Ray KK, Landmesser U, Leiter LA, Kallend D, Dufour R, Karakas M, Hall T, Troquay RP, Turner T, Visseren FL, Wijngaard P, Wright RS, Kastelein JJ. Inclisiran in patients at high cardiovascular risk with elevated LDL cholesterol. N Engl J Med. 2017;376(15):1430–40.

59. Crooke ST, Geary RS. Clinical pharmacological properties of mipomersen (Kynamro), a second generation antisense inhibitor of apolipoprotein B. Br J Clin Pharmacol. 2013;76(2):269–76.
60. Crosby J, Peloso GM, Auer PL, Crosslin DR, Stitziel NO, Lange LA, Lu Y, Tang ZZ, Zhang H, Hindy G, Masca N, Stirrups K, Kanoni S, Do R, Jun G, Hu Y, Kang HM, Xue C, Goel A, Farrall M, Duga S, Merlini PA, Asselta R, Girelli D, Olivieri O, Martinelli N, Yin W, Reilly D, Speliotes E, Fox CS, Hveem K, Holmen OL, Nikpay M, Farlow DN, Assimes TL, Franceschini N, Robinson J, North KE, Martin LW, DePristo M, Gupta N, Escher SA, Jansson JH, Van Zuydam N, Palmer CN, Wareham N, Koch W, Meitinger T, Peters A, Lieb W, Erbel R, Konig IR, Kruppa J, Degenhardt F, Gottesman O, Bottinger EP, O'Donnell CJ, Psaty BM, Ballantyne CM, Abecasis G, Ordovas JM, Melander O, Watkins H, Orho-Melander M, Ardissino D, Loos RJ, McPherson R, Willer CJ, Erdmann J, Hall AS, Samani NJ, Deloukas P, Schunkert H, Wilson JG, Kooperberg C, Rich SS, Tracy RP, Lin DY, Altshuler D, Gabriel S, Nickerson DA, Jarvik GP, Cupples LA, Reiner AP, Boerwinkle E, Kathiresan S. Loss-of-function mutations in APOC3, triglycerides, and coronary disease. New England J Med. 2014;371(1):22–31.
61. Huff MW, Hegele RA. Apolipoprotein C-III: going back to the future for a lipid drug target. Circ Res. 2013;112(11):1405–8.
62. Baldi S, Bonnet F, Laville M, Morgantini C, Monti L, Hojlund K, Ferrannini E, Natali A. Influence of apolipoproteins on the association between lipids and insulin sensitivity: a cross-sectional analysis of the RISC study. Diabetes Care. 2013;36(12):4125–31.
63. Graham MJ, Lee RG, Brandt TA, Tai LJ, Fu W, Peralta R, Yu R, Hurh E, Paz E, McEvoy BW, Baker BF, Pham NC, Digenio A, Hughes SG, Geary RS, Witztum JL, Crooke RM, Tsimikas S. Cardiovascular and metabolic effects of ANGPTL3 antisense oligonucleotides. N Engl J Med. 2017;377(3):222–32.
64. Dewey FE, Gusarova V, O'Dushlaine C, Gottesman O, Trejos J, Hunt C, Van Hout CV, Habegger L, Buckler D, Lai KM, Leader JB, Murray MF, Ritchie MD, Kirchner HL, Ledbetter DH, Penn J, Lopez A, Borecki IB, Overton JD, Reid JG, Carey DJ, Murphy AJ, Yancopoulos GD, Baras A, Gromada J, Shuldiner AR. Inactivating variants in ANGPTL4 and risk of coronary artery disease. N Engl J Med. 2016;374(12):1123–33.
65. Capoulade R, Chan KL, Yeang C, Mathieu P, Bosse Y, Dumesnil JG, Tam JW, Teo KK, Mahmut A, Yang X, Witztum JL, Arsenault BJ, Despres JP, Pibarot P, Tsimikas S. Oxidized phospholipids, lipoprotein(a), and progression of calcific aortic valve stenosis. J Am Coll Cardiol. 2015;66(11):1236–46.
66. Wiesner P, Tafelmeier M, Chittka D, Choi SH, Zhang L, Byun YS, Almazan F, Yang X, Iqbal N, Chowdhury P, Maisel A, Witztum JL, Handel TM, Tsimikas S, Miller YI. MCP-1 binds to oxidized LDL and is carried by lipoprotein(a) in human plasma. J Lipid Res. 2013;54(7):1877–83.
67. Robciuc MR, Maranghi M, Lahikainen A, Rader D, Bensadoun A, Oorni K, Metso J, Minicocci I, Ciociola E, Ceci F, Montali A, Arca M, Ehnholm C, Jauhiainen M. Angptl3 deficiency is associated with increased insulin sensitivity, lipoprotein lipase activity, and decreased serum free fatty acids. Arterioscler Thromb Vasc Biol. 2013;33(7):1706–13.
68. Rodriguez CR, Seman LJ, Ordovas JM, Jenner J, Genest MS Jr, Wilson PW, Schaefer EJ. Lipoprotein(a) and coronary heart disease. Chem Phys Lipids. 1994;67-68:389–98.
69. Waldeyer C, Makarova N, Zeller T, Schnabel RB, Brunner FJ, Jorgensen T, Linneberg A, Niiranen T, Salomaa V, Jousilahti P, Yarnell J, Ferrario MM, Veronesi G, Brambilla P, Signorini SG, Iacoviello L, Costanzo S, Giampaoli S, Palmieri L, Meisinger C, Thorand B, Kee F, Koenig W, Ojeda F, Kontto J, Landmesser U, Kuulasmaa K, Blankenberg S. Lipoprotein(a) and the risk of cardiovascular disease in the European population: results from the BiomarCaRE consortium. Eur Heart J. 2017;38(32):2490–8.
70. Sugihara C, Freemantle N, Hughes SG, Furniss S, Sulke N. The effect of C-reactive protein reduction with a highly specific antisense oligonucleotide on atrial fibrillation assessed using beat-to-beat pacemaker Holter follow-up. J Interv Card Electrophysiol. 2015;43(1):91–8.
71. Noveck R, Stroes ES, Flaim JD, Baker BF, Hughes S, Graham MJ, Crooke RM, Ridker PM. Effects of an antisense oligonucleotide inhibitor of C-reactive protein synthesis on the endotoxin challenge response in healthy human male volunteers. J Am Heart Assoc. 2014;3(4):e001084.
72. Pena JM, MacFadyen J, Glynn RJ, Ridker PM. High-sensitivity C-reactive protein, statin therapy, and risks of atrial fibrillation: an exploratory analysis of the JUPITER trial. Eur Heart J. 2012;33(4):531–7.
73. Liu J, Fang PH, Dibs S, Hou Y, Li XF, Zhang S. High-sensitivity C-reactive protein as a predictor of atrial fibrillation recurrence after primary circumferential pulmonary vein isolation. Pacing Clin Electrophysiol. 2011;34(4):398–406.
74. Marcus GM, Smith LM, Ordovas K, Scheinman MM, Kim AM, Badhwar N, Lee RJ, Tseng ZH, Lee BK, Olgin JE. Intracardiac and extracardiac markers of inflammation during atrial fibrillation. Heart Rhythm. 2010;7(2):149–54.
75. Boos CJ. Relationship between C-reactive protein concentrations during glucocorticoid therapy and recurrent atrial fibrillation. Eur Heart J. 2004;25(19):1761–2.
76. Strandberg TE, Tilvis RS. C-reactive protein, cardiovascular risk factors, and mortality in a prospective study in the elderly. Arterioscler Thromb Vasc Biol. 2000;20(4):1057–60.
77. Aguirre A, Sancho-Martinez I, Belmonte JCI. Reprogramming toward heart regenera-

tion: stem cells and beyond. Cell Stem Cell. 2013;12(3):275–84.
78. Giacca M, Zacchigna S. Harnessing the microRNA pathway for cardiac regeneration. J Mol Cell Cardiol. 2015;89:68–74.
79. Clevers H. Stem cells, asymmetric division and cancer. Nat Genet. 2005;37(10):1027.
80. De Windt LJ, Giacca M. Non-coding RNA function in stem cells and regenerative medicine. Non-coding RNA Res. 2018;3(2):39.
81. Luginbühl J, Sivaraman DM, Shin JW. The essentiality of non-coding RNAs in cell reprogramming. Non-coding RNA Res. 2017;2(1):74–82.
82. Pijlman GP, Funk A, Kondratieva N, Leung J, Torres S, van der Aa L, Liu WJ, Palmenberg AC, Shi P-Y, Hall RA. A highly structured, nuclease-resistant, noncoding RNA produced by flaviviruses is required for pathogenicity. Cell Host Microbe. 2008;4(6):579–91.
83. Daou N, Lecolle S, Lefebvre S, della Gaspera B, Charbonnier F, Chanoine C, Armand A-S. A new role for the calcineurin/NFAT pathway in neonatal myosin heavy chain expression via the NFATc2/MyoD complex during mouse myogenesis. Development. 2013;140(24):4914–25.
84. Gonçalves TJ, Armand A-S. Non-coding RNAs in skeletal muscle regeneration. Non-coding RNA Res. 2017;2(1):56–67.
85. Martinet C, Monnier P, Louault Y, Benard M, Gabory A, Dandolo L. H19 controls reactivation of the imprinted gene network during muscle regeneration. Development. 2016;143(6):962–71.
86. Santolini M, Ferry A, Hakim V, Maire P. Six homeoproteins and a linc-RNA at the fast MYH locus lock fast myofiber terminal phenotype. PLoS Genet. 2014;10(5):e1004386.
87. van Rooij E, Quiat D, Johnson BA, Sutherland LB, Qi X, Richardson JA, Kelm RJ Jr, Olson EN. A family of microRNAs encoded by myosin genes governs myosin expression and muscle performance. Dev Cell. 2009;17(5):662–73.
88. Choong OK, Lee DS, Chen C-Y, Hsieh PC. The roles of non-coding RNAs in cardiac regenerative medicine. Non-coding RNA Res. 2017;2(2):100–10.
89. Ebrahimi B. In vivo reprogramming for heart regeneration: a glance at efficiency, environmental impacts, challenges and future directions. J Mol Cell Cardiol. 2017;108:61–72.
90. Eschenhagen T, Bolli R, Braun T, Field LJ, Fleischmann BK, Frisén J, Giacca M, Hare JM, Houser S, Lee RT. Cardiomyocyte regeneration: a consensus statement. Circulation. 2017;136(7):680–6.
91. Garreta E, Prado P, Belmonte JCI, Montserrat N. Non-coding microRNAs for cardiac regeneration: exploring novel alternatives to induce heart healing. Non-coding RNA Res. 2017;2(2):93–9.
92. Roberts EG, Lee EL, Backman D, Buczek-Thomas JA, Emani S, Wong JY. Engineering myocardial tissue patches with hierarchical structure–function. Ann Biomed Eng. 2015;43(3):762–73.
93. Di Mauro V, Barandalla-Sobrados M, Catalucci D. The noncoding-RNA landscape in cardiovascular health and disease. Non-coding RNA Res. 2018;3(1):12–9.
94. Ali I, Salim K, A Rather M, A Wani W, Haque A. Advances in nano drugs for cancer chemotherapy. Curr Cancer Drug Targets. 2011;11(2):135–46.
95. Blanco E, Shen H, Ferrari M. Principles of nanoparticle design for overcoming biological barriers to drug delivery. Nat Biotechnol. 2015;33(9):941–51.
96. Moghimi SM, Hunter AC, Murray JC. Nanomedicine: current status and future prospects. FASEB J. 2005;19(3):311–30.
97. Petros RA, DeSimone JM. Strategies in the design of nanoparticles for therapeutic applications. Nat Rev Drug Discov. 2010;9(8):615–27.
98. Riehemann K, Schneider SW, Luger TA, Godin B, Ferrari M, Fuchs H. Nanomedicine—challenge and perspectives. Angew Chem Int Ed. 2009;48(5):872–97.
99. Biray Avci C, Ozcan I, Balci T, Ozer O, Gunduz C. Design of polyethylene glycol-polyethylenimine nanocomplexes as non-viral carriers: mir-150 delivery to chronic myeloid leukemia cells. Cell Biol Int. 2013;37(11):1205–14.
100. Wu Y, Crawford M, Mao Y, Lee RJ, Davis IC, Elton TS, Lee LJ, Nana-Sinkam SP. Therapeutic delivery of MicroRNA-29b by cationic Lipoplexes for Lung Cancer. Mol Ther Nucleic Acids. 2013;2:e84.
101. Di Mauro V, Iafisco M, Salvarani N, Vacchiano M, Carullo P, Ramirez-Rodriguez GB, Patricio T, Tampieri A, Miragoli M, Catalucci D. Bioinspired negatively charged calcium phosphate nanocarriers for cardiac delivery of MicroRNAs. Nanomedicine (Lond). 2016;11(8):891–906.
102. Montgomery RL, Hullinger TG, Semus HM, Dickinson BA, Seto AG, Lynch JM, Stack C, Latimer PA, Olson EN, Van Rooij E. Therapeutic inhibition of miR-208a improves cardiac function and survival during heart failure. Circulation. 2011;124(14):1537–47.
103. Pan Z-w, Lu Y-j, Yang B-f. MicroRNAs: a novel class of potential therapeutic targets for cardiovascular diseases. Acta Pharmacol Sin. 2010;31(1):1.
104. Thum T, Gross C, Fiedler J, Fischer T, Kissler S, Bussen M, Galuppo P, Just S, Rottbauer W, Frantz S. MicroRNA-21 contributes to myocardial disease by stimulating MAP kinase signalling in fibroblasts. Nature. 2008;456(7224):980.
105. Liu G, Friggeri A, Yang Y, Milosevic J, Ding Q, Thannickal VJ, Kaminski N, Abraham E. miR-21 mediates fibrogenic activation of pulmonary fibroblasts and lung fibrosis. J Exp Med. 2010;207(8):1589–97.
106. Zhong X, Chung AC, Chen H-Y, Meng X-M, Lan HY. Smad3-mediated upregulation of miR-21 promotes renal fibrosis. J Am Soc Nephrol. 2011;22(9):1668–81.
107. Fleissner F, Jazbutyte V, Fiedler J, Galuppo P, Mayr M, Ertl G, Bauersachs J, Thum T. The endogenous

NO synthase inhibitor asymmetric dimethylarginine impairs angiogenic progenitor cell function in patients with coronary artery disease through a microRNA dependent mechanism. Cardiovasc Res. 2010;87:138–43.
108. Kumarswamy R, Volkmann I, Jazbutyte V, Dangwal S, Park D-H, Thum T. Transforming growth factor-β–induced endothelial-to-mesenchymal transition is partly mediated by microRNA-21. Arterioscler Thromb Vasc Biol. 2012;32(2):361–9.
109. Ji R, Cheng Y, Yue J, Yang J, Liu X, Chen H, Dean DB, Zhang C. MicroRNA expression signature and antisense-mediated depletion reveal an essential role of MicroRNA in vascular neointimal lesion formation. Circ Res. 2007;100(11):1579–88.
110. Anderson ME, Mohler PJ. MicroRNA may have macro effect on sudden death. Nat Med. 2007;13(4):410.
111. Thum T, Galuppo P, Kneitz S, Wolf C, Van Laake L, Engelhardt S, Ertl G, Bauersachs J. 40 MicroRNAs in the human heart: a clue to fetal gene reprogramming in heart failure. Eur J Heart Fail Suppl. 2007;6:1–1.
112. Roy S, Khanna S, Hussain S-RA, Biswas S, Azad A, Rink C, Gnyawali S, Shilo S, Nuovo GJ, Sen CK. MicroRNA expression in response to murine myocardial infarction: miR-21 regulates fibroblast metalloprotease-2 via phosphatase and tensin homologue. Cardiovasc Res. 2009;82(1):21–9.
113. Cheng Y, Ji R, Yue J, Yang J, Liu X, Chen H, Dean DB, Zhang C. MicroRNAs are aberrantly expressed in hypertrophic heart: do they play a role in cardiac hypertrophy? Am J Pathol. 2007;170(6):1831–40.
114. Elmén J, Lindow M, Schütz S, Lawrence M, Petri A, Obad S, Lindholm M, Hedtjärn M, Hansen HF, Berger U. LNA-mediated microRNA silencing in non-human primates. Nature. 2008;452(7189):896.
115. Adam O, Löhfelm B, Thum T, Gupta SK, Puhl S-L, Schäfers H-J, Böhm M, Laufs U. Role of miR-21 in the pathogenesis of atrial fibrosis. Basic Res Cardiol. 2012;107(5):278.
116. Yan M, Chen C, Gong W, Yin Z, Zhou L, Chaugai S, Wang DW. miR-21-3p regulates cardiac hypertrophic response by targeting histone deacetylase-8. Cardiovasc Res. 2014;105(3):340–52.
117. Ikeda S, He A, Kong SW, Lu J, Bejar R, Bodyak N, Lee K-H, Ma Q, Kang PM, Golub TR. MicroRNA-1 negatively regulates expression of the hypertrophy-associated calmodulin and Mef2a genes. Mol Cell Biol. 2009;29(8):2193–204.
118. Care A, Catalucci D, Felicetti F, Bonci D, Addario A, Gallo P, Bang M-L, Segnalini P, Gu Y, Dalton ND. MicroRNA-133 controls cardiac hypertrophy. Nat Med. 2007;13(5):613.
119. Yang B, Lin H, Xiao J, Lu Y, Luo X, Li B, Zhang Y, Xu C, Bai Y, Wang H. The muscle-specific microRNA miR-1 regulates cardiac arrhythmogenic potential by targeting GJA1 and KCNJ2. Nat Med. 2007;13(4):486.
120. Sayed D, Hong C, Chen I-Y, Lypowy J, Abdellatif M. MicroRNAs play an essential role in the development of cardiac hypertrophy. Circ Res. 2007;100(3):416–24.
121. Zhao Y, Ransom JF, Li A, Vedantham V, von Drehle M, Muth AN, Tsuchihashi T, McManus MT, Schwartz RJ, Srivastava D. Dysregulation of cardiogenesis, cardiac conduction, and cell cycle in mice lacking miRNA-1-2. Cell. 2007;129(2):303–17.
122. Costantini DL, Arruda EP, Agarwal P, Kim K-H, Zhu Y, Zhu W, Lebel M, Cheng CW, Park CY, Pierce SA. The homeodomain transcription factor Irx5 establishes the mouse cardiac ventricular repolarization gradient. Cell. 2005;123(2):347–58.
123. Zhao Y, Samal E, Srivastava D. Serum response factor regulates a muscle-specific microRNA that targets Hand2 during cardiogenesis. Nature. 2005;436(7048):214.
124. Karakikes I, Chaanine AH, Kang S, Mukete BN, Jeong D, Zhang S, Hajjar RJ, Lebeche D. Therapeutic cardiac-targeted delivery of miR-1 reverses pressure overload–induced cardiac hypertrophy and attenuates pathological remodeling. J Am Heart Assoc. 2013;2(2):e000078.
125. Da Costa Martins PA, De Windt LJ. MicroRNAs in control of cardiac hypertrophy. Cardiovasc Res. 2012;93(4):563–72.
126. Li Q, Lin X, Yang X, Chang J. NFATc4 is negatively regulated in miR-133a-mediated cardiomyocyte hypertrophic repression. Am J Phys Heart Circ Phys. 2010;298(5):H1340–7.
127. Ren J, Samson WK, Sowers JR. Insulin-like growth factor I as aÈCardiac hormone: physiological and pathophysiological implications in heart disease. J Mol Cell Cardiol. 1999;31(11):2049–61.
128. Elia L, Contu R, Quintavalle M, Varrone F, Chimenti C, Russo MA, Cimino V, De LM, Frustaci A, Catalucci D. Reciprocal regulation of microRNA-1 and insulin-like growth factor-1 signal transduction cascade in cardiac and skeletal muscle in physiological and pathological conditions. Circulation. 2009;120(23):2377–85.
129. Dong D-L, Chen C, Huo R, Wang N, Li Z, Tu Y-J, Hu J-T, Chu X, Huang W, Yang B-F. Reciprocal repression between microRNA-133 and calcineurin regulates cardiac hypertrophy: a novel mechanism for progressive cardiac hypertrophy. Hypertension. 2010;55(4):946–52.
130. Feng B, Chen S, George B, Feng Q, Chakrabarti S. miR133a regulates cardiomyocyte hypertrophy in diabetes. Diabetes Metab Res Rev. 2010;26(1):40–9.
131. Xiao J, Luo X, Lin H, Zhang Y, Lu Y, Wang N, Zhang Y, Yang B, Wang Z. MicroRNA miR-133 represses HERG K+ channel expression contributing to QT prolongation in diabetic hearts. J Biol Chem. 2007;282(17):12363–7.
132. Duisters RF, Tijsen AJ, Schroen B, Leenders JJ, Lentink V, van der Made I, Herias V, van Leeuwen RE, Schellings MW, Barenbrug P. miR-133 and

miR-30 regulate connective tissue growth factor: implications for a role of microRNAs in myocardial matrix remodeling. Circ Res. 2009;104(2):170–8.
133. Luo X, Lin H, Pan Z, Xiao J, Zhang Y, Lu Y, Yang B, Wang Z. Down-regulation of miR-1/miR-133 contributes to re-expression of pacemaker channel genes HCN2 and HCN4 in hypertrophic heart. J Biol Chem. 2008;283(29):20045–52.
134. Hua Y, Zhang Y, Ren J. IGF-1 deficiency resists cardiac hypertrophy and myocardial contractile dysfunction: role of microRNA-1 and microRNA-133a. J Cell Mol Med. 2012;16(1):83–95.
135. Townley-Tilson WD, Callis TE, Wang D. MicroRNAs 1, 133, and 206: critical factors of skeletal and cardiac muscle development, function, and disease. Int J Biochem Cell Biol. 2010;42(8):1252–5.
136. Bagnall RD, Tsoutsman T, Shephard RE, Ritchie W, Semsarian C. Global microRNA profiling of the mouse ventricles during development of severe hypertrophic cardiomyopathy and heart failure. PLoS One. 2012;7(9):e44744.
137. Drawnel FM, Wachten D, Molkentin JD, Maillet M, Aronsen JM, Swift F, Sjaastad I, Liu N, Catalucci D, Mikoshiba K. Mutual antagonism between IP3RII and miRNA-133a regulates calcium signals and cardiac hypertrophy. J Cell Biol. 2012;199(5):783–98.
138. Villar AV, Merino D, Wenner M, Llano M, Cobo M, Montalvo C, García R, Martín-Durán R, Hurlé JM, Hurlé MA. Myocardial gene expression of microRNA-133a and myosin heavy and light chains, in conjunction with clinical parameters, predict regression of left ventricular hypertrophy after valve replacement in patients with aortic stenosis. Heart. 2011;97(14):1132–7.
139. Hogan PG, Chen L, Nardone J, Rao A. Transcriptional regulation by calcium, calcineurin, and NFAT. Genes Dev. 2003;17(18):2205–32.
140. Wang K, Lin Z-Q, Long B, Li J-H, Zhou J, Li P-F. Cardiac hypertrophy is positively regulated by MicroRNA miR-23a. J Biol Chem. 2012;287(1):589–99.
141. Guo J, Gertsberg Z, Ozgen N, Steinberg SF. p66Shc links α1-adrenergic receptors to a reactive oxygen species-dependent AKT-FOXO3A phosphorylation pathway in cardiomyocytes. Circ Res. 2009;104(5):660–9.
142. van Rooij E, Sutherland LB, Qi X, Richardson JA, Hill J, Olson EN. Control of stress-dependent cardiac growth and gene expression by a microRNA. Science. 2007;316(5824):575–9.
143. Lin Z, Murtaza I, Wang K, Jiao J, Gao J, Li P-F. miR-23a functions downstream of NFATc3 to regulate cardiac hypertrophy. Proc Natl Acad Sci. 2009;106(29):12103–8.
144. Yang J, Nie Y, Wang F, Hou J, Cong X, Hu S, Chen X. Reciprocal regulation of miR-23a and lysophosphatidic acid receptor signaling in cardiomyocyte hypertrophy. Biochim Biophys Acta (BBA)-Mol Cell Biol Lipids. 2013;1831(8):1386–94.
145. Van Rooij E, Sutherland LB, Thatcher JE, DiMaio JM, Naseem RH, Marshall WS, Hill JA, Olson EN. Dysregulation of microRNAs after myocardial infarction reveals a role of miR-29 in cardiac fibrosis. Proc Natl Acad Sci. 2008;105(35):13027–32.
146. Boon RA, Seeger T, Heydt S, Fischer A, Hergenreider E, Horrevoets AJ, Vinciguerra M, Rosenthal N, Sciacca S, Pilato M. MicroRNA-29 in aortic dilation: implications for aneurysm formation. Circ Res. 2011;109(10):1115–9.
147. Bonauer A, Carmona G, Iwasaki M, Mione M, Koyanagi M, Fischer A, Burchfield J, Fox H, Doebele C, Ohtani K. MicroRNA-92a controls angiogenesis and functional recovery of ischemic tissues in mice. Science. 2009;324(5935):1710–3.
148. Yang WJ, Yang DD, Na S, Sandusky GE, Zhang Q, Zhao G. Dicer is required for embryonic angiogenesis during mouse development. J Biol Chem. 2005;280(10):9330–5.
149. Suárez Y, Fernández-Hernando C, Yu J, Gerber SA, Harrison KD, Pober JS, Iruela-Arispe ML, Merkenschlager M, Sessa WC. Dicer-dependent endothelial microRNAs are necessary for postnatal angiogenesis. Proc Natl Acad Sci. 2008;105(37):14082–7.
150. Fish JE, Santoro MM, Morton SU, Yu S, Yeh R-F, Wythe JD, Ivey KN, Bruneau BG, Stainier DY, Srivastava D. miR-126 regulates angiogenic signaling and vascular integrity. Dev Cell. 2008;15(2):272–84.
151. van Solingen C, Seghers L, Bijkerk R, Duijs JM, Roeten MK, van Oeveren-Rietdijk AM, Baelde HJ, Monge M, Vos JB, de Boer HC. Antagomir-mediated silencing of endothelial cell specific microRNA-126 impairs ischemia-induced angiogenesis. J Cell Mol Med. 2009;13(8a):1577–85.
152. Wang S, Aurora AB, Johnson BA, Qi X, McAnally J, Hill JA, Richardson JA, Bassel-Duby R, Olson EN. The endothelial-specific microRNA miR-126 governs vascular integrity and angiogenesis. Dev Cell. 2008;15(2):261–71.
153. Bernardo BC, Gao X-M, Winbanks CE, Boey EJ, Tham YK, Kiriazis H, Gregorevic P, Obad S, Kauppinen S, Du X-J. Therapeutic inhibition of the miR-34 family attenuates pathological cardiac remodeling and improves heart function. Proc Natl Acad Sci. 2012;109(43):17615–20.
154. Nalls D, Tang S-N, Rodova M, Srivastava RK, Shankar S. Targeting epigenetic regulation of miR-34a for treatment of pancreatic cancer by inhibition of pancreatic cancer stem cells. PLoS One. 2011;6(8):e24099.
155. Zemljic-Harpf AE, Miller JC, Henderson SA, Wright AT, Manso AM, Elsherif L, Dalton ND, Thor AK, Perkins GA, McCulloch AD. Cardiac-myocyte-specific excision of the vinculin gene disrupts cellular junctions, causing sudden death or dilated cardiomyopathy. Mol Cell Biol. 2007;27(21):7522–37.

156. Okamura Y, Saga Y. Pofut1 is required for the proper localization of the notch receptor during mouse development. Mech Dev. 2008;125(8):663–73.
157. Nakagawa Y, Takamatsu H, Okuno T, Kang S, Nojima S, Kimura T, Kataoka TR, Ikawa M, Toyofuku T, Katayama I. Identification of semaphorin 4B as a negative regulator of basophil-mediated immune responses. J Immunol. 2011;186(5):2881–8.
158. Molkentin JD. Calcineurin and beyond: cardiac hypertrophic signaling. Circ Res. 2000;87(9):731–8.
159. Takeda Y, Yoneda T, Demura M, Usukura M, Mabuchi H. Calcineurin inhibition attenuates mineralocorticoid-induced cardiac hypertrophy. Circulation. 2002;105(6):677–9.
160. Xing W, Zhang T-C, Cao D, Wang Z, Antos CL, Li S, Wang Y, Olson EN, Wang D-Z. Myocardin induces cardiomyocyte hypertrophy. Circ Res. 2006;98(8):1089–97.
161. Alcendor RR, Kirshenbaum LA, Imai S-i, Vatner SF, Sadoshima J. Silent information regulator 2α, a longevity factor and class III histone deacetylase, is an essential endogenous apoptosis inhibitor in cardiac myocytes. Circ Res. 2004;95(10):971–80.
162. Rane S, He M, Sayed D, Yan L, Vatner D, Abdellatif M. An antagonism between the AKT and beta-adrenergic signaling pathways mediated through their reciprocal effects on miR-199a-5p. Cell Signal. 2010;22(7):1054–62.
163. Haghikia A, Missol-Kolka E, Tsikas D, Venturini L, Brundiers S, Castoldi M, Muckenthaler MU, Eder M, Stapel B, Thum T. Signal transducer and activator of transcription 3-mediated regulation of miR-199a-5p links cardiomyocyte and endothelial cell function in the heart: a key role for ubiquitin-conjugating enzymes. Eur Heart J. 2010;32(10):1287–97.
164. da Costa Martins PA, Salic K, Gladka MM, Armand A-S, Leptidis S, El Azzouzi H, Hansen A, Coenen-de Roo CJ, Bierhuizen MF, Van Der Nagel R. MicroRNA-199b targets the nuclear kinase Dyrk1a in an auto-amplification loop promoting calcineurin/NFAT signalling. Nat Cell Biol. 2010;12(12):1220.
165. Ali T, Shaheen F, Mahmud M, Waheed H, Jan MI, Javed Q, Murtaza I. Serotonin-promoted elevation of ROS levels may lead to cardiac pathologies in diabetic rat. Arch Oral Biol. 2015;67(2):655–61.
166. Jan MI, Khan RA, Ali T, Bilal M, Bo L, Sajid A, Malik A, Urehman N, Waseem N, Nawab J. Interplay of mitochondria apoptosis regulatory factors and microRNAs in valvular heart disease. Arch Biochem Biophys. 2017;633:50–7.
167. Murtaza I, Wang H-X, Feng X, Alenina N, Bader M, Prabhakar BS, Li P-F. Down-regulation of catalase and oxidative modification of protein kinase CK2 lead to the failure of apoptosis repressor with caspase recruitment domain to inhibit cardiomyocyte hypertrophy. J Biol Chem. 2008;283(10):5996–6004.
168. Murtaza I, Wang H-X, Mushtaq S, Javed Q, Li P-F. Interplay of phosphorylated apoptosis repressor with CARD, casein Kinase-2 and reactive oxygen species in regulating Endothelin-1–induced Cardiomyocyte hypertrophy. Iran J Basic Med Sci. 2013;16(8):928.
169. Ali T, Mushtaq I, Maryam S, Farhan A, Saba K, Jan MI, Sultan A, Anees M, Duygu B, Hamera S. Interplay of N acetyl cysteine and melatonin in regulating oxidative stress-induced cardiac hypertrophic factors and microRNAs. Arch Biochem Biophys. 2019;661:56–65.
170. Caporali A, Meloni M, Völlenkle C, Bonci D, Sala-Newby GB, Addis R, Spinetti G, Losa S, Masson R, Baker AH. Deregulation of microRNA-503 contributes to diabetes mellitus–induced impairment of endothelial function and reparative angiogenesis after limb ischemia. Circulation. 2011;123(3):282–91.
171. McArthur K, Feng B, Wu Y, Chen S, Chakrabarti S. MicroRNA-200b regulates vascular endothelial growth factor–mediated alterations in diabetic retinopathy. Diabetes. 2011;60(4):1314–23.
172. Porrello ER, Mahmoud AI, Simpson E, Hill JA, Richardson JA, Olson EN, Sadek HA. Transient regenerative potential of the neonatal mouse heart. Science. 2011;331(6020):1078–80.
173. Van Rooij E, Sutherland LB, Liu N, Williams AH, McAnally J, Gerard RD, Richardson JA, Olson EN. A signature pattern of stress-responsive microRNAs that can evoke cardiac hypertrophy and heart failure. Proc Natl Acad Sci. 2006;103(48):18255–60.
174. Thum T. MicroRNA therapeutics in cardiovascular medicine. EMBO Mol Med. 2012;4(1):3–14.
175. Marquart TJ, Allen RM, Ory DS, Baldán Á. miR-33 links SREBP-2 induction to repression of sterol transporters. Proc Natl Acad Sci. 2010;107(27):12228–32.
176. Boettger T, Beetz N, Kostin S, Schneider J, Krüger M, Hein L, Braun T. Acquisition of the contractile phenotype by murine arterial smooth muscle cells depends on the Mir143/145 gene cluster. J Clin Invest. 2009;119(9):2634–47.
177. Thom T. American Heart Association statistics committee and stroke statistics subcommittee: heart disease and stroke statistical-2006 update: a report from the American Heart Association statistics committee and stroke statistics subcommittee. Circulation. 2006;113:e85–e151.
178. Freeman RV, Otto CM. Spectrum of calcific aortic valve disease: pathogenesis, disease progression, and treatment strategies. Circulation. 2005;111(24):3316–26.
179. Lloyd-Jones D, Adams R, Brown T, Carnethon M, Dai S, De Simone G, Ferguson T, Ford E, Furie K, Gillespie C. American Heart Association statistics committee and stroke statistics subcommittee. Executive summary: heart disease and stroke statistics–2010 update: a report from the American Heart Association. Circulation. 2010;121(7):948–54.
180. Butcher JT, Penrod AM, García AJ, Nerem RM. Unique morphology and focal adhesion devel-

opment of valvular endothelial cells in static and fluid flow environments. Arterioscler Thromb Vasc Biol. 2004;24(8):1429–34.
181. Nigam V, Srivastava D. Notch1 represses osteogenic pathways in aortic valve cells. J Mol Cell Cardiol. 2009;47(6):828–34.
182. Cushing MC, Mariner PD, Liao J-T, Sims EA, Anseth KS. Fibroblast growth factor represses Smad-mediated myofibroblast activation in aortic valvular interstitial cells. FASEB J. 2008;22(6):1769–77.
183. Zhang M, Liu X, Zhang X, Song Z, Han L, He Y, Xu Z. MicroRNA-30b is a multifunctional regulator of aortic valve interstitial cells. J Thorac Cardiovasc Surg. 2014;147(3):1073–80. e1072
184. Speer MY, Yang H-Y, Brabb T, Leaf E, Look A, Lin W-L, Frutkin A, Dichek D, Giachelli CM. Smooth muscle cells give rise to osteochondrogenic precursors and chondrocytes in calcifying arteries. Circ Res. 2009;104(6):733–41.
185. Leopold JA. Vascular calcification: mechanisms of vascular smooth muscle cell calcification. Trends Cardiovasc Med. 2015;25(4):267–74.
186. Nakashima A, Katagiri T, Tamura M. Cross-talk between Wnt and bone morphogenetic protein 2 (BMP-2) signaling in differentiation pathway of C2C12 myoblasts. J Biol Chem. 2005;280(45):37660–8.
187. Itoh T, Takeda S, Akao Y. MicroRNA-208 modulates BMP-2-stimulated mouse preosteoblast differentiation by directly targeting V-ets erythroblastosis virus E26 oncogene homolog 1. J Biol Chem. 2010;285(36):27745–52.
188. Hu R, Liu W, Li H, Yang L, Chen C, Xia Z-Y, Guo L-J, Xie H, Zhou H-D, Wu X-P. A Runx2/miR-3960/miR-2861 regulatory feedback loop during mouse osteoblast differentiation. J Biol Chem. 2011;286(14):12328–39.
189. Carabello BA. Modern management of mitral stenosis. Circulation. 2005;112(3):432–7.
190. Cooley N, Cowley MJ, Lin RC, Marasco S, Wong C, Kaye DM, Dart AM, Woodcock EA. Influence of atrial fibrillation on microRNA expression profiles in left and right atria from patients with valvular heart disease. Physiol Genomics. 2011;44(3):211–9.
191. Nishi H, Sakaguchi T, Miyagawa S, Yoshikawa Y, Fukushima S, Saito S, Ueno T, Kuratani T, Sawa Y. Impact of microRNA expression in human atrial tissue in patients with atrial fibrillation undergoing cardiac surgery. PLoS One. 2013;8(9):e73397.
192. Yetkin E, Waltenberger J. Molecular and cellular mechanisms of aortic stenosis. Int J Cardiol. 2009;135(1):4–13.
193. Villar AV, García R, Merino D, Llano M, Cobo M, Montalvo C, Martín-Durán R, Hurlé MA, Nistal JF. Myocardial and circulating levels of microRNA-21 reflect left ventricular fibrosis in aortic stenosis patients. Int J Cardiol. 2013;167(6):2875–81.
194. Cheng Y, Zhu P, Yang J, Liu X, Dong S, Wang X, Chun B, Zhuang J, Zhang C. Ischaemic preconditioning-regulated miR-21 protects heart against ischaemia/reperfusion injury via anti-apoptosis through its target PDCD4. Cardiovasc Res. 2010;87(3):431–9.
195. Gabriely G, Wurdinger T, Kesari S, Esau CC, Burchard J, Linsley PS, Krichevsky AM. MicroRNA 21 promotes glioma invasion by targeting matrix metalloproteinase regulators. Mol Cell Biol. 2008;28(17):5369–80.
196. Kassiri Z, Defamie V, Hariri M, Oudit GY, Anthwal S, Dawood F, Liu P, Khokha R. Simultaneous transforming growth factor β-tumor necrosis factor activation and cross-talk cause aberrant remodeling response and myocardial fibrosis in Timp3-deficient heart. J Biol Chem. 2009;284(43):29893–904.
197. Yao Q, Cao S, Li C, Mengesha A, Kong B, Wei M. Micro-RNA-21 regulates TGF-β-induced myofibroblast differentiation by targeting PDCD4 in tumor-stroma interaction. Int J Cancer. 2011;128(8):1783–92.
198. Duffy HS. The ever shrinking world of cardiac ion channel remodeling: the role of microRNAs in heart disease. Heart Rhythm. 2009;6(12):1810.
199. Liu H, Chen G-x, Liang M-y, Qin H, Rong J, Yao J-p, Wu Z-k. Atrial fibrillation alters the microRNA expression profiles of the left atria of patients with mitral stenosis. BMC Cardiovasc Disord. 2014;14(1):10.
200. Girmatsion Z, Biliczki P, Bonauer A, Wimmer-Greinecker G, Scherer M, Moritz A, Bukowska A, Goette A, Nattel S, Hohnloser SH. Changes in microRNA-1 expression and IK1 up-regulation in human atrial fibrillation. Heart Rhythm. 2009;6(12):1802–9.
201. Di Leva G, Calin GA, Croce CM. MicroRNAs: fundamental facts and involvement in human diseases. Birth Defects Res C Embryo Today. 2006;78(2):180–9.
202. Griffiths-Jones S. The microRNA registry. Nucleic Acids Res. 2004;32(suppl_1):D109–11.
203. Ikeda S, Kong SW, Lu J, Bisping E, Zhang H, Allen PD, Golub TR, Pieske B, Pu WT. Altered microRNA expression in human heart disease. Physiol Genomics. 2007;31(3):367–73.
204. Mowbray AL, Kang D-H, Rhee SG, Kang SW, Jo H. Laminar shear stress up-regulates peroxiredoxins (PRX) in endothelial cells PRX 1 as a mechanosensitive antioxidant. J Biol Chem. 2008;283(3):1622–7.
205. Holliday CJ, Ankeny RF, Jo H, Nerem RM. Discovery of shear-and side-specific mRNAs and miRNAs in human aortic valvular endothelial cells. Am J Phys Heart Circ Phys. 2011;301(3):H856–67.
206. Caroli A, Cardillo MT, Galea R, Biasucci LM. Potential therapeutic role of microRNAs in ischemic heart disease. J Cardiol. 2013;61(5):315–20.
207. Li L-M, Hou D-X, Guo Y-L, Yang J-W, Liu Y, Zhang C-Y, Zen K. Role of microRNA-214–targeting phosphatase and tensin homolog in advanced glycation

end product-induced apoptosis delay in monocytes. J Immunol. 2011;186(4):2552–60.
208. van Mil A, Grundmann S, Goumans M-J, Lei Z, Oerlemans MI, Jaksani S, Doevendans PA, Sluijter JP. MicroRNA-214 inhibits angiogenesis by targeting quaking and reducing angiogenic growth factor release. Cardiovasc Res. 2012;93(4):655–65.
209. Taylor RS, Brown A, Ebrahim S, Jolliffe J, Noorani H, Rees K, Skidmore B, Stone JA, Thompson DR, Oldridge N. Exercise-based rehabilitation for patients with coronary heart disease: systematic review and meta-analysis of randomized controlled trials. Am J Med. 2004;116(10):682–92.
210. Wisløff U, Loennechen JP, Currie S, Smith GL, Ellingsen Ø. Aerobic exercise reduces cardiomyocyte hypertrophy and increases contractility, Ca2+ sensitivity and SERCA-2 in rat after myocardial infarction. Cardiovasc Res. 2002;54(1):162–74.
211. Cardin S, Guasch E, Luo X, Naud P, Le Quang K, Shi Y, Tardif J-C, Comtois P, Nattel S. Role for MicroRNA-21 in atrial profibrillatory fibrotic remodeling associated with experimental postinfarction heart failure. Circ Arrhythm Electrophysiol. 2012;5(5):1027–35.
212. Ardite E, Perdiguero E, Vidal B, Gutarra S, Serrano AL, Muñoz-Cánoves P. PAI-1–regulated miR-21 defines a novel age-associated fibrogenic pathway in muscular dystrophy. J Cell Biol. 2012;196(1):163–75.
213. Yuan J, Chen H, Ge D, Xu Y, Xu H, Yang Y, Gu M, Zhou Y, Zhu J, Ge T. Mir-21 promotes cardiac fibrosis after myocardial infarction via targeting Smad7. Cell Physiol Biochem. 2017;42(6):2207–19.
214. Sayed D, He M, Hong C, Gao S, Rane S, Yang Z, Abdellatif M. MicroRNA-21 is a downstream effector of AKT that mediates its antiapoptotic effects via suppression of Fas ligand. J Biol Chem. 2010;285(26):20281–90.
215. Brudecki L, Ferguson DA, McCall CE, El Gazzar M. MicroRNA-146a and RBM4 form a negative feed-forward loop that disrupts cytokine mRNA translation following TLR4 responses in human THP-1 monocytes. Immunol Cell Biol. 2013;91(8):532–40.
216. Huang W, Tian S-S, Hang P-Z, Sun C, Guo J, Du Z-M. Combination of microRNA-21 and microRNA-146a attenuates cardiac dysfunction and apoptosis during acute myocardial infarction in mice. Mol Ther-Nucleic Acids. 2016;5:e296.
217. Hullinger TG, Montgomery RL, Seto AG, Dickinson BA, Semus HM, Lynch JM, Dalby CM, Robinson K, Stack C, Latimer PA. Inhibition of miR-15 protects against cardiac ischemic injury. Circ Res. 2012;110(1):71–81.
218. Boon RA, Dimmeler S. MicroRNAs in myocardial infarction. Nat Rev Cardiol. 2015;12(3):135.
219. Qian L, Van Laake LW, Huang Y, Liu S, Wendland MF, Srivastava D. miR-24 inhibits apoptosis and represses Bim in mouse cardiomyocytes. J Exp Med. 2011;208(3):549–60.
220. Fiedler J, Jazbutyte V, Kirchmaier BC, Gupta SK, Lorenzen J, Hartmann D, Galuppo P, Kneitz S, Pena JT, Sohn-Lee C. MicroRNA-24 regulates vascularity after myocardial infarction. Circulation. 2011;124(6):720–30.
221. Port JD, Walker LA, Polk J, Nunley K, Buttrick PM, Sucharov CC. Temporal expression of miRNAs and mRNAs in a mouse model of myocardial infarction. Physiol Genomics. 2011;43(19):1087–95.
222. Park S-Y, Lee JH, Ha M, Nam J-W, Kim VN. miR-29 miRNAs activate p53 by targeting p85α and CDC42. Nat Struct Mol Biol. 2009;16(1):23.
223. Ye Y, Hu Z, Lin Y, Zhang C, Perez-Polo JR. Downregulation of microRNA-29 by antisense inhibitors and a PPAR-γ agonist protects against myocardial ischaemia–reperfusion injury. Cardiovasc Res. 2010;87(3):535–44.
224. Doebele C, Bonauer A, Fischer A, Scholz A, Reiss Y, Urbich C, Hofmann W-K, Zeiher AM, Dimmeler S. Members of the microRNA-17-92 cluster exhibit a cell-intrinsic antiangiogenic function in endothelial cells. Blood. 2010;115(23):4944–50.
225. Harris TA, Yamakuchi M, Ferlito M, Mendell JT, Lowenstein CJ. MicroRNA-126 regulates endothelial expression of vascular cell adhesion molecule 1. Proc Natl Acad Sci. 2008;105(5):1516–21.
226. Long G, Wang F, Duan Q, Chen F, Yang S, Gong W, Wang Y, Chen C, Wang DW. Human circulating microRNA-1 and microRNA-126 as potential novel indicators for acute myocardial infarction. Int J Biol Sci. 2012;8(6):811.
227. López-Novoa JM, Bernabeu C. The physiological role of endoglin in the cardiovascular system. Am J Phys Heart Circ Phys. 2010;299(4):H959–74.
228. Nattel S. Targeting MicroRNA-208a to suppress adverse postmyocardial infarction remodelling related to RNA activation of endoglin gene expression. Can J Cardiol. 2015;31(5):591–2.
229. Liu N, Olson EN. MicroRNA regulatory networks in cardiovascular development. Dev Cell. 2010;18(4):510–25.
230. Liu N, Bezprozvannaya S, Williams AH, Qi X, Richardson JA, Bassel-Duby R, Olson EN. microRNA-133a regulates cardiomyocyte proliferation and suppresses smooth muscle gene expression in the heart. Genes Dev. 2008;22(23):3242–54.
231. Zile MR, Mehurg SM, Arroyo JE, Stroud RE, DeSantis SM, Spinale FG. Relationship between the temporal profile of plasma microRNA and left ventricular remodeling in patients after myocardial infarction. Circ Cardiovasc Genet. 2011;4(6):614–9.
232. Wang K-C, Garmire LX, Young A, Nguyen P, Trinh A, Subramaniam S, Wang N, Shyy JY, Li Y-S, Chien S. Role of microRNA-23b in flow-regulation of Rb phosphorylation and endothelial cell growth. Proc Natl Acad Sci. 2010;107(7):3234–9.
233. Devaux Y, Vausort M, Goretti E, Nazarov PV, Azuaje F, Gilson G, Corsten MF, Schroen B, Lair M-L, Heymans S. Use of circulating microRNAs to

diagnose acute myocardial infarction. Clin Chem. 2012;58(3):559–67.
234. Oury C, Servais L, Bouznad N, Hego A, Nchimi A, Lancellotti P. MicroRNAs in valvular heart diseases: potential role as markers and actors of valvular and cardiac remodeling. Int J Mol Sci. 2016;17(7):1120.
235. Olivieri F, Antonicelli R, Lorenzi M, D'Alessandra Y, Lazzarini R, Santini G, Spazzafumo L, Lisa R, La Sala L, Galeazzi R. Diagnostic potential of circulating miR-499-5p in elderly patients with acute non ST-elevation myocardial infarction. Int J Cardiol. 2013;167(2):531–6.
236. Rossi AC, Mammucari C, Argentini C, Reggiani C, Schiaffino S. Two novel/ancient myosins in mammalian skeletal muscles: MYH14/7b and MYH15 are expressed in extraocular muscles and muscle spindles. J Physiol. 2010;588(2):353–64.
237. Wilson KD, Hu S, Venkatasubrahmanyam S, Fu J-D, Sun N, Abilez OJ, Baugh JJ, Jia F, Ghosh Z, Li RA. Dynamic microRNA expression programs during cardiac differentiation of human embryonic stem cells: role for miR-499. Circ Cardiovasc Genet. 2010;3(5):426–35.
238. Cheng C, Wang Q, You W, Chen M, Xia J. MiRNAs as biomarkers of myocardial infarction: a meta-analysis. PLoS One. 2014;9(2):e88566.
239. Zhang J, Jiao J, Cermelli S, Muir K, Jung KH, Zou R, Rashid A, Gagea M, Zabludoff S, Kalluri R. miR-21 inhibition reduces liver fibrosis and prevents tumor development by inducing apoptosis of CD24+ progenitor cells. Cancer Res. 2015;75(9):1859–67.
240. Wang J-X, Jiao J-Q, Li Q, Long B, Wang K, Liu J-P, Li Y-R, Li P-F. miR-499 regulates mitochondrial dynamics by targeting calcineurin and dynamin-related protein-1. Nat Med. 2011;17(1):71.
241. Hosoda T, Zheng H, Cabral-da-Silva M, Sanada F, Ide-Iwata N, Ogórek B, Ferreira-Martins J, Arranto C, D'Amario D, Del Monte F. Human cardiac stem cell differentiation is regulated by a mircrine mechanism. Circulation. 2011;12:1287–96.
242. Li K, Lin T, Chen L, Wang N. MicroRNA-93 elevation after myocardial infarction is cardiac protective. Med Hypotheses. 2017;106:23–5.
243. Bayoumi AS, Teoh J-P, Aonuma T, Yuan Z, Ruan X, Tang Y, Su H, Weintraub NL, Kim I-M. MicroRNA-532 protects the heart in acute myocardial infarction, and represses prss23, a positive regulator of endothelial-to-mesenchymal transition. Cardiovasc Res. 2017;113(13):1603–14.
244. Sun C, Liu H, Guo J, Yu Y, Yang D, He F, Du Z. MicroRNA-98 negatively regulates myocardial infarction-induced apoptosis by down-regulating Fas and caspase-3. Sci Rep. 2017;7(1):7460.
245. Zhang X, Wang X, Zhu H, Zhu C, Wang Y, Pu WT, Jegga AG, Fan G-C. Synergistic effects of the GATA-4-mediated miR-144/451 cluster in protection against simulated ischemia/reperfusion-induced cardiomyocyte death. J Mol Cell Cardiol. 2010;49(5):841–50.
246. Zhang Z, Li H, Chen S, Li Y, Cui Z, Ma J. MicroRNA-122 regulates caspase-8 and promotes the apoptosis of mouse cardiomyocytes. Braz J Med Biol Res. 2017;50(2):e5760.
247. Mishima Y, Stahlhut C, Giraldez AJ. miR-1-2 gets to the heart of the matter. Cell. 2007;129(2):247–9.
248. Ai J, Zhang R, Li Y, Pu J, Lu Y, Jiao J, Li K, Yu B, Li Z, Wang R. Circulating microRNA-1 as a potential novel biomarker for acute myocardial infarction. Biochem Biophys Res Commun. 2010;391(1):73–7.
249. Fichtlscherer S, Zeiher AM, Dimmeler S. Circulating microRNAs: biomarkers or mediators of cardiovascular diseases? Arterioscler Thromb Vasc Biol. 2011;31(11):2383–90.
250. Han M, Toli J, Abdellatif M. MicroRNAs in the cardiovascular system. Curr Opin Cardiol. 2011;26(3):181–9.
251. Liu J, Sun F, Wang Y, Yang W, Xiao H, Zhang Y, Lu R, Zhu H, Zhuang Y, Pan Z. Suppression of microRNA-16 protects against acute myocardial infarction by reversing beta2-adrenergic receptor down-regulation in rats. Oncotarget. 2017;8(12):20122.
252. Pan Z, Sun X, Shan H, Wang N, Wang J, Ren J, Feng S, Xie L, Lu C, Yuan Y. MicroRNA-101 inhibited postinfarct cardiac fibrosis and improved left ventricular compliance via the FBJ osteosarcoma oncogene/transforming growth factor-β1 pathway. Circulation. 2012;126(7):840–50.
253. Shen Y, Shen Z, Miao L, Xin X, Lin S, Zhu Y, Guo W, Zhu YZ. miRNA-30 family inhibition protects against cardiac ischemic injury by regulating cystathionine-γ-lyase expression. Antioxid Redox Signal. 2015;22(3):224–40.
254. Gupta SK, Foinquinos A, Thum S, Remke J, Zimmer K, Bauters C, de Groote P, Boon RA, de Windt LJ, Preissl S. Preclinical development of a microRNA-based therapy for elderly patients with myocardial infarction. J Am Coll Cardiol. 2016;68(14):1557–71.
255. Fan ZG, Qu XL, Chu P, Gao YL, Gao XF, Chen SL, Tian NL. MicroRNA-210 promotes angiogenesis in acute myocardial infarction. Mol Med Rep. 2018;17(4):5658–65.
256. Fan F, Sun A, Zhao H, Liu X, Zhang W, Jin X, Wang C, Ma X, Shen C, Zou Y. MicroRNA-34a promotes cardiomyocyte apoptosis post myocardial infarction through down-regulating aldehyde dehydrogenase 2. Curr Pharm Des. 2013;19(27):4865–73.
257. Fan G-C, Ren X, Qian J, Yuan Q, Nicolaou P, Wang Y, Jones WK, Chu G, Kranias EG. Novel cardioprotective role of a small heat-shock protein, Hsp20, against ischemia/reperfusion injury. Circulation. 2005;111(14):1792–9.
258. Wu Z, Qi Y, Guo Z, Li P, Zhou D. miR-613 suppresses ischemia-reperfusion-induced cardiomyocyte apoptosis by targeting the programmed cell death 10 gene. Biosci Trends. 2016;10(4):251–7.
259. Abonnenc M, Nabeebaccus AA, Mayr U, Barallobre-Barreiro J, Dong X, Cuello F, Sur S, Drozdov I, Langley SR, Lu R. Extracellular matrix secretion

by cardiac fibroblasts: role of microRNA-29b and microRNA-30c. Circ Res. 2013;113(10):1138–47.
260. Zhang Y, Huang X-R, Wei L-H, Chung AC, Yu C-M, Lan H-Y. miR-29b as a therapeutic agent for angiotensin II-induced cardiac fibrosis by targeting TGF-β/Smad3 signaling. Mol Ther. 2014;22(5):974–85.
261. Lorenzen JM, Schauerte C, Hübner A, Kölling M, Martino F, Scherf K, Batkai S, Zimmer K, Foinquinos A, Kaucsar T. Osteopontin is indispensible for AP1-mediated angiotensin II-related miR-21 transcription during cardiac fibrosis. Eur Heart J. 2015;36(32):2184–96.
262. Vegter EL, van der Meer P, de Windt LJ, Pinto YM, Voors AA. MicroRNAs in heart failure: from biomarker to target for therapy. Eur J Heart Fail. 2016;18(5):457–68.
263. Bujak M, Frangogiannis NG. The role of TGF-β signaling in myocardial infarction and cardiac remodeling. Cardiovasc Res. 2007;74(2):184–95.
264. Van Rooij E, Olson EN. Searching for miR-acles in cardiac fibrosis. Am Heart Assoc; 2009;104(2):138–40.
265. Zhu H, Fan G-C. Role of microRNAs in the reperfused myocardium towards post-infarct remodelling. Cardiovasc Res. 2011;94(2):284–92.
266. Jan MI, Khan RA, Malik A, Ali T, Bilal M, Bo L, Sajid A, Urehman N, Waseem N, Nawab J. Data of expression status of miR-29a and its putative target mitochondrial apoptosis regulatory gene DRP1 upon miR-15a and miR-214 inhibition. Data Brief. 2018;16:1000–4.
267. Ke Z-P, Xu P, Shi Y, Gao A-M. MicroRNA-93 inhibits ischemia-reperfusion induced cardiomyocyte apoptosis by targeting PTEN. Oncotarget. 2016;7(20):28796.
268. He S, Liu P, Jian Z, Li J, Zhu Y, Feng Z, Xiao Y. miR-138 protects cardiomyocytes from hypoxia-induced apoptosis via MLK3/JNK/c-jun pathway. Biochem Biophys Res Commun. 2013;441(4):763–9.
269. Wang J, Liew OW, Richards AM, Chen Y-T. Overview of microRNAs in cardiac hypertrophy, fibrosis, and apoptosis. Int J Mol Sci. 2016;17(5):749.
270. Song C-L, Liu B, Diao H-Y, Shi Y-F, Zhang J-C, Li Y-X, Liu N, Yu Y-P, Wang G, Wang J-P. Downregulation of microRNA-320 suppresses cardiomyocyte apoptosis and protects against myocardial ischemia and reperfusion injury by targeting IGF-1. Oncotarget. 2016;7(26):39740.
271. Liang W, Guo J, Li J, Bai C, Dong Y. Downregulation of miR-122 attenuates hypoxia/reoxygenation (H/R)-induced myocardial cell apoptosis by upregulating GATA-4. Biochem Biophys Res Commun. 2016;478(3):1416–22.
272. Zou Y, Liu W, Zhang J, Xiang D. miR-153 regulates apoptosis and autophagy of cardiomyocytes by targeting Mcl-1. Mol Med Rep. 2016;14(1):1033–9.
273. Wang J-X, Gao J, Ding S-L, Wang K, Jiao J-Q, Wang Y, Sun T, Zhou L-Y, Long B, Zhang X-J. Oxidative modification of miR-184 enables it to target Bcl-xL and Bcl-w. Mol Cell. 2015;59(1):50–61.
274. Bo L, Su-Ling D, Fang L, Lu-Yu Z, Tao A, Stefan D, Kun W, Pei-Feng L. Autophagic program is regulated by miR-325. Cell Death Differ. 2014;21(6):967.
275. Wang K, Liu F, Zhou L, Ding S, Long B, Liu C, Sun T, Fan Y, Sun L, Li P. miR-874 regulates myocardial necrosis by targeting caspase-8. Cell Death Dis. 2013;4(7):e709.
276. Higashi K, Yamada Y, Minatoguchi S, Baba S, Iwasa M, Kanamori H, Kawasaki M, Nishigaki K, Takemura G, Kumazaki M. MicroRNA-145 repairs infarcted myocardium by accelerating cardiomyocyte autophagy. Am J Phys Heart Circ Phys. 2015;309(11):H1813–26.
277. Chen Y-W, Chou H-C, Lin S-T, Chen Y-H, Chang Y-J, Chen L, Chan H-L. Cardioprotective effects of quercetin in cardiomyocyte under ischemia/reperfusion injury. Evid-Based Complement Altern Med. 2013;2013:1–16.
278. Pandey R, Yang Y, Jackson L, Ahmed RP. MicroRNAs regulating meis1 expression and inducing cardiomyocyte proliferation. Cardiovasc Reg Med. 2016;3:e1468.
279. Eulalio A, Mano M, Dal Ferro M, Zentilin L, Sinagra G, Zacchigna S, Giacca M. Functional screening identifies miRNAs inducing cardiac regeneration. Nature. 2012;492(7429):376.
280. Liang D, Li J, Wu Y, Zhen L, Li C, Qi M, Wang L, Deng F, Huang J, Lv F. miRNA-204 drives cardiomyocyte proliferation via targeting Jarid2. Int J Cardiol. 2015;201:38–48.
281. Porrello ER, Mahmoud AI, Simpson E, Johnson BA, Grinsfelder D, Canseco D, Mammen PP, Rothermel BA, Olson EN, Sadek HA. Regulation of neonatal and adult mammalian heart regeneration by the miR-15 family. Proc Natl Acad Sci. 2013;110(1):187–92.
282. Yin VP, Lepilina A, Smith A, Poss KD. Regulation of zebrafish heart regeneration by miR-133. Dev Biol. 2012;365(2):319–27.
283. Katz MG, Fargnoli AS, Kendle AP, Hajjar RJ, Bridges CR. The role of microRNAs in cardiac development and regenerative capacity. Am J Phys Heart Circ Phys. 2015;310(5):H528–41.
284. Tao G, Wang J, Martin JF. Small RNA: from development to regeneration. Sci Transl Med. 2015;7:212.
285. Tian Y, Liu Y, Wang T, Zhou N, Kong J, Chen L, Snitow M, Morley M, Li D, Petrenko N. A microRNA-hippo pathway that promotes cardiomyocyte proliferation and cardiac regeneration in mice. Sci Transl Med. 2015;7(279):279ra238.
286. Camelliti P, Borg TK, Kohl P. Structural and functional characterisation of cardiac fibroblasts. Cardiovasc Res. 2005;65(1):40–51.
287. Jayawardena TM, Egemnazarov B, Finch EA, Zhang L, Payne JA, Pandya K, Zhang Z, Rosenberg P, Mirotsou M, Dzau VJ. MicroRNA-mediated in vitro and in vivo direct reprogramming of car-

diac fibroblasts to cardiomyocytes. Circ Res. 2012;110(11):1465–73.
288. Santulli G, Iaccarino G, De Luca N, Trimarco B, Condorelli G. Atrial fibrillation and microRNAs. Front Physiol. 2014;5:15.
289. Romaine SP, Tomaszewski M, Condorelli G, Samani NJ. MicroRNAs in cardiovascular disease: an introduction for clinicians. Heart. 2015;101(12):921–8.
290. Marques FZ, Romaine SP, Denniff M, Eales J, Dormer J, Garrelds IM, Wojnar L, Musialik K, Duda-Raszewska B, Kiszka B. Signatures of miR-181a on the renal transcriptome and blood pressure. Mol Med. 2015;21(1):739–48.
291. Marques F, Booth S, Charchar F. The emerging role of non-coding RNA in essential hypertension and blood pressure regulation. J Hum Hypertens. 2015;29(8):459.
292. Corsten MF, Dennert R, Jochems S, Kuznetsova T, Devaux Y, Hofstra L, Wagner DR, Staessen JA, Heymans S, Schroen B. Circulating MicroRNA-208b and MicroRNA-499 reflect myocardial damage in cardiovascular disease. Circ Cardiovasc Genet. 2010;3(6):499–506.
293. Zhang Y, Zhang M, Li X, Tang Z, Wang X, Zhong M, Suo Q, Zhang Y, Lv K. Silencing microRNA-155 attenuates cardiac injury and dysfunction in viral myocarditis via promotion of M2 phenotype polarization of macrophages. Sci Rep. 2016;6:22613.
294. Corsten M, Heggermont W, Papageorgiou A-P, Deckx S, Tijsma A, Verhesen W, van Leeuwen R, Carai P, Thibaut H-J, Custers K. The microRNA-221/-222 cluster balances the antiviral and inflammatory response in viral myocarditis. Eur Heart J. 2015;36(42):2909–19.
295. Schober A, Nazari-Jahantigh M, Wei Y, Bidzhekov K, Gremse F, Grommes J, Megens RT, Heyll K, Noels H, Hristov M. MicroRNA-126-5p promotes endothelial proliferation and limits atherosclerosis by suppressing Dlk1. Nat Med. 2014;20(4):368.
296. O'Connell RM, Taganov KD, Boldin MP, Cheng G, Baltimore D. MicroRNA-155 is induced during the macrophage inflammatory response. Proc Natl Acad Sci. 2007;104(5):1604–9.
297. Jan MI, Khan RA, Sultan A, Ullah A, Ishtiaq A, Murtaza I. Analysis of NT-proBNP and uric acid due to left ventricle hypertrophy in the patients of aortic valve disease. Pak J Med Sci. 2019;35(1):183.

The manufacturer's authorised representative in the EU is Springer Nature Customer Service Centre GmbH, Europaplatz 3, 69115 Heidelberg, Germany. If you have any concerns regarding our products, please contact ProductSafety@springernature.com

Printed and bound by CPI Group (UK) Ltd, Croydon, CR0 4YY
30/09/2026
02225248-0020